Dystonia: Etiology, Clinical Features, and Treatment

Dystonia: Etiology, Clinical Features, and Treatment

MITCHELL F. BRIN

University of California, Irvine, Irvine, California, and Allergan, Inc., Irvine, California.

CYNTHIA COMELLA

Rush-Presbyterian Medical Center, Chicago, Illinois.

JOSEPH JANKOVIC

Baylor College of Medicine, Houston, Texas.

LIPPINCOTT WILLIAMS & WILKINS
A **Wolters Kluwer** Company
Philadelphia • Baltimore • New York • London
Buenos Aires • Hong Kong • Sydney • Tokyo

Managing Editors: Joy Bartnett and Richard Robinson of WE MOVE
Custom Publishing Manager: Jennifer Jett
Typesetter: Peirce Graphic Services, LLC
Printer: Edwards Brothers

© **2004 by LIPPINCOTT WILLIAMS & WILKINS**
530 Walnut Street
Philadelphia, PA 19106-3780 USA
LWW.com

Printed in USA

ISBN: 0-7817-4114-9

Care has been taken to confirm the accuracy of the information presented and to describe generally accepted practices. However, the authors, editors, and publisher are not responsible for errors or omissions or for any consequences from application of the information in this book and make no warranty, expressed or implied, with respect to the currency, completeness, or accuracy of the contents of the publication. Application of this information in a particular situation remains the professional responsibility of the practitioner.

The authors, editors, and publisher have exerted every effort to ensure that drug selection and dosage set forth in this text are in accordance with current recommendations and practice at the time of publication. However, in view of ongoing research, changes in goverment regulations, and the constant flow of information relating to drug therapy and drug reactions, the reader is urged to check the package insert for each drug for any change in indications and dosage and for added warnings and precautions. This is particularly important when the recommended agent is a new or infrequently employed drug.

Some drugs and medical devices presented in this publication have Food and Drug Administration clearance for limited use in restricted research settings. It is the responsibility of the health care provider to ascertain the Food & Drug Administration status of each drug or device planned for use in their clinical practice.

00 01 02 03
2 3 4 5 6 7 8 9 10

Contents

Introduction

Dystonia: Clinical Features, Etiology, and Treatment was written and edited by people devoted to understanding the pathophysiology of dystonia, identifying its causes and developing the best possible treatments. Many were inspired by the work of Stanley Fahn and David Marsden and have dedicated their professional lives to assisting individuals and families affected by this disabling condition. This book was also written to honor the families, friends, and caregivers who, despite their constant fears and daily obstacles, provide unconditional love and support to people with dystonia.

This book presents the fundamental aspects of the classification, etiology, and differential diagnosis of this uncommon neurologic condition and provides a summary of the genetics and neurophysiology of dystonia. The remaining focus is on the practical aspects of nonmedical, medical, surgical, and chemodenervation therapies. Relevant to the office-based presentation of dystonia, additional breadth is provided covering management considerations for each of the focal dystonias and dystonia-related conditions.

Until approximately 20 years ago, dystonia was considered a rare, untreatable disorder. Little was understood about its etiology and pathophysiology. Subsequently, 13 dystonia genes have been mapped, and many structurally and functionally abnormal protein products have been identified. Important contributions to understanding pathophysiology have come from the application of neurophysiologic and brain imaging techniques. Investigators now have an extensive armamentarium of neuroscientific tools to assist them in unlocking the many mysteries of dystonia. New therapeutic advances have altered the outlook for dystonia patients by providing an effective means of symptom improvement. In particular, the introduction and acceptance of botulinum toxin as a treatment for focal dystonia in the 1980s fundamentally changed the way clinicians approached dystonia and secondarily stimulated research into all aspects of the disorder.

Dystonia: Clinical Features, Etiology, and Treatment is a tribute to all of the patients, public and private charities, foundations, advocacy organizations, and commercial corporations engaged in deciphering the complexities of the central nervous system and providing better treatments for those affected with dystonia. The editors wish to thank the WE MOVE team, including Joy Bartnett, Richard Robinson, and especially Judy Blazer, for their hard work and patience in bringing this book into being. We hope this volume will serve as a useful guide for those who provide care for and those whose lives are touched by this disorder.

Mitchell F. Brin
Cynthia L. Comella
Joseph Jankovic
co-editors

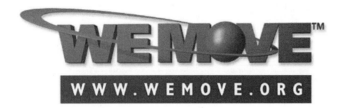

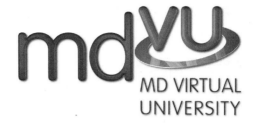

WE MOVE

Information You Need
From a Source You Can Trust

Serving the movement disorder community since 1991, WE MOVE's mission is to facilitate the communication of emerging clinical advances and therapeutic approaches to the management and treatment of movement disorders.

WE MOVE's award-winning Web site at www.wemove.org is the recognized virtual hub of online activities for the movement disorder community. WE MOVE recently launched the Movement Disorder Virtual University (MDVU) at www.mdvu.org, the new online home for all WE MOVE physician-directed educational information and activities. WE MOVE is a not-for-profit (501 3c) organization and an ACCME-accredited provider of continuing medical education courses for medical professionals.

Dystonia Rating Scales and Office Forms are available for download at www.mdvu.org.

PART I

Clinical Features

CHAPTER 1

Pathophysiology of Dystonia

Mitchell F. Brin and Cynthia L. Comella

CLINICAL FEATURES AND CLASSIFICATION

Dystonia is a neurologic syndrome dominated by involuntary muscle contractions that may be sustained (tonic), spasmodic (rapid or clonic), patterned, or repetitive. The muscle movements frequently cause abnormal postures including twisting, flexing or extending, and adducting or abducting movements. There may be overlying spasms that can resemble tremor. A feature that sets dystonia apart from tremor is the directional preponderance of the movement.

Dystonia is notable for its dynamic character. Changes in activity or posture may alter the clinical symptoms. For example, pure writer's cramp is a dystonia that appears only with the specific act of writing and is not present during any other activity of the hand. Musician's dystonia is another example of a task-specific dystonia, in which playing an instrument results in the appearance of dystonia, while other activities, including writing, are normal. Cervical dystonia may be severe when sitting in a chair or walking but completely resolve when lying down. A foot dystonia may be present when walking forward or bicycling, and be absent when walking backwards.

Pain may also occur in some patients with dystonia. An uncomfortable tightness or pulling may occur in the forearm of a patient with writer's cramp or the calf of a patient with a foot dystonia. More severe pain may accompany cervical dystonia, often localized to the area of the neck with the most severe muscle spasm.[1,2] Recently, investigators[3] have noted that in some patients, the pain associated with cranial-cervical dystonia is either chronic muscle-tension-type headache or migraine headache, suggesting that headache is common in this population.[4–6] Another common feature of dystonia is the presence of a sensory trick or *geste antagoniste*, which reduces or eliminates the dystonic posture.

Mitchell F. Brin: University of California, Irvine, Irvine, California, and Allergan, Inc., Irvine, California. The author is an employee of Allergan.

Cynthia Comella: Rush-Presbyterian Medical Center, Chicago, Illinois. The author has received research grants from Allergan, Inc., Elan Biopharmaceuticals, and Ipsen, Ltd.

Dystonia may involve any voluntary muscle. Because the movements and resulting postures are often unusual and the condition is rare, it is one of the most frequently misdiagnosed neurologic conditions.[7]

As a clinical syndrome, dystonia may be classified according to clinical distribution and symptomatology, age at onset, and etiology (Table 1-1). Classifying a patient's dystonia may be important as it may offer clues about prognosis and approach to management.

Based upon clinical and genetic epidemiological studies, the distribution of age of onset of dystonia may be divided into three categories. Infantile onset, occurring before the age of 2, is unusual for the primary dystonias. These individuals typically have injury, metabolic, or other secondary etiologies. Childhood onset is defined as occurring from ages 2 to 26. In this age group, onset of symptoms frequently occurs in the leg and may generalize to involve the entire body. Onset in the arm may also occur; in these patients, spread of symptoms is less common. Onset in the neck or face in this age group is distinctly unusual for primary dystonia, and a secondary etiology should be sought. As with infantile onset, in cases in which the initial presentation of posturing is of the head and neck, the cause may not be dystonia at all but rather a structural abnormality of the cervical vertebrae such as a subluxation.

Adult-onset dystonia begins after the age of 26 years and may involve the arms, neck, and face. In this age group, onset of dystonia in the leg is rare for primary dystonia; therefore, other etiologies should be assessed. In particular, onset in the leg may arise from structural brain lesions contralateral to the dystonia or as a presenting symptom of young-onset Parkinson's disease.

When classified by distribution, patients are categorized as having focal, segmental, or generalized symptoms. Focal dystonia symptoms involve one body region. Common examples of focal dystonia include blepharospasm (forced, involuntary eye closure), oromandibular dystonia (face, jaw, or tongue), torticollis or cervical dystonia (neck), writer's cramp (action-induced dystonic contraction of hand muscles), and spasmodic dysphonia (vocal cords). Segmental dystonia involves contiguous body regions. Examples include Meige's

TABLE 1-1. *Classification of Dystonia*[a]

I. Age at onset
  A. Infantile (< 2 yr)
  B. Early, or Childhood (2–26 yr)
  C. Late, or Adult (> 26 yr)
II. Etiology
  A. Primary
    1. With hereditary pattern
      a. Autosomal dominant
        (1) Classic types
          (a) Childhood-onset dystonia
          (b) Focal dystonia
        (2) Variant types
          (a) Dopa-responsive dystonia
          (b) Myoclonic dystonia
      b. X-linked recessive
    2. Sporadic (without a documented hereditary pattern)
      a. Classic types
      b. Variant types
  B. Symptomatic
    1. Associated with hereditary neurologic syndromes and with known enzyme defect (chromosomal location; gene product; OMIM #)
      a. Wilson's disease (13q14.3-q21.1; copper-transporting ATPase; 277900)
      b. GM1 gangliosidosis (3p21.33; β-galactosidase deflclency; 230500)
      c. GM2 gangliosidosis type 1 (Tay-Sachs disease) (15q23-q24; hexosaminidase A deficiency; 272800)
      d. Hexosaminidase A and B deficiency (5q31.3-q33.1; GM2 activator deficiency; 272750)
      e. Metachromatic leukodystrophy (22q13.31-qter; arylsulfatase A; 250100)
      f. Lesch-Nyhan syndrome (Xq26-q27.2; hypoxanthine guanine phosphoribosyltransferase; 300322)
      g. Homocystinuria (21q22.3; cystathionine beta-synthase; 236200)
      h. Glutaric acidemia (19p13.2; glutaryl-CoA dehydrogenase; 231670)
      i. Triosephosphate isomerase deficiency (12p13; Triosephosphate isomerase; 190450)
      j. Methylmalonic aciduria (6p21; Methylmalonyl-CoA mutase; 251000)
      k. Pantothenate Kinase-Associated Neurodegeneration (Hallervorden-Spatz disease) (20p13-p12.3; pantothenate kinase; 234200)
      l. Ataxia-telangiectasia (11q22.3; ATM protein; 208900)
      m. Pelizaeus-Merzbacher disease (Xq22; proteolipid protein-1; 312080)
      n. Huntington's disease (4p16.3; huntingtin; 143100)
      o. Rett syndrome (Xq28; methyl-CpG-binding protein-2; 312750)
      p. Machado-Joseph's disease (14q24.3-q31; ataxin-3; 109150)
      q. Juvenile neuronal ceroid-lipofuscinosis (16p.12.2; CLN3; 204200)
    2. Associated with probable hereditary neurologic syndromes, without known enzyme defect, but with a chemical marker (chromosomal location; OMIM #)
      a. Leigh's disease (multiple loci; 256000)
      b. Familial basal ganglia calcifications (Fahr's disease) (14q; 213600)
      c. Neuroacanthocytosis (choreoacanthocytosis) (heterogenous, 0q21;100500)
      d. Hartnup's disease (5p15; 234500)
      e. Hereditary bilateral optic atrophy with dystonia (mitochondrial) (MTND6, MTND4;500001)
    3. Associated with hereditary neurologic syndromes, without known enzyme defect or chemical marker
      a. Hereditary juvenile dystonia-parkinsonism
      b. Progressive pallidal degeneration (260200)
      c. Spinocerebellar degenerations
      d. Olivopontocerebellar atrophies
      e. Hereditary spastic paraplegia with dystonia
    4. Due to known environmental cause
      a. Perinatal cerebral injury
      b. Athetoid cerebral palsy
      c. Delayed-onset dystonia
      d. Encephalitis and postinfectious
        (1) Reye's syndrome
        (2) Subacute sclerosing leucoencephalopathy
        (3) Wasp sting
        (4) Creutzfeldt-Jakob disease

TABLE 1-1. *Classification of Dystonia^a (Continued)*

    e. Head trauma
    f. Thalamotomy
    g. Brainstem lesion, including pontine myelinolysis
    h. Focal cerebral vascular injury
    i. Arteriovenous malformation
    j. Brain tumor
    k. Multiple sclerosis
    l. Cervical cord injury
    m. Peripheral injury
    n. Drugs: D2 receptor antagonists, levodopa, ergotism, anticonvulsants
    o. Toxins: Mn, CO, carbon disulfide, cyanide, methanol, disulfiram
    p. Metabolic: hypoparathyroidism
    q. Dystonia associated with parkinsonism
    r. Psychogenic dystonia
    s. Pseudodystonia
    t. Sandifer syndrome
    u. Stiff-man syndrome
    v. Rotational atlanto-axial subluxation
    w. Soft tissue nuchal mass
    x. Bone disease
    y. Ligamentous absence, laxity or damage
    z. Congenital muscular torticollis
    aa. Congenital postural torticollis
    bb. Congenital Klippel-Feil syndrome
    cc. Posterior fossa tumor
    dd. Syringomyelia
    ee. Arnold Chiari malformation
    ff. Trochlear nerve palsy
    gg. Vestibular torticollis
III. Distribution
  A. Focal; examples include:
    1. Blepharospasm (forced, involuntary eye-closure)
    2. Oromandibular dystonia (face, jaw, or tongue)
    3. Torticollis (neck)
    4. Writer's cramp (action-induced dystonic contraction of hand muscles)
    5. Spasmodic dysphonia (vocal cords)
  B. Segmental (cranial/axial/crural)
  C. Generalized (ambulatory, nonambulatory)

^aThis table is expanded from those presented by Fahn, et al.[14] and by Calne and Lang.[15] OMIM, Online Mendelian Inheritance in Man
    ATPase, adenosine triphosphatase; Mn, manganese; CO, carbon monoxide.

syndrome (involvement of eyes and lower face and/or jaw), cervical dystonia plus writer's cramp, or blepharospasm plus cervical dystonia. Generalized dystonia is defined as dystonia with involvement of one leg, trunk, and one other body region or both legs and one other body region. Childhood-onset primary dystonia usually begins as a focal dystonia in the leg or foot, but typically spreads to become generalized dystonia. In adult-onset dystonia with initial arm, neck, or face involvement, progression to generalized dystonia is rare.

According to the etiologic classification, patients with idiopathic disease (primary dystonia) have no evidence by history, examination, or laboratory studies of any identifiable cause for the dystonic symptoms. The clinical phenomenology will often be a clue to etiology. Primary dystonia is typically action-induced; symptoms are enhanced with use of the affected body part and the region may appear normal at rest. Secondary dystonia may present as dystonia at rest or as a fixed posture.

The presence of extensive dystonia limited to one side of the body (hemidystonia) suggests a secondary etiology.

However, patients may have factors in their history that precipitate the onset of dystonic symptoms.[8,9] For primary dystonia, therefore, there must be normal perinatal and early developmental histories, no prior history of neurologic illness, or exposure to drugs known to cause acquired dystonia (e.g., phenothiazines). There must also be normal intellectual, pyramidal, cerebellar and sensory examinations, and diagnostic studies.[10,11] Patients who have abnormalities noted above are classified as having symptomatic dystonia.

EPIDEMIOLOGY

The prevalence of the condition is unknown, but it is estimated that there are at least 250,000 cases of idiopathic dystonia in the United States.[12,13] Approximately 1 in 3,000 people is diagnosed with dystonia but the true prevalence is probably much higher. The epidemiology of cervical dystonia (CD or torticollis) has not been studied, but the prevalence of all focal dystonias has been estimated at 300 per million, which is 9 times the prevalence of generalized dystonia.[13] CD is probably the most commonly diagnosed form of focal dystonia, but graphospasm (writer's cramp) may be the most prevalent form of dystonia in the general population.

LABORATORY AND NEUROPATHOLOGIC STUDIES

Laboratory investigations are typically normal in patients with idiopathic dystonia. Patients with secondary dystonia will have laboratory findings consistent with the underlying disorder.

Studies with positron emission tomography (PET) have suggested abnormalities in the sensory[16,17] or motor[18] cortex in classic idiopathic disease, and motor cortex[19] in X-linked dystonia-parkinsonism (Lubag [20,21]). However, there are no consistent findings across all forms of dystonia.

There are no consistent brain pathologic findings in patients with idiopathic dystonia. Among the various reviews[22–26] of primarily idiopathic dystonia, the most frequently cited lesions are in the basal ganglia, including the putamen, head of caudate, and upper brain stem. Hedreen et al.[27] proposed that the putamen and the striatopallidal-thalamo-cortical circuit appear to be the most likely sites in which to search for the unknown defect in primary dystonia.

In a review of the behavioral and motor consequences of focal lesions of the basal ganglia, Bhatia and Marsden[28] found that putaminal and globus pallidus (lentiform nuclei) lesions were frequent causes of dystonia. There are a number of reports of metabolic disorders, particularly those affecting mitochondrial function, causing dystonic symptoms. For instance, in 1986, Novotny and coworkers[29] reported families with Leber's disease and dystonia. Berkovic and colleagues[30] reported three unrelated patients with generalized dystonia and bilateral striatal hypodensities on computed tomography, suggesting a mitochondrial etiology. Nigro and colleagues[31] reported a partial cytochrome b deficiency in a patient with dystonia and myopathy and bilateral hypodense putaminal lesions. Bruyn et al.[32] reviewed a family with "hereditary spastic dystonia," a large kindred with either Leber's hereditary optic atrophy, dystonia, or both, with putaminal necrosis. Donnet et al.[33] reported a patient with a dystonic right arm, ptosis, complete ophthalmoplegia, a cataract, ragged-red fibers on muscle biopsy, and defects in abnormal complex III and IV activity. Benecke and coworkers[34] reported abnormal complex I activity in patients with dystonia, observing a defect that was more pronounced in patients with segmental or generalized dystonia compared to those with focal dystonia. Jun et al.[35] then reported a specific mitochondrial mutation (np 14459) in their patients with hereditary optic atrophy.[29] We[36] described a patient with severe primary bilateral putaminal degeneration as shown on neuroimaging; this finding was subsequently correlated with neuropathologic findings of gliosis, spongiform degeneration, and cavitation. These findings support the concept that disturbed putaminal function, including that caused by molecular defects, may be important in the genesis of the dystonia phenotype.

There is also little known about the precise biochemistry of dystonia. Some patients derive benefit from pharmacotherapy with anticholinergics, benzodiazepines, baclofen, dopamine depletors, or dopamine-blocking agents. However, from the few available autopsies,[37] there is normal choline acetyltransferase in the cortex and striatum. In examples of secondary dystonia,[38] there is a marked and consistent elevation of norepinephrine in several regions of brain stem. In dopa-responsive dystonia (DRD), a rare form of childhood-onset dystonia, there is reduced biological half-life of dopamine, suggesting impaired storage is responsible for diurnal fluctuations. In the case of primary putaminal degeneration reported by Walker et al.,[36] the substantia nigra pars compacta contained a normal number of neurons but decreased tyrosine hydroxylase immunoreactivity.

Rajput et al.[39,40] published the first neurochemical and pathologic studies of a patient with DRD. They found normal numbers of hypopigmented substantia nigra neurons, normal tyrosine hydroxylase (TH) immunoreactivity, and no evidence of a neurodegenerative process in the striatum. There was reduced dopamine in the substantia nigra and striatum. In the striatum, TH protein and TH activity were reduced, with a loss more pronounced in the putamen than caudate. The absence of gliosis or other histologic evidence for a major nerve terminal loss supported either an incomplete arborization of striatal dopamine terminals, accompanied by a lack of melanization in the nigral perikarya, or a reduced dopamine synthetic capacity of the nigrostriatal neurons. With the additional observations by Ichinose et al.,[41] the hypothesis of reduced dopamine synthetic capacity seems more likely.

CONTRIBUTIONS OF THE SENSORY SYSTEMS TO THE PATHOPHYSIOLOGY OF DYSTONIA

Sensory tricks often ameliorate dystonic movements and postures and such maneuvers can be effective in different parts of the body. Such a sensory trick is also known as a *geste antagoniste* or *gegendruckphanomen*. Patients with CD often find that gently touching the chin, back of the head, or the top of the head will relieve symptoms. The use of sensory tricks to keep the head in the body midline position was reported by 88.9% of patients in one series.[42] The physiology of sensory tricks remains unknown. In a recent study, 13 of 25 patients with idiopathic CD had markedly reduced electromyographic (EMG) activity (50% or more) even during arm movement, but before the arm touched the skin, while performing a sensory trick.[43] Some patients have been reported to have reduced dystonia while thinking about a sensory trick.[44]

Botulinum toxin type A (BTX-A) may also modify the sensory feedback loop to the central nervous system, and this mechanism may be partially responsible for its beneficial effect in treating dystonia. Ludlow et al.[45] and Zwirner et al.[46] proposed that reduced muscle activity and therefore feedback to laryngeal motoneuron pools may be a primary mechanism of action of BTX-A. Brin et al.[47] offered the possibility that toxin might have a direct effect on sensory afferents by blocking intrafusal fibers, resulting in decreased activation of muscle spindles. This would effectively change the sensory afferent system by reducing the Ia traffic. Filippi et al.[48] supported this hypothesis by establishing that local injections of BTX-A directly reduce afferent Ia fibers traffic, and therefore exert a modulatory effect on sensory feedback. This may also account for the clinical observation that injections of BTX-A have an effect on regional noninjected muscles, most striking in spastic limbs.[49]

Support for this mechanism derives from the cumulative work of Kaji and colleagues.[50–55] They showed that the increase in severity of dystonic writer's cramp associated with enhancing Ia muscle spindle activity with the tonic vibration maneuver may be decreased by intramuscular injections of dilute lidocaine, which preferentially affects the afferent innervation of the muscle spindle. Both ethanol and lidocaine block sodium channels; however, the former blocks the channels for a longer duration than the anesthetic. Kaji has coined the term muscle afferent block (MAB) for this combination treatment of lidocaine plus ethanol, and has shown an effect in neck, jaw,[54] and limb dystonia,[50–51] and spasticity.[53–55] The benefit for each treatment only lasts a few weeks, and therefore is of limited use in most dystonic and spastic situations. However, this model of blocking Ia afferents supports the proposed mechanism of action with BTX-A on conditions associated with excessive muscle contraction. These studies support the importance of the afferent system in the clinical manifestations of dystonia.[56]

TRAUMA AND DYSTONIA

Trauma is generally accepted as a factor that may trigger dystonia,[9,57–59] although this matter is debated by some clinicians.[60] The incidence of head/neck trauma has been reported in 5 to 21% of cervical dystonia cases.[2,61–64] Patients with spasmodic dysphonia may report the onset of symptoms immediately after a laryngeal/pharyngeal trauma, most often following a viral infection. Approximately 20% of our patients have a clear family history of dystonia, and therefore a genetic predisposition to the development of symptoms. However, some of the "sporadic" cases may be genetically susceptible or "primed"; after exposure to the appropriate environmental factors ("trigger factors") such as exposure to infections or trauma, symptoms manifest. Limb dystonia[65–67] and jaw dystonia[68,69] have been reported to occur after peripheral traumas. Similar models have been proposed for other movement disorders.[70] There is a growing body of experimental evidence that the appropriately predisposed patient may develop dystonia with overactivity.[71,72]

In some patients, the putative triggering injury is relatively mild or chronic or repetitive, as had been noted by Schott.[73] The dystonia typically occurs in the traumatized body part or region and in many cases is associated with pain. Sometimes the dystonic posture evolves as the pain improves.

ACKNOWLEDGMENTS

This work was supported, in part, by the Bachmann-Strauss Dystonia and Parkinson Foundation, and the United States Public Health Grant FD-R-001452

REFERENCES

1. Chan J, Brin MF, Fahn S. Idiopathic cervical dystonia: clinical characteristics. Mov Disord 1991;6:119–126.
2. Jankovic J, Leder S, Warner D, et al. chwartz K. Cervical dystonia: Clinical findings and associated movement disorders. Neurology 1991;41:1088–1091.
3. Galvez-Jimenez N, Lampuri C, Patino-Piecirilo R, et al. Dystonia and deadaches: the response to botulinum toxin (BTx) therapy [Abstract]. Mov Disord 2002;17:1141.
4. Csala B, Deuschl G. [Craniocervical dystonia. Pragmatic general concept or nosologic entity?] Nervenarzt 1994;65:75–94.
5. Gobel H, Heinze A, Heinze-Kuhn K, et al. Botulinum toxin A in the treatment of headache syndromes and pericranial pain syndromes. Pain 2001;91:195–199.
6. Friedman J, Standaert DG. Dystonia and its disorders. Neurol Clin 2001;19:681–705.
7. Fahn S. The varied clinical expressions of dystonia. Neurol Clin 1984;2:541–554.
8. Jankovic J. Post-traumatic movement disorders: central and peripheral mechanisms. Neurology 1994;44:2006–2014.
9. Jankovic J. Can peripheral trauma induce dystonia and other movement disorders? Yes! Mov Disord 2001;16:7–12.
10. Marsden CD, Harrison MJG. Idiopathic torsion dystonia (dystonia musculorum deformans). A review of forty-two patients. Brain 1974;97:793–810.
11. Burke RE, Brin MF, Fahn S, et al. Analysis of the clinical course of non-Jewish, autosomal dominant torsion dystonia. Mov Disord 1986; 1:163–178.
12. National Institutes of Health. Dystonia Workshop. 1993. Bethesda, MD.
13. Nutt JG, Muenter MD, Aronson A, et al. Epidemiology of focal and generalized dystonia in Rochester, Minnesota. Mov Disord 1988; 3:188–194.
14. Fahn S, Marsden CD, Calne DB. Classification and investigation of dystonia. In: Marsden CD, Fahn S, eds. Movement Disorders 2. London: Butterworths, 1987:332–358.
15. Calne DB, Lang AE. Secondary dystonia. Adv Neurol 1988;50:9–33.
16. Tempel LW, Perlmutter JS. Abnormal vibration-induced cerebral blood flow responses in idiopathic dystonia. Brain 1990;113:691–707.
17. Perlmutter JS, Raichle ME. Pure hemidystonia with basal ganglion abnormalities on positron emission tomography. Ann Neurol 1984; 15:228–233.
18. Playford ED, Rassingham RE, Marsden CD, et al. Abnormal activation of striatum and dorsolateral prefontal cortex in dystonia [Abstract]. Neurology 1992;42 (Suppl 3):377.
19. Takahashi H, Snow B, Waters C, et al. Evidence for nigrostriatal lesions in Lubag (X-linked dystonia- parkinsonism in the Philippines) [Abstract]. Neurology 1992;42 (Suppl 3):441.
20. Fahn S, Moskowitz C. X-Linked recessive dystonia and parkinsonism in Filipino males [Abstract]. Ann Neurol 1988;24:179.
21. Wilhelmsen KC, Weeks DE, Nygaard TG, et al. Genetic mapping of the "Lubag" (X-linked dystonia-parkinsonism) in a Filipino kindred to the pericentromeric region of the X chromosome. Ann Neurol 1991;29:124–131.

22. Obeso JA, Gimenez Roldan S. Clinicopathological correlation in symptomatic dystonia. Adv Neurol 1988;50:113–122.

23. Marsden CD, Obeso JA, Zarranz JJ, et al. The anatomical basis of symptomatic hemidystonia. Brain 1985;108:463–483.

24. Narbona J, Obeso JA, Tunon T, et al. Hemidystonia secondary to localized basal ganglia tumour. J Neurol Neurosurg Psychiatry 1984;47:704–709.

25. Jankovic J, Patel SC. Blepharospasm associated with brain stem lesions. Neurology 1983;33:1237–1240.

26. Zweig RM, Hedreen JC, Jankel WR, et al. Pathology in brainstem regions of individuals with primary dystonia. Neurology 1988;38:702–706.

27. Hedreen JC, Zweig RM, DeLong MR, et al. Primary dystonias: a review of the pathology and suggestions for new directions of study. Adv Neurol 1988;50:123–132.

28. Bhatia KP, Marsden CD. The behavioural and motor consequences of focal lesions of the basal ganglia in man. Brain 1994;117:859–876.

29. Novotny EJ Jr, Singh G, Wallace DC, et al. Leber's disease and dystonia: a mitochondrial disease. Neurology 1986;36:1053–1060.

30. Berkovic SF, Karpati G, Carpenter S, et al. Progressive dystonia with bilateral putaminal hypodensities. Arch Neurol 1987;44:1184–1187.

31. Nigro MA, Martens ME, Awerbuch GI, et al. Partial cytochrome b deficiency and generalized dystonia. Pediatr Neurol 1990;6:407–410.

32. Bruyn GW, Vielvoye GJ, Went LN. Hereditary spastic dystonia: a new mitochondrial encephalopathy? Putaminal necrosis as a diagnostic sign. J Neurol Sci 1991;103:195–202.

33. Donnet A, Guinot H, Pellissier JF, et al. [Segmental dystonia and mitochondrial encephalomyopathy]. Rev Neurol (Paris) 1992;148:51–53.

34. Benecke R, Strumper P, Weiss H. Electron transfer complex I defect in idiopathic dystonia. Ann Neurol 1992;32:683–686.

35. Jun AS, Brown MD, Wallace DC. A mitochondrial DNA mutation at np 14459 of the ND6 gene associated with maternally inherited Leber's hereditary optic neuropathy and dystonia. Proc Natl Acad Sci USA 1994;91:6206–6210.

36. Walker RH, Purohit DP, Good PF, et al. Severe generalized dystonia due to primary putaminal degeneration: case report and review of the literature. Mov Disord 2002;17:576–584.

37. Jankovic J, Svendsen CN, Bird ED. Brain neurotransmitters in dystonia. N Engl J Med 1987;316:278–279.

38. de Yebenes JG, Brin MF, Mena MA, et al. Neurochemical findings in neuroacanthocytosis. Mov Disord 1988;3:300–312.

39. Rajput AH, Gibb WR, Zhong XH, et al. Dopa-responsive dystonia: pathological and biochemical observations in a case [see comments]. Ann Neurol 1994;35:396–402.

40. Calne DB. DOPA-responsive dystonia. Ann Neurol 1994;35:381–382.

41. Ichinose H, Ohye T, Takahashi E, et al. Hereditary progressive dystonia with marked diurnal fluctuation caused by mutations in the GTP cyclohydrolase I gene. Nat Genet 1994;8:236–242.

42. Jahanshahi M. Factors that ameliorate or aggravate spasmodic torticollis. J Neurol Neurosurg Psychiatry 2000;68:227–229.

43. Wissel J, Muller J, Ebersbach G, et al. Trick maneuvers in cervical dystonia: investigation of movement- and touch-related changes in polymyographic activity. Mov Disord 1999;14:994–999.

44. Greene PE, Bressman S. Exteroceptive and interoceptive stimuli in dystonia. Mov Disord 1998;13:549–551.

45. Ludlow CL, Hallett M, Sedory SE, et al. The pathophysiology of spasmodic dysphonia and its modification by botulinum toxin. In: Berardelli A, Benecke R, Manfredi M, Marsden CM, eds. Motor Disturbances II. New York: Academic Press, 1990:273–288.

46. Zwirner P, Murry T, Swenson M, et al. Effects of botulinum toxin therapy in patients with adductor spasmodic dysphonia: acoustic, aerodynamic, and videoendoscopic findings. Laryngoscope 1992;102:400–406.

47. Brin MF, Blitzer A, Stewart C, et al. Treatment of spasmodic dysphonia (laryngeal dystonia) with local injections of botulinum toxin: review and technical aspects. In: Blitzer A, Brin MF, Sasaki CT, Fahn S, Harris KS, eds. Neurological Disorders of the Larynx. New York: Thieme, 1992:214–228.

48. Filippi GM, Errico P, Santarelli R, et al. Botulinum-A Toxin Effects on Rat Jaw Muscle Spindles. Acta Oto-Laryngol 1993;113:400–404.

49. Borg-Stein J, Pine ZM, Miller JR, et al. Botulinum toxin for the treatment of spasticity in multiple sclerosis. New observations. Am J Phys Med Rehabil 1993;72:364–368.

50. Kaji R, Rothwell JC, Katayama M, et al. Tonic vibration reflex and muscle afferent block in writer's cramp. Ann Neurol 1995;38:155–162.

51. Kaji R, Kohara N, Katayama M, et al. Muscle afferent block by intramuscular injection of lidocaine for the treatment of writer's cramp. Muscle Nerve 1995;18:234–235.

52. Kaji R, Shibasaki H, Kimura J. Writer's cramp: a disorder of motor subroutine? [editorial; comment]. Ann Neurol 1995;38:837–838.

53. Kaji R, Mezaki T, Kubori T, et al. [Treatment of spasticity with botulinum toxin and muscle afferent block]. Rinsho Shinkeigaku 1996;36:1334–1335.

54. Yoshida K, Kaji R, Kubori T, et al. Muscle afferent block for the treatment of oromandibular dystonia. Mov Disord 1998;13:699–705.

55. Mezaki T, Kaji R, Hirota N, et al. Treatment of spasticity with muscle afferent block. Neurology 1999;53:1156–1157.

56. Hallett M. Physiology of dystonia. Adv Neurol 1998;78:11–18.

57. Brin MF, Fahn S, Bressman SB, et al. Dystonia precipitated by peripheral trauma. Neurology 1986;36 (Suppl 1):119.

58. Jankovic J, Van der Linden C. Dystonia and tremor induced by peripheral trauma: predisposing factors. J Neurol Neurosurg Psychiatry 1988;51:1512–1519.

59. Gordon M, Brin MF, Giladi N, et al. Dystonia precipitated by peripheral trauma [Abstract]. Mov Disord 1990;5 (Suppl 1):236.

60. Weiner WJ. Can peripheral trauma induce dystonia? No! Mov Disord 2001;16:13–22.

61. Chan J, Brin M, Fahn S. Idiopathic cervical dystonia: clinical characteristics. Mov Disord 1991;6:119–126.

62. Rondot P, Marchand MP, Dellatolas G. Spasmodic torticollis: review of 220 patients. Can J Neurol Sci 1991;18:143–151.

63. Lowenstein DH, Aminoff MJ. The clinical course of spasmodic torticollis. Neurology 1988;38:530–532.

64. Samii A, Pal PK, Schulzer M, et al. Post-traumatic cervical dystonia: a distinct entity? Can J Neurol Sci 2000;27:55–59.

65. Frucht S, Fahn S, Ford B. Focal task-specific dystonia induced by peripheral trauma. Mov Disord 2000;15:348–350.

66. Hollinger P, Burgunder J. Posttraumatic focal dystonia of the shoulder. Eur Neurol 2000;44:153–155.

67. Thyagarajan D, Kompoliti K, Ford B. Post-traumatic shoulder 'dystonia': persistent abnormal postures of the shoulder after minor trauma. Neurology 1998;51:1205–1207.

68. Schrag A, Bhatia KP, Quinn NP, et al. Atypical and typical cranial dystonia following dental procedures. Mov Disord 1999;14:492–496.

69. Sankhla C, Lai EC, Jankovic J. Peripherally induced oromandibular dystonia. J Neurol Neurosurg Psychiatry 1998;65:722–728.

70. Barbeau A. Etiology of Parkinson's disease: a research strategy. Can J Neurol Sci 1984;11:24–28.

71. Byl N, Wilson F, Merzenich M, et al. A sensory dysfunction associated with repetitive strain injuries of tendinitis and focal hand dystonia: a comparative study. J Orthop Sports Phys Ther 1996;23:234–244.

72. Byl NN, Merzenich MM, Jenkins WM. A primate genesis model of focal dystonia and repetitive strain injury: I. Learning-induced dedifferentiation of the representation of the hand in the primary somatosensory cortex in adult monkeys. Neurology 1996;47:508–520.

73. Schott GD. The relationship of peripheral trauma and pain to dystonia. J Neurol Neurosurg Psychiatry 1985;48:698–701.

CHAPTER 2

Genetics of Dystonia

Susan B. Bressman, Michele Tagliati, and Christine Klein

INTRODUCTION TO DYSTONIA: ITS MANY CLINICAL AND GENETIC SUBTYPES

Dystonia or torsion dystonia refers to sustained muscle contractions that cause twisting and repetitive movements and postures.[1] There are many causes for dystonia, including many genetic causes, and two broad etiologic categories are used. These categories are primary or idiopathic dystonia and secondary or symptomatic dystonia (Table 2-1). In primary torsion dystonia (PTD), an exogenous or acquired cause, such as trauma, neuroleptic intake, or birth asphyxia cannot be identified. PTD is distinguished from most secondary dystonias by the absence of any sign other than dystonia. The laboratory evaluation of patients with PTD is normal; there are no consistent morphologic changes upon pathologic examination. Postmortem neurochemical analyses have yielded limited insight into the pathogenesis of PTD. No single treatment is consistently effective for PTD or many secondary dystonias. However, several secondary dystonias have specific effective therapies, including Wilson's disease and dopa-responsive dystonia (DRD). Current treatments for dystonia include anticholinergic medications, botulinum toxin injections, and surgical interventions such as pallidotomy or pallidal stimulation. In some patients, these may provide significant improvement of symptoms.

The clinical spectrum of dystonia is remarkably variable; age at onset ranges from early-childhood to the eighth decade. Muscle involvement varies from a single muscle to generalized contractions of the limb, axial, and cranial muscles. For PTD, the age-at-onset distribution is bimodal, with modes at age 9 (early onset) and 45 (late onset); this distribution is di-

vided by a nadir at age 27 years.[2] Furthermore, there is a relationship between the age at symptom onset, body region first affected, and clinical progression of signs. When PTD begins in childhood or adolescence, it often starts in a leg or arm, and then progresses to involve multiple body regions. When PTD begins during the adult years, symptoms first involve the neck, cranial, or arm muscles; however, dystonia tends to remain localized.[3] This relationship between age, site-onset, and spread appears to be less strong in secondary dystonia.[4]

The clinical/etiologic classification of dystonia is outlined in Table 2-1. In Table 2-2, the different forms of hereditary dystonia are genetically categorized. Currently, at least 14 forms of dystonia syndromes have been distinguished on a genetic basis as *DYT* or dystonia loci.[5,6] However, this genetic classification includes a mix of primary and secondary dystonias. They also include the paroxysmal dystonias, which are generally categorized separately under episodic dyskinetic syndromes that may have dystonic contractions (Table 2-2).[7] Also, while a chromosomal location has been identified for many forms of dystonia included in this list of 14, only three genes have been shown to be mutated. Thus, most genes that cause primary dystonia have not been identified.

Primary Torsion Dystonia

The prevalence of PTD is difficult to estimate because of the variation in its expression and the tendency for mild cases to go undiagnosed. In Rochester, Minnesota, prevalence was calculated to be approximately 330 per million, with late-onset focal PTD being 10 times more common than early-onset generalized PTD.[8] Ethnic differences in disease frequency are also reported. Several large studies found that early-onset PTD is 5 to 10 times more common in Ashkenazi Jews than in non-Jews or non-Ashkenazi Jews.[9,10]

Early-Onset Primary Torsion Dystonia

From its earliest descriptions, a genetic etiology for early-onset PTD, also termed dystonia musculorum deformans or Oppenheim's disease, was suspected.

Susan Bressman: Department of Neurology, Beth Israel Medical Center, New York, New York, and Albert Einstein College of Medicine, Bronx, New York.

Michele Tagliati: Department of Neurology, Beth Israel Medical Center, New York, New York, and Albert Einstein College of Medicine, Bronx, New York.

Christine Klein: Department of Neurology, Medical University of Lübeck, Germany.

The authors have not provided disclaimer information.

TABLE 2-1. *Classification of Dystonia*

I. By Age at Onset
- *Early-onset* (≤ 26 years); usually starts in a leg or arm and frequently progresses to involve other limbs and the trunk
- *Late-onset* (>26 years); usually starts in the neck, cranial muscles (including vocal cords) or arm and tends to remain localized with restricted spread to adjacent muscles

II. By Distribution
- *Focal*—single body region (e.g., writer's cramp, blepharospasm, torticollis, spasmodic dysphonia)
- *Segmental*—contiguous body regions (e.g., face plus jaw or Meige's syndrome, torticollis plus brachial dystonia)
- *Multifocal*—noncontiguous body regions (e.g. arm plus leg, blepharospasm plus writer's cramp)
- *Generalized*—both legs plus at least one other body region, usually one or both arms

III. By Cause
  A. Primary (or idiopathic)—dystonia is the only sign and evaluation does not reveal an identifiable exogenous cause or other inherited or degenerative disease
    1. *Childhood or adolescent limb-onset:* Often spreads to other limbs, infrequent cranial involvement. Many cases due to TOR1A (*DYT1*) GAG deletion
    2. *Mixed phenotype:* Child or adult onset in limb, neck, or cranial muscles, dysarthria/dysphonia common. Mapped to chromosome 8 (*DYT6*) in Swiss Mennonite families
    3. *Early and adult-onset segmental cervical/cranial:* Child or early adult-onset in cervical/cranial and cervical/brachial muscles (*DYT13*)
    4. *Adult cervical, cranial, or brachial-onset:* Dystonia usually localized. Mapped to chromosome 18p (*DYT7*) in a German family with torticollis. Other similar families excluded from locus
  B. Secondary dystonia
    1. Associated with hereditary neurologic syndromes
      a. Dystonia Plus
        Dopa-responsive dystonia
          GCHI mutations (*DRD* or *DYT5*)
          Tyrosine hydroxylase mutations
          Other biopterin deficient states
          Dopamine agonist-responsive dystonia due to decarboxylase deficiency
        Myoclonus—dystonia
          Due to epsilon sarcoglycan mutations on chromosome 7 (DYT11)
          Due to other genes (DYT15 on chromosome 8p)
      b. Other inherited disorders
        Autosomal dominant
          Rapid-onset dystonia-parkinsonism (*DYT12*)
          Huntington's disease
          Machado-Joseph's disease/SCA3 disease
          Other SCA subtypes
          DRPLA
          Familial basal ganglia calcifications
        Autosomal recessive
          Wilson's disease
          Gangliosidoses
          Metachromatic leukodystrophy
          Homocystinuria
          Hartnup's disease
          Glutaric acidemia
          Methylmalonic aciduria
          Pantothenate kinase associated neurodegeneration
          Dystonic lipidosis
          Ceroid-lipofuscinosis
          Ataxia-telangiectasia
          Neuroacanthocytosis
          Intraneuronal inclusion disease
          Juvenile parkinsonism (parkin)
        X-linked recessive
          Lubag (X-linked dystonia-parkinsonism, DYT3)
          Lesch-Nyhan syndrome
          Deafness/Dystonia
        Mitochondrial
          MERRF/MELAS
          Leber's disease
    2. Due to acquired/exogenous causes
          Perinatal cerebral injury
          Encephalitis, infectious and post-infectious
          Head trauma
          Pontine myelinolysis

TABLE 2-1. *Classification of Dystonia (Continued)*

    Primary antiphospholipid syndrome
    Stroke
    Tumor
    Multiple sclerosis
    Cervical cord injury or lesion
    Peripheral injury
    Drugs (e.g., due to dopamine receptor blockers, acute and tardive)
    Toxins
    Psychogenic
3. Dystonia due to degenerative parkinsonian disorders of unknown etiology
    PD (Parkinson's disease)
    PSP (Progressive supranuclear palsy)
    CBGD (Corticobasal ganglionic degeneration)
4. Dystonia as a feature of other dyskinetic disorders)
    Tics
    Paroxysmal disorders
        PKD (*DYT10/EKD1, EKD2*)
        PNKD (*DYT8*)
        CSE (*DYT9*)

TABLE 2-2. *Molecular Classification of Dystonia*

Dystonia type	Mode of inheritance/*OMIM*[*a]	Chromosomal location	Gene product and mutation
DYT1 Early-onset generalized TD	Autosomal dominant *128100*	9q34	3-base pair (GAG) deletion in the *DYT1* gene results in the loss of one glutamic acid residue in the ATP-binding protein TorsinA
DYT2 Autosomal recessive TD	Autosomal recessive *224500*	Unknown	Unknown
DYT3 X-linked dystonia-parkinsonism "Lubag"	X-linked *314250*	Xq13.1	Unknown
DYT4 "Non-DYT1" TD Whispering dystonia in one family	Autosomal dominant *128101*	Unknown	Unknown
DYT5 Dopa-responsive dystonia and parkinsonism; Segawa syndrome	Autosomal dominant *128230*	14q22.1-q22.2	Mutations in the GTP cyclohydrolase I gene
DYT6 Adolescent and early adult-onset TD of mixed phenotype	Autosomal dominant *602629*	8p21–8p22	Unknown
DYT7 Late-onset focal dystonia	Autosomal dominant *602124*	18p	Unknown
DYT8 Paroxysmal nonkinesigenic dyskinesia or dystonic choreoathetosis	Autosomal dominant *118800*	2q33-q25	Unknown
DYT9 Paroxysmal choreoathetosis with episodic ataxia and spasticity	Autosomal dominant *601042*	1p21-p13.3	Unknown
DYT10 Paroxysmal kinesiogenic dyskinesia/choreoathetosis	Autosomal dominant *128200*	16p11.2-q12.1	Unknown
DYT11 Myoclonus-dystonia	Autosomal dominant *159900*	7q21–31	Mutations in the epsilon sarcoglycan gene
DYT12 Rapid-onset dystonia-parkinsonism	Autosomal dominant *128235*	19q	Unknown
DYT13 Early and adult onset cranial cervical brachial	Autosomal dominant *607671*	1p36.32-p36.13	Unknown
DYT14 Dopa responsive dystonia	Autosomal dominant *128230*	14q22.1—q22.2	Unknown

[a]OMIM: Online Mendelian Inheritance in Man; Available at: http://www.ncbi.nlm.nih.gov/entrez/query.fcgi?db=OMIM
TD, torsion dystonia; ATP, adenosine triphosphate.

INHERITANCE PATTERN

In the early years of the twentieth century, the initial reports regarding early-onset primary dystonia described two important features that were not fully appreciated for many decades. This form of dystonia is familial,[11] and more common in Jews of Eastern European ancestry.[9] In 1970, Eldridge[12] proposed that early-onset primary dystonia was inherited as an autosomal recessive trait in Jews, and an autosomal dominant trait in non-Jews. For nearly 20 years, this view was widely accepted. Then studies from Israel[10] and the United States,[2,13] as well as reanalysis of Eldridge's original data,[14] indicated that the disorder is not autosomal recessive in Jews. Studies showed that in this population, the disorder is autosomal dominant with reduced penetrance (30%). The age-adjusted risk for first-degree relatives is approximately 15.5% and 6.5% for second-degree relatives. Parent, offspring, and sibling risks were not significantly different, which is consistent with dominant inheritance. Furthermore, there is no evidence for sporadic cases or new mutations; that is, all cases are inherited.[2,13] The study by Bressman and colleagues[2] found that the range of clinical features in the relatives of early-onset Ashkenazi probands is limited. When relatives were compared to probands, the disease was somewhat milder, more localized, and slightly later in age-at-onset. Most relatives shared a similar phenotype of early limb-onset dystonia; symptom onset after age 40 and onset in cranial muscles were rare.[2] With the subsequent discovery of a founder mutation in this population as well as cloning of the DYT1 gene, the above family study findings have been confirmed and explained. In other words, a single founder mutation underlies the great majority of early-onset primary dystonia in Ashkenazim. This mutation is, for the most part, limited (early limb-onset) in its expression.

Early-onset dystonia in the non-Jewish Caucasian population is also inherited as an autosomal dominant trait with markedly reduced penetrance.[9,14-16] A systematic analysis[15] of non-Jewish British probands was conducted. These patients had generalized, multifocal, or segmental dystonia (most with early-onset dystonia). Researchers concluded that approximately 85% of cases were inherited as an autosomal dominant trait with reduced penetrance of 40%; the remaining 15% were likely to be nongenetic phenocopies. Increased paternal age of singleton cases was found and approximately 14% of genetic cases were thought to be new mutations. As in the study of Ashkenazi families, there was variable and often milder expression in affected relatives. Unlike the Ashkenazi population, a larger proportion of non-Jewish affected family members (i.e., 10 to 15%) had late onset (i.e., >44 years). A proposed explanation for the genetic and clinical differences between these populations was that in Jews, the disorder is genetically homogenous; among non-Jews, there is a likelihood of genetic heterogeneity of dystonia.[13] The presence of a single founder mutation and genetic drift are the most plausible reasons for the higher frequency of early-onset dystonia, which is a dominant disorder, in Jews[13]; thus, most cases would be the result of the same mutational event and clinical homogeneity would be expected. In non-Jews, a heterogeneous population with a lower incidence of disease, the disorder is likely to result from mutation/selection balance. Thus, multiple mutations, including new mutations, would be expected. In addition, this greater etiologic heterogeneity among non-Jews might then explain the greater clinical heterogeneity observed in this population. Again, recent linkage studies, as well as the cloning of DYT1, confirm this hypothesis.

GENETIC LINKAGE STUDIES

In 1989, Ozelius et al.[17] mapped the first primary dystonia locus, termed DYT1. These researchers studied a large North American, non-Jewish family of French Canadian ancestry. The gene was localized to the 9q32–34 region. Subsequently, Kramer and colleagues[18] found linkage of dystonia in 12 Ashkenazi families with markers in the same region. Clinical features were similar in the non-Jewish and 12 Jewish families; in both groups, the onset was early (e.g., average 14.4 ± 3 years and 13.2 ± 1 years, respectively). In 86% of the non-Jewish family, symptoms began in a limb; in 90% of the 12 Jewish families, symptoms also began in a limb.

After the initial linkage findings, studies of European,[19] non-Jewish North American,[16] and Ashkenazi[20,21] families confirmed that DYT1 is a common cause of early-onset primary dystonia; however, DYT1 is not responsible for dystonia in all early-onset families.[19]

LINKAGE DISEQUILIBRIUM OF DYT1 WITH 9Q MARKERS IN ASHKENAZI JEWS

Soon after the discovery of linkage for early-onset primary dystonia with 9q markers in Ashkenazi families, it became apparent that the Ashkenazi families shared a common 9q haplotype.[20] However, no such linkage was observed among non-Jewish 9q-linked PTD families.[17] The sharing of a particular haplotype of alleles more frequently than would be expected by chance is called linkage disequilibrium. For markers that are tightly linked to the disease gene, such an association of linked alleles and the disease gene implies the disease is largely the result of a single mutation event or founder mutation. Strong linkage disequilibrium between the DYT1 gene and a haplotype at the 9q marker loci ABL and ASS was found.[20] This was then extended to include four additional polymorphic markers: D9S62a, D9S62b, D9S63, and D9S64.[22]

The presence of strong linkage disequilibrium at the relatively large genetic distance of at least a few centiMorgans (cM) also suggests that the mutation is recent. Risch and colleagues[22] calculated that the mutation was introduced into the Ashkenazi population approximately 350 years ago. The mutation probably originated in Lithuania or Byelorussia. Risch et al.[22] also argued that the high current prevalence of the disease in Ashkenazim was the result of the tremendous growth of this population during the eighteenth century. In addition, this growth occurred from a small founder population. The current prevalence in this population is estimated to be approximately 1:3,000 to 1:9,000 with a gene frequency of about 1:2,000 to 1:6,000.[22] A founder mutation and genetic drift (i.e., changes in gene frequency caused by chance events such as migrations, population expansions, etc.), rather than a heterozygote advantage (i.e., nonpenetrant *DYT1* carriers with some advantage that leads to carriers being more prevalent) is probably responsible for the high frequency of *DYT1* dystonia in Ashkenazim. This same mechanism probably also accounts for the high frequency of other genetic diseases (e.g., familial dysautonomia, Bloom's syndrome, BRCA1 [breast/ovarian cancer]) in Ashkenazim.

IDENTIFICATION OF *DYT1*

In 1997, Ozelius and coworkers identified the *DYT1* gene, named *TOR1A*.[23,24] This was done by using the finding of linkage disequilibrium and haplotype analyses in Ashkenazi cases, narrowing the region to a 150-kb interval.[25] A heterozygous GAG deletion in the coding sequence in one of four genes within the candidate region was identified. It is the only disease mutation in *TOR1A* identified to date, except for an 18-base pair deletion found in one individual with PTD myoclonus and a mutation in epsilon sarcoglycan.[26] In addition to Ashkenazi cases, the GAG deletion has also been found in non-Jewish individuals as well as families with diverse ethnic backgrounds.[27-30]

Analyses of haplotypes indicate that current deletions in the non-Jewish population originate from multiple independent mutation events. Further, although the GAG deletion in the great majority of Ashkenazim derives from the same founder mutation, a small number of Ashkenazim harbor GAG deletions arising from different mutation events.[22] PTD cases caused by *de novo* GAG deletion events have also been described.[31]

The GAG deletion results in the loss of one residue of a pair of glutamic acid residues near the carboxy terminus of the deduced 332 amino acid novel protein, termed torsinA.[23] TorsinA has an adenosine triphosphate (ATP)-binding domain with distant similarity to the AAA/heat shock protein (HSP)/Clp-ATPase superfamily of chaperone-like proteins. This protein family is distinguished by ATP-binding and/or ATPase activity and oligomeric associations with other proteins. Mutations in the carboxy region of these proteins can block binding to companion proteins and function in a dominant-negative manner. Thus, it is hypothesized that the glutamic acid deletion in torsinA may act in a dominant-negative fashion by disrupting activity of a multimeric complex.[24] Expression of torsinA has been examined in normal adult brain.[32,33] TorsinA is widely distributed, with intense expression in dopamine neurons of the substantia nigra compacta, cerebellar dentate nucleus, Purkinje cells, basis pontis, locus

ceruleus, numerous thalamic nuclei, the pedunculopontine nucleus, the oculomotor nuclei, the hippocampal formation, and frontal cortex. Expression appears to be restricted to neurons.[33] The intense expression in nigral neurons suggests there may be dysfunction in dopamine transmission.[34] When transfected into mammalian cells, both wild-type and mutant torsinA behave as lumenally oriented glycoproteins.[35] Overexpression of wild-type and mutant torsinA shows a different pattern of distribution for the proteins. Wild-type protein is localized to the cytoplasm and neurites, most likely in the endoplasmic reticulum. Mutant protein forms multiple large spheroid inclusions in the cytoplasm around the nucleus.[36] The relationship of overexpressed mutant protein to the disease process is not known.

The clinical expression of the *DYT1 TOR1A* GAG deletion is generally similar across ethnic groups.[28,29,37,38] The great majority of people with the *TOR1A* GAG deletion have early-onset dystonia (i.e., before 26 years of age); one or more limbs are usually affected and more than 95% have an affected arm. The trunk and neck may also be affected; however, the cranial muscles are less likely to be involved (<15%). In rare cases, affected family members may have late-onset dystonia. The most common adult forms of dystonia are focal and segmental arm dystonia. Because of the founder effect, the *TOR1A* GAG deletion is more prominent in the Ashkenazi population. In this population, this GAG deletion accounts for approximately 90% of early limb-onset cases. In comparison, only 40 to 65% of non-Jewish individuals with early limb-onset PTD carry the mutation.[39] That is, as expected, there is genetic heterogeneity; mutations other than the *TOR1A* GAG deletion may produce a phenotype of early-limb-onset PTD among non-Jews. Interestingly, asymptomatic carriers of the *TOR1A* GAG deletion show abnormal regional metabolic covariance patterns on positron emission tomography (PET) scans, indicating that the penetrance of the gene is greater than previously assumed.[40]

The finding that some cases with the *DYT1*-phenotype lack the GAG deletion might suggest the presence of other, unidentified *TOR1A* gene mutations. However, extensive screening for other mutations in *TOR1A* has revealed only a single family with another mutation[24,26] implicating other loci for both the GAG-negative early-limb–onset DYT 1-like phenotype, as well as the late-onset and cervical-cranial phenotypes. This evidence derives from linkage studies excluding the *DYT1* locus in families with and without the *DYT1* phenotype, and also more recent mapping studies of other PTD loci. At least four similar genes, including *TOR1A*, exist in the human genome[24] and represent candidate genes for early-onset cases without the GAG deletion or other types of dystonia.

Late-Onset Primary Torsion Dystonia

Late-onset PTD is more complex genetically than early-onset and the role of genes in etiology in the various adult clinical subtypes is not fully established. Similar to early-onset primary dystonia, late-onset, focal, or cervical-cranial primary dystonia also appears to be inherited in an autosomal dominant fashion.[41-45] However, unlike early-onset dystonia, most studies show that penetrance is even more reduced (approximately 12 to 15% compared to 30% for early onset); alternatively, penetrance may be higher in a subset with the remainder nongenetic. Consistent with the notion that penetrance may be higher in a subset are the descriptions of large non-Jewish families with more highly penetrant autosomal dominant late-onset or cervical-cranial predominant dystonia.

MAPPING GENES FOR LATE-ONSET AND CERVICAL/CRANIAL PRIMARY TORSION DYSTONIA

A second PTD locus (*DYT6*) on chromosome 8 in two families of Mennonite and Amish origin[46] was identified, including one family previously excluded from *DYT1*.[47] Other loci (*DYT7* and *DYT13*) were mapped in North German and Italian families.[48,64] In addition, inborn errors of the mitochondrial respiratory chain (complex I function) have been implicated in the etiology of sporadic focal dystonia.[49]

The locus name assignments for the PTD loci were given by the Human Genome Organization/Genome Database (HUGO/GDB) (Table 2-2). The skip from *DYT1* to *DYT6* is confusing but historically based on the inclusion of dystonic disorders that are either not considered primary (i.e., X-linked dystonia-parkinsonism assigned *DYT3*[50,51] and dopa-responsive dystonia assigned *DYT5*, see below), or only clinically described and not subjected to genetic analyses (autosomal recessive dystonia in the Gypsy population assigned *DYT2*[52] and dystonia with whispering dysphonia assigned *DYT4*[53,54]). Some authors also use *DYT4* as an umbrella term to categorize all forms of autosomal dominant non-*DYT1* PTD.[5]

DYT6

The two Mennonite families with linkage to *DYT6* are clinically similar to each other and initially were not known to be related, although subsequent genealogical investigation revealed a common ancestor (unpublished data). Penetrance appears to be approximately 30% and the clinical picture in these families is broad or mixed. Approximately one-half of the 15 affecteds have onset of symptoms in childhood; body regions first affected include arm, leg, neck, larynx, tongue and facial muscles, and almost all have had some degree of spread or progression of dystonia to other body regions but again this varied widely. Most have both limb and cervical/cranial involvement, and for the majority the greatest disability stems from dystonia of the neck and cranial muscles, including speech involvement. The PTD locus in these families maps to chromosome 8 (maximum 2-point logarithm of odds [LOD] score = 5.80 at the anonymous locus D8S1797).[46] The delimited region bearing the disease gene spans 40 cM, with identical haplotypes segregating with PTD in both families, consistent with the common ancestor.

DYT7

DYT7 was initially mapped in a family from northwest Germany with seven members affected primarily with late-onset torticollis, although mild facial and arm involvement and spasmodic dysphonia were also noted. The gene localized to a 30 cM region on chromosome 18p between D18S1153 and 18pter.[48] Subsequently the same group reported allelic association for several chromosome 18 markers in sporadic and familial torticollis suggesting a founder mutation for adult-onset torticollis in the northwest German and the central European population.[55,56] However, other investigators could not replicate the finding of allelic association in a group of German patients with focal dystonia and reanalysis of the original data set questioned the results.[57] The original investigators then attempted to confirm their findings assessing a highly polymorphic microsatellite with an estimated distance of 50 kb from D18S1098; no allelic association was found and the authors called into question the validity of their primary finding of an association.[58] Although a common founder of focal dystonia cases of northern German or central European origin appears to be ruled out, a second finding supports the presence of a dystonia gene on chromosome 18p, because patients with a deletion of the short arm of chromosome 18 (18p-syndrome) may also present with dystonic symptoms.[59,60]

The extent to which *DYT6* and *DYT7* account for adult and cervical/cranial-onset primary dystonia remains unclear, and there is evidence indicating other yet-unmapped loci. That is, linkage analyses in 6 large non-*DYT1* families with phenotypes that overlap *DYT6* and *DYT7* have excluded both *DYT6* and *DYT7*.[61-63]

DYT13

This locus on chromosome 1 was mapped in an Italian family with 11 definitely affected members. A mixed phenotype that appears to be somewhat more indolent compared to *DYT6* was observed.[64] The age of onset ranged from 5 to 40 years (average, 15.6 years). All patients had juvenile or early-adult onset, with neck or arm involvement. Mild course and occasional generalization was reported. Similar to *DYT1* and *DYT6*, mode of inheritance is autosomal dominant with reduced penetrance. The novel PTD locus (*DYT13*) is within a 22-cM interval on the short arm of chromosome 1, with a maximum LOD score of 3.44 ($\theta = 0$) between the disease and marker D1S2667.[64]

OTHER GENETIC CAUSES OF DYSTONIA

Dystonia-Plus

There are two classes of inherited nonprimary dystonia that have been segregated into a category of dystonia-plus: dopa-responsive dystonia and myoclonus-dystonia. They are separated from the other inherited secondary dystonias because they so closely resemble primary dystonia clinically and because, like primary dystonia, they have no evidence of neural degeneration.

Dopa-Responsive Dystonia

Typically, dopa-responsive dystonia (DRD) presents in mid-childhood (i.e., 5 to 6 years of age) with dystonia affecting the gait. Arm dystonia, hyperreflexia, and parkinsonism are also common features.[65] Over the years the clinical spectrum of this disorder has broadened and includes adult-onset parkinsonism,[66,67] adult-onset oromandibular dystonia,[68] spontaneously remitting dystonia,[69] developmental delay and spasticity mimicking cerebral palsy,[70] and limb dystonia that is not only diurnal but clearly related to exercise.[71] The hallmark feature for all clinical subtypes of DRD is a dramatic and sustained response to low-dosage levodopa, although rarely (especially those with compound heterozygous mutations and adult-onset cases) the dose required may be substantial [Nygaard, personal communication].[68,72,73] Some DRD patients also may have an excellent response to anticholinergics (e.g., trihexyphenidyl).[74]

The genetic basis for many cases of DRD are heterozygous mutations in the GTP cyclohydrolase-1 (GCH1) gene located on chromosome 14 (DYT5).[76-78] New mutations appear to occur commonly, and for unclear reasons clinical expression is more common in females.[79] GCH1 is the first and rate-limiting enzyme in the synthesis of tetrahydrobiopterin, which is an essential cofactor for tyrosine (and phenylalanine and tryptophan) hydroxylase and thus dopamine synthesis.[75,76] It is now evident that some cases of DRD are caused by compound heterozygous mutations in GCH1[74] and homozygous mutations in other enzymes involved in dopamine synthesis including tyrosine hydroxylase[80-82] and 6-pyruvoyltetrahydropterin synthase (6-PTS).[83] The clinical picture in these homozygous conditions often is more severe and includes signs other than dystonia (e.g., hypotonia, severe bradykinesia, drooling, ptosis). One important homozygous condition that mimics DRD and needs to be considered in the differential diagnosis is dystonia caused by mutations in the parkin gene.[84] Generally, the presence of early prominent parkinsonism and severe dyskinesias favors parkin mutations.

In order to confirm the diagnosis of DRD (and to distinguish its specific genetic etiology), various imaging and biochemical tests have been investigated as genetic analysis is complex. That is, no common mutation in GCH1 has been found so that sequencing of all six exons may be necessary, and even with sequencing, a proportion of cases have no identified mutation.[75,85] One test that has been used to distinguish DRD from juvenile parkinsonism is fluorodopa PET, which is normal in DRD. Similarly, single-photon emission tomography using [123I]β-CIT, a sensitive marker of dopamine uptake sites, is also normal in DRD.[86] In contrast, PET with [11C]-raclopride to measure D2 dopamine-receptor binding,[87] shows increased binding in both symptomatic and asymptomatic gene carriers, suggesting either upregulation or reduced competition for ligand as a consequence of decreased dopamine in gene carriers, regardless of clinical signs. One test that has been advocated as sensitive and specific for both affected and nonmanifesting GCH1 gene carriers is phenylalanine loading.[88,89] Biopterin is necessary for the hydroxylation of phenylalanine to tyrosine in the liver. Thus, challenging patients with DRD with phenylalanine (they have normal baseline levels of phenylalanine and tyrosine) results in abnormal elevations of serum phenylalanine, decreased tyrosine, and elevated phenylalanine/tyrosine ratios at 1, 2, and 4 hours postload. This test, however, does not distinguish DRD from phenylketonuria (PKU) carriers, which requires measurement of biopterin (which is decreased) or repeating the challenge after giving biopterin (which corrects the defect in DRD).

Myoclonus-Dystonia

From early descriptions of dystonia, it was evident that in some patients dystonic movements or jerks may be quite rapid, approximately 100 milliseconds (ms), and resemble myoclonus.[90,91] This may occur in DYT1 and other forms of primary dystonia,[91] but it may also be the most prominent feature inherited.[92] In families with myoclonus dystonia (M-D), affected individuals have myoclonus, dystonia, or commonly, both.[93,94] Symptom onset is usually in the first or second decade; males and females are equally affected in most, but not all, families; and the pattern of inheritance appears autosomal dominant with reduced penetrance and variable expression. The neck and arms are involved most commonly, followed by the trunk and bulbar muscles, with less common involvement of the legs. The disorder tends to plateau in adulthood and affected adults often report that the muscle jerks respond dramatically to alcohol.[90,92,94]

In 1999, a missense change (Val54Ile) in a conserved region of the dopamine D2 receptor (DRD2) on 11q23 was found to cosegregate with M-D in one family.[95] However this change has not been identified in other families or singleton cases, and there is no evidence of linkage to 11q23 in other M-D families.[95-98] Furthermore, receptor binding and signal transduction assays of the D2 dopamine mutant and wild-type receptors reveal identical agonist and antagonist affinities and functional responses.[96] Thus, the role of this mutation, including the molecular mechanisms through which it may contribute to M-D, remains to be determined.

Concurrently with the above finding, a M-D locus on chromosome 7q21 (DYT11) was mapped in another M-D

North American family with 10 affected individuals and clinical features typical for this disorder.[99] Obligate recombinations restricted the disease to an interval of about 28 cM. This locus has been confirmed in other M-D families and the region containing DYT11 has been narrowed to 14 cM.[97] Three candidate genes were screened (metabotropic glutamate receptor type 3 and two γ-subunits of guanine nucleotide-binding proteins)[97,99] and did not reveal any mutations. More recently, mutations in the gene coding for epsilon-sarcoglycan (SGCE) on chromosome 7q21 have been reported in many identified familial cases.[100]

RAPID-ONSET DYSTONIA-PARKINSONISM

Rapid-onset dystonia parkinsonism (RDP) was first described by Dobyns et al.[101] in a large family with an autosomal dominant form of dystonia-parkinsonism with an unusually rapid course of the disease. To date, four unrelated families with clinically typical RDP have been reported.[101-104] Mode of inheritance is autosomal dominant with reduced penetrance. In this disorder, there is usually early (adolescent and early adult) onset of waxy dystonia with prominent dysarthria and grimacing, and also bradykinesia, postural instability and hyperreflexia. Motor signs may, however, be restricted to focal or segmental dystonia only. Depression and intermittent hemidystonia and dysarthria associated with stress and anxiety have also been described in one family.[104] Symptoms either come on rapidly (over hours to days) or there is an episode of rapid progression from mild to severe disability.[105] After the worsening, symptoms tend to plateau but there is no significant improvement with medical therapies including levodopa. Some patients showed decreased levels of the dopamine metabolite, homovanillic acid (HVA) in cerebrospinal fluid.[106] Imaging of the dopamine re-uptake system using [11C]β-CFT revealed slightly elevated values, indicating that there is no degeneration of striatal dopamine terminals or loss of dopamine reuptake sites in RDP.[107]

A gene for RDP was mapped to chromosome 19q13 (DYT12) with a highest multipoint LOD score of 5.77 across two of the four families at the marker D19S198 and with obligate recombination events at the markers D19S587 and D19S900, defining a candidate region of approximately 8 cM.[108] Pittock et al. independently showed linkage to the same chromosome 19 locus in a family with eight affected individuals.[104]

OTHER DYSKINESIA SYNDROMES WITH DYSTONIA: INHERITED PAROXYSMAL DYSKINESIAS

Paroxysmal dystonias/dyskinesias are rare conditions, clinically characterized by various combinations of paroxysmal hyperkinesias, including dystonia, chorea, athetosis, and ballism.[109] In 1967, Kertesz[110] distinguished between nonkinesigenic and kinesigenic forms of paroxysmal dystonia/dyskinesia (PNKD and PKD, respectively); Lance[111] added an

intermediate form that is marked by dystonia that is not strictly on movement or kinesigenic but comes on after prolonged exercise.

PNKD (formerly termed paroxysmal dystonic choreoathetosis or PDC) was first described by Mount and Reback[112] in a large family with autosomal dominantly inherited paroxysmal dystonia. Symptoms usually begin in infancy but may also manifest in childhood or adolescence. Attacks may be precipitated by a variety of factors including emotional stress, fatigue, chocolate, coffee, or alcohol intake but not sudden movement. Attacks last from minutes to hours and typically last one hour; they may occur several times each day or infrequently. The disorder was independently mapped in two different families of Italian and Polish descent to a locus, DYT8, on chromosome 2q,[113,114] with maximum LOD scores of 4.64 and 4.77, respectively. Linkage studies of a third unrelated family narrowed the DYT8 region to 4 cm between the markers D2S295 and D2S377[115] with a LOD score of 5.08 for the marker D2S163. Subsequently, this PNKD locus has been confirmed in additional families[116,117] and the candidate region refined to 3.6 cm between the markers D2S164 and D2S2359.[117]

Paroxysmal kinesigenic dyskinesia/choreoathetosis is the most frequent type of the paroxysmal dyskinesias. The familial form is also inherited in an autosomal dominant fashion[110,118] with an unexplained male predominance.[118] Symptoms begin in early childhood to early adulthood and are precipitated by sudden movements (such as arising suddenly), startle, or hyperventilation. Attacks usually last less than five minutes, may occur over 100 times per day (but are usually less frequent), and respond to treatment with low dosages of anticonvulsants, especially carbamazepine.[110,119] A locus for PKD (DYT10) was first mapped in eight Japanese families to the pericentromeric region of chromosome 16 (16p11.2-q12.1) with a maximum multipoint LOD score of 11.51 at the marker D16S3081.[120] The critical interval (12.4 cM) was localized between the markers D16S3093 and D16S416.[120] This region overlaps by 6.0 cM with a region for infantile convulsions and paroxysmal dyskinesias (ICCA syndrome), a recently identified neurological disorder with benign infantile convulsions and paroxysmal dyskinesias.[121]

Because there is an increased frequency of afebrile infantile convulsions in the Japanese families with PKD, it was hypothesized that these disorders are allelic. Linkage to an overlapping region was then found by a second group in an African American kindred with PKD.[122] In this family, the obligate region overlapped the Japanese PKD region by 9.8 cm and the ICCA region by 3.4 cm, suggesting that indeed one gene may be responsible for the disorder in all three populations. However, most recently the notion of one gene for all PKD and ICCA has been rejected by linkage finding in a large Indian family with PKD.[123] Linkage analysis in this family identified a locus on the long arm of chromosome 16 that overlaps with the PKD locus identified in the African American family, but not that found among Japanese families with PKD. The second PKD locus [EKD2] is between D16S685 and D16S503 and does not overlap the ICCA locus.

It is suggested that there may be a cluster of genes on human chromosome 16 responsible for these similar syndromes.[123]

Finally, Auburger et al.[124] described a family with autosomal dominant paroxysmal choreoathetosis with episodic ataxia and constant spasticity (*DYT9*). The disease gene was localized in a 12-cm region on chromosome 1p, between the markers D1S443 and D1S197. The maximum LOD score was 7.2.[124]

CONCLUSIONS

Clinical Application of Genetic Advances to Practice

Because of the extremely reduced penetrance and variable expression of primary dystonia and dystonia plus syndromes and because mild cases may remain undiagnosed, it is common to obtain a negative family history in the office. Based on current findings, it is reasonable to assume a genetic etiology for most cases of early-onset primary dystonia, regardless of family history. Many cases are caused by *DYT1*. At least a proportion of late-onset primary dystonia is also genetic. Because almost all dystonia with involvement of the *DYT1* gene appears to be due to the same GAG deletion, screening is relatively easy. The test is available commercially and is considered the first diagnostic test for all patients with primary dystonia whether Ashkenazi or non-Jewish. This includes patients with an onset by age 26 years or those with onset later in life but who have a relative with early onset (<26 years).[39] Before diagnostic testing is done, it is preferable to have genetic counseling performed. In this way, the implications of a positive or negative test result may be explained.

For example, even if the test is negative, a genetic etiology is not excluded and this must be discussed. If the test is positive, a diagnosis is secured; however, this diagnosis affects other at-risk family members. These family members, even if asymptomatic, may desire to have carrier testing, and immediate genetic counseling for all asymptomatic family members is also recommended. The psychological and social implications of a disorder with autosomal dominant inheritance that has markedly reduced penetrance and extremely variable expression are complex.

At present, there is no commercial testing for other genetic causes of primary dystonia. In large families, linkage to *DYT6*, *DYT7*, *DYT12*, or any other known loci, may be performed on a research basis only. For example, this is true for sequencing of the *GCH1* gene in DRD patients. Linkage studies for genes that are not yet identified may help to narrow the chromosomal regions of the respective loci, and thus may facilitate the search for these various dystonia genes.

SUMMARY

There is accumulating evidence for genetic heterogeneity, and specifically for locus heterogeneity in PTD and the dystonia plus syndromes. In PTD, distinct though overlapping phenotype-genotype entities have emerged, including:

- Early limb onset—*DYT1*
- Mixed early-onset—*DYT6*
- Late cervical onset—*DYT7*
- Mixed juvenile or early-adult onset—*DYT13*
- There is also evidence for more than one locus for each of these phenotypes. The same concept holds true for many of the non-PTD syndromes. The relationships of these loci to disease mechanisms are currently unknown.

The close correlation between age at onset and body regions affected, along with the clinical differences among loci (e.g., *DYT1*, *DYT6*, and *DYT7*), support gene defects with distinct anatomic and temporal brain expression. However, the apparent presence of multiple loci with similar if not identical phenotypes also implies that mutations in different genes may produce a common disturbance of motor control.

REFERENCES

1. Fahn S, Marsden CD, Calne DB. Classification and investigation of dystonia. In: Marsden CD, Fahn S, eds. Movement Disorders 2. London: Butterworth, 1987:332–358.
2. Bressman SB, de Leon D, Brin MF, et al. Idiopathic torsion dystonia among Ashkenazi Jews: Evidence for autosomal dominant inheritance. Ann Neurol 1989;26:612–620.
3. Greene P, Kang UJ, Fahn S. Spread of symptoms in idiopathic torsion dystonia. Mov Disord 1995;10:143–152.
4. Bressman SB, Fahn S. Childhood Dystonia. In: Watts RL, Koller WC, eds. Movement Disorders: Neurologic Principals and Practice. New York, McGraw Hill, 1997:419–428.
5. Müller U, Steinberger D, Nemeth AH. Clinical and molecular genetics of primary dystonias. Neurogenetics 1997;1:165–177.
6. Klein C, Brin MF, de leon D, et al. De novo mutations (GAG deletion) in the DYT1 gene in two non-Jewish patients with early-onset dystonia. Hum Mol Genet 1998;7:1133–1136.
8. Nutt JG, Muenter MD, Aronson A, et al. Epidemiology of focal and generalized dystonia in Rochester, Minnesota. Mov Disord 1988; 3:188–194.
9. Zeman W, Dyken P. Dystonia musculorum deformans; clinical, genetic and pathoanatomical studies. Psychiatr Neurol Neurochir 1967;70: 77–121.
10. Zilber N, Korczyn AD, Kahana E, et al. Inheritance of idiopathic torsion dystonia among Jews. J Med Genet 1984;21:13–26.
11. Schwalbe W. Eine eigentümliche tonische Krampfform mit hysterischen Symptomen [Thesis]. Berlin, 1908.
12. Eldridge RA. The torsion dystonias: literature review, genetic and clinical studies. Neurology 1970;20(Suppl2):1–78.
13. Risch N, Bressman SB, de Leon D, et al. Segregation analysis of idiopathic torsion dystonia in Ashkenazi Jews suggests autosomal dominant inheritance. *Am J Hum Genet* 1990;46:533–538.
14. Pauls DL, Korczyn AD. Complex segregation analysis of dystonia pedigrees suggests autosomal dominant inheritance. Neurology 1990;40:1107–1110.
15. Fletcher NA, Harding AE, Marsden CD. A genetic study of idiopathic torsion dystonia in the United Kingdom. Brain 1990;113:379–396.
16. Kramer PL, Heiman GA, Gasser T, et al. The DYT1 gene on 9q34 is responsible for most cases of early limb-onset idiopathic torsion dystonia in non-Jews. Am J Hum Genet 1994;55:468–475.
17. Ozelius L, Kramer P, Moskowitz CB, et al. Human gene for torsion dystonia located on chromosome 9q32–34. Neuron 1989;2:1427–1434.
18. Kramer LP, de Leon D, Ozelius L, et al. Dystonia gene in Ashkenazi Jewish population located on chromosome 9q32–34. Ann Neurol 1990;27:114–120.
19. Warner T, Fletcher NA, Davis MB, et al. Linkage analysis in British families with idiopathic torsion dystonia. Brain 1993;116:739–744.

20. Ozelius LJ, Kramer PL, de Leon D, et al. Strong allelic association between the torsion dystonia gene (DYT1) and loci on chromosome 9q34 in Ashkenazi Jews. Am J Hum Genet 1992;50:619–628.

21. Bressman SB, de Leon D, Kramer PL, et al. Dystonia in Ashkenazi Jews: clinical characterization of a founder mutation. Ann Neurol 1994a;35:771–771.

22. Risch N, deLeon D, Ozelius L, et al. Genetic analysis of idiopathic torsion dystonia in Ashkenazi Jews and their recent descent from a small founder population. Nat Genet 1995;9:152–159.

23. Ozelius LJ, Hewett JW, Page C, et al. The early-onset torsion dystonia gene (DYT1) encodes an ATP-binding protein. Nat Genet 1997a; 17:40–48.

24. Ozelius LJ, Page CE, Klein C, et al. The TOR1A (DYT1) gene family and role in early onset torsion dystonia. Genomics, 1999;62:377–384.

25. Ozelius LJ, Hewett J, Kramer P, et al. Fine localization of the torsion dystonia gene (DYT1) on human chromosome 9q34:YAC map and linkage disequilibrium. Genome Res 1997b;7:483–494.

26. Leung JC, Klein C, Friedman J, et al. Novel mutation in the TOR1A (DYT1) gene in atypical early onset dystonia and polymorphisms in dystonia and early onset parkinsonism. Neurogenetics 2001;3:133–143.

27. Ikeuchi T, Shimohata T, Nakano R, et al. A case of primary torsion dystonia in Japan with the 3-bp (GAG) deletion in the DYT1 gene with a unique clinical presentation. Neurogenetics 1999;2:189–190.

28. Valente EM, Warner TT, Jarman PR, et al. The role of primary torsion dystonia in Europe. Brain 1998;121:2335–2339.

29. Slominski PA, Markova ED, Shadrina MI, et al. A common 3-bp deletion in the DYT1 gene in Russian families with early-onset torsion dystonia. Hum Mutat 1999;14:269.

30. Lebre AS, Durr A, Jedynak P, et al. A DYT1 mutation in French families with idiopathic torsion dystonia. Brain 1999;122:41–45.

31. Hjermind LE, Werdelin LM, Sorensen SA. Inherited and de novo mutations in sporadic cases of DYT1-dystonia. Eur J Hum Genet 2002;10:213–216.

32. Augood SJ, Penney JB, Friburg IK, et al. Expression of early-onset torsion dystoni gene (DYT1) in human brain. Ann Neurol 1998;43:669–673.

33. Shashidharan P, Kramer BC, Walker RH, et al. Immunohistochemical localization and distribution of torsinA in normal human and rat brain. Brain Res 2000;853:197–206.

34. Augood SJ, Martin DM, Ozelius LJ, et al. Distribution of the mRNAs encoding torsinA and torsinB in the normal adult brain. Ann Neurol 1999;46:761–769.

35. Kustedjo K, Bracey MH, Cravatt BF. Torsin A and its torsion dystonia-associated mutant forms are lumenal glycoproteins that exhibit distinct subcellular localizations. J Biol Chem 2000;275:27933-27939.

36. Hewett J, Gonzalez-Agosti C, Slater D, et al. Mutant torsinA, responsible for early-onset torsion dystonia, forms membrane inclusions in cultured neural cells. Hum Mol Genet 2000;9:1403–1413.

37. Klein C, Friedman J, Bressman S, et al. Genetic testing for early-onset torsion dystonia (DYT1): introduction of a simple screening method, experiences from testing of a large patient cohort, and ethical aspects. Genet Test 1999;3:323–328.

38. Bressman SB, Sabatti C, Raymond D, et al. The DYT1 phenotype and guidelines for diagnostic testing. Neurology 2000;54:1746–1752.

39. Bressman SB, Heiman GA, Nygaard TG, et al. A study of idiopathic torsion dystonia in a non-Jewish family:evidence for genetic heterogeneity. Neurology 1994;44:283–287.

40. Eidelberg D, Moeller JR, Antonini A, et al. Functional brain networks in DYT1 dystonia. Ann Neurol 1998;44:303–312.

41. Defazio G, Livrea P, Guanti G, et al. Genetic contribution to idiopathic adult-onset blepharospasm and cranial-cervical dystonia. Eur Neurol 1993;33:345–350.

42. Bressman SB, Rassnick H, Almasy L, et al. Inheritance of late-onset idiopathic torsion dystonia. Neurology 1995;45(suppl4):A457[abstract].

43. Waddy HM, Fletcher NA, Harding AE, et al. A genetic study of idiopathic focal dystonias. Ann Neurol 1991;29:320–324.

44. Stojanovic M, Cvetkovic D, Kostic VS. A genetic study of idiopathic focal dystonias. J Neurol 1995;242:508–511.

45. Leube B, Kessler KR, Goecke T, et al. Frequency of familial inheritance among 488 index patients with idiopathic focal dystonia and clinical variability in a large family. Mov Disord 1997;12:1000–1006.

46. Almasy L, Bressman SB, Kramer PL, et al. Idiopathic torsion dystonia linked to chromosome 8 in two Mennonite families. Ann Neurol 1997;42:670–673.

47. Bressman SB, Hunt AL, Heiman G, et al. Exclusion of the DYT1 locus in a non- Jewish family with early onset dystonia. Mov Disord 1994;9:626–632.

48. Leube B, Doda R, Ratzlaff T, et al. Idiopathic torsion dystonia: assignment of a gene to chromosome 18p in a German family with adult onset, autosomal inheritance and purely focal distribution. Hum Mol Genet 1996;5:1673–1677.

49. Schapira AHV, Warner T, Gash MT, et al. Complex I function in familial and sporadic dystonia. Ann Neurol 1997;41:556–559.

50. Kupke KG, Lee LV, Viterbo GH, et al. X-linked recessive torsion dystonia in the Philippines. Am J Med Genet 1990;36:237–242.

51. Nemeth AH, Nolte D, Dunne E, et al. Refined linkage disequilibrium and physical mapping of the gene locus for X-linked dystonia-parkinsonism (DYT3). Genomics 1999;60:320–329.

52. Giménez-Roldán S, Delgado G, Marín M, et al. Hereditary torsion dystonia in gypsies. Adv Neurol 1988;50:73–81.

53. Parker N. Hereditary whispering dysphonia. J Neurol Neurosurg Psychiatry 1985;48:218–224.

54. Ahmad F, Davis MB, Waddy HM, et al. Evidence for locus heterogeneity in autosomal dominant torsion dystonia. Genomics 1993; 15:9–12.

55. Leube B, Hendgen T, Kessler KR, et al. Sporadic focal dystonia in Northwest Germany: molecular basis on chromosome 18p. Ann Neurol 1997;42:111–114.

56. Leube B, Hendgen T, Kessler KR, et al. Evidence for DYT7 being a common cause of cervical dystonia (torticollis) in Central Europe. Am J Med Genet 1997;74:529–532.

57. Klein C, Ozelius L, Hagenah J, et al. Search for a founder mutation in idiopathic focal dystonia from Northern Germany. Am J Hum Genet 1998b;63:1777–1782.

58. Leube B, Auburger G. Questionable role of adult-onset focal dystonia among sporadic dystonia patients. Ann Neurol 1998;44:984–985.

59. Klein C, Page CE, LeWitt P, et al. Genetic analysis of three patients with an 18p- syndrome and dystonia. Neurology 1999;52:649–651.

60. Tezzon F, Zanoni T, Passarin MG, et al. Dystonia in a patient with deletion of 18p. Ital J Neurol Sci 1998;19:90–93.

61. Jarman P, Valente EM, Leube B, et al. Primary torsion dystonia: the search for genes is not over. J Neurol Neurosurg Psychiatry 1999;67:395–397.

62. Klein C, Pramstaller PP, Castellan CC, et al. Clinical and genetic evaluation of a family with a mixed dystonia phenotype from South Tyrol. Ann Neurol 1998c;44:394–398.

63. Münchau A, Valente EM, Davis MB, et al. A Yorkshire family with adult-onset cranio-cervical primary torsion dystonia. Mov Disord 2000;15:954–959.

64. Valente EM, Bentivoglio AR, Cassetta E, et al. DYT13, a novel primary torsion dystonia locus, maps to chromosome 1p36.13–36.32 in an Italian family with cranial-cervical or upper limb onset. Ann Neurol 2001;49:662–666 .

65. Nygaard TG, Marsden CD, Fahn S. Dopa-responsive dystonia: long-term treatment response and prognosis. Neurology 1991;41:174–181.

66. Nygaard TG, Takahashi H, Heiman GA, et al. Long-term treatment response and fluorodopa positron emission tomographic scanning of parkinsonism in a family with dopa-responsive dystonia. Ann Neurol 1992;32:603–608.

67. Saunders-Pullman R, Eidelberg D, Nygaard T, et al. Typical parkinsonism in dopa-responsive dystonia [Abstract]. Ann Neurol 1997;42:447.

68. Steinberger D, Topka H, Fischer D, et al. GCH1 mutation in a patient with adult-onset oromandibular dystonia. Neurology 1999;52:877–879.

69. Di Capua M, Bertini E. Remission in dihydroxyphenylalanine-responsive dystonia. Mov Disord 1995;10:223.

70. Nygaard TG, Waran SP, Levine RA, et al. Dopa-responsive dystonia simulating cerebral palsy. Pediatr Neurol 1994;11:236–240.

71. Deonna T, Roulet E, Ghika J, et al. Dopa-responsive childhood dystonia: a formes frustes with writer's cramp, triggered by exercise. Dev Med Child Neurol 1997;39:49–53.

72. Saunders-Pullman R, Braun I, Bressman S. Pediatric movement disorders. Child Adolesc Psychiatr Clin North Am 1999;8:747–765.

73. Furukawa Y, Kish SJ, Bebin EM, et al. Dystonia with motor delay in compound heterozygotes for GTP cyclohydrolase I gene mutations. Ann Neurol 1998a;44:10–16.

74. Jarman PR, Bandmann O, Marsden CD, et al. GTP cyclohydrolase 1 mutations in patients with dystonia responsive to anticholinergic drugs. J Neurol Neurosurg Psychiatry 1997;63:304–308.

75. Ichinose H, Ohye T, Takahiashi E, et al. Hereditary progressive dystonia with marked diurnal fluctuation caused by mutations in the GTP cyclohydrolase gene. Nat Genet 1994;8:236–242

76. Furukawa Y, Shimadzu M, Rajput AH, et al. GTP cyclohydrolase 1 mutations in hereditary progressive and dopa responsive dystonia. Ann Neurol 1996;39:609–617.

77. Ichinose H, Nagatsu T. Molecular genetics of dopa-responsive dystonia. Adv Neurol 1999;80:195–198.

78. Ichinose H, Inagaki H, Suzuki T, et al. Molecular mechanisms of hereditary progressive dystonia with marked diurnal fluctuation, Segawa's disease. Brain Dev 2000;22 (Suppl 1):107–110.

79. Furukawa Y, Land AE, Trugman JM, et al. Gender-related penetrance and de novo GTP-cyclohydrolase I gene mutations in dopa-responsive dystonia. Neurology 1998;50:1015–1020.

80. Knappskog PM, Flatmark T, Mallet J, et al. Recessively inherited l-dopa responsive dystonia caused by a point mutation (Q381K) in the tyrosine hydroxylase gene. Hum Mol Genet 1995;4:1209–1212.

81. Lüdecke B, Knappskog PM, Clayton PT, et al. Recessively inherited L-DOPA-responsive parkinsonism in infancy caused by a point mutation (L205P) in the tyrosine hydroxylase gene. Hum Mol Genet 1996;5:1023–1028.

82. van den Heuvel LP, Luiten B, Smeitink JA, et al. A common point mutation in the tyrosine hydroxylase gene in autosomal recessive L-DOPA-responsive dystonia in the Dutch population. Hum Genet 1998;102:644–646.

83. Hanihara T, Inoue K, Kawanishi C, et al. 6-pyrovoyl-tetrahydropterin synthase deficiency with generalized dystonia and diurnal fluctuation of symptoms: a clinical molecular study. Mov Disord 1997;12:408–411.

84. Tassin J, Dürr A, Bonnet A-M, Gil R, et al. Levodopa-responsive dystonia: GTP cyclohydrolase I or parkin mutations? Brain 2000;123:1112–1121.

85. Bandmann O, Nygaard TG, Surtees R, et al. Dopa-responsive dystonia in British patients: New mutations of the GTP-cyclohydrolase 1 gene and evidence for genetic heterogeneity. Hum Mol Genet 1996;5:403–406.

86. Naumann M, Pirker W, Reiners K, et al. [123]beta-CIT single photon emission tomography in dopa-responsive dystonia. Mov Disord 1997;12:448–451.

87. Kishore A, Nygaard TG, de la Fuente-Fernandez R, et al. Striatal D2 receptors in symptomatic and asymptomatic carriers of dopa-responsive dystonia measured with [11C]-raclopride and positron emission tomography. Neurology 1998;50:1028–1032.

88. Hyland K, Fryburg JS, Wilson WG, et al. Oral phenylalanine loading in dopa-responsive dystonia: a possible diagnostic test. Neurology 1997;48:1290–1297.

89. Hyland K, Arnold LA, Trugman JM. Defects of biopterin metabolism and biogenic amine biosynthesis: clinical diagnostic, and therapeutic aspects. Adv Neurol 1998;78:301–308.

90. Mahloudji M, Pikielny RT. Hereditary essential myoclonus. Brain 1967;90:669–674.

91. Obeso JA, Rothwell JC, Lang AE, et al. Myoclonic dystonia. Neurology 1983;33:825–830.

92. Quinn NP. Essential myoclonus and myoclonic dystonia. Mov Disord 1996;11:119–124.

93. Gasser T. Inherited myoclonus-dystonia syndrome. Adv Neurol 1998;78:325–334.

94. Kyllerman M, Forsgren L, Sanner G, et al. Alcohol responsive myoclonic dystonia in a large family. Dominant inheritance and phenotypic variation. Mov Disord 1990;5:270–279.

95. Klein C, Brin MF, Kramer P, et al. Association of a missense change in the D2 dopamine receptor with myoclonus dystonia. Proc Natl Acad Sci USA 1999;96:5173–5176.

96. Klein C, Gurvich N, Sena-Esteves M, et al. Evaluation of the role of the D2 dopamine receptor in myoclonus-dystonia. Ann Neurol 2000;47:369–373.

97. Klein C, Schilling K, Saunders-Pullman RJ, et al. A major locus for myoclonus-dystonia maps to chromosome 7q in eight families. Am J Hum Genet 2000b;67:1314–1319.

98. Durr A, Tassin J, Vidailhet M, et al. D2 dopamine receptor gene in myoclonic dystonia and essential myoclonus. Ann Neurol 2000;48:127–128.

99. Nygaard TG, Raymond D, Chen C, et al. Localization of a gene for myoclonus dystonia to chromosome 7q21–31. Ann Neurol 1999;46:794–798.

100. Zimprich A, Grabowski M, Asmus F, et al. Mutations in the gene encoding epsilon-sarcoglycan cause myoclonus-dystonia syndrome. Nat Genet 2001;29:66–69.

101. Dobyns WB, Ozelius LJ, Kramer PL, et al. Rapid-onset dystonia-parkinsonism. Neurology 1993;43:2596–2602.

102. Brashear A, DeLeon D, Bressman SB, et al. Rapid-onset dystonia-parkinsonism in a second family. Neurology 1997;48:1066–1069.

103. Webb DW, Broderick A, Brashear A, et al. Rapid onset dystonia-parkinsonism in a 14-year-old girl. Eur J Paediatr Neurol 1999;3:171–173.

104. Pittock SJ, Joyce C, O'Keane V, et al. Rapid-onset dystonia-parkinsonism: a clinical and genetic analysis of a new kindred. Neurology 2000;55:991–995.

105. Brashear A, Farlow MR, Butler IJ, et al. Variable phenotype of rapid-onset dystonia-parkinsonism. Mov Disord 1996;11:151–156.

106. Brashear A, Butler IJ, Hyland K, et al. Cerebrospinal fluid homovanillic acid levels in rapid-onset dystonia-parkinsonism. Ann Neurol 1998;43:521–526.

107. Brashear A, Mulholland GK, Zheng Q-H, et al. PET imaging of the presynaptic dopamine uptake sites in rapid-onset dystonia-parkinsonism (RDP). Mov Disord 1999;14:132–137.

108. Kramer PL, Mineta M, Klein C. Rapid-onset dystonia-parkinsonism: linkage to chromosome 19q13. Ann Neurol 1999;46:176–182.

109. Fahn S. The paroxysmal dyskinesias. In: Marsden CD, Fahn S (eds.) Movement Disorders 3. Cambridge: Butterworth-Heinemann, 1994:310–345.

110. Kertesz A. Paroxysmal kinesigenic choreoathetosis. Neurology 1967;17:680–690.

111. Lance JW. Familial paroxysmal dystonic choreoathetosis and its differentiation from related syndromes. Ann Neurol 1977;2:285–293.

112. Mount LA, Reback S. Familial paroxysmal choreoathetosis: preliminary report on a hitherto undescribed clinical syndrome. Arch Neurol Psychiatry 1940;44:841–847.

113. Fouad GT, Servidei S, Durcan S, et al. A gene for familial paroxysmal dyskinesia (FPD1) maps to chromosome 2q. Am J Hum Genet 1996;59:135–139.

114. Fink JK, Rainer S, Wilkowski J, et al. Paroxysmal dystonic choreoathetosis: tight linkage to chromosome 2q. Am J Hum Genet 1996;59:140–145.

115. Jarman PR, Davis MB, Hodgson SV, et al. Paroxysmal dystonic choreoathetosis. Genetic linkage studies in a British family. Brain 1997;120:2125 2130.

116. Raskind WH, Bolin T, Wolff J, et al. Further localization of a gene for paroxysmal dystonic choreoathetosis to a 5-cM region on chromosome 2q34. Hum Genet 1998;102:93–97.

117. Hofele K, Benecke R, Auburger G. Gene locus FPD1 of the dystonic Mount-Reback type of autosomal dominant paroxysmal choreoathetosis. Neurology 1997;49:1252–1256.

118. Nagamitsu S, Matsuishi T, Hshimoto K. Multicenter study of paroxysmal dyskinesias in Japan: clinical and pedigree analysis. Mov Disord 1999;14:658–663.

119. Fahn S. The early history of paroxysmal dyskinesias. Adv Neurol 2002;89:377–385.

120. Tomita H-a, Nagamitsu S, Wakui K, et al. Paroxysmal kinesigenic choreoathetosis locus maps to chromosome 16p11.2-q12.1. Am J Hum Genet 1999;65:1688–1697.

121. Lee WL, Tay A, Ong HT, et al. Association of infantile convulsions with paroxysmal dyskinesias (ICCA syndrome): confirmation of linkage to human chromosome 16p12-q12 in a Chinese family. Hum Genet 1998;103:608–612.

121. Bennett LB, Roach ES, Bowcock AM. A locus for paroxysmal kinesigenic dyskinesia maps to human chromosome 16. Neurology 2000;54:125–130.

123. Valente EM, Spacey SD, Wali GM, et al. A second paroxysmal kinesigenic choreoathetosis locus (EKD2) mapping on 16q13-q22.1 indicates a family of genes which give rise to paroxysmal disorders on human chromsome 16. Brain 2000;123:2040–45.

124. Auburger G, Ratzlaff T, Lunkes A, et al. A gene for autosomal dominant paroxysmal choreoathetosis/spasticity (CSE) maps to the vicinity of a potassium channel gene cluster on chromosome 1p, probably within 2 cM between D1S443 and D1S197. Genomics 1996;31:90–94.

CHAPTER 3

Genetic Testing and Genetic Counseling

Dana O. Doheny, Deborah de Leon, and Deborah Raymond

INTRODUCTION

In 1975, the American Society of Human Genetics adopted the following definition of genetic counseling:

> Genetic counseling is the communication process that deals with the human problems associated with the occurrence, or the risk of an occurrence, of a genetic disorder in the family. This process involves an attempt by one or more appropriately trained persons to help the individual or family to (1) comprehend the medical facts, including the diagnosis, probable course of the disorder, and the available management; (2) appreciate the way heredity contributes to the disorder, and the risk of recurrence in specified relatives; (3) understand the alternatives for dealing with the risk of occurrence; (4) choose the course of action which seems to them appropriate in view of their risk, their family goals, and their ethical and religious standards, and to act in accordance with that decision; and (5) to make the best possible adjustment to the disorder in an affected family member and/or to the risk of recurrence of that disorder.[1]

During the last 25 years, the field of genetic counseling has expanded rapidly to include not only reproductive risks and related issues but also issues related to DNA predictive and diagnostic testing. When counseling individuals with dystonia and their families, the genetic counselor must be knowledgeable about the disorder, including the subtypes and inheritance patterns, available testing options, and support resources.

CLASSIFICATION OF DYSTONIA

Historically, dystonia has been a poorly understood and often misdiagnosed condition even among neurologists. In general terms, dystonia is "the simultaneous, sustained contraction of

Dana O. Doheny: Mount Sinai School of Medicine, Department of Human Genetics, New York, New York.

Deborah de Leon: Irvine, California, private practice.

Deborah Raymond: Beth Israel Medical Center, Department of Neurology, New York, New York.

The authors have no commercial relationship with the funder.

opposing muscles that twist the involved body region into an unnatural position." Dystonic movements are repetitive and may be rhythmic. Sometimes these movements are accompanied by tremors, which may range from slow and athetotic, to rapid and jerky. Dystonic movements are not typically associated with pain except in the case of cervical dystonia, which most often is not the result of the *DYT1* GAG deletion. Voluntary movement often aggravates the contractions of primary dystonia. Such voluntary movements may be either nonspecific or task-specific, such as writing but not feeding, or walking forward but not backward. Symptoms may also worsen with fatigue or stress, and alternately, may be alleviated with relaxation, hypnosis, or sleep. Tactile sensory techniques, or "sensory tricks," such as touching the cheek or the chin (as in patients with cervical dystonia) may also help to alleviate the dystonic posturing.

Dystonia may be classified as primary torsion dystonia (PTD), secondary dystonia, and dystonia plus. In PTD, dystonia is the only symptom. The primary dystonias may be further categorized based on clinical criteria, including the age of symptom onset, distribution of symptoms, and dopa-responsiveness.[3] Secondary or symptomatic dystonia occurs in association with other neurologic findings or results from an environmental insult. The "dystonia plus" syndromes include two classes of inherited nonprimary dystonia, myoclonus-dystonia and dopa-responsive dystonia (DRD), which clinically resemble the primary dystonias and show no evidence of neural degeneration. Therefore, as part of the differential diagnosis of dystonia, it is important to distinguish dystonia from other inherited disorders that may present clinically with dystonic features. Some of these disorders have diagnostic tests available, such as the spinocerebellar ataxias (SCAs), Wilson's disease, and the gangliosidoses.

As a result of the identification of gene loci, the clinical classification is rapidly being replaced by genetic classifications.[4,5] Continued investigation of these gene loci and their association with specific dystonias will provide a better understanding of the clinical picture, as well as reliable diagnostic and carrier testing options. Table 3-1 outlines the clinical and molecular genetic subtypes of dystonia.

23

TABLE 3-1. *Clinical and Molecular Genetic Classification of the Dystonias*[27a]

Disease Name	Gene Symbol/ Product	Chromosome Location	Mode of Inheritance	Phenotype	DNA Testing	OMIM
Idiopathic torsion dystonia (ITD); dystonia musculorum deformans; Oppenheim's disease	DYT1/TorsinA	9q34	AD	Childhood and adolescent onset; limb onset with generalization within 3 years	Clinical	128100
Torsion dystonia 2	DYT2	Unknown	AR	In Spanish gypsies; not confirmed	None	224500
Lubag disease, X-linked dystonia-parkinsonism	DYT3	Xq13.1	XLR	Dystonia with parkinsonism; average onset mid-30s; predominantly in Panay, Philippines	Research	314250
Torsion dystonia 4, whispering dysphonia	DYT4	Unknown	AD	One Australian family; adolescent and adult onset; whispering speech	None	128101
Dopa-responsive dystonia (DRD)	DYT5/ GTPCH-1	14q22.1-q22.2	AD	Childhood onset; one limb involvement progresses to all limbs within 5 years; diurnal variation; dopa-responsive	Clinical/ Research	128230
Torsion dystonia 6, Adult-onset ITD of mixed type	DYT6	8p21-p22	AD	Mennonite/Amish dystonia with mixed face, eyes, neck, or limb onset; childhood or adult onset; cranial or cervical involvement predominates	Research	602629
Torsion dystonia 7, Adult-onset focal torsion dystonia	DYT7	18p	AD	German families; adult onset; neck, face, or hand onset; neck involvement predominates	Research	602124
Paroxysmal dystonic choreoathetosis (PDC), Mount-Reback syndrome, Dystonia 8	DYT8	2q33-q35	AD	Recurrent episodes of involuntary movements with dystonic postures; often precipitated by coffee, alcohol, hunger, fatigue, tobacco; variable age of onset; may be the same as DYT10	Research	118800
Paroxysmal choreoathetosis with episodic ataxia (CSE), Kinesigenic choreoathetosis with episodic ataxia and spasticity, Dystonia 9	DYT9	1p	AD	Recurrent episodes of involuntary movements with dystonic postures, imbalance or spastic paraplegia, dysarthria, double vision, headache; often precipitated by exercise, stress, fatigue, alcohol; childhood and adolescent onset	Research	601042
Paroxysmal kinesigenic choreoathetosis (PKC), Familial paroxysmal dystonia, Dystonia 10	DYT10	16p11.2-q12.1	AD	Recurrent brief episodes of involuntary movements with dystonic postures; anticonvulsant-responsive; may be the same as DYT8	None	128200
Hereditary alcohol-responsive myoclonus dystonia	DYT11	7q21	AD	Muscle jerks and/or torsion dystonia, aggravated by fatigue, stress, alleviated by alcohol; childhood and adolescent onset	Research	159900

TABLE 3-1. *Clinical and Molecular Genetic Classification of the Dystonias[27a] (Continued)*

Disease Name	Gene Symbol/ Product	Chromosome Location	Mode of Inheritance	Phenotype	DNA Testing	OMIM
Rapid-onset dystonia-parkinsonism (RDP)	*DYT12*	19q13	AD	Adolescent and adult-onset; dystonia with parkinsonism; abrupt onset with rapid progression of hours to weeks; non-dopa-responsive	Research	128235
Leber's hereditary optic neuropathy (LHON)	*LDYT*	MtDNA (18 missense mutations identified)	mt	Mid-life central vision loss leading to central scotoma and blindness	Research	535000

AD, autosomal dominant; AR, autosomal recessive; XLR, X-linked recessive; MT, mitochondrial.
Updated January 2001.

MOLECULAR DIAGNOSIS

Many cases of early-onset generalized primary torsion dystonia (PTD) are caused by a 3-basepair GAG deletion in the coding sequence in one allele of the *DYT1* (TorsinA) gene on chromosome 9q34.[6] Diagnosis may be confirmed by molecular testing.[6–8] Among individuals with early limb-onset (< 26 years) PTD, the *DYT1* GAG deletion was found in 80 to 90% of Ashkenazi Jewish populations and 40 to 60% of non-Jewish populations.[8,9] Among individuals who did not meet the clinical diagnostic criteria for *DYT1* dystonia, 10 to 12%, including 0.1% of individuals with late-onset focal/segmental dystonia, were found to carry the GAG deletion.[6,9] This demonstrates the genetic heterogeneity of PTD. Individuals presenting with PTD found not to carry the GAG deletion may hypothetically carry a different mutation in the *DYT1* gene or a mutation in another dystonia gene, or the symptoms may be because of nongenetic factors.[9] The negative result in the *DYT1* GAG deletion genetic test, therefore, does not eliminate the possibility that the individual has a hereditary dystonia, because the individual may not carry this specific deletion in *DYT1*.

Most cases of DRD are caused by mutations in the GTP cyclohydrolase-1 (GTPCH-1 or GCH-1) gene on chromosome 14q22.[10] GTPCH-1 is the critical enzyme in the biosynthesis of tetrahydrobiopterin (BH4), which is the cofactor involved in the conversion of tyrosine to dopamine. Most of the 60 GTPCH-1 mutations identified to date have occurred only once in an ethnic group, suggesting that there is a high spontaneous mutation rate.[11] This makes clinical genetic testing both costly and labor intensive, because it requires complete sequencing of the gene. Additionally, approximately 30 to 40% of individuals with DRD do not have a mutation that is presently identifiable. Reports show that some mutation-negative patients have either large deletions that are not revealed through conventional sequencing,[12] or mutations in noncoding regulatory regions of the gene (5′, 3′, and intronic regulatory regions),[13–15] or mutations in other genes such as tyrosine hydroxylase,[16] parkin,[13] and 6-pyruvoyltetrahydropterin synthase.[17,18] A clinically available biochemical screen for DRD, called phenylalanine loading, was initially thought to be a more sensitive alternative to mutation screening[19] but the sensitivity and specificity of this test are unclear.[20] For all of these reasons, dramatic therapeutic response to a low dose of levodopa remains the diagnostic gold standard for DRD.

Genetic analysis for the other dystonias is in the research phase and is not diagnostic. At this time, genetic counseling for non-*DYT1* dystonia and non-DRD is limited to providing information about the apparent mode of inheritance based on literature review and pedigree information, and discussion of nongenetic issues and support resources. The genetic counselor may encourage DNA banking, provide brain donation information, and review research study participation options. As additional genes responsible for dystonias are identified and direct DNA-based genetic testing for these genes becomes available, more specific genetic counseling may be provided.

The duty to recontact former patients about advances in research that might be relevant to them is not presently a part of standard care. Among genetic service providers, recontacting patients is an ethically or legally desirable goal, although considered not feasible within the confines of the current health care system.[21] Individuals who seek genetic counseling should be encouraged to periodically check back with their genetic service providers (e.g., every 6 months to 1 year). Patients should also recontact the counselor if there is a change in clinical status or family history, or for an update on research developments, including available testing options. The genetic counselor may also provide patients with Internet sites and information on support groups and research organizations, encouraging them to join such groups to receive newsletters and updated information. It is also important to identify those individuals who do not wish to be recontacted, documenting such informed preference in their chart.[21]

DYSTONIA

Prevalence

It is estimated that the *DYT1* GAG deletion is responsible for more than 50% of cases of early limb-onset, primary dystonia among non-Jewish populations and approximately 90%

among Ashkenazi Jewish populations.[22,23] The frequency of early limb-onset primary dystonia is estimated to range from 1 in 5,000 to 1 in 15,000 among Ashkenazi Jews.[22] The prevalence among non-Ashkenazi Jewish and non-Jewish populations has not been confirmed; however, earlier studies estimated a frequency of 1 in 160,000 in the general population. Based on additional studies among Ashkenazi Jewish populations, this may be an underestimate.

MODE OF INHERITANCE

DYT1 dystonia is inherited in an autosomal dominant pattern with reduced penetrance of approximately 30% and variable expression.[25,26] The carrier of this mutation has a 50% chance, with each pregnancy, of passing the mutant allele onto his or her offspring. This 50% risk is the same whether individuals are symptomatic or asymptomatic or whether they have a *de novo* mutation. Reduced penetrance means that some individuals may carry the mutant allele but do not have symptoms. In the case of *DYT1* dystonia, an estimated 30% of carriers of this dominant mutation manifest symptoms and 70% of carriers do not display visible symptoms.[26] Variable expression refers to the broad clinical range among families and even within a single family. The factors that influence penetrance and expression are not yet known.[27]

The Clinical Picture

The most commonly recognized symptoms of dystonia are writer's cramp or foot inversion. The average age of symptom onset of *DYT1* dystonia is 12 years, with a range from 4 to 44 years;[2] symptom onset rarely occurs after the age of 26. In 95% of individuals with early-onset primary dystonia caused by the *DYT1* GAG deletion, onset of symptoms occurs in a limb. Approximately half of these patients initially experience symptoms in a leg and approximately half initially have symptoms in an arm; the remaining 5% of patients have symptom onset in the neck or a cranial muscle, such as the larynx. There have been no cases of *DYT1* dystonia reported with cranial onset. Progression and age of symptom onset appear to differ, depending on site of onset.[2]

In leg onset:

- In most patients initially manifests as an inversion of the foot or gait abnormality;
- Has an average age of symptom onset of 9 years (range, 4 to 23 years);[23] and
- Typically progresses within a few months to several years to generalized dystonia involving other limbs, the trunk, or both. Some patients remain segmental.

In arm onset:

- Has a later average age of symptom onset (i.e., 15 years, range, 7 to 44 years);[23]
- Is more variable in its progression; and

- Approximately 50% of patients progress to generalized dystonia.

In neck- and larynx onset:

- Manifests variable progression;
- Has an even later age of onset;
- Has a variable average age of onset dependent on the specific site of onset: when the neck is the initial site, the average age of onset is 26.7 with a range of 21 to 34 years; when the larynx is the initial site the average age of onset is 15 with a range of 12 to 18 years;[23,27] and
- Is unlikely to spread downward or generalize. [23,27]

It is estimated that more than 60% of dystonias caused by the *DYT1* GAG deletion progress to generalized dystonia involving other limbs and the trunk. The cranial muscles are involved in only 11 to 18% of patients.[2] There are no known cognitive changes associated with *DYT1* dystonia. Life span is not reduced, although severely affected individuals may be extremely disabled and possibly wheelchair-bound.[23]

Clinical Criteria

A study has confirmed a genotype-phenotype correlation in early-onset primary dystonia. The study recommends utilization of strict clinical criteria; this will allow accurate prediction of carrier status in two-thirds of individuals with this type of dystonia.[9] The spectrum of dystonia produced by the *DYT1* GAG deletion is broad with respect to age of symptom onset and disease progression.[9] Among known deletion carriers, both childhood- and adult-onset cases exist. There is variable expression of symptoms, from focal to generalized and with a wide range of expression, even within a family. However, most carriers manifest a characteristic phenotype. This characteristic phenotype of symptomatic *DYT1* GAG deletion carriers includes onset in a limb, usually before the age of 24 years; frequent spread to other limbs; occasional spread to the neck; and rare spread to the cranial muscles.[27]

Within the framework of the characteristic phenotype, the following findings suggest a clinical diagnosis of early-onset primary dystonia (*DYT1*) and a recommendation for direct DNA-based *DYT1* GAG deletion testing:[2,9] onset in a limb, usually spreading to another limb; age of symptom onset less than 26 years, except in familial cases of early-onset PTD; or absence of additional neurological abnormalities, except tremor.

The following findings suggest that the dystonia is unlikely to be *DYT1*:[28]

- Focal or segmental cervical-cranial dystonia of any age of onset. Focal dystonias include:
  - cervical dystonia (CD) or spasmodic torticollis characterized by involuntary tilting of the neck;
  - spasmodic dysphonia (SD) characterized by wavering or halting speech or a voice is that reduced to a breathless whisper;

- blepharospasm or involuntary closure of the eyelids, which occurs for extended periods of time in patients with more severe disease; and
- oromandibular dystonia involving involuntary opening, closing, or deviation of the jaw
- Writer's cramp (involuntary contractions or extensions of the hand and finger muscles when writing making writing difficult or impossible) beginning after the age of 44 years
- Dramatic improvement with levodopa therapy (suggestive of DRD)
- Abnormal brain computed tomography (CT) or magnetic resonance imaging (MRI)
- Additional abnormalities on neurological examination, indicating a more complex neurologic disorder such as Wilson's disease, Huntington's disease, spinocerebellar ataxia, or multiple sclerosis
- A history that suggests secondary dystonia, such as head trauma, encephalitis, exposure to certain drugs (particularly neuroleptics) or toxins, perinatal anoxia, or brain tumor
- Presence of inconsistent weakness, nonphysiologic sensory findings, or incongruous movements that suggest a psychogenic basis.

Obtaining Family History

To assess the risk of dystonia to other family members accurately, it is important to obtain a detailed family history and construct a pedigree. The family history may be obtained from the affected individual or another family member identified as an accurate historian. Appropriate information to obtain includes ethnicity, date of birth, history of neurologic abnormalities or symptoms of a movement disorder, history of psychiatric disorder or cognitive deficit, current symptoms of movement disorders, and date and cause of death.

It should be noted that a negative family history does not necessarily exclude the presence of the *DYT1* GAG deletion or another dystonia mutation. First, as discussed previously, *DYT1* dystonia has a 30% penetrance, which means that there may be many individuals who are asymptomatic. Secondly, rare *de novo DYT1* GAG deletions have been identified in several families,[29] although the mutation rates are unknown. Other possible reasons for an apparent negative family history may be less obvious but nonetheless important. The parent of the affected individual may have died at an early age, before manifestation of symptoms. The parent may be undiagnosed, misdiagnosed, or even asymptomatic. Perhaps a family member "always wrote funny" or "had a hoarse voice." These findings were not considered a neurologic disorder or problematic and appropriate medical attention was not sought. Other issues to consider when reviewing the family history are nonpaternity, adoption, and limitations of information, as in the case of Holocaust survivors or estranged family members.

Because of the variable expression of dystonia within a single family, the affected status of each individual in the family must be thoroughly reviewed. The historian may not have adequate information or contact with all family members. When necessary to obtain adequate historical details, other family members may consent to be contacted for information. This is done with the permission of the affected individual or, in the case of a minor child, with the consent of the parent or guardian.

To obtain the most accurate history of movement disorders within a family, it is necessary to ask specific questions pertaining to the varied symptomatology of dystonia. The following is a list of questions that may be asked. Affirmative responses to any of these questions do not indicate definitively the presence of a movement disorder but may indicate the need for further investigation. Such questions may include: do you experience any of the following?

- Increased blinking or inability to keep eyes open, especially in bright lights
- Feeling of sand in the eyes
- Intermittent and frequent puckering of the mouth or lips
- Involuntary chewing movements or tongue popping
- Repetitive pulling up or down of the jaw
- Abnormal movements or "tics" of the face or other parts of the body
- Difficulty swallowing solids, liquids, or saliva (drooling)
- Frequent choking or coughing when eating
- Stuttering
- Tremulous voice, choking when talking, or any difficulty speaking
- Running out of breath when speaking with a soft voice
- Turning, tilting, or shifting of the head in any direction
- Shaking or jerking of the head
- Lifting or pulling up or down of the shoulders
- Stiffness or pain in the neck
- Twisting of the body when lying, sitting, standing, or walking
- Scoliosis or abnormal deviation of the spine
- Tremors of the hands or feet
- Arms or legs twist or move involuntarily when using the hands or walking
- Difficulty with grasping, writing, or drawing
- History of clumsiness
- Cramps or painful muscles at rest or with the use of the arms or legs
- Toes go up or down involuntarily
- "Pigeon-toed"
- Slow runner or slower on physical activities than others
- Clubfoot or a foot that turns in

If a family member is reported to have a movement disorder, medical records or a neurologic examination may be requested.

Risks to Family Members and Genetic Testing Issues

The availability of specific genetic testing for early-onset primary torsion dystonia has advantages and disadvantages. As a diagnostic tool, genetic testing is accurate and disease-specific. Testing eliminates some costs as well as anxiety related to differential diagnosis.[9] Determining carrier status, even in asymptomatic individuals, may be applicable in reproductive decision-making. Genetic testing in either scenario should be considered only with appropriate pretest and posttest genetic counseling. In this way, the individual considering testing may make an informed decision and fully understand the meaning of the test results.

In addition to the disorder-specific genetic issues, general issues of genetic counseling pertaining to genetic testing should be addressed. These include patient confidentiality, genetic discrimination risk related to insurance and employment, and the logistics of information transfer.[9] Individuals seeking genetic testing should be informed that in rare instances, genetic test results, or even the act of having the test performed, may have financial implications for retirement planning as well as for obtaining life, disability, and health insurance.[30–33] The potential for genetic discrimination, as well as federal and state legislation to protect against such discrimination, may be further explored with reference to the Health Insurance Portability and Accountability Act (HIPAA) and state-specific legislation.

Additionally, there needs to be a discussion about dissemination of information to others—who to tell and who not to tell. Caution should be exercised in the communication and documentation of test results.[24] Individuals seeking genetic testing should be apprised of the sensitive nature of the test results and the potential issues that surrounding the sharing of that information with third parties, such as insurance carriers, employers, or other family members. This is true especially in the case of asymptomatic testing. Pertaining to family members, there needs to be a discussion about informing other at-risk family members. Pedigree information will enable the genetic counselor to make a list of individuals who are at-risk and could be contacted. Some individuals may be reticent to discuss their private affairs with other family members; however, they should be advised of the appropriateness of allowing other family members to be aware of their at-risk status and to make an informed decision regarding genetic testing. Furthermore, individuals need to respect the autonomy of other family members regarding their decisions. The individual may feel uncomfortable discussing the disorder or incompetent when explaining the genetic implications. In such a situation, the genetic counselor may offer assistance by providing literature, being available for discussion, or possibly assisting the individual in drafting a letter of explanation to other family members.

Parents

In assessing the risk of the parents of affected individuals, it is necessary to consider the following possibilities:

1. One parent carries the *DYT1* GAG deletion and is asymptomatic. Seventy percent of gene carriers are without symptoms.

2. One parent carries the mutant allele and is symptomatic. Thirty percent of gene carriers manifest symptoms.

3. Neither parent carries the mutation and the affected individual has a *de novo* mutation.

Therefore, it is appropriate for both parents of an affected individual, who is shown to carry the *DYT1* GAG deletion, to consider being tested for the mutant allele and being evaluated for dystonic symptoms.[2] For genetic counseling purposes, this is helpful to determine whether the mutation has been maternally or paternally inherited. This information may be useful in assessing which other family members may be at risk for carrying the gene deletion, and guiding those who should be offered testing.

Siblings and Other Family Members

The risk to siblings and other family members of carriers of the *DYT1* GAG deletion depends on the genetic status of the parents. The gene status of the parents, including those who are asymptomatic, may be determined by genetic testing. If the parent of the affected *DYT1*-positive individual is found to carry the *DYT1* GAG deletion allele, siblings of the affected individual have a 50% chance of also carrying the mutant allele. If both parents are *DYT1*-negative, the siblings are at no greater risk than that of the general (or Ashkenazi Jewish) population. In rare patients, however, nonpaternity involving the tested parents may be an issue.

Offspring

All individuals with the *DYT1* GAG deletion have a 50% chance of transmitting the mutant allele to their offspring. This risk is true regardless of whether the individual is symptomatic or asymptomatic or if the individual's mutation is *de novo*. The penetrance of *DYT1* dystonia is approximately 30%, which means that approximately 30% of offspring who acquire the mutation will manifest symptoms of the disorder and 70% will not.[26] As a result of the variable expression of *DYT1* dystonia, even within a family, the severity of the disorder in those individuals who carry the mutation and do manifest symptoms cannot be predicted.

Prenatal Testing

Prenatal testing is available for fetuses at 50% risk, provided the presence of the *DYT1* GAG deletion has been confirmed in one of the parents. Genetic testing for the *DYT1* GAG deletion can be performed on fetal cells obtained by chorionic villi sampling (CVS) at 9 to 11 weeks gestation or amniocentesis at 16 to 18 weeks gestation.

CVS testing should be considered with caution. It is the role of the genetic counselor to educate and counsel prospective parents about testing options; however, the decision whether to proceed with testing must be made by the parents.[34] Before prenatal testing, the genetic counselor should discuss:

- possible results,
- advantages of having this information,
- disadvantages of having this information, and
- if the information will be useful to them.

Motivation for testing should also be addressed. Prospective parents seeking prenatal counseling should be advised that because of the reduced penetrance and variable expression of *DYT1* dystonia, mutation status cannot predict whether the child will be affected. In addition, if the child is affected, the potential severity of symptoms cannot be predicted. If termination of a mutation-carrying fetus is acceptable to the parents, a family of unaffected children can be planned. If termination is not an option, prospective parents should also consider whether the decision to test should be reserved for the child to make when he or she reaches adulthood.[34–36]

Other Reproductive Options

Other options available for prospective parents are preimplantation genetic diagnosis (PGD) and gamete donation. Both options are available only if the presence of the *DYT1* GAG deletion has been confirmed in one of the parents. PGD involves *in vitro* fertilization (IVF) techniques, and micromanipulation and genetic analysis of the embryo. Preimplantation genetic diagnosis:

- allows for the selected transfer of unaffected (non-*DYT1* mutation) embryos;
- avoids the possibility of a termination after conventional prenatal diagnosis later during a pregnancy; and
- allows a couple to have their own biologic children.

Gamete donation involves IVF in the case of a donated ovum, or artificial insemination in the case of donated sperm, depending on which prospective parent is the mutation carrier. These options are complex psychologically, costly, and require thorough consideration before the decision to proceed is made. Couples interested in pursuing such reproductive options should be referred to an IVF center.

Asymptomatic Testing

For asymptomatic carrier testing, pretest and post-test counseling is mandatory. The pretest counseling sessions should provide the individual with the appropriate information regarding the risks and benefits of testing. This will enable the individual to make an informed decision regarding carrier testing. The counseling session must include explanations of the genetic aspects of the disorder as well as the psychosocial issues. The results of such genetic testing may have implications for major life issues. These include decisions regarding education, marriage, children, employment, and career choices, as well as availability of health, disability, and life insurance. Test results may also affect family relationships and self-image issues. Psychological screening may be appropriate to assess the individual's ability to deal

with the decision-making process and possible ramifications of test results.

Equally important is the post-test counseling. During such sessions, the test results should be explained, the interpretation of the test results should be reviewed, and psychosocial issues should be addressed. In the case of a mutation-positive result, the penetrance and variable expression of the disorder, as well as the genetic issues should be reviewed. The carrier individual must understand that mutation status is not predictive. Because of reduced penetrance and the broad clinical spectrum of *DYT1* dystonia, the presence of the *DYT1* deletion cannot predict whether an individual will manifest symptoms or how severe those symptoms will be. Issues of blame and guilt may need to be addressed, particularly when an asymptomatic parent is found to be a carrier. With a mutation-negative result, the individual may be relieved of the uncertainty, but may also experience "survivor guilt," based on the knowledge that one or more of his or her loved ones have or may develop this disorder. If the psychological effects of the testing are beyond the scope of the genetic counselor, a referral for psychological evaluation and counseling should be made.

Asymptomatic parents

As explained previously, testing of asymptomatic parents of affected individuals shown to carry the *DYT1* GAG deletion is appropriate for genetic counseling purposes to determine maternal-paternal transmission. Such testing is not considered predictive testing as symptoms will not likely occur after the age of 30.[22] However, pretest and posttest genetic counseling is important to review the genetic implications of the test results, as well as the psychological issues that may arise.

Asymptomatic children

The testing of unaffected at-risk children younger than the age of 18 is not recommended. This standpoint is supported by policy statements from the National Society of Genetic Counselors[34] and the American Society of Human Genetics.[35] The reasons for this position are as follows:

1. There is no preventive treatment for gene carriers.
2. There is concern about the effect of test results on family dynamics, whether test results will negatively affect the family's view of the child as well as the child's self-image and self-esteem.
3. There is a question of the child's autonomy or competence in making such a decision versus a parent's request.[34-36]

Conversely, childhood testing may allow more time to cope with the results and avoid the trauma of learning genetic status at the time of reproductive decision-making.[9] Individual situations should be assessed and counseled accordingly, with the caveat that testing of minors be carefully considered, and always include psychological screening. As with prenatal testing, testing during childhood allows the parent, rather than the child being tested, to provide informed consent for testing. Such testing should be considered cautiously, and motivation should be evaluated. When possible, children should be involved in the decision whether to undergo testing.[34] Parents should consider whether the decision to test should be reserved for children to make when they attain adulthood.[34,35]

Other at-risk asymptomatic family members

Testing of other at-risk family members may be offered with appropriate pretest and post-test genetic counseling. Such individuals seeking genetic testing should be informed that, in rare instances, genetic test results may have financial implications for retirement planning and for obtaining life, disability, and health insurance.[32,33]

DOPA-RESPONSIVE DYSTONIA

Prevalence

Dopa-responsive dystonia (DRD) does not appear to exhibit any ethnic predilection. Studies in England and Japan have estimated the prevalence at 0.5 per million.[37]

Mode of Inheritance

As described above for *DYT1* dystonia, DRD is an autosomal dominant condition with reduced penetrance. Most cases are the result of a heterozygous mutation in GTPCH-1. However, penetrance in DRD is "gender influenced." That is, expression of the gene depends on the gender of the individual. Anywhere from 2.5[15] to 4.3[14] times more females than males have DRD. Studies estimate penetrance in females to be 87 to 100% and 38 to 55% in males.[14,15] However, these estimates include individuals with mild symptoms that would be clinically insignificant. Thus, previously published, more conservative penetrance estimates of 45% in women and 15% in men may be more relevant for genetic counseling.[38] In one report, up to 50% of sporadic cases of DRD have *de novo* GTPCH-1 mutations.[39]

The Clinical Picture

DRD typically begins with childhood-onset limb dystonia often accompanied by parkinsonian features. In a large review of 86 patients with DRD the average age of onset was 6 years, with a range of 9 months to 16 years. Ninety-three percent of patients began with leg dystonia; symptom onset occurred only rarely in the arm or neck.[40] In approximately 14% of patients, parkinsonian signs such as rest tremor, bradykinesia, hypomimia, postural instability, and cogwheel rigidity were present, but the authors felt that these signs may be a feature of DRD in up to 50% of patients.[40] The dystonia was progressive; the arms were involved in 69% of patients;

the neck was involved in 26% of patients.[40] Sixty-seven percent of individuals with DRD experienced diurnal variation of symptoms. Symptoms were better in the morning and worsened by the end of the day. Other clinical studies have resulted in similar findings.[12] There is a great deal of clinical overlap between DRD and conditions such as *DYT1* dystonia, diplegic cerebral palsy, sporadic spastic paraplegia, and juvenile-onset parkinsonism (JOPD) caused by parkin mutations. DRD and JOPD both show marked improvement of symptoms with levodopa therapy. In patients with DRD, the response is sustained; however, patients with JOPD usually experience medication-induced fluctuations on low doses of levodopa, including wearing off and dyskinesias.

An alternative phenotype of DRD is adult-onset parkinsonism, which may be clinically indistinguishable from Parkinson's disease.[12,14] However, its course is usually benign and there is little or no wearing off, suggesting that the neurons remain intact.[41] There does not seem to be any relationship between the type of GTPCH-1 mutation and age at onset or presentation of symptoms.[13]

Clinical Criteria

The criteria for the characteristic DRD phenotype are similar to those for *DYT1* with the exception that index cases might have a family history or diagnosis of DRD, primary torsion dystonia, cerebral palsy, spastic paraplegia, or parkinsonism.

Risks to Family Members and Genetic Testing Issues

As discussed, genetic and biochemical testing for DRD is costly and not 100% sensitive. Commercial testing is available but is expensive because the entire gene needs to be sequenced. For straightforward diagnosis, a short trial of levodopa is much simpler and more sensitive. However, in patients with incomplete dopa responsiveness or possible recessive inheritance, genetic testing may help to distinguish between or rule out DRD caused by GTPCH1 or tyrosine hydroxylase (TH) mutations and young-onset PD due to parkin mutations. Because DRD is treatable with little or no residual morbidity, asymptomatic carrier testing is rarely, if ever, an issue in reproductive decision-making. Nevertheless, individuals wishing to understand their genetic risk and explore genetic testing options should have genetic counseling.

As discussed, genetic counseling should include a discussion of the potential for genetic discrimination and of sharing diagnosis and testing information with other at-risk family members. Sharing information is particularly important in DRD, because it can expedite diagnosis and initiation of treatment in newly affected children. Additionally, such communication can aid in the management of relatives with adult-onset parkinsonism who may have been diagnosed with idiopathic Parkinson's disease and, thus, presented with a graver prognosis. Such individuals could be treated with low-dose levodopa indefinitely with relatively low chances of the wearing off and dyskinesias commonly experienced by patients with Parkinson's disease.

The risk of DRD to family members is as described for *DYT1*, with the exception that clinically significant DRD is approximately 15% penetrant in men and approximately 45% penetrant in women.

Asymptomatic Testing

Because there is no detectable GTPCH-1 mutation in up to 40% of patients with DRD, genetic testing of asymptomatic family members is inappropriate unless a mutation has been identified in an affected family member. When a family mutation is known, screening other family members for the mutation is available commercially and may be done at minimal cost. Pretest and posttest counseling is still essential for asymptomatic carrier testing and should include many or all the issues addressed above. Many asymptomatic carriers are also unaware that they are at increased risk for adult-onset parkinsonism.

Asymptomatic parents

Parents may elect to have genetic testing to define the risk of symptoms better in themselves and their children and determine which side of the family may be at risk. In sporadic cases, there is up to a 50% chance that neither parent carries a mutation.

Asymptomatic children

Testing of asymptomatic children is not recommended for the reasons stated and because therapy can be initiated with the first sign of symptoms.

RARE VARIANTS OF DOPA-RESPONSIVE DYSTONIA

In rare cases, a patient with DRD may have a pair of GTPCH-1 mutations or mutations in other autosomal recessively inherited genes, such as tyrosine hydroxylase and 6-pyruvyltetrahy-dropterin synthase.[17,18] In autosomal recessive inheritance, an affected individual receives a nonworking gene from each parent. The parents who have only one copy each of this gene are completely asymptomatic and are not at risk for developing symptoms. Offspring of such couples have a 25% chance of inheriting both nonworking genes and manifesting symptoms.

These rare forms of DRD are typically characterized by severe neurologic dysfunction including mental retardation, delayed milestones, convulsions, truncal hypotonia, limb hypertonia, dystonia, or abnormal eye movements. Symptoms begin during the first 6 months of life.[42] There is one report of a patient with tyrosine hydroxylase deficiency mimicking spastic paraplegia.[16] Some patients respond well to levodopa therapy, while others do not respond. Thus, the phenotypic spectrum has yet to be fully defined. A handful

of mutations have been identified.[16,18,43] Most are novel mutations; it is not yet clear whether there is any genotype-phenotype correlation.

Genetic testing is available, provided that the mutations have been identified in the affected child or the carrier parents. Thus, prenatal diagnosis is an option for couples who have an affected child and are considering an additional pregnancy.

It is not yet known whether levodopa may be used prophylactically to prevent mental retardation and other symptoms. If levodopa could be used in this manner, then testing of asymptomatic children, particularly infants, would become critical.[14]

REFERENCES

1. Resta R. Genetic Counseling: Coping with the human impact of genetic disease [online]. Available at: *www.accessexcellence.org/AE/AEC/CC/counseling_background.html. Accessed January 3, 2001.*
2. Fahn S, Bressman SB, Marsden CD. Classification of dystonia. Adv Neurol 1998;78:1–10.
3. Muller U, Steinberger D, Nemeth AH. Clinical and molecular genetics of primary dystonias. Neurogenetics 1998;1:165–177.
4. Klein C, Breakefield XO, Ozelius LJ. Genetics of primary dystonia. Semin Neurol 1999;19:271–280.
5. Ozelius LJ, Hewett JW, Page CE, et al. The early-onset torsion dystonia gene (*DYT1*) encodes an ATP-binding protein. Nat Genet 1997; 17:40–48.
6. Warner TT, Jarman P. The molecular genetics of the dystonias. J Neurol Psychiatry 1998;64:427–429.
7. Valente EM, Warner TT, Jarman PR, et al. The role of primary torsion dystonia in Europe. Brain 1998;121:2335–2339.
8. Klein C, Friedman J, Bressman SB, et al. Genetic testing for early-onset torsion dystonia (*DYT1*): introduction of a simple screening methods, experiences from testing of a large patient cohort, and ethical aspects. Genet Test 1999;3:323–328.
9. Furukawa Y, Shimadzu M, Rajput AH, et al. GTP-Cyclohydrolase I gene mutation in hereditary progressive and dopa-responsive dystonia. Ann Neurol 1996;39:609–617.
10. Nishiyama N, Yukishita S, Hagiwara H, et al. Gene mutation in hereditary progressive dystonia with marked diurnal fluctuation (HPD), strictly defined dopa-responsive dystonia. Brain Dev 2000;22(Suppl 1):102–106.
11. Furukawa Y, Guttman M, Sparagana SP, et al. Dopa-responsive dystonia due to a large deletion in the GTP cyclohydrolase I gene. Ann Neurol 2000;47:517–520.
12. Tassin J, Durr A, Bonnet AM, et al. Levodopa-responsive dystonia GTP cyclohydrolase I or parkin mutations? Brain 2000;123:1112–1121.
13. Furukawa Y, Lang AE, Trugman JM, et al. Gender-related penetrance and de novo GTP-cyclohydrolase I gene mutations in dopa-responsive dystonia. Neurology 1998;50:1015–1020.
14. Steinberger D, Weber Y, Korinthenberg R, et al. High penetrance and pronounced variation in expressivity of GCH1 mutations in five families with dopa-responsive dystonia. Ann Neurol 1998;43:634–639.
15. Furukawa Y, Graf WD, Wong H, et al. Dopa-responsive dystonia simulating spastic paraplegia due to tyrosine hydroxylase (TH) gene mutations. Neurology. 2001;56:260–263.
16. Hanihara T, Inoue K, Kawanishi C, et al. 6-Pyruvoyltetrahydropterin synthase deficiency with generalized dystonia and diurnal fluctuation of symptoms: a clinical and molecular study. Mov Disord 1997; 12:408–411.
17. Wevers RA, de Rijk-Van Andel JF, et al. A review of biochemical and molecular genetic aspects of tyrosine hydroxylase deficiency including a novel mutation (291delC). J Inher Metab Dis 1999;22:364–373.
18. Hyland K, Fryburg JS, Wolson WG, et al. Oral phenylalanine loading in dopa-responsive dystonia: a possible diagnostic test. Neurology 1997;48:1290–1297.
19. Saunders-Pullman R, Hyland K, Raymond D, et al. Markers of disease in dopa-responsive dystonia. Mov Disord 1998;13:285.

20. Fitzpatrick JL, Hahn C, Costa T, et al. The duty to recontact: attitudes of genetic service providers. Am J Hum Genet 1999;64:852–860.
21. Risch N, de Leon D, Ozelius LJ, et al. Genetic analysis of idiopathic torsion dystonia in Ashkenazi Jews and their recent decent from a small founder population. Nat Genet 1995;9:152–159.
22. Bressman, SB, de Leon D, Kramer PL, et al. Dystonia in Ashkenazi Jews: clinical characterization of a founder mutation. Ann Neurol 1994;36:771–777.
23. Zeman W, Dyken P. Dystonia musculorum deformans: clinical, genetic, and pathoanotomical studies. Psychiatr Neurol Neurochir 1967;70:77–121.
24. Risch N, Bressman SB, deLeon D, et al. Segregation analysis of idiopathic torsion dystonia in Ashkenazi Jews suggests autosomal dominant inheritance. Am J Hum Genet 1990;46:533–538.
25. Bressman SB, de Leon D, Brin MF, et al. Idiopathic dystonia among Ashkenazi Jews: evidence for autosomal dominant inheritance. *Ann Neurol*. 1989;26:612–620.
26. Bressman SB, Sabatti C, Raymond D, et al. The *DYT1* phenotype and guidelines for diagnostic testing. Neurology 2000;54:1746–1752.
27. De Leon D, Bressman SB. Early onset primary dystonia (*DYT1*). In: GeneClinics 1999 [online]. Available at: *http://www.Geneclinics.org*. Accessed January 2, 2001.
28. Bressman SB, de Leon D, Raymond D, et al. Secondary dystonia and the *DYT1* gene. Neurology 1997;48:1571–1577.
29. Klein C, Brin MF, de Leon D, et al. De novo mutations (GAG deletion) in the *DYT1* gene in two non-Jewish patients with early-onset dystonia. Am J Hum Genet 1998;7:1133–1136.
30. Jacobs LA, Deatrick JA. The individual, the family, and genetic testing. J Prof Nurs 1999;5:313–324.
31. Hudson KI, Rothenberg KH, Andrew LB, et al. Genetic discrimination and health insurance: an urgent need for reform. Science 1995; 270:391–393.
32. Mehlman MJ, Kodish ED, Whitehouse P, et al. The need for anonymous genetic counseling and testing. Am J Hum Genet 1996; 58:393–397.
33. Rothenberg KH. Genetic discrimination and health insurance: a call for legislative action. J Am Med Womens Assoc 1997;52:43–44.
34. National Society of Genetic Counselors, Policy Statement: Prenatal and Childhood Testing for Adult-onset Disorders [Adopted 1995].
35. ASHG/ACMG Report. Points to Consider: Ethical, Legal, and Psychosocial Implications of Genetic Testing in Children and Adolescents, 1995.
36. Wertz DC, Fanos JH, Reilly PR. Genetic testing for children and adolescents. Who decides? JAMA 1994;272:875–881.
37. Nygaard TG. Dopa-responsive dystonia: delineation of the clinical syndrome and clues to pathogenesis. Adv Neurol 1993;60:577–585.
38. Nygaard TG. An analysis of North American families with dopa-responsive dystonia. In: Segawa M, ed. Hereditary Progressive Dystonia with Marked Diurnal Fluctuation. Carnforth, UK: Parthenon; 1993: 97–104.
39. Nygaard, TG, Snow BJ, Fahn S, et al. Dopa-responsive dystonia: clinical characteristics and definition. In: Segawa M, ed. Hereditary Progressive Dystonia with Marked Diurnal Fluctuation. Carnforth, UK: Parthenon; 1993:21–35.
40. Nygaard TG, Marsden CD, Duvoisin RC. Dopa-responsive dystonia. Adv Neurol 1988;50:377–384.
41. Nygaard TG, Marsden CD, Fahn S. Dopa-responsive dystonia: long-term treatment response and prognosis. Neurology 1991;41:174–181.
42. Furukawa Y, Kish SJ. Dopa-responsive dystonia: recent advances and remaining issues to be addressed. Mov Disord 1999;14:709–715.
43. Lonlay DE, Nassogne MC, van Gennip AH, et al. Tyrosine hydroxylase deficiency unresponsive to l-dopa treatment with unusual clinical and biochemical presentation. J Inherit Metab Dis 2000;23: 819–825.

CHAPTER 4

Physiology of Dystonia

Alfredo Berardelli, Ryuji Kaji, and Antonio Currà

INTRODUCTION

Dystonia is defined as a syndrome of sustained muscle contractions frequently causing twisting or repetitive movements or abnormal postures. Examples of focal dystonias include blepharospasm, cervical dystonia, and writer's cramp. One clinical feature of dystonia is the sensory trick, namely a tactile or proprioceptive sensory input to a nearby body part. This sensory input dramatically improves abnormal posture or movement. For example, in patients with blepharospasm, the wearing of sunglasses to avoid bright light is effective in reducing contractions in the orbicularis oculi muscles. The effectiveness of sensory tricks in improving dystonia suggests a sensory-motor mismatch in motor control.

Another important feature in dystonia is that it often affects only a specific task or, in other words, it is task-specific. For example, writer's cramp usually begins as a task-specific disorder affecting writing only; however, it may later involve other tasks as well. Other task-specific dystonias include musician's cramp (e.g., pianist's cramp), typist's cramp, and telegrapher's cramp. These dystonia all affect activities involving frequently used or repetitive motor acts. Task-specific cramps cause stereotypical symptoms. For example, the abnormal pattern of muscle contraction in writer's cramp typically remains the same over time. These findings suggest that dystonia is a disorder of a frequently used motor program or subroutine[1] in which motor output is matched to a fixed sensory input. The physiologic mechanisms underlying primary dystonia are reviewed here.

Alfredo Berardelli: Dipartimento di Scienze Neurologiche, Universita' di Roma "La Sapienza," Rome, Italy; Istituto Neurologico Mediterraneo Neuromed IRCCS, Pozzilli, IS, Italy.

Ryuji Kaji: Department of Neurology, Tokushima University School of Medicine, Tokushima City, Japan.

Antonio Currà: Dipartimento di Scienze Neurologiche, Universita' di Roma "La Sapienza," Rome, Italy; Istituto Neurologico Mediterraneo Neuromed IRCCS, Pozzilli, IS, Italy.

The authors have no commercial relationship with the funder.

PHYSIOLOGIC MECHANISMS UNDERLYING PRIMARY DYSTONIA

Peripheral Abnormalities

Evidence indicates that trauma to the peripheral nerves or structures, after variable periods, predisposes an individual to the development of dystonia.[2-4] Peripheral trauma may alter the normal input-output relationship for controlling a frequently used motor act, thus causing sensory-motor mismatch.

Brain Stem Reflexes

Brain stem reflexes may be studied by testing the blink reflex and masseter inhibitory reflex. Both techniques explore the function of trigeminal-facial pathways in the brainstem.[5] In normal subjects, the blink reflex consists of an early response (R1) is followed by a late bilateral response (R2). In patients with cranial dystonia, the excitability of the late bilateral R2 component of the blink reflex, conditioned by electrical and photic stimuli, is enhanced.[6,7] The abnormality elicited by photic conditioning stimuli probably reflects these patients' clinically observed sensitivity to bright light.[8] The R2 component of the blink reflex recovery cycle is also abnormal in patients with dystonia without blepharospasm.[9]

The masseter inhibitory reflex consists of an early phase or SP1, followed by a late phase or SP2 of inhibition in the ongoing electromyographic (EMG) activity. The recovery cycle of the late phase of the masseter inhibitory reflex is enhanced in patients with cranial dystonia, even in those without jaw-closing dystonia.[10] The abnormalities described with these techniques suggest that in cranial dystonia there is an abnormality of both excitatory and inhibitory interneurons, possibly the result of an enhanced facilitation of the excitatory and inhibitory interneurons subserving these brain stem reflexes.

Spinal Reflexes

In a positron emission tomography (PET) study, Tempel and Perlmutter[11] reported an abnormal regional cerebral blood flow response after vibratory stimulation of the hand in patients with hand dystonia. During the study, these investigators also found a vibratory, stimulation-induced dystonic cramp in the stimulated arm or hand in patients. This was not noted in normal subjects. In an attempt to study the mechanism underlying sensory tricks in cervical dystonia, Leis and colleagues[12] examined the clinical effects of vibratory or electric stimulation over the head and neck region. These investigators found that vibration over the specific skin area affected dystonic contractions.

Vibration over the muscle tendon is an effective means of stimulating muscle spindle afferents (group Ia), and in normal subjects evokes a tonic contraction of the stimulated muscle after a long latency period. This response, known as the tonic vibration reflex (TVR), is mediated by pathways through the brain stem center. In patients with hand dystonia, this reflex was abnormal. Rather than causing delayed activation of the stimulated muscle, vibratory stimulation reproduced dystonic contractions in other muscles after a short latency period.[13]

Conversely, blocking the muscle afferent with diluted lidocaine not only abolished vibration-induced abnormal muscle activation but also relieved the dystonic symptoms. These findings indicate an abnormal link between muscle afferents and efferents in dystonia. In patients with hand dystonia, Grunewald and colleagues[14] examined vibration-induced, illusory kinesthetic sense in the affected hand. This was accomplished by matching the movement of the unaffected hand. Despite having normal positional sense, patients' kinesthetic sense was severely impaired. This finding strengthens the notion of an abnormal sensory-motor link in dystonia. Long-latency reflexes (LLRs) may be recorded from thenar muscles under isometric contraction; this is accomplished by electrically stimulating the median nerve. Naumann and Reiners[15] reported abnormal LLR components. Although the pathophysiologic importance of their finding remains unknown, the investigators suggested disinhibited thalamocortical outflow to the supplementary motor area.

Spinal Inhibitory Circuits: Reciprocal Inhibition

Reciprocal inhibition between agonist and antagonist muscles in the forearm consists of an initial short-lasting disynaptic Ia inhibitory phase. This is followed by a longer lasting phase, caused by presynaptic inhibition of large proprioceptive afferent fibers. In patients with writer's cramp, the late phase of inhibition, and sometimes both the early and late phases, are reduced.[16,17] In dystonia, the abnormalities in the presynaptic phase of reciprocal inhibition usually return to normal after botulinum toxin injection.[18] Reciprocal inhibition is also abnormal in the unaffected arms of patients with writer's cramp as well as in patients with cervical dystonia. The finding of abnormal reciprocal inhibition implies that the Ia input to the spinal cord is processed abnormally in dystonia. The normalization of presynaptic inhibition after botulinum toxin is thought to be mediated by

changes in the intrafusal fibers that decrease the muscle spindle input to the spinal cord.

The more advanced technique of tendon stimulation makes it possible to study group III-elicited presynaptic inhibition of group I afferents.[19] Use of this technique has shown that group III fibers elicit an abnormal presynaptic inhibition on Ia fibers in patients with dystonia.[20] Dystonia causes widespread dysfunction of presynaptic inhibitory mechanisms in the spinal cord; therefore, group III afferents are also involved. Overall, the abnormalities in presynaptic inhibition could originate from abnormal supraspinal control of the interneurons that mediate presynaptic inhibition. Alternatively, presynaptic inhibition abnormalities could reflect an abnormal spinal input.

Cortical Abnormalities: Somatosensory Evoked Potentials

Somatosensory evoked potentials (SEPs) may be used to investigate the central processing of sensory input. Many studies have examined the frontal N30 component in patients with dystonia; however, the results have been conflicting. Reilly et al.[21] studied SEPs in patients with writer's cramp. These investigators used a stimulation rate of 1 Hz and reported increased amplitudes of frontal N30. Conversely, Grissom et al.[22] used a slow rate of stimulation of 0.2 Hz and demonstrated a substantial reduction of the N30 amplitude. They found a markedly reduced amplitude of N30 in patients with hand dystonia. In patients with cervical dystonia, Mazzini et al.[23] reported that the amplitude of N30 was reduced, whereas Nardone et al.[24] found it to be normal. Kanovsky et al.[25] examined the effect of head position in patients with cervical dystonia on median SEPs. They found that botulinum toxin injection substantially reduced the peak-to-peak P22/N30 amplitude.

The relationship between sensory input and motor strategy was studied in focal hand dystonia. The study analyzed the attenuation of SEPs or gating before a movement.[26] The previous studies on SEP gating during movement were affected by the competition between the sensory stimuli and the afferents activated by the movement itself (i.e., peripheral gating). This latter study used a reaction-time model in which electric stimulation to the median nerve triggered the movement of the stimulated hand. Under these experimental conditions, the SEPs evoked within the first 50 milliseconds after the stimulus could not be affected by peripheral gating. The actual movement began at least 70 milliseconds after the sensory stimulation or premovement gating. This method is therefore useful for assessing possible changes in sensory input to the motor cortices that are induced by the motor preparation or central gating. Normal subjects had a substantial gating of frontal N30 components, whereas dystonic patients had practically no gating of these components. This finding again suggests an abnormal control of sensory input in dystonia.[27,28]

Altered control is of interest because the tuning of sensory input is already abnormal before the movement. This alteration of control is probably related to the observations of abnormal movement-related cortical potentials preceding the movement in dystonia.[1,29] Other evidence was obtained using the analysis of spatial and temporal summations of dual SEP inputs. These summations were less inhibited in patients with dystonia than in normal subjects.[30,31] Hence, basal ganglia may have an important role in sensory gating at various cortical and subcortical levels.[32]

Transcranial Stimulation

In normal subjects, transcranial magnetic and electrical stimulation excites the motor cortex and produces muscle responses as a result of activation of the corticospinal system. Studies with electrical stimulation first showed that patients with primary dystonia have normal conduction along the corticospinal tract.[33] This finding was later confirmed, also with magnetic stimulation.[34] In these patients, the threshold intensity for magnetic stimuli required to elicit motor-evoked potentials (MEPs) is normal.

Transcranial magnetic stimulation (TMS) is used successfully for testing the excitability of the cortical motor areas. In patients with dystonia, some investigators have assessed the changes in the size of the MEPs at different stimulation intensities.[34,35] With increasing stimulus intensity, there is a relatively greater increase in MEPs in dystonic patients than in normal subjects. This abnormal input-output relationship of the corticomotoneuronal system in dystonia suggests an abnormally high cortical output. This defect possibly contributes to the excessive motor output that is typically present during action in these patients.

Cortical excitability is also commonly investigated by studying the cortical silent period (SP). In contracting muscles, single magnetic shocks evoke an MEP, followed by a silence of the EMG activity (cortical SP). This EMG silence is considered largely the result of the activation of inhibitory interneurons in the cortical motor areas. A shortened cortical SP has been described in upper limb muscles,[34–36] and more prominently in cranial muscles.[37] A short facial-muscle SP is of particular interest because unlike the SP in limb-muscles, the SP recorded in the facial muscle originates solely from intracortical inhibitory mechanisms.[38] The more prominent shortening of the SP in facial muscles probably depends on the exclusive cortical origin of this response.

Filipovic et al.[39] found that the SP during a dystonic muscle contraction in the forearm was shorter than that recorded during a similar, voluntarily exerted muscle contraction. A short SP suggests that the dystonic motor pattern is disengaged from normal inhibitory mechanisms acting in the motor cortex during voluntary action. In general, the reduced excitability of cortical inhibitory interneurons may arise from lesions in the motor cortex or reduced facilitation from subcortical or other cortical structures. In patients with primary dystonia, there is no evidence of damage to the motor cortex; however, PET scans disclose reduced blood flow during movement.[40] Therefore, the re-

duced cortical SP indicates a reduced activation of the primary motor area. Perhaps this is due to the dysfacilitation operated by overactive prefrontal motor planning centers via cortico-cortical connections.[41]

Cortical excitability may also be tested by administering paired magnetic shocks at varying interstimulus intervals (ISIs) in a conditioning-test design. At short ISIs of 1 millisecond to 6 milliseconds, a subthreshold conditioning stimulus inhibits the test response. This inhibition is the result of the activation of intracortical GABAergic circuits. In patients with dystonia, Ridding et al.[42] found less inhibition of the test response when patients were studied at rest. The investigators attributed this reduced inhibition to a lack of focusing of the motor command within the motor cortex. This impairment may contribute to the overflow of muscle activity in dystonia.

Paired stimuli may be delivered with long ISIs of 60 milliseconds to 200 milliseconds and suprathreshold conditioning shocks. With this method, the conditioning shock elicits an inhibition of the test response. The intracortical neurons activated with this model probably differ from the interneurons subserving the intracortical inhibition obtained with short ISIs. With paired stimuli delivered at long ISIs, an abnormal suppression of the test response has been reported in patients with dystonia.[36,43]

Mapping studies of motor cortex projections to the upper limb muscles in patients with writer's cramp have provided evidence of an altered corticomotor representation.[44] Experiments investigating the effect of botulinum toxin injection on the topography of the primary motor cortex showed that botulinum toxin injection reversed the cortical changes and concurrently improved hand dystonia. Following this line, Gilio et al.[45] studied the effect of botulinum toxin on the intracortical inhibition tested with TMS at short ISIs. Before toxin injection, patients had less inhibition of the test response than normal subjects did. One month afterwards, patients had test response inhibition similar to normal subjects, and 3 months afterwards, they again had less inhibition than normal subjects did. These findings show that botulinum toxin may alter the excitability of the cortical motor areas by reorganizing the inhibitory and excitatory circuits.

Sensory Abnormalities

Several studies have reported clinically detectable sensory abnormalities in dystonia. Patients with hand dystonia were substantially worse on graphesthesia and manual form perception.[46] Patients also performed lower than normal subjects on somatosensory discrimination tasks.[47] In an animal study, monkeys were trained to perform a precision grip task in a stressful condition.[48] After a few months of repeated use of the hand, disabilities of the hand developed that were similar to dystonia. Monkeys with these dystonia-like disabilities underwent acute surgical explorations of the primary sensory cortex (S1). These investigations disclosed noteworthy disorganization of the hand representation in S1.

This abnormality would explain clinical sensory deficits in human dystonia.

Motor Abnormalities: Kinematics and EMG Studies

In normal subjects, rapid arm movements performed at a single joint are characterized by a stereotyped EMG sequence of alternating bursts in the agonist and antagonist muscles.[49] Patients with dystonia complete rapid elbow movements in an abnormally slow manner. EMG activity shows longer AG1 burst and cocontraction activity between agonist and antagonist muscles. Patients' movements also have variable amplitude; EMG recordings show extra activity in muscles not directly involved in the desired movement.[50] Overall, these abnormalities suggest an overflow of muscle activation in dystonia.

Studies of arm-reaching movements have also shown slowness and increased variability of movement. Some reports also describe a prolonged deceleration phase.[51] In a study of sequential movements, patients with dystonia were slower than controls in accomplishing individual movements. In addition, these patients took longer than controls to switch from one submovement to the next.[52] Currà et al.[54] investigated the effect of movement cueing on the motor performance in patients with dystonia. These investigators studied two different conditions. In the externally triggered condition, subjects initiated movement execution in response to a visual cue. In the self-initiated task, subjects initiated movements at will. Patients with dystonia had a general impairment in the execution of sequential movement; however, these patients were slower in executing self-initiated movement than externally triggered trajectories.

Only a few studies have investigated the reaction time in patients with dystonia. The reaction time appeared to be normal during simple arm-reaching movements,[51] head rotation and finger extension,[1] and single pointing movements.[53] Conversely, when tested on consecutive motor responses, a slowness of reaction time has been described in patients with generalized dystonia.[53]

In summary, the abnormalities that are typically seen in dystonic patients during voluntary movements are an overflow of muscle activity. There is pronounced movement slowness, with major difficulty in accomplishing self-initiated movements.

CONCLUSIONS

The physiologic changes described in patients with dystonia range from the increased excitability of brain stem reflex pathways to failure of reciprocal inhibition and prolonged stretch reflexes to changes in cerebral cortical activity at rest and during movement. Most neurophysiologic studies demonstrate a common pathophysiologic mechanism of reduced inhibition (i.e., increased facilitation) at various levels of the motor system, including the spinal cord, brain stem, and cortical motor areas, probably at the level of interneuron function. Increasing evidence emphasizes the role of disturbed central processing of sensory input in the generation, maintenance, or even suppression of dystonic movements. This abnormality may be particularly evident in patients with focal dystonias. Although the primary cause for changes of the interneuron function remains unclear, multilevel involvement in dystonia suggests an abnormality of a control structure. The most suitable candidates to exert this complex modulatory activity are the basal ganglia as they indirectly influence:

- The cortical motor areas via the thalamus;
- The sensory cortices via their connections to cortical projections; and
- The brain stem and spinal cord motor circuitry by direct descending pathways.

The results of functional imaging studies and evaluation of most patients with secondary dystonia support the notion that altered basal ganglia motor output is a factor responsible for dystonia. This functional abnormality also explains the presence of bradykinesia in dystonia. Voluntary movement, similar to the dystonic movement, is characterized by cocontraction combined with overflow of activity to muscles that are not normally involved in the task. In addition, during complex motor tasks, the time taken to switch between submovements is prolonged. Basal ganglia play an important role in setting the pattern of excitability in the motor system; this applies to both immediate and future movements. Moreover, Brotchie et al.[54] showed that as monkeys became more familiar with a simple arm-movement task, the discharge rate of pallidal neurons varied accordingly. By conferring automaticity to the motor execution, the basal ganglia exert a specific role in skilled learned movements. The motor skill is achieved by optimizing the processes that, during movement, enhance one motor action and inhibit others. This function of the basal ganglia may explain why dystonia frequently manifests as a task-specific disturbance.

REFERENCES

1. Kaji R, Ikeda A, Ikeda T, et al. Physiological study of cervical dystonia. Task-specific abnormality in contingent negative variation. Brain 1995;118:511–522.
2. Jankovic J. Post-traumatic movement disorders: central and peripheral mechanisms [see comments]. Neurology 1994;44:2006–2014.
3. Ross MH, Charness ME, Lee D, et al. Does ulnar neuropathy predispose to focal dystonia? Muscle Nerve 1995;18:606–611.
4. Schrag A, Bhatia KP, Quinn NP, et al. Atypical and typical cranial dystonia following dental procedures [see comments]. Mov Disord 1999;14:492–496.
5. Ongerboer de Visser BW, Cruccu G, Manfredi M, et al. Effects of brainstem lesions on the masseter inhibitory reflex. Functional mechanisms of reflex pathways. Brain 1990;113:781–792.
6. Berardelli A, Rothwell JC, Day BL, et al. Pathophysiology of blepharospasm and oromandibular dystonia. Brain 1985;108:593–608.
7. Tolosa E, Montserrat L, Bayse A. Blink reflex studies in focal dystonias: enhanced excitability of brainstem interneurons in cranial dystonia and spasmodic torticollis. Mov Disord 1988;3:61–69.
8. Katayama M, Kohara N, Kaji R, et al. Effect of photic conditioning on blink reflex recovery function in blepharospasm. Electroencephalogr Clin Neurophysiol 1996;101:446–452.

9. Pauletti G, Berardelli A, Cruccu G, et al. Blink reflex and the masseter inhibitory reflex in patients with dystonia. Mov Disord 1993;8: 495–500.

10. Cruccu G, Pauletti G, Agostino R, et al. Masseter inhibitory reflex in movement disorders, Huntington's chorea, Parkinson's disease, dystonia, and unilateral masticatory spasm. Electroencephalogr Clin Neurophysiol 1991;81:24–30.

11. Tempel LW, Perlmutter JS. Abnormal vibration-induced cerebral blood flow responses in idiopathic dystonia. Brain 1990;113:691–707.

12. Leis AA, Dimitrijevic MR, Delapasse JS, et al. Modification of cervical dystonia by selective sensory stimulation. J Neurol Sci 1992; 110:79–89.

13. Kaji R, Rothwell JC, Katayama M, et al. Tonic vibration reflex and muscle afferent block in writer's cramp. Ann Neurol 1995;38:155–162.

14. Grunewald RA, Yoneda Y, Shipman JM, et al. Idiopathic focal dystonia: a disorder of muscle spindle afferent processing? Brain 1997;120:2179–2185.

15. Naumann M, Reiners K. Long-latency reflexes of hand muscles in idiopathic focal dystonia and their modification by botulinum toxin. Brain 1997;120:409–416.

16. Panizza M, Lelli S, Nilsson J, Hallett M. H-reflex recovery curve and reciprocal inhibition of H-reflex in different kinds of dystonia. Neurology 1990;40:824–828.

17. Nakashima K, Rothwell JC, Day BL, et al. Reciprocal inhibition between forearm muscles in patients with writer's cramp and other occupational cramps, symptomatic hemidystonia and hemiparesis due to stroke. Brain 1989;112:681–697.

18. Priori A, Berardelli A, Mercuri B, et al. Physiological effects produced by BoNT treatment of upper limb dystonia. Changes in reciprocal inhibition between forearm muscles. Brain 1995;118:801–807.

19. Priori A, Berardelli A, Inghilleri M, et al. Electrical stimulation over muscle tendons in humans. Evidence favouring presynaptic inhibition of Ia fibres due to the activation of group III tendon afferents. Brain 1998;121:373–380.

20. Lorenzano C, Priori A, Currà A, et al. Impaired EMG inhibition elicited by tendon stimulation in dystonia. Neurology 2000;26;55:1789–1793.

21. Reilly JA, Hallett M, Cohen LG, et al. The N30 component of somatosensory evoked potentials in patients with dystonia. Electroencephalogr Clin Neurophysiol 1992;84:243–247.

22. Grissom JR, Lackland AFB, Toro C, et al. The N30 and N140-P190 median somatosensory evoked potential waveforms in dystonia involving the upper extremity. Neurology 1995;45(Suppl 4):A458.

23. Mazzini L, Zaccala M, Balzarini C. Abnormalities of somatosensory evoked potentials in spasmodic torticollis. Mov Disord 1994;9:426–430.

24. Nardone A, Mazzini L, Zaccala M. Changes in EMG response to perturbations and SEPs in a group of patients with idiopathic spasmodic torticollis. Mov Disord 1992;7(Suppl 1):25.

25. Kanovsky P, Streitova H, Dufek J, et al. Change in lateralization of the P22/N30 cortical component of median nerve somatosensory evoked potentials in patients with cervical dystonia after successful treatment with botulinum toxin A. Mov Disord 1998;13:108–117.

26. Murase N, Kaji R, Shimazu H, et al. Abnormal premovement gating of somatosensory input in writer's cramp. Brain 2000;123:1813–1829.

27. Hallett M. Is dystonia a sensory disorder [editorial]? Ann Neurol 1995;38:139–140.

28. Hallett M. Disorder of movement preparation in dystonia [editorial]. Brain 2000;123:1765–1766.

29. Deuschl G, Toro C, Matsumoto J, et al. Movement related cortical potential in writer's cramp. Ann Neurol 1995;38:862–868.

30. Tinazzi M, Priori A, Bertolasi L, et al. Abnormal central integration of a dual somatosensory input in dystonia. Evidence for sensory overflow. Brain 2000;123:42–50.

31. Frasson E, Priori A, Bertolasi L, et al. Somatosensory disinhibition in dystonia. Mov Disord 2001;16:674–682.

32. Kaji R, Murase N. Sensory function of basal ganglia. Mov Disord 2001;16:593–594.

33. Thompson PD, Dick JP, Day BL, et al. Electrophysiology of the corticomotoneurone pathways in patients with movement disorders. Mov Disord 1986;1:113–117.

34. Mavroudakis N, Caroyer JM, Brunko E, et al. Abnormal motor evoked responses to transcranial magnetic stimulation in focal dystonia. Neurology 1995;45:1671–1677.

35. Ikoma K, Samii A, Mercuri B, et al. Abnormal cortical motor excitability in dystonia. Neurology 1996;46:1371–1376.

36. Rona S, Berardelli A, Vacca L, et al. Alterations of motor cortical inhibition in patients with dystonia. Mov Disord 1998;13:118–124.

37. Currà A, Romaniello A, Berardelli A, et al. Shortened cortical silent period in facial muscles of patients with cranial dystonia. Neurology 2000;54:130–135.

38. Cruccu G, Inghilleri M, Berardelli A, et al. Cortical mechanisms mediating the inhibitory period after magnetic stimulation of the facial motor area. Muscle Nerve 1997;20:418–424.

39. Filipovic SR, Ljubisavljevic M, Svetel M, et al. Impairment of cortical inhibition in writer's cramp as revealed by changes in electromyographic silent period after transcranial magnetic stimulation. Neurosci Lett. 1997;222:167–170.

40. Ceballos-Baumann AO, Passingham RE, Warner T, et al. Overactive prefrontal and underactive motor cortical areas in idiopathic dystonia. Ann Neurol 1995;37:363–372.

41. Dum RP, Strick PL. Premotor areas: nodal points for parallel efferent systems involved in the central control of movements. In: Humphrey DR, Freund HJ, eds. Motor Control: Concepts and Issues. New York, NY: Wiley, 1991:383–397.

42. Ridding MC, Sheean G, Rothwell JC, et al. Changes in the balance between motor cortical excitation and inhibition in focal, task specific dystonia. J Neurol Neurosurg Psychiatry 1995;53:493–498.

43. Chen R, Wassermann EM, Canos M, et al. Impaired inhibition in writer's cramp during voluntary muscle activation. Neurology 1997; 49:1054–1059

44. Byrnes ML, Thickbroom GW, Wilson SA, et al. The corticomotor representation of upper limb muscles in writer's cramp and changes following botulinum toxin injection. Brain 1998;121:977–988.

45. Gilio F, Currà A, Lorenzano C, et al. Effects of botulinum toxin type A on intracortical inhibition in patients with dystonia. Ann Neurol 2000;48:20–26.

46. Byl N, Wilson F, Merzenich M, et al. Sensory dysfunction associated with repetitive strain injuries of tendonitis and focal hand dystonia: a comparative study. J Orthop Sports Phys Ther 1996;23:234–244.

47. Bara-Jimenez W, Shelton P, Sanger TD, et al. Sensory discrimination capabilities in patients with focal hand dystonia. Ann Neurol 2000; 47:377–380.

48. Byl NN, Merzenich MM, Jenkins WM. A primate genesis model of focal dystonia and repetitive strain injury: I. Learning-induced dedifferentiation of the representation of the hand in the primary somatosensory cortex in adult monkeys. Neurology 1996;47:508–520.

49. Berardelli A, Hallett M, Rothwell JC, et al. Single-joint rapid arm movements in normal subjects and in patients with motor disorders. Brain 1996;119:661–674.

50. van der Kamp W, Berardelli A, Rothwell JC, et al. Rapid elbow movements in patients with torsion dystonia. J Neurol Neurosurg Psychiatry 1989;52:1043–1049.

51. Inzelberg R, Flash T, Schechtman E, et al. Kinematic properties of upper limb trajectories in idiopathic torsion dystonia. J Neurol Neurosurg Psychiatry 1995;58:312–319.

52. Agostino R, Berardelli A, Formica A, et al. Sequential arm movements in patients with Parkinson's disease, Huntington's disease and cystonia. Brain 1992;115:1481–1495.

53. Currà A, Berardelli A, Agostino R, et al. Movement cueing and motor execution in dystonia. Mov Disord 2000;15:103–112.

54. Brotchie P, Iansek R, Horne MK. Motor function of the monkey globus pallidus. 2. Cognitive aspects of movement and phasic neuronal activity. Brain 1991;114:1685–1702.

PART II

Therapeutics

CHAPTER 5A

Nonpharmacologic Therapies

Nancy N. Byl

INTRODUCTION

Neuroplasticity and Learning

Although humans have an almost infinite number of degrees of freedom and permutations of movement variability, many functional activities performed in everyday life are repetitive. New skills are constantly learned. With practice, old skills are perfected. Some activities are performed so repetitively, they become habitual, nearly automatic, stable, reproducible, and secure (e.g., righting ourselves with gravity, swallowing, talking, running, writing, typing, etc.). Neural adaptation is the foundation of learning, not only in children but also in adults. Changes in structure and function of the nervous system are driven throughout life by engaging in highly attended, repetitive, progressive rewarded behaviors.[1–8]

Selective spatial and spectral cell assemblies have sharp segregation and result in more complex, efficient, voluntary behaviors. These event-by-event complex signal representations are highly plastic and modified by development, the environment, and goal-directed practice.[2,4,9–13] Challenged, attended, engaging, repetitive behaviors can slow down the negative effects of aging, as well as enable restoration of function after neural insults such as anoxia, traumatic head injury, stroke, surgery, or disease.

With advanced technology, researchers are able to confirm structural adaptations in the nervous system. There is evidence that positive feedback and behavioral rewards drive increases in myelination, acetylcholine, dopamine, and other modulatory neurotransmitters which can lead to continual positive neural adaptation.[5,6,14-28] Adaptive learning may also be measured by an increase in the size and an improvement in the distinct orderly somatotopic representation; a reduction in the size of the cutaneous receptive fields; an increase in the density of the receptive fields; and change in the latency, amplitude or density of sensory and motor-evoked field responses.

Nancy N. Byl: Department of Physical Therapy and Rehabilitation Science, School of Medicine, University of California, San Francisco, California.

The author has on commercial relationship with the funder.

The parts of the body that require the most distinct sensory processing and fine motor control have a disproportionately large somatotopic representation on the sensory and motor cortices (e.g., lips, mouth, tongue, larynx, and hand).[29] This not only alters the sensitivity of these parts and the ability to perform skilled movements; in addition, it may lead to more disability after an injury.[30,31]

The hand has been the target of many somatosensory and motor neuroplasticity studies because of its high degree of differentiation and distinct representation on the brain. However, the principles of neural adaptation are applicable well beyond the hand. Postural mechanisms for righting the head and trunk require the integration of reflex and differentiated movements as do other sophisticated tasks such as talking, chewing, swallowing, and airway control.

Neural Adaptation and Voluntary Movements

Goal-directed movements require the transformation of environmental sensory representations into muscle control signals (sensorimotor transformation). There are three broad categories of voluntary movement: reflex responses, rhythmic motor responses, and fine motor movements.[31] Reflex movements are predictable, automatic, and fixed; they are usually produced by a sensory stimulus. A type of pattern generator that produces a pattern of nearly automatic movement (e.g., contact with a moving surface on the bottom of the feet may stimulate stepping) may drive rhythmic motor movements which become habituated. Voluntary movements are mediated by direct connections between the cortex and spinal cord, along with important afferent somatosensory and nociceptive information gathered from the skin, muscles, tendons, and joints of the limbs and trunk. Movements involve multiple joints as well as sequential and temporal pattern activation of multiple muscles.

Although the simplest motor behaviors are triggered by sensory stimuli and are obligatory, motor neurons also receive strong sensory inputs from the limbs whose muscles they control on a voluntary basis. The primary purpose of somatosensory information is to guide directed movements.[31]

All movements activate sensory receptors in the muscles, joints, and skin. The sensory feedback provided by these receptors is low at rest and increases with exploratory movements, learning a new motor task, and increased attention or arousal. Twenty-five percent of the neurons fire equally with passive or active touch.[32,33] A continuous stream of tactile, visual, and proprioceptive information is required to make voluntary movements both accurate and properly sequenced. Depending on the task, sensory feedback will be scaled up or down, with the gain control system acting through the effect of motor pathways. This is also applicable to feedback from joint receptors.[34] Movement itself stimulates other perturbations and counter-responses. In addition, some joint afferents and cutaneous mechanoreceptors can also act like nociceptors, which are primarily sensitive to the extremes of the range of motion rather than midrange movement detection.[35,36]

The submodalities of somatic function, such as touch, pain, and position sense are processed through different pathways leading to the thalamus, which acts like a gatekeeper for information to the cerebral cortex.[31] Initially, sensory information is unimodal; however, ultimately, it becomes multimodal and assists in producing a unified percept and the memory of that percept. Sensory information ascends in serial and parallel pathways. One of the primary purposes of somatosensory information is to guide directed movement. Although individuals may try to guide movement with their eyes, this system is too slow to enable rapid fine motor movements.

The response properties of light tactile input from the skin and proprioceptive inputs from the muscles and joints are integrated at the cortical level, creating direction, movement, and orientation sensitive units.[37–47] Muscle spindles are most sensitive to changes in length of a muscle while tendon organs are most sensitive to changes in muscle tension associated with muscle contraction. Contraction of the muscle makes the muscle spindle too short, while simultaneously creating a stretch of the Golgi tendon organ. In combination with changes in length, the corticospinal neurons encode force and the rate of change in load. That change in force may provide more important information about limb movement than change in position.[48] The prioprioceptors along with the tactile receptors are also responsible for shaping the hand for functional use. Unexpected mechanical loads have been correlated with a change in the latency of firing (70 to 80 milliseconds), which is consistent with the supraspinal pathways involving the somatosensory cortex. Grip adjustments for predictable loads occur with force changes. These mechanical events also inform the central nervous system (CNS) about the completeness of the succinct phases of the task, which in turn, trigger preprogrammed corrective action.

Paradoxically, voluntary movement may reduce the transmission of tactile inputs to the primary sensory cortex (movement-related gating of sensory transmission). This gating limits the amount of afferent input that must be processed at higher levels. Interestingly, movement itself is not essential to produce gating since it is also noted in isometric contractions.[49] The modulation is nonspecific in terms of direction of movement and can be modified by selective attention, behavioral context, motivational state and reward. The motor cortex seems the major source of the centrally originating gating signal.[49] Neurons also stop firing when the sensory information is not relevant to a texture task or the motor task.

Inhibition and excitation are found both in the higher and lower order neurons. Feedback inhibitory afferents provide redundant information. Inhibitory feedback allows active output neurons to limit activity and creates rings of less active neurons. Inhibitory interneurons may also be activated at more distant sites, such as the cortex. For example, when reading Braille, Merkel and Meissner corpuscles transmit the neural image of the pattern to the primary sensory cortex (3b), signaling shape and sharpening the shape as a result of a pause in firing (excitatory and inhibitory).

Perception of an object (e.g., weight, surface friction, texture, position) also involves peripheral and centrally mediated activity, especially during object prehension and manipulation.[50–53] A smooth object automatically facilitates a frictional force to overcome the load lifted against gravity. The force generated to lift a smooth object is greater than the force automatically generated to lift the same object (same size and weight) with a rough surface. When the surface is smooth, the object is perceived as heavier, even if the weight is the same.[52]

Set-related anticipatory trunk movements occur in the primary motor cortex and the supplementary motor area before movement is executed.[53] This anticipatory mode of motor control is part of the feed-forward control system. Set-related activity is associated predominantly with sensory stimuli that detect imminent perturbations and initiate proactive, protective strategies. Feed-forward information from the spindle is used by the motor system to control posture and movement. When catching a ball, feed-forward mechanisms allow the body to "compute" the time for the ball to arrive. There is also an anticipatory contraction. When the ball hits the hand, the sudden muscle stretch produces a contraction of both the agonist and antagonist. Feed-forward information is essential for rapid action. Feed-forward processing depends on the nervous system's ability to predict the consequences of sensory events and may be used to modify the operations of feedback mechanisms.

During feedback, the neurons are informed about the consequences of the movement. The signals from the sensors are compared with a desired state, providing a reference signal or error signal. Feedback systems are characterized by their gain. A high-gain system (e.g., approaching 1) fires vigorously to minimize deviations from the optimal target state. However, these firings are unstable, particularly if there are long delays (e.g., to change the contractility). Muscle spindles as well as the cutaneous afferents also provide critical feedback.[54–56]

Novel voluntary behaviors require processing in multiple motor pathways and are continuously monitored for errors.

As the behavior becomes more accurate, the need for sampling the sensory inflow and updating the motor program decreases. After practice, the behavior becomes faster, more accurate and more automatic. At that point activity in the supplementary motor area decreases. Higher cortical functions such as motivation, emotions, planning, preparing, sequencing, executing, and modifying movement can enhance or disrupt fine motor performance.

Hebb[57] noticed that individual motor actions shared important characteristics even when performed in a different manner. This is called motor equivalence. That is, while writing with the dominant hand, the writing has a characteristic appearance. When writing with the nondominant hand or holding the pen in the teeth or performed with the big toe, the characteristics of the writing remain the same. Writing activates the functional representation of writing in the sensorimotor and premotor areas of the brain.[58] The extremity that is used activates another area of the brain consistent with the somatotopic representation. This concept can be important when rehabilitating a patient who cannot perform a task normally because of an impairment. This phenomenon also suggests that to facilitate neuroadaptation, it may be possible to use a nonaffected limb to restore the functional representation and then transfer the learning to the affected limb.

FOCAL HAND DYSTONIA

Focal dystonia is a painless, task-specific disorder of movement. Task-specific dystonias involving the hand include occupational hand cramp, writer's cramp, keyboarder's cramp, musician's cramp or golfer's yip. In each case, involuntary movements are imposed on a specific voluntary task.[59–75] In 1861, Duchenne[76] described hand cramps as a functional spasm of the muscles. In 1888, Gowers[77] described hand cramps as a neurotic illness. Today, focal dystonia is thought to be a neurologic impairment of inhibition and excitation resulting from dysfunction in circuitry or integration involving the basal ganglia, sensory thalamus, somatosensory cortex, or sensorimotor cortex.[78–91] Detailed neurophysiologic theories on etiology are covered in detail in earlier chapters. However, relevant to conservative treatment, some clinicians and researchers suggest that aberrant learning may be an important etiology of focal hand dystonia. This could be a consequence of peripheral trauma, psychological state, or a finite limitation of temporal integration in neural adaptation, disrupting sensory motor processing.

Focal hand dystonia has been reported after musculoskeletal injury, peripheral nerve trauma, central neural trauma, disease, anatomic restriction or severe pain.[61,78,92–109] Although there are no prospectively collected epidemiologic data on the development of posttraumatic movement disorders, some patients with focal dystonia demonstrate strong temporal-anatomic relationships between trauma and the onset of movement disorder symptoms. Jankovic[96] suggests that peripherally induced movement disorders should be considered when:

1. Trauma is severe enough to cause persistent local symptoms (e.g., symptoms persist at least 2 weeks and may even cause the patient to seek late medical attention);
2. The anatomic site of the original injury is the same site as the initial manifestation of the movement disorder; and
3. The movement disorder develops within days or months, for up to 1 year after the injury.[96]

Historically, patients with posttraumatic, peripherally induced movement dysfunction exhibit dystonic movements similar to patients with primary dystonia. However, those with trauma more commonly have underlying contractures and limitations of passive movement with a fixed posture. Usually sensory tricks are not effective.

Conversely, Weiner argues that peripheral trauma is not a likely cause of focal dystonia. If all peripheral traumas are considered, a very small proportion of those injured develop dystonia. For example, there are many people who perform repetitive tasks in their job; however, only a few develop dystonia. In addition, in the case of head injuries, the absence of dystonia is more common than the presence of dystonia.[97] Weiner suggests that individuals developing focal dystonia associated with a peripheral trauma may be those who have known risk factors for dystonia irrelevant to the injury itself (e.g., a family history of dystonia).

Patient personality such as perfectionism and perseveration, anxiety, phobias, stress, or emotional instability might also lead to focal hand dystonia.[110–114] Generally, it is not uncommon that people who present with job-related, repetitive, fine motor control problems also report increased stress, anxiety, increased time on task, and persistent attention to improve quality or quantity of their work.[110] Initially, the increased investment of time is associated with enhanced outcomes and improved performance. The critical factor may relate to a change, such as a modification of the equipment, application of new techniques, a threat against job security, an increase in job complexity, or personal stress. Often with this history, time-on-task increases; but, fatigue and deterioration of performance, rather than improvement are noted. Patients sense some emergent uncoordination, and ultimately, the fingers seem to develop a life of their own, curling or extending involuntarily when the patient attempts to perform the target task. Patients may also develop focal dystonia without obvious psychological stress. It is unlikely there is a single cause of focal dystonia; rather, an accumulation of anatomic, physiologic, neurologic, musculoskeletal, and emotional factors may stress the nervous system beyond its point of stability.[103,115]

Finite Limits of Neural Adaptation

Neural plasticity is not infinite. At some point, competition between neural structures for isolated and shared functions, timing, refractory periods, hard-wired programs, neurochemical processes, and cellular mechanisms limit expansion of new dendritic branching and synaptic information.

Consequently, there may be times when highly attended, repetitive behaviors could indeed exceed the capacity of neural processing. Within a given cortical area, cortical pyramidal cells cannot be reexcited effectively by another perturbation for tens to hundreds of milliseconds. These integration times are dictated primarily by the time for recovery from inhibition, which dominates post-stimulus excitability. The cortex continues to define its representation of the temporal aspects of behaviorally important inputs by generating more synchronous representations of sequenced input perturbations or events. These time constants govern and limit the cortex's ability to "chunk," or separately represent by distributed, coordinated discharge, successive events within its processing channels. Reorganization and merging of distinct somatotopic differentiation may interfere with normal, voluntary fine motor control. This could happen if attended repetitive behaviors become stereotypical and nearly simultaneous in time. The nervous system could lose the ability to distinctly record individual inputs or generate precise outputs. This may interfere with normal sensorimotor feedback and motor control. The question is whether such limits in neural adaptation could lead to aberrant learning in conditions such as focal hand dystonia.

In 1996, Byl et al.[82] proposed that focal hand dystonia might be a consequence of aberrant learning. The sensorimotor learning hypothesis was proposed: attended, rapid, repetitive, stereotypical movements may lead to near simultaneous, stereotypical inputs to the skin, joint receptors, and muscle afferents, dedifferentiating the somatosensory hand representation and degrading fine motor control. Since then, evidence of aberrant somatosensory organization and abnormal somatosensory responses in patients with hand dystonia has been documented by others.[81,83,116–120]

Based on both the theories of neuroadaptivity and sensorimotor physiology, Sanger et al.[121] and Merzenich and DeCharms[4] outlined a computational model of focal dystonia that may explain several common features of focal dystonia. These include:

• Symptoms develop in otherwise healthy individuals in response to highly attended repetitive movements;
• Evolution of symptoms is variable in terms of time;
• Symptoms appear only during the performance of a target-specific task;
• Dystonic movements persist despite stopping the task;
• Symptoms may be decreased but not remediated with dopamine-depleting drugs or botulinum toxin; and
• Evidence of abnormalities in motor and sensory cortical representations of the dystonic limb.

In this model, gain could be increased by expanding or even shrinking the sensory cortical representation of a limb due to adaptation as a result of repetitive use, increasingly more simultaneous firing, coupling of multiple sensory signals, or voluntary coactivation of muscles.[2,4,6,7,9,11–13,21–26,122–124] The loop through the deep nuclei to the cortex, basal ganglia, and thalamus combines with the sensorimotor loop gain and contributes to instability.[125,126] If only certain mechanical models of the sensorimotor loop are unstable, then a focal dystonia rather than a generalized dystonia develops.

The computational analysis suggests there are three distinct phases for the development of dystonia: incipient, unstable, and sustained.[126] Incipient dystonia implies that the loop gain is approaching 1; however, clinical symptoms are not yet apparent. It would be helpful to measure the loop gain as it approaches 1 but before motor activity becomes prominently sustained. This increase in motor and supplementary motor cortical excitability has been demonstrated with electrophysiologic mapping and magnetic source imaging. Unstable dystonia represents the epoch of early symptoms of dystonia. It is correlated hypothetically with trigger loop instability. However, it may be possible to accomplish the movements without instability by using sensory tricks to minimize the deviation. Interventions that cause only slight changes in loop gains may be able to resolve symptoms completely because only a small change in sensory processing would be needed to reduce the gain below 1. Sustained dystonia refers to a dystonia in which symptoms may worsen rapidly as the sensory cortical representation either expands or degrades. The loop gain may increase well beyond 1 and clinical intervention may be ineffective. As the gain continues to increase, increased numbers of triggering postures or movements would be expected, and more muscle groups would be affected.

This model further suggests that the appropriate treatment should result in a decrease in the imbalance in the loop gain that could occur at any point in either the sensorimotor or extrapyramidal loops. A permanent solution requires use of cortical plasticity to redifferentiate cortical and subcortical representations. Retraining may not be possible in the context of severe dystonia without temporarily breaking the cycle. One approach is to increase the variability of practiced movements so that there are many uncorrelated movement components, each with only a few relevant sensory neurons. This is comparable to behaviors directed to uncoupling the pathologically coupled modes. It may also be possible to temporarily modify the loop by using pharmaceutical agents, such as botulinum toxin, and then pair the treatment with retraining.

Assessment

As part of the assessment process for patients with focal dystonia, physical performance parameters should be measured and objectively recorded. It is important to examine the involved and uninvolved limbs.[127,128] It is also imperative to observe the patient performing the target task. A complete neurologic evaluation should be performed. In addition, measurements that should be recorded include:

• Posture;
• Range of motion (e.g., shoulder elevation and rotation, forearm supination and pronation, finger spread, etc.)[9,103,129];

- neurovascular entrapment[100];
- Peripheral nerve entrapments[60,93,95,130,131];
- Sympathetic signs (e.g., temperature, sweating, color);
- Selected strength of intrinsic muscles (lumbricals and interossei) and extrinsic muscles (e.g., wrist extension, finger flexion and extension)[132];
- Sensory discrimination: graphesthesia, kinesthesia, localization, and stereognosis[82,122,126,133–135];
- Fine-motor speed and motor accuracy (e.g., Purdue test [Lafayette Instruments][133]; PAR Tapper [Digital Reaction Time])[136,137];
- Voluntary fine motor control at the target task should be videotaped and then scored on an ordinal scale for quality and severity (Arm Dystonia Disability Scale)[135]; and
- Functional independence (e.g., CAFÉ 40).[138]

A rating scale should be used to score the severity of the movement disorder.[135,139–141] The Arm Dystonia Disability Scale (ADD) is rated on a four-point scale as follows: 0 = normal; 1 = mild difficulty in playing/writing; 2 = moderate difficulty; and 3 = marked difficulty in playing and writing. The Tubiana and Chamagne Scale (TCS)[142] is rated on a six-point scale: 0 = unable to play; 1 = plays several notes but stops because of blockage or lack of facility; 2 = plays short sequences without rapidity and with unsteady fingering; 3 = plays easy pieces but is unable to perform more technically challenging pieces; 4 = plays almost normally but avoids difficult passages for fear of motor problems; 5 = returns to concert performance. It is also important to analyze task-specific motor performance to determine which normal movements have been preserved. Preserved simple movements may serve as the starting point for restoring selective fine motor control.

Dynamic electromyography may be performed as part of the assessment. Electromyography can be used to confirm the classic cocontraction of antagonists and agonists or lack of reflex inhibition and to document the variability in force and amplitude between the muscles recruited. Electromyography could also document the time required to turn off muscle firing.[61,143,144] With multiple channels, it is possible to determine which muscles are firing first. Even though the fingers may be flexing, the extensors may have been the first to contract.

Brain imaging can be ordered to rule out other possible causes of the dystonic movements, however, these tests are most commonly used in research. Positive emission tomography (PET)[91,145–148]; functional magnetic resonance imaging (fMRI); magnetoencephalography and transcranial magnetic stimulation[81,83,149,150] have been used to analyze CNS responsiveness, blood flow patterns, and somatotopic organization. High-speed three-dimensional video images, force, and acceleration data have also been used to characterize the dystonia. Computer technology (e.g., MIDI) is gaining acceptance in motor research laboratories to document timing and forces.[102,127,151]

Principles of Current Nonpharmacologic Treatment Approaches for Focal Hand Dystonia

As a rule, the specific conservative therapies for focal hand dystonia are primarily empiric and only partially successful. Most patients arrive with a long list of previous, usually ineffective therapies. Most conservative programs include muscle strengthening, modification of musical or computer instruments, drugs to deplete or enhance dopamine, injections of botulinum toxin, special diets, hypnosis, biofeedback, behavioral therapies, or surgery. Although evidence to support the different strategies is increasing, in 1990, Hochberg et al.[66] concluded that no single treatment modality had yet proven to be effective with predictability. However, what is clear is that individuals who are focused and committed to recover must modify life stresses and methodically begin a retraining program.

General Guidelines

All affected individuals should be educated about the suspected contribution of aberrant learning to the development of the dystonia. Effective intervention strategies for patients with focal dystonia must create an environment for positive learning and recovery. These strategies should minimize stressors, enhance patient self-esteem, and build self-confidence. Patients with focal dystonia should be encouraged to establish a foundation of positive health and wellness (good nutrition, hydration, strength, endurance, postural alignment, and flexibility) to facilitate normal healing and repair before embarking on a specific rehabilitation program. All unnecessary emotional stress and anxiety must be minimized. Patients must stop the abnormal movements and focus on getting better. Each person must believe that they have control over their recovery and be willing to take the responsibility to get better. Hand use strategies must be changed. Each patient must learn to use the hand in a functional position with movement initiated proximally (e.g., from the trunk, shoulder, and elbow) with controlled digit movements also shifted away from the extrinsic muscles to the intrinsic muscles of the hand.

The basic foundation for recovery begins with a strong foundation of health and wellness, including the following:

- Establish a regular fitness program (30 to 60 minutes per day of moderate exercise 3 to 5 days per week).
- Eat a healthy diet.
- Stay well-hydrated to maximize oxygen delivery to heavily used tissues (at least 10 to 12 glasses of noncaffeinated fluids).
- Obtain adequate, restful sleep.
- Seek counseling as needed to build confidence, self-esteem, and reduce anxiety.
- Adapt strategies to reduce the effects of stress on neurovascular entrapments, such as balancing the posture with gravity, diaphragmatic breathing, and neural mobilization.
- Reduce unnecessary biomechanical trauma to the hands by using stress-free hand techniques in all activities of daily living including the target task (Table 5-1).

TABLE 5-1. *Healthy Hands: Stress-Free Functional Activities*

I. Reducing Stress on the Trunk and Upper Limb

A. Balance the Posture with Gravity

1. The position of the trunk is a critical foundation for using the arm. The trunk must be balanced with gravity to provide a stable base for the hand to work. The trunk must be aligned with gravity.
   a. Stand with your back near a wall, heels approximately 2 inches away from the wall. Put a towel around your neck and tuck in your chin (like saying "yes") and balance your head over your shoulders. Note how far your head and shoulders are from the wall.
   b. Bend and straighten your knees slowly; let your lower back flatten against the wall and feel your head getting closer to the wall. Look straight ahead with the eyes open and then repeat with the eyes closed.
   c. As you glide up and down the wall, find the position in which your head seems well centered over your trunk without feeling strain.
   d. With your head in neutral and the back of your head lightly and comfortably touching the wall, glide both arms up over your head.

2. Imagine being in a quiet, peaceful place as you work on breathing/relaxing. Take the stress out of your neck, shoulders and trunk by breathing with your diaphragm. Use the muscles of the abdominal wall to breathe rather than the neck muscles.
   a. Lie on your back with your knees bent.
   b. Let the abdominal wall relax as you take a breath of air in while letting your back go into extension (increase the arch of your back by anteriorly rotating you pelvis). Keep your neck muscles quiet.
   c. Then blow out and rock your pelvis posteriorly, flattening your back and pulling your chest wall down towards your feet. Blow your stress away as you flatten your back.
   d. Take your air in through your nose and blow the air out through your mouth. Practice breathing this way for at least 5 minutes. Start and end the day by taking the time to evaluate your breathing. Integrate this diaphragmatic breathing throughout your day.
   e. After you are comfortable with the breathing exercises:
      i) Put a rolled towel perpendicular to the spine at the level of your lower back and repeat the diaphragmatic breathing. This will help you arch your back and flatten the back.
         a) Roll a larger towel and place along the midline of the spine (parallel to the spine).
         b) Repeat the breathing. Now the shoulders are a little extended.
      ii) Improve the mobility of the shoulders and the neurovascular tissue around the shoulder and the axilla. The arteries and veins can get congested when you are stressed and you tighten the muscles around your neck and axilla.
         a) To increase the mobility of the neurovascular bundle, it is necessary to avoid end range stretching. The nerves and the blood vessels do not like to be stretched. Instead, it is best to "pump" the arm, taking the muscles, nerves, vascular tissue, and fascia to comfortable and variable lengths.
         b) Lie on the floor on your back, knees bent. Depress your shoulders (let them glide down toward your feet). Then glide the shoulder out to the side. Only take your arm out to the side in the pain-free, tension-free range. The elbow should be at approximately a right angle. Wave good-bye with the hand/wrist. Make the waving smooth. Keep the hand/wrist in a neutral position and straighten and bend the elbow.
         c) Make the fingers straight and bend the wrist back toward the forearm (the palm facing towards the wall). Now, bend and straighten the elbow. Repeat this series of exercises for approximately 5 minutes).

3. Gently increase the freedom of movement of the shoulder.
   a. Make large circling movements of the shoulder; do not feel any tension around the scapula.
   b. Practice the large circling movements at different speeds and different ranges of motion.
   c. Bring the hand to the target surface by making large circling movements and then dropping your hand to the instrument, letting it fall with gravity.
   d. Sit facing a table, hands and arms on the table. Practice moving the trunk on the arm to increase stress-free mobility at the shoulder. Do the same thing again, except place arm out to the side approximately 70° and lean the trunk over your arm.

B. Health and Wellness Program: Aerobics

1. Participate in an aerobics program three times per week: walking, treadmill, stationary bike, stair climbing, and bike riding.
2. Participate in fitness activities while keeping the pressure off your hands/arms (do not use heavy gripping).
   a. Do not heavily grip on the bars of the stair climber or treadmill. Simply rest your hands on a bar to keep your balance.
   b. Spend 20–30 minutes with your heart rate at 70–80% of maximum depending on your age.
   c. Ask your doctor or your therapist what your training heart rate should be.

C. Maintaining Healthy Tissues to Perform our Work

1. Drink plenty of water and fluids (10–12 glasses per day). If you have a glass of wine, coffee, or diet soda, you must replace this fluid with another glass of water or juice. The flow of blood in your body is like the oil in your car. If you are going to use your arms heavily in your work, you must keep the tissues gliding smoothly on each other. In addition, you constantly need oxygen to maintain tissue health.
2. If you are still practicing, playing, or working, remember to take frequent breaks and use your hands for short intervals of time (e.g., 5–15 minutes and take a break).
3. Convert some of your physical practice playing your instrument to mental practice. If you are working on a computer, practice changing your techniques at the computer when you are not at work (See Keyboard section).
4. Keep the hand balanced (looking round). Allow the intrinsic muscles (inside the hand) to support the normal arches of the hand and avoid overuse of the extrinsic muscles (those arising on the forearm).

TABLE 5-1. *Healthy Hands: Stress-Free Functional Activities (Continued)*

D. Stress-Free Hand Use

1. Strengthen the small muscles inside the hand (intrinsics) to facilitate the maintenance of the functional position of the hand and the stability of the arches of the hand complex.
   a. Spread your fingers apart (try not to use muscles that straighten the fingers; these include the long tendons on the top of your hand). With your fingers spread apart, give some resistance by trying to use your other hand to bring them together.
   b. Now try to hold the fingers together while you use your other hand to try and spread them apart.
   c. Bend the fingers to 90° at the large knuckle joints (metacarpal-phalangeal joints) by placing the back of your hand against the edge of a table (with the wrist neutral and the metacarpal-phalangeal joint bent to 90°) and take a finger from the other hand and press the interphalageal joints down towards the palm and use the muscles inside the hand to keeping the fingers straight.
      i) Now, one finger at a time, try to keep the fingers straight as you use the other hand to try and bend the finger.
      ii) Give resistance at the distal segments of the finger.
      iii) Use a rubber band for resistance.
2. Use the small muscles inside the hand to do activities of daily living (e.g., precision gripping) while keeping the muscles of the forearm quiet. To prepare for this, it is necessary to strengthen the muscles inside the hand.
   a. Initiate bending the fingers at the base of the fingers (the large metacarpal-phalangeal joint); try to do this without bending the other joints of the fingers (e.g., the finger joints should maintain a slight bend from 5–15°), but the base joint could move to 90°).
   b. Do not practice gripping exercises. Heavy gripping should be avoided.
      i) Do not squeeze the steering wheel when you are driving. You only need to create a controlling power grip when you are turning.
      ii) Do not hold free weights and ball. Do not participate in fitness exercises that require holding on to free weights, squeezing a ball, or specifically strengthening the grip in other ways.
      iii) Use a precision grip (3 point or spherical grip that includes keeping your fingers round and bringing the pads of your thumb and second and third finger together) to pick up objects and to hold your key).
      iv) Avoid using a key grip (side of thumb pressed against side of the index finger) when using a key. This grip will tend to stress the stability of the base joint of your thumb.
   c. When reaching for an object, keep the hand relaxed. When the object makes contact with the hand, let the sensory information (sense of touch) from the surface of the object open the hand.
   d. Strengthen the base joint of your thumb by bringing it away from the palm of your hand and giving resistance to the first phalanx (bone closest to the joint).
3. When playing the piano or using the computer keyboard:
   a. Have your hand relaxed and drop it onto the keyboard; let the keyboard open the hand. It is not necessary to actively spread the fingers to try to reach an octave. You will reach further by letting the surface open your hand.
   b. Avoid rapid, forceful finger flexion and extension movements during all of the tasks you perform with your hands. Most specifically, stop using individual finger flexion and extension on the keyboard. Transfer the work from the fingers to the forearm.
      i) Lift the fingers off the keyboard by rotating the forearm into supination (palm up, lifting the thumb and index finger and then rotate the forearm into more pronation by letting the elbow leave the side of your trunk and lifting the fourth and fifth digit from the keyboard).
      ii) When the hand is pronated (palm down), let the elbow swing away from the side a little if necessary to keep the hand relaxed and down on the keyboard. When the elbow swings away from the trunk, internal rotation of the shoulder can take the stress off the forearm at the end of the range of pronation. This is especially a good technique if you do not have full pronation. You can not keep your arm next to your trunk and turn your palm down parallel to the floor.
4. When playing a string instrument, get into a comfortable position. Make yourself tall with gravity by lifting the rib cage high. Balance your head over your shoulders.
5. Use the hand in a natural functional position:
   a. Make the palm round from the base of the thumb to the base of the 5th finger and round from the pads of the fingers to the base of the thumb. Thus, all of the finger joints should be slightly bent, the palm is round and the wrist is extended approximately 15°. When you are standing with your arms are at your side, this will usually be the natural position of the hand. Look in a mirror.
   b. Do not let the fingers collapse or hyperextend (overly extend) when placing your hands on any surface; let them rest down.
      i) Practice dropping the hand onto a surface and maintaining the roundness of the hand (a small soft ball could be taped into the palm for assistance). Once learned, remove the ball and try to maintain the same round appearance of the hand arches. (You might want to take a picture of the appearance of the hand with the ball in the palm so you can maintain this shape when the ball is removed).
      ii) Lean lightly onto the hand while it is on a flat surface and maintain the natural, round shape of the hand (normal arches).
      iii) Thread the fingers of one hand through the fingers of the other hand to help stabilize the hand when placing weight onto the hand.
6. With a soft, flexible, ball approximately 2 inches in diameter on the table, roll the palm of the hand over the ball and let the finger pads drop onto the surface. Then repeat to get the idea that the palm is round.

TABLE 5-1. *Healthy Hands: Stress-Free Functional Activities (Continued)*

7. Try to comfortably achieve full, stress-free range of motion of the cervical spine and upper extremity.
   a. Lie on your back, with your knees bent.
   b. Turn your head to the left and to the right. Side bend your head to the left and the right. Practice nodding with your chin like you are saying yes, only moving from the very top joint of the neck.
   c. Keep your abdominal wall tightly tucked and the back flat. Keep the pelvis stable and lift one leg up to 90° of hip flexion and keep it there while you lift the other leg. Do not let the abdominal wall move as you do this. If you cannot do that, put a few pillows under your feet and repeat until you can do this by keeping the abdominal wall stable. Then keep one leg up at 90° and let the other leg go out straight and come back. Do this while keeping the abdomen still. Then do the same with the other leg. Then keep one leg up at 90° and let the other leg go out straight and come back. Do this while keeping the abdomen still. Then do the same with the other leg
8. Gently take your hands through a normal and comfortable range of motion.
   a. Go to each finger web and gently massage in the web space and then on both the palmar and dorsal side of your hand
   b. Passively, gently spread open each digit and hold at the end range for a few minutes
   c. Put the palm of your hands together
   d. With palms together, gently move the wrists back and forth (parallel to the floor in flexion and extension) and then move towards and away from the thumb (ulnar and radial deviation).
   e. Put your hands down on the surface and move them away from each other (ulnar deviation) and then bring them back towards each other

E. Using the Computer Keyboard Safely
1. Sit in a stable position
   a. Sit with feet flat on the floor. Sit tall with hips about 90° (vary this posture throughout the day). Consider using a wedge in the chair to balance the spine in neutral.
   b. Do not let your head or shoulders be forward; use your lower abdominal muscles to keep your rib cage high. This will help balance your head over your shoulders.
   c. When you are at work, change your posture frequently and take frequent breaks (e.g., every 20 minutes).
2. When you are spending time trying to change your techniques on the keyboard, practice with your eyes closed. It is good to start out by just placing your fingers on the keyboard and feeling smoothly across the board.
3. Place the computer screen at or slightly below eye level. Look straight ahead (even ask a coworker to look at your alignment and give you feedback). Consider purchasing special antiglare glasses for computer terminal display work or use a screen glare protector.
   a. Place the monitor approximately 2 feet away from the eyes for the majority of work; pull the screen closer as necessary for close work.
   b. Keyboard height should be adjusted to maintain elbow flexion at about 80° (positioned in approximately 100° of extension). Forearms should be angled toward the floor, and not resting on the table. If it is difficult to let your hands rest lightly on the keyboard with the wrist free, it may be helpful to have a pillow on your lap or a pillow between your trunk and your arm where the forearms receive positive sensory information from the pillow to help them relax.
   c. Look at the contour of the hand when it is at your side; maintain that position as the hand is dropped on the keyboard.
   d. Keep the wrist in neutral (0–15° extension) when using the keyboard. Do not rest your wrist on a "wrist rest." Resting the wrist and forearm on the work surface will increase the pressure in the carpal tunnel and force all of the work to be done with the fingers. If you have a wrist pad, think of the pad as a sensory tickle to let you know that your wrists should be "floating" above the rest.
   e. Do not curl the fingers when striking the keys. Avoid using the tips but rather the pads of the fingers. Initiate the movement at the base joint of the fingers. Imagine that you are using muscles inside your hand and not the long muscles that bend the fingers. Watch your forearm. All muscles should be quiet. Let all of the fingers rest down lightly on the keyboard the pads of the fingers. Do not let any of your fingers fly up. Continue this resting down even when one finger is engaged in depressing a key. Do not allow the adjacent fingers to extend to get them away from the active finger.
   f. It is not necessary to actively lift the fingers following pressing down. It is enough simply to release the pressure down.
   g. Change the fulcrum of movement from the fingers of the hand to the elbow and shoulder.
      i) Allow the elbow to move freely in flexion and extension.
      ii) Use the large muscles of the shoulder and the trunk to move up and down the keyboard.
      iii) Avoid reaching one finger out in isolation of the others.
4. Do not squeeze the mouse; drape your hand around the mouse.
   a. Keep your wrist in neutral.
   b. Do not activate the mouse button by lifting and bending the index finger.
   c. Use rotation of the forearm to activate the button on the mouse.
   d. Make sure the mouse is close to you and that the arm is not extended out to the side. Use a cover over the number keys if necessary to keep the arm closer to your trunk. Then use the mouse on the cover.
5. Take regular breaks. During these breaks, either walk around or do some exercises to relieve the stress.
   a. Try to do the diaphragmatic breathing initially while sitting quietly. Then try to continue the breathing while working
   b. Do gentle mobilization exercises as you breathe by bringing arms up and down along with your breathing.
   c. Place your arms on the desk and gently bend your trunk over the arms. Let all the movements be made by the trunk, not the arms.

TABLE 5-1. *Healthy Hands: Stress-Free Functional Activities (Continued)*

6. Consider obtaining a public software program that forces you to take a break from the computer. Usually there is a forced screen break.

E. Writing

1. The fulcrum for the movement for writing should be the shoulder and elbow, not the fingers. The hand should be resting down on the table.
2. The hand should be round and relaxed. Avoid the excessive squeezing of the thumb, index and third finger around the pen. Also avoid writing by flexing and extending the fingers.
   a. If you continue to write using the typical grip, put Velcro on the pen. The rough surface will stimulate you to place less force on the pen and still feel security of control. However, still try to write with the elbow off the table, moving from the elbow and the shoulder with rhythmical movements.
   b. Let the arm rest lightly on the table and comfortably against the side. Avoid resting the elbow on the surface. If it is hard to get the palm down, allow the shoulder to move out a little away from your trunk into abduction (arm out to side and internal rotation).
3. Put some Velcro on the pen and try holding the pen lightly between the second and third fingers rather than the thumb and index finger. First just practice this way of holding the pen. The hand should be open, with the fingers and the thumb resting down.
   a. Move the pen from the elbow and shoulder; keep the wrist and fingers quiet. Practice rhythmical circling movements making loops.
   b. Practice writing in shaving cream, finger paints or water.
   c. Practice picking up the pen and laying it down without feeling any tension.
   d. Mentally review relaxed writing before beginning to write with new technique.
   e. Let all fingers rest down. Do not hold any fingers up off the pen.
   f. Place a mirror between the unaffected hand and the affected hand. For example, place your non-writing hand (left) in front of the mirror. Look at the mirror image and note that it looks like the right hand.
      i) Now pick up a pen and put it down. Have the opposite hand behind the mirror and copy what you see in the mirror. In other words, make the involved hand look exactly like the mirror image.
      ii) Notice if your hand appears relaxed. The knuckles should not be white.
      iii) Pick up other objects and put them down or manipulate them in front of the mirror, copying everything with the affected side.
      iv) Write in different ways with different pens.
      v) Try to increase the time you can write without tension. Progressively increase this time frame.
         a) If you have access to biofeedback, put the electrodes on the flexor and extensor muscles of the forearm.
         b) Practice just picking up the pen and putting it down and moving it between your fingers while keeping the biofeedback quiet.
         c) Practice writing circles and moving across the page with movements from the shoulder and the elbow, not the wrist or digits.

F. Driving

1. Use a lumbar roll or a wedge in the seat of your car.
2. Pull the seat close to the steering wheel so you do not have to stretch out your foot to reach the pedal.
3. Sit tall.
4. Keep your arms comfortably at your side. You can put a pillow in your lap to support your arm.
5. Mentally rehearse and review calm alert driving.
6. Do not squeeze the wheel in a "death grip." Hold the steering wheel by gently pushing your arms together. You only need to hold the wheel with a palmar squeeze when turning. You may want to put an ergonomic cover on the steering wheel.
7. When you need to turn your head from one side to the other, use the trunk to turn. Shift your weight to the right hip when you want to turn to the left. Shift your weight to the left hip when you want to turn to the right.
8. Do not grip the shift bar with excessive force; simply press the palm of your hand down on the shift bar to shift. Move your trunk to follow your arm if necessary.

G. Using a Key

1. Avoid holding the key with a lateral pinch grip (key grip squeezing the key against the index finger with the thumb).
2. Use a three point precision grip with your thumb and the second and third digits to gently hold the key.

- Maintain general flexibility of muscles, fascia, and tendons.
- Initiate self-massage and soft tissue mobilization (for reduced mobility of muscles and fascia).
- Modify work ergonomics and appropriately modify the design.
- Determine if modifications can be made for the instrument interface.
- Carefully evaluate the benefit of an orthosis (a device to position the fingers and wrist, a freestanding pen, tape, pairing fingers together) to keep the hand in a functional position while controlling abnormal movements.
- Put rough surfaces on objects manipulated with the hand to decrease stress (e.g., pen, pencil, keys, keyboard).
- Remove any splints or orthoses if dystonic movements are exaggerated.
- Begin a sensorimotor retraining program to restore fine motor control that includes normalizing the representation of the hand (Appendices 5A and 5B).
- Integrate safe, stress-free strategies for hand on the target interfaces

Patients must learn to let the surface of an object provide the sensory stimulus to open the hand and grade the force needed. Patients must learn to avoid heavy gripping by using a precision grip. They must also learn to move from proximal (e.g., trunk, shoulder, elbow) rather than distal joints (e.g., fingers). Some activities that should be practiced include: lifting a glass, using a utensil, brushing teeth, cooking, cleaning house, lifting objects of the same size and weight with different surfaces, washing dishes, writing, using a keyboard, manipulating small objects, playing a musical instrument (the target instrument or another instrument), turning a key, opening doors, and driving a car.

Desensitization

In France, Tubiana and Chamagne[152] developed a four-stage treatment program for musicians. This program is based on desensitization or deprogramming of the acquired bad habits. During this program, there is an attempt to "restructure the body-image," selectively improve muscle differentiation and relaxation, individually retrain the muscles, and then provide technical retraining at the instrument. Usually, postural and shoulder imbalances are identified along with the specific hand dystonia. Patients also participate in counseling if needed. Tubiana and Chamagne[152] regard rehabilitation as a long-term, cooperative, supportive relationship if success is to be achieved and estimate that it takes 1 year for appropriate treatment. These investigators have seen a large population of subjects. Of 438 patients, 95 returned to concert performance, 57 did not improve, and there was partial improvement in the remainder of patients.

Negative Reinforcement

Leversedge and Sylvester[153] developed a negative reinforcement protocol for the treatment of typists with writer's cramp. They focused on breaking down the primary manifestations of the motor dysfunction to identify the sensorimotor aspects that require treatment. The patients hold a metal stylus and insert it into holes of increasingly smaller size, trace a flat zigzag on a metal plate, or write with a pen that reacts to excessive pressure from the thumb. When a mistake is made, an electric shock is delivered to the palm. An apparatus was rigged for typists so that a shock was delivered when the fingers curled into their palms. In one study, six patients were treated and experienced substantial improvement that was maintained for varying periods (i.e., weeks to months of follow-up). A similar approach was described by Tecce et al.[154]

Use of Orthoses

Writer's cramp generally affects the dominant hand[155] and may interfere with the ability to perform one's job as well personal activities of daily living. Sometimes the writer's cramp extends to other tasks such as keyboarding. Inevitably, the dystonia leads to excessive and uncontrollable gripping of the pen, often with flexion and ulnar deviation of the wrist leading to excessive pressure on the pen and the paper. Writing is not continuous but often broken by hesitations, picking up the pen and restarting, and slowness in writing. In a series of five patients, Tas et al.[155] reported on the effect of a thermoplastic hand orthosis for patients with writer's cramp. All of the patients had normal neurological examinations. All were teachers who had to do a lot of writing. The orthosis was individually constructed for each patient, but generally provided a mechanism to hold the pen, keep the fingers in flexion and control the wrist in extension. After the patients learned to write with the orthoses, all were able to write without discomfort. Their writing was legible while the orthosis was worn and they could write without interruption for approximately an hour. Without the device, the patients could only write for a few minutes.

Similar results were reported by Ranawaya and Lang[146] using a Blackburn writing system that included a tripod design. This was a mobile device with two legs mounted in ball bearings and the pen serving as the third leg. The pen was inserted into the holder. The patient placed the device under the palm and glided it over the paper using proximal muscles. After 4 weeks, 15 patients showed improvement in their writing ability. However, only 30% obtained useful benefits. The device was awkward and they preferred using alternate methods. In a case of arthritis, Koller and Vetere-Overfield[157] had patients use a pen that was inserted through a small cubic block making grasping easier. Now there are some writing devices that allow the pen to be independently positioned and free-standing on the paper. Different mechanisms are included for the patient to access the pen.

While writing orthoses may be helpful in assisting patients to continue to be functional despite hand cramps, they do not remediate hand dystonia. Orthoses should be used on an as-needed basis to facilitate functional activities while preventing abnormal dystonic movements. A retraining program designed to restore normal hand function is still necessary. Sometimes orthoses allow patients to continue to function and delay the beginning of needed rehabilitation.

Music Lessons

There are music teachers who specialize in working with musicians with a variety of musculoskeletal, peripheral nerve, postural, and neural injuries including focal hand dystonia.[135] Teachers have learned stress-free techniques because they may have suffered an injury themselves or they have incorporated basic biomechanics and clinical kinesiology into playing techniques. Music teachers are interested in teaching individuals to perform with efficiency and effectiveness and want to help their students prevent injuries. They may also teach students about the upper anatomy and kinesiology of the limb.

Although there are many technical differences involved in playing different instruments, there are some guidelines to follow to create a safe foundation for performance. The musician should:

- Use good postural alignment.
- Maintain a neutral position of the wrist and fingers (along the third metacarpal) with all fingers resting down (adjacent fingers are not held off the instrument).
- Let the weight of the hand drop onto the surface;
- Do not let any joint collapse when contacting the instrument; maintain the functional position of the hand (round, lined up with the center of the hand along the middle digit).
- Avoid adducting the thumb across the palm of the hand.
- Contact the surface with the pads of the digits and not the tips.
- Avoid unnecessary rapid alternating digital movements using the long finger flexors and extensors.
- Move from proximal joint at the shoulder and elbow rather than the digits.
- use forearm pronation and supination instead of finger extension to lift the fingers.
- Release the pressure down rather than forcefully lifting the digit up off the surface.
- When you need to use individual fingers for a passage, initiate the pressure down from the metacarpal phalangeal joint using the intrinsic muscles of the hand (the intrinsic muscles serve individual digits while the extrinsic flexors and extensors serve multiple digits, forcing cocontractions of flexors and extensors)
- Imagine playing the instrument normally without the dystonia.
- When playing is resumed, use mental practice rather than physical practice to learn the music and improve techniques.

Some teachers recommend that patients with focal hand dystonia temporarily stop playing. When the patient can begin to play the instrument without triggering the abnormal movements, the patient is encouraged to play for a limited time frame (initially only 5-minute intervals), performing simple activities such as dropping the hand onto the keyboard without collapsing at any location or feeling any abnormal muscle contractions. When the musician begins to play again, the teacher may recommend starting with new repertoire. As a general rule, all musicians and those using the computer should take a break every 30 minutes and stay well-hydrated, warm, and rested when playing frequently.

Limb Immobilization

In 2001, Priori et al.[158] reported on the use of limb immobilization as a conservative management strategy for patients with focal hand dystonia. This intervention strategy was based on the assumption that occupational dystonia of the upper limb was related to an enlargement and overlap of cortical areas representing the dystonic digits[81,90,105,159,160] and prolonged limb immobilization was associated with a shrinkage of the motor cortical representation in nondystonic subjects.[161,162] This study recruited one woman and seven men with primary musician's cramp involving the fingers and wrist. All had to interrupt their professional activity because of the dystonia; none were taking medication for dystonia. All had failed to improve with conventional treatment.

Each patient was placed in a cast with a plastic splint immobilizing the fingers and joints on the dystonia side. Patients wore the splint for 5 weeks, 24 hours per day with removal once a week for less than 10 minutes for local hygiene. Two of the patients were immobilized for 4 weeks and 3 for 5 weeks. After removal of the splint the patients gradually resumed daily activities including the target, progressing from 20 minutes per day for the first week, to 30 minutes three times per day for 3 weeks, and then 1 hour three times a day for the next month. Musicians were also asked to practice basic technical exercise for beginning musicians. After the third month post-splint removal the musicians could play as long as they wanted as long as they did not trigger dystonic movements.

All patients were videotaped and assessed at 1, 4, 12, and 24 weeks after cast removal. Two neurologists rated the patients clinically according to the Arm Dystonia Disability Scale (ADDS). Musicians were assessed with the Tubiana and Chamagne Scale (TCS). Patients were also asked to assess the effectiveness of the intervention (percent of improvement compared to their status before casting).

The day the cast was removed and for approximately 1 week, patients complained of clumsiness and weakness with difficulty controlling the hand with minor local subcutaneous and joint edema. Some had pain in the immobilized joint but none had contractures. After a week, their motor performance slightly improved and 4 weeks later, all patients had regained normal voluntary control of the hand with normal strength and reduced dystonic movements. Improvement in the ADDS and TCS scores were measured. These improvements persisted and remained significant even after

12 to 24 weeks. At 24 weeks, the improvement on the ADDS varied from 20 to 100% from baseline. Moderate improvement (20 to 33%) was measured in three of the seven patients and marked improvement (>70%) was measured in four of the patients. All patients attended follow-up assessments. Over this time, motor improvements remained consistent. Three patients played a public concert. The greatest improvement was measured in the most severely involved ($r = -0.746$ correlation). No patients were worse but one patient only retained the benefit for 6 months.

These results are exciting. Unfortunately, the number of subjects was very small and the subjects only were reported to have dystonia an average of 3.62 years (ranging from 1 to 8 years). Patients may possibly recover even more completely if a retraining program based on the principles of neuroplasticity is incorporated postimmobilization. One question is whether the results will be equally effective for patients who have suffered focal dystonia for more extended periods of time. Second, if the etiology of the dystonia is the result of aberrant learning that not only leads to an increased representation of the hand, but a disorganized representation (e.g., overlapping representations of the digits), then how would immobilization alone shrink as well as normalize the organization of the digits? Third, it is not clear there is agreement on whether the size of the representation is larger or smaller than normal in patients with focal dystonia. The authors referenced the work of Byl et al.[122] and Topp et al.[109] to substantiate the enlargement of the cortical representation. These researchers reported disorganization as well as a decreased area of representation in nonhuman primate studies. In human studies (primarily musicians), the area of representation of the dystonic hand was reduced compared to the nondystonic representation.[116] Bara-Jiminez et al.[83] also reported a reduction in the size of the somatosensory representation of the hand for the dystonic hand compared to the nondystonic hand and compared to controls. Last, some patients may not be able to tolerate the casting. The cast may stimulate involuntary movement and the movement disorder could move more proximal (e.g., shoulder and neck). Some patients may find the hand stiff, swollen, or painful well after the cast is removed.

Constraint-Induced Paradigm

Constraint-induced paradigms (CI) were initially promoted in stroke rehabilitation programs.[163] CI therapy has also been applied to patients with focal hand dystonia. Based on the principles of neuroplasticity, the idea is that when the unaffected side is constrained, the patient is forced to use the affected side. In this forced-use situation, patients must engage the involved hand in meaningful ways. As was originally reported in the 1980s,[164] effectiveness was reported in case studies and small pilot studies.[163,165,166]

In a paradigm designed by Candia et al.,[166,167] patients with focal dystonia followed the principles of constraint-induced movement therapy (now referred to as sensory motor retuning). The basic principles of the therapy are to:

1. Determine the most dystonic digit.
2. Avoid constraining the most dystonic finger.
3. Identify the fingers that constrain the independent use of the dystonic finger.
4. Constrain the fingers in a position that is similar to the normal resting angle used in performing the target task.
5. Carry out selected exercises of the dystonic finger.
6. Progressively increase the speed at which the dystonic finger is required to move in concert with the other fingers of the hand and then progressively decrease expecting more exacting requirements (shaping).
7. Generalize the daily practice needed to sustain patient motivation to the target task.
8. Practice intensively (i.e., massed practice) but not to the point it creates excessive fatigue or increases the dystonic movement postures.
9. Outline a home practice program.

In the Candia paradigm,[166,167] the movement of the affected extremity was restricted for 2 weeks with a splint designed to control abnormal movement of adjacent digits. While the unaffected limb was restricted, the most affected extremity received intensive training for 6 hours per day for the 10 weekdays. The treatment involved identifying one finger as being the main dystonic digit and one or two other digits as being involved in performing the target-specific task. A splint was then created to free the digit exhibiting the main dystonic symptoms. The splint had the flexibility of releasing other digits to participate with the dystonic finger as well. One or several other digits were immobilized and extensive practice was directed toward performing individual movements of the dystonic finger that coordinated with movements of the other fingers. When a given finger was confirmed as the most dystonic, other digits were immobilized and the subject was required to carry out sequences of movements with the finger. The immobilization of adjacent fingers was simply a means of enabling independent movement of the most involved digit.

During fixation, the finger is positioned appropriately to accomplish the target task. Then, the involved finger should begin to carry out alternating, individual finger movements with all possible permutations of the other fingers of the dystonic hand. This should include sequential movements of one finger, and then alternating movements of adjacent two or three digits including the most dystonic digit. The patient does this for 10 minutes in an ascending and then descending order with continuous repetitions. Then, a 2-minute rest is instituted after the sequence of movements of two or three fingers. Five such blocks were carried out in an hour.

Performance was paced by a metronome, starting at a medium tempo (60 bpm), and then increased and decreased in rate. The speed sequencing was then reinitiated with the goal of having the subject generate faster and faster, then slower and slower, alternating movements in successive sequences (shaping). This was fatiguing. After completion of the first five blocks, the splint was removed and subjects were given a 10-minute rest period. Then patients received four more 10-minute blocks of exercises with 2 minutes of rest between blocks. Various permutations of possible finger movement were used.

After specific motor training, the subjects were encouraged to play their instruments without the splint. They played approximately 10 bars from a self-selected musical piece (15 to 30 seconds). If they could not do this, they were encouraged to try again. After two successful repetitions, they were asked to play a different 10-bar segment and then asked to play portions of musical pieces for longer and longer durations, until they had played for a period of 15 minutes (excluding rest intervals). Subjects were fearful of having the dystonic movement return; however, they were encouraged to continue. The complexity and duration of the practice within the unsplinted performance period were based on the therapist's judgment. Success encouraged more success and continued performance. After a rest of 5 minutes, if the subject was not too fatigued, the splint was replaced and a second series of alternating digital maneuvers was carried out for half the time taken by the first series. This regimen was continued for 8 consecutive days.

On the last treatment day, the subjects were given the splint that was constructed for them and asked to practice for 1 hour each day over a period of 1-year post-therapy. They were also instructed to do the unsplinted repertoire for 10% of the time that was their usual custom. This period was increased by 10% in each succeeding month, assuming there was not deterioration in the level of motor control.

Some subjects have been followed for up to 24 months. This rehabilitation routine has improved the function of the affected limb in a series of 80 patients. However, a controlled trial of treatment is only reported on 5 subjects. The researchers used a dexterity-displacement device, which continuously recorded digital displacement during metronome-paced movements of two fingers, and a spectral analysis of the record reporting on smoothness of the movements. A Dystonic Evaluation Scale (DES) was used, in which the patients rated how well they were performing movement sequences and passages from their repertoire without the splint. The DES was administered at the beginning of each treatment day. A one-way analysis of variance revealed that the scores at pretreatment, posttreatment, and 1-month follow-up were significantly different from one another. Post hoc testing indicated that the pretreatment scores were significantly different from posttreatment scores at 1-month follow-up. One patient did not do the home program and relapsed. The others did the home program and remained stable for up to 14 months.

Comprehensive Sensorimotor and Selective Sensory Motor Training Based on the Principles of Neuroplasticity

With the increase in evidence regarding somatosensory degradation in patients with focal hand dystonia, the challenge is to determine the best way to remediate the underlying sensory dedifferentiation and to document whether improvement in somatosensory processing improves motor control. If the somatosensory cortex is adaptable and highly attended, repetitive, stereotypic behaviors can degrade the representation of the hand, then specific attended, repetitive but variable activities should be able to restore normal sensory representation of the hand, rebalance the sensorimotor feedback loop, and facilitate the recovery of normal fine motor control (see Appendices 5A and 5B for details).

The comprehensive sensorimotor learning program is fundamentally based on the principles of neuroplasticity and the activities must be consistent with the assumptions about strengthening the central and peripheral pathways connecting the hand to the brain and integrating the sensory and motor systems. In addition, the intervention program must follow the principles of neuroplasticity. Finally, the intervention must be sequenced in a logical fashion that challenges patients to perform tasks, perhaps incompletely, but normally without any abnormal movements. Ultimately, the level of task complexity progresses until the whole target task can be completed in a normal fashion. This may require beginning with good postural alignment, diaphragmatic breathing, and large, rhythmical proximal movements from the shoulder. Neural adaptation should proceed in a progressive manner but gains may not be linear.

The philosophy of retraining must be clearly explained to the patient. Initially, patients may hear that the problem is "all in their head." The hand-brain connections and the principles of neuroplasticity must be carefully outlined to obtain maximum patient compliance. When patients admit there are noteworthy psychosocial or work-related stresses that persist in their lives that could get in the way of recovery, then they should be encouraged to pursue counseling.

The challenge is to develop a progressive program of attended, successful, repetitive, but nonstereotypical sensory and motor behaviors that can be performed normally. If the demands of the task exceed what the nervous system can do normally, then the patient is at risk for negative rather than positive learning (e.g., if a patient simply puts the palm of the hand on a surface and the fingers and wrist curl, then it may be necessary to work with the hand midway between pronation and supination).

Before initiating therapy, objective measurements of physical, sensory, and motor performances should be documented. These skills should be reassessed at baseline, during treatment, and at the end of treatment. The primary goals of a rehabilitation program based on the principles of neuroplasticity are to:

1. Create a healthy foundation for learning.
2. Empower the patient to re-educate the nervous system.
3. Use the principles of neuroplasticity to maximize learning (attended, repetitive, normal, progressive, rewarded movements).
4. Restore the normal somatotopic representation of the hand (thalamus, basal ganglia, somatosensory cortex, motor cortex, sensorimotor cortex).

5. Use visual, mental, and mirror imagery to learn to perform the affected tasks correctly.
6. Restore reflex inhibition (e.g., stop the co-contractions of extensors and flexors).
7. Restore normal, graded, coordinated movements of the hand.
8. Restore normal patterns of voluntary fine motor movement (e.g., only perform the parts of the task that can be done correctly, progressing the complexity of movements as able).
9. Restore fine motor control at the target and other similar tasks.

When the patient cannot perform any aspect of the target task without triggering the dystonia and/or if thinking about performing the task triggers abnormal movement, then using mental imagery to try and imagine doing the task normally may be one of the first steps toward recovery. Mental imagery may also be used to help restore self-esteem and self-confidence. When patients lose control of independence in a familiar task, patients may experience a serious loss of well-being. Mental imagery can focus on positive thinking, successful recovery, and resumption of normal activities. Mental imagery should also include performing the target task. Imagery may recruit up to 30% of the neurons that would normally be recruited if the task was actually being performed.[168] When the focus is on imaging a sequence of tasks, the neuronal activity will be enhanced more specifically in the supplementary motor cortex more than in other areas.

Before beginning aggressive motor retraining, the patient should improve accuracy of sensory discrimination and control of graded hand movements. All of the activities performed with the affected hand should be focused on the sensory aspects of the task, not the motor aspects of the task (e.g., while driving, feel everything about the steering wheel or when finding change, try to feel the desired coin). If the affected hand is sensitive (e.g., tactile inputs set off abnormal motor responses), then sensory training may actually begin on the unaffected side. Identify the most dystonic finger and begin sensory retraining on the adjacent and then the target digit. The sensory retraining should progress from the pads of the digits, to the lateral and medial surfaces between adjacent digits. During sensory activities, the patient should be blindfolded or asked to keep their eyes closed. The sensorimotor retraining program should: comprise all common sensory modalities, such as light touch, deep touch, vibration, temperature, muscle stretch, surface orientation, and static and dynamic joint position sense; enhance the accuracy of the sensorimotor feedback loop; incorporate active and passive stimulation, with and without movement; deliver stimuli in both the temporal and spatial domains; be carefully progressed; integrate a mechanism to provide reward for accuracy; comprise single stimuli and progress to discriminating two stimuli that are either spatially or temporally distinct; and be innovative and creative.

Based on the physiological sensory findings, the retraining will improve cortical segregation and redifferentiation if:

- Heavily attended sensory signals are presented to a limited skin surface; this serves as signal that leads to redifferentiation of the hand representation in the primary sensory cortex (e.g., tasks that depend on slowly adaptive afferents include roughness estimation,[169] reading braille or embossed letters or performing grating-orientation discrimination and tasks involving primarily rapidly adaptive afferents include flutter discrimination and recognition of small surface asperities[168–171]
- Two mechanoreceptor systems are engaged that have small receptive fields and low mechanical thresholds;
- Psychophysical tasks are presented in a context that is heavily attended, driving coincident delivery neuromodulators with a neural signal about which the cortex can reorganize;
- Stimuli are presented to a limited skin surface within each training session so that the other processes (i.e., the processes leading to segregation) have cues only from a limited portion of the skin surface at any given time;
- Sensory tasks are practiced heavily before reengaging the patient in tasks involving controlled, fine motor skills;
- Sensory stimuli are applied concurrent with the motor tasks that led to the dystonia;
- All training behaviors are goal directed, highly attended, interesting or engaging and progressive but not stereotypical;
- Timely feedback is provided regarding performance;
- Sensory experiences are included within practical, functional activities;
- Training is provided to the affected and unaffected sides; and
- Sensory stimuli are of adequate intensity that can be received and processed but do not reach the intensity that they trigger abnormal movements (e.g., in some cases the sensory stimulus leads to an exaggerated motor response and in other cases the stimulus is not adequate to be accurately discriminated).

The sensory training should be done in a variety of positions to access all possible sensory maps. Reading braille involves sensory discrimination. Learning to read a novel in braille would be ideal for learning. Playing the card game solitaire with braille cards can be helpful. Ideally, only one finger should be used to explore a sensory stimulus. If, there is increased muscle firing while using the most involved dystonic finger, it may be necessary to start learning to read braille with the unaffected side or with a less involved finger. Patients can also practice trying to recognize raised letters such as embossed lettering, alphabet soup letters pasted on cardboard, stickers or buttons pasted on the wall, or matching magnetic letters. The letters should initially be large (e.g., start with letters 8-mm high, and decrease to 4 mm or less. Each session should focus on two specific digits and then rotate the target digits. Patients can also be encouraged to play games such as dominoes or Scrabble with the eyes closed. In a study of 10 patients with focal hand dystonia, Zeuner et al.[170] showed that reading braille for 30 to 60 minutes daily for 8 weeks improved spatial acuity and dystonia.

Once sensory processing is improved and it is possible to perform sensory activities without increased abnormal motor response, selective fine motor training should begin.[172] The sensory training ultimately needs to progress to the target instrument, and be implemented in the target position during performance of the target task. First, identify a position in which the target task may be performed in a normal manner. If this position can be found, then patients may begin to practice the target task in that position. If the position cannot be found, then identify that particular component of the task can be performed in a normal fashion. Initially, the patient may be asked to palpate the target instrument and not perform any aspect of the target task. The palpation of the target instrument should be performed out of the playing position and progressed to the playing position.

It is then essential to be able to balance or grade movements. This includes being able to lightly maintain contact with a surface without unnecessary downward pressure. This can be accomplished by placing the hand on the moving belt of a treadmill. This should be done with the hand in different orientations to the belt and then trying to manipulate objects on the belt. It can also be accomplished by holding the digits (together or one at a time) on a moving record without changing the quality of the sound.

Normal movement, albeit a limited version of the full task, can be reinforced with visual imagery (i.e., practicing in the patient's mind, watching oneself perform the task) and motor imagery (i.e., mentally going through each component of the motor task).[58,168,173–176] The target task and other similar target tasks may be rehearsed accurately and smoothly at different speeds with different degrees of complexity (e.g., playing a single note on a keyboard versus a chord, versus running a melody within a chord).

When subjects cannot perform the target task without triggering the abnormal movement, the patients should then attempt to perform the task with the unaffected side, the foot, or while using both hands together. The maps of well-learned, nearly automatic rhythmic tasks (e.g., walking, writing, etc.) and well-learned complex voluntary tasks (e.g., playing a musical instrument, typing, etc.) must be remapped on the cortex, both by function as well as geographic location.[58] When the contralateral limb can be trained to perform the target task normally or bimanual tasks can be performed in midtrunk position, stress may be reduced and performance of the task on the affected side may be enhanced. Ultimately, the goal is to restore normal movement on the affected side. Then, all activities must focus on normalizing the involved digits.

All the selective, fine motor movements should involve specific well-controlled, smooth contractions practiced at variable speeds. A metronome may be used to guide increases in the speed of the movements. Guiding movement retraining may be assisted by placing digits on a surface. In this way, patients are able to remain quiet and may concentrate on the specific, selective movements of each individual, involved digit. A variety of activities can be included in fine motor training. Some of these activities include:

- Practicing large rhythmic movements with the affected limb.
- Practicing going to a target and holding at the target without abnormal movements.
- Working on graded movements (e.g., place the hand on a treadmill or a record player).
- Manipulating objects (e.g., retrieve objects of varying size from cups, progressing from large to small, manipulate small pegs in and out of different holes[177]).
- Performing activities that require the thumb paired with the involved digits.
- Achieving accuracy and then increasing speed.
- Initially focusing on moving from proximal muscles (e.g., the shoulder).
- Taking advantage of the natural weight of the arm.
- Teaching patients how to use the intrinsic muscles of the hand for functional activities.
- Learning to hold objects lightly (e.g., can take the pen out of a subject's hand without resistance).
- Avoiding power gripping.
- Practicing performing activities similar to the target task.
- Ultimately moving to perform activities with the target instrument.
- Learning to perform the target task without the dystonia.

Biofeedback may be helpful to facilitate motor learning. Biofeedback may also be used to determine the muscle firing patterns that drive the abnormal movement at the target task. The therapist needs to determine whether the primary movers drive the firing of the antagonist muscles or if the antagonists drive the firing of the agonist (e.g., if the flexors drive the contraction of the extensors or vice versa). It is surprising that in some cases, the antagonist may fire first, even though the finger is curling. Biofeedback can be as simple as taping the digit (e.g., providing increased sensory input to increase awareness) or may be an auditory or visual signal driven by the sensitivity of the electrode to pick up active muscle firing. Biofeedback may provide information regarding muscle activity while at rest as well as during functional activities.

A two-channel unit is recommended. The patient should be taught to place one electrode on the flexor surface of the forearm and the second on the extensor surface. In addition, patients need to be shown how to use tape as a biofeedback mechanism. For example, if the finger is curling excessively, tape on the extensor surface will be stretched, giving the subject information about excessive flexion. Ideally, if using electrodes as sensors of muscle contraction, patients should take the biofeedback unit home to heighten their awareness of using the hands in a stress-free manner for all functional activities. Electrical stimulation to the wrist extensor, can be paired with biofeedback over flexor tendons at wrist to assess co-contraction of flexors and extensors. Biofeedback can be used to teach patients to:

- Inhibit co-contractions of agonists and antagonists, particularly the extrinsic finger extensors and flexors;
- Use the intrinsic muscles of the hand to initiate flexion at the MP joint without recruiting the finger flexors;
- Abduct the fingers and extend the interphalangeal joints using the intrinsic muscles, while keeping the extensor communis quiet;
- Release digit-downward pressure without lifting and extending the finger with the extensor digitorum;
- Alternate and sequence adjacent digits by using the interossei and the lumbricals (on as well as off their instrument); and
- Complete personal care and household activities, writing, keyboarding, and the target-specific task using the intrinsic muscles inside the hand and minimizing the use of the extrinsic muscles.

Audio and audiovisual training tapes may be made for the subjects to use in helping them to develop the skills of imagery. The subject should be encouraged to image without the assistance of the tapes as soon as possible because self-imagery provides the most viable image. The tapes should focus on tension-free movement of the involved limb; healing and relaxation; balancing the posture with gravity; decreasing muscle tension; relieving stress from all hand functions related to work, activities of daily living and recreation; normalizing sensory processing, such as the ability to discriminate all textures, letters, figures; eliminating abnormal movements; freely moving the upper limb using proximal shoulder and elbow joints; and normalizing the target task (e.g., such as writing, computer work, or instrumental play).

Mirrors may also be used to reinforce learning to change the strategy for writing, keyboard techniques, and instrumental play. Ramachandran et al.[178] and Yang and colleagues[179] studied somatosensory reorganization in patients with amputations. Mirrors were used as a type of virtual reality to restore the somatosensory function of the amputated limb in patients with phantom limb pain. In the mirror-box study, patients reported having sensations of movement in the phantom limb when the normal limb was moved. Patients with painful spasms in the phantom limb experienced relief when the mirror was used to facilitate movement in the phantom limb.[178]

When mirrors are used, the affected hand is placed out of view (e.g., behind the mirror). The subject concentrates on the mirror image (e.g., the right hand looks like the left hand in the mirror). The subject attempts to replicate the mirror image. The mirrors are made out of picture frames that can be placed on a table surface, a keyboard, or the target instrument. Activities that relate to the development of controlled movements should be performed in the mirror. If a patient is having trouble with both hands, then it is possible to have another person place their hand in front of the mirror to try and simulate the normal mirror image.

Training activities must be structured, even though the site of training may vary. Ideally, concentrate attention on a particular task for 5 to 15 minutes, with modifications of the task as skill improves; and repeating similar sessions on different tasks repeated throughout the day to accumulate at least 1.5 to 2.0 hours of total daily training. In other words, rigorous attention and accurate feedback over time is necessary to assure appropriate decision making and learning. However, it is possible to train in different environments. For example, people should be encouraged to carry games, objects, coins, puzzles, and shapes in their pockets to challenge sensory exploration and discrimination. For each task, there must be a purpose for manipulating the objects, either to use functionally, to match objects, to assemble objects (i.e., puzzles) or play somatosensory games with the eyes closed. In general, when performing sensory discrimination tasks, patients must not be using vision or cognition to guide decision-making (see Appendices 5A and 5B).

This somatosensory rehabilitation training strategy has been evaluated through preliminary studies involving case studies, single case designs repeated over several subjects, and repeated measures follow-up studies. These pilot studies provide initial evidence that somatosensory reeducation can be effective in restoring fine motor control in patients with focal hand dystonia.[135,149,180–182] The major constraints to the implementation of this clinical paradigm based on the sensorimotor learning hypothesis are related to patient compliance, poor mentoring, and lack of objective data from randomized clinical trials. Sometimes patients cannot stop the abnormal movement because they need to perform their job. Others have difficulty "taking a break" from the target task especially when the target task is part of their work. Still others are challenged to use their hand in a stress-free way and many are challenged to make a commitment to carry out goal-directed, specific, progressive, repetitive rewarded activities at the intensity needed to drive changes in neural structure. Further, when treatment must be provided within the constraints of reimbursement guidelines and the time frame defined as appropriate by the healthcare system, patients may be denied access to the frequency and duration of therapy that is needed.

SUMMARY

Research is still needed to improve our understanding about the etiology of different types of focal dystonia. However, at the same time, randomized clinical trials across multiple sites are needed to confirm the effectiveness of different nonpharmacologic intervention strategies. These trials must not only focus on the nonpharmacologic approaches to treatment, but combine pharmaceutical and nonpharmacologic treatments (e.g., compare pharmaceutical management with desensitization, constraint, orthoses, limb immobilization, sensitization, or learning-based sensorimotor training). In addition, traditional and experimental treatment interventions should be studied when paired with and without psychological counseling. Clinical research studies need to pair different clinical disciplines as well as facilitate partnerships with clinicians and basic scientists. Based on the principles of neural plasticity and aberrant learning, the potential to restore function, in the case of isolated focal hand dystonia originating after a defined situation of stressful, overuse, is possible in a directed, committed patient who can decompress the job requirements, reduce physical and emotional stress, and integrate strategies based on neural adaptation and learning to restore normal motor control. We need to continue to gather evidence to understand the complete pathophysiology of the disorder of focal dystonia fully, particularly of the hand.

ACKNOWLEDGMENTS

Research was funded by several different sources including: REAC Funds, School of Medicine, UCSF; Academic Senate Research Grant, UCSF; and National Institutes of Health grant PO1 NS 34835.

REFERENCES

1. Merzenich MM, Jenkins WM. Cortical representation of learned behaviors. In: Andersen P, Hvalby O, Paulsen O, Hockfelt B, eds. Memory Concepts. Amsterdam, The Netherlands: Elsevier; 1993:467.
2. Merzenich MM, Jenkins WM. Cortical plasticity, learning and learning dysfunction. In: Jules B, Kovacs I, eds. Maturational Windows and Adult Cortical Plasticity. New York, NY: Addison-Wesley, 1995:247–272.
3. Merzenich MM, Wright B, Jenkins WM, et al. Cortical plasticity underlying perceptual, motor and cognitive skill development: implications for neurorehabilitation. Cold Springs Harb Symp Quant Biol 1996;61:1–8.
4. Merzenich MM, DeCharms, RC. Neural representations, experience and change. In: Llinas R, Churchland P, eds. The Mind-Brain Continuum. Boston, MA: MIT Press, 1996:61–81.
5. Nagarajan SS, Blake D, Wright BA, et al. Practice-related improvements in somatosensory, integral discrimination are temporally specific but generalize across skin location, hemisphere and modality. J Neurosci 1999;18:1559–1663.
6. Nudo R, Wise B, Fuentes F, et al. Neural substrates for the effects of rehabilitation training on motor recovery after ischemic infarct. Science 1996;272:1791–1795.
7. Nudo RJ, Millikin GW. Reorganization of movement representations in primary motor cortex following focal ischemic infarcts in adult squirrel monkeys. J Neurosci 1996;75:2140–2149.
8. Spengler F, Roberts TPL, Poeppel D, et al. Learning transfer and neuronal plasticity in humans trained in tactile discrimination. Neurosci Lett 1997;232:151–154.
9. Merzenich MM, Kaas JH, Wall J, et al. Topographic reorganization of somatosensory cortical areas 3b and 1 in adult monkeys following restricted deafferentiation. Neuroscience 1983;8:33–55.
10. Merzenich MM, Kaas JH, Wall J, et al. Progression of change following median nerve section in the cortical representation of the hand in areas 3b and 2 in adult owl and squirrel monkeys. Neuroscience 1983;10:639–665.
11. Merzenich MM, Nelson R, Stryker M, et al. Somatosensory cortical map changes following digit amputation in adult monkeys. J Comp Neurol 1984;224:591–605.
12. Merzenich MM. Development and maintenance of cortical somatosensory representations: functional 'maps" and neuroanatomic repertoires. In: Barnard KE, Brazelton TB, eds. Touch: The Foundation of Experience. Madison, WI: International University Press, 1991:47–71.
13. Merzenich MM, Allard T, Jenkins WM. Neural ontogeny of higher brain function: implications of some recent neurophysiological findings. In: Franzen O, Westman P, eds. Information Processing in the Somatosensory System. London, England: McMilland Press, 2001:193–211.
14. Allard T, Clark SA, Jenkins WM, et al. Reorganization of somatosensory area 3b representations in adult owl monkeys after digit syndactyly. J Neurophysiol 1991;66:1048–1058.
15. Jenkins W, Merzenich M. Reorganization of neocortical representations after brain injury: a neurophysiological model of the bases of recovery from stroke. Prog Brain Res 1987;71:249–266.
16. Jenkins W, Allard T, Nudo R. Cortical representational plasticity. In: Raskic P, Singer W, eds. Neurobiology of the Neocortex. New York, NY: John Wiley and Sons, 1988:41–67.
17. Jenkins W, Merzenich M, Ochs M, et al. Functional reorganization of primary somatosensory cortex in adult owl monkeys after behaviorally controlled tactile stimulation. J Neurophysiol 1990;63:82–104.
18. Jenkins WM, Merzenich MM, Ochs MT, et al. Functional reorganization of primary somatosensory cortex in adult owl monkeys after behaviorally controlled tactile stimulation. J Neurophysiol 1990;53:82–104.
19. Juliano SL, Ma W, Eslin D. Cholinergic depletion prevents expansion of topographic maps in somatosensory cortex. Proc Natl Acad Sci USA 1991;88:780–784.
20. Kaas JH, Merzenich MM, Killackey HP. The reorganization of somatosensory cortex following peripheral nerve damage in adult and developing mammals. Ann Rev Neurosci 1983;6:325–356.
21. Recanzone G, Jenkins W, Hradek G, et al. Progressive improvement in discriminative abilities in adult owl monkeys performing a tactile frequency discrimination task. J Neurophysiol. 1992;67:1015–1030.
22. Recanzone GH, Merzenich MM, Jenkins WM, et al. Topographic reorganization of the hand representation in cortical area 3b of owl monkeys trained in a frequency-discrimination task. J Neurophysiol 1992;67:1031–1056.
23. Recanzone GH, Merzenich MM, Jenkins WM. Frequency discrimination training engaging a restricted skin surface results in an emergence of a cutaneous response zone in cortical area 3a. J Neurophysiol 1992;67:1057–1070.
24. Recanzone GH, Merzenich MM, Jenkins WM. Frequency discrimination training engaging a restricted skin surface results in an emergence of a cutaneous response zone in cortical area 3a. J Neurophysiol 1992;67:1047–1056.
25. Wang X, Merzenich MM, Sameshima K, et al. Afferent input integration and segregation in learning are input timing dependent. Neurosci Abstr. 1994;20:1427 Society for Neuroscience.
26. Wang X, Merzenich MM, Sameshima K, et al. Remodeling of hand representation in adult cortex determined by timing of tactile stimulation. Nature 1995;378:71–75.
27. Xerri, C, Coq JO, Merzenich MM, et al. Experience-induced plasticity of cutaneous maps in the primary somatosensory cortex of adult monkeys and rats. J Physiol Paris 1996;90:277–287.
28. Bassareo V, DiChiara G. Differential influence of associative and nonassociative learning: mechanisms on the responsiveness of prefrontal and accumbal dopamine transmission to food stimuli in rats fed ad libitum. J Neurosci 1997;17:851–861.
29. Penfield W, Rasmussen T. The Cerebral Cortex of Man: A Clinical Study of Localization of Function. New York, NY: MacMillan, 1950.
30. Ghez C, Vicario O. Discharge of the red nucleus neurons during voluntary muscle contraction activity patterns and correlation with isometric forces. J Physiol Paris 1978;74:283–285.
31. Kandel ER, Schwartz JH, Jessel TM. Principles of Neural Science, 4th ed. New York, NY: Elsevier Science, 1991.
32. Jiang W, Chapman CE, Lamarre Y. Modulation of cutaneous responsiveness of neurones in the primary somatosensory cortex during conditioned arm movements in the monkey. Exp Brain Res 1991;84:342–354.
33. Knecht S, Kunesch E, Buchner H, et al. Facilitation of somatosensory evoked potentials by exploratory finger movements. Exp Brain Res. 1993;95:330–338.
34. Grigg P. Mechanical factors influencing response of joint afferent neurons from cat knee. J Neurophysiol 1975;38:1473–1483.
35. Burgess PR, Perl ER. Cutaneous mechnoreceptors and nociceptors. In: Iggo A, ed. Handbook of Sensory Physiology: Volume 2. Somatosensory System. New York, NY: Springer, 1973:29–78.
36. Burgess PR, Wei JY, Clark FS, et al. Signaling of the kinesthesis information by peripheral sensory receptors. Annal Rev Neurosci 1988;5:171–187.
37. Costanzo RM, Gardner EP. A quantitative analysis of responses of direction-sensitive neurons in somatosensory cortex of awake monkeys. J Neurophysiol 1980;43:1319–1341.
38. Hyvarinen J, Poranen A. Function of the parietal associative area 7 as revealed from cellular discharges in alert monkeys. Brain 1974;97:673–692.

39. Hyvarinen J, Poranen A. Movement-sensitive and direction and orientation-selective cutaneous receptive fields in the hand area of the post-central gyrus in monkeys. J Neurophysiol 1978;283:523–537.

40. Hyvarinen J, Poranen A, Jokinen Y. Influence of attentive behavior on neuronal responses to vibration in primary somatosensory cortex of the monkey. J Neurophysiol 1980;43:870–883.

41. Iwamura Y. Dynamic and hierarchical processing in the monkey somatosensory cortex. Biomed Res 1983;14:107–111.

42. Iwamura Y, Tanaka M, Sakamoto M, et al. Functional subdivisions representing different finger regions in area 3 of the first somatosensory cortex of the conscious monkey. Exp Brain Res 1983;51:315–326.

43. Iwamura Y, Tanaka M, Sakamoto M, et al. Rostrocaudal gradients in the neuronal receptive field complexity in the finger region of the alert monkey's postcentral gyrus. Exp Brain Res 1993;92:360–368.

44. Warren S, Hamalainen HA, Gardner EP. Objective classification of motion-and direction-sensitive neurons in primary somatosensory cortex of awake monkeys. J Neurophysiol 1986;56:598–622.

45. Whitsel BL, Roppola JR, Werner G. Cortical information processing of stimulus motion on primate skin. J Neurophysiol 1972;35:691–717.

46. Hyvarinen J, Poranen A. Receptive field integration and submodality convergence in the hand area of the post-central gyrus of the alert monkey. J Neurophysiol 1978;283:539–556.

47. Livingstone E, Livingstone S. Upper limb. In: Kapanji IA, ed. The Physiology of the Joints, vol. 2. London, UK; Churchill Livingstone, 1970:170–174.

48. Evarts EV. Relation of pyramidal tract activity to force exerted during voluntary movements. J Neurophysiol 1968;31:14–27.

49. Jiang W, Lamarre Y, Chapman CE. Modulation of cutaneous cortical evoked potentials during isometric and isotonic contractions in the monkey. Brain Res 1990;536:69–78.

50. Jeannerod M. The timing of natural prehension movements. J Motor Behav 1984;26:235–254.

51. Jeannerod M. Object oriented action. In: Bennett KMB, Castillo U, eds. Insights into the Reach to Grasp Movement. Amsterdam, The Netherlands: Elsevier/North-Holland, 1994:3–15.

52. Johansson RS. How is grasping modified by somatosensory input? In: Humphrey DR, Freund JH, eds. Dablem Workshop on Motor Control: Concepts and Issues. Chichester, UK: Wiley, 1991:331–335.

53. Johansson RS. Sensory control of dexterous manipulation in humans. In: Wing AM, Haggard P, Flanagan JR, eds. Hand and Brain. The Neurophysiology and Psychology of Hand Movements. San Diego, CA: Academic Press, 1996:381–414.

54. Burke D, Hagbarth KE, Lofstedt L. Muscle spindle activity in man during shortening and lengthening contractions. J Physiol 1978;277:131–142.

55. Burke D, Gandevia SC, Macefield G. Responses to passive movement of receptors in joint, skin and muscle of the human hand. J Physiol 1988;402:347–361.

56. Wannnier TMJ, Maier MA, Hopp-Raymond MC. Contrasting properties of monkey somatosensory and motor cortex neurons activated during the control of force in precision grip. J Neurophysiol 1991;65:572–587.

57. Hebb DO. The Organization of Behaviors: A Neuropsychological Therapy. New York, NY: Wiley, 1949.

58. Rijntjes M, Dettmers C, Buchel C, et al. A blueprint for movement: functional and anatomical representations in the human motor system. J Neurosci 1999;19:8043–8048.

59. Altenmueller E. Causes and cures of focal limb dystonia in musicians. In: Scott R, Black J, eds. Health and the Musician: Proceedings of the 1997 York Conference. London, UK: BAPAM Publications, 1997:G.1–1–12.

60. Chen R, Hallett M. Focal dystonia and repetitive motion disorders. Clin Orthop 1998;351:102–106.

61. Cohen L, Hallett M. Hand cramps: clinical features and electromyographic patterns in focal dystonia. Neurology. 1988;38:1005–1012.

62. Crossman AR, Brotchie JM. Pathophysiology of dystonia. Adv Neurol 1998;78:19–26.

63. Critchley M. Occupational palsies in musical performers. In: Critchley M, Henson RA, eds. Music and the Brain. London, UK: Wm. Heinermann Medical Books, LTD., 1977;365–377.

64. Hays B. "Painless" hand problems of string pluckers. Med Prob Perf Art 1987;2:39–40.

65. Hochberg FH, Leffert RD, Heller MD, et al. Hand difficulties among musicians. JAMA 1983;249:1869–1872.

66. Hochberg F, Harris S, Blartert T. Occupational hand cramps: professional disorders of motor control. Hand Injury Sports Perform Arts. 1990;6:427–428.

67. McDaniel KD, Cummings JL, Shain S. The "ypi's": a focal dystonia of golfers. Neurology 1989;39:192–195.

68. Marsden CN, Sheehy MP. Writer's cramp (Review). Trends Neurosci 1990;13:148–153.

69. Marsden CD, Fahn S, eds. Movement Disorders 2. London, UK: Butterworths, 1987:332–353.

70. Panizza M, Hallett M, Nilsson J. Reciprocal inhibition in patients with hand cramps. Neurology 1989;39:85–89.

71. Rhoad R, Stern P. Writer's cramp—a focal dystonia: etiology, diagnosis, and treatment. J Hand Surg (Am) 1993;18:541–544.

72. Rothwell J, Obeso J, Day B, et al. Pathophysiology of dystonias. Adv Neurol 1983;39:851–863.

73. Sheehy M, Marsden C. Writer's cramp: a focal dystonia. Brain. 1982;105:461–480.

74. Sheehy MP, Rothwell JC, Marsden CD. Writer's cramp. Adv Neurol 1998;50:4457–4472.

75. Utti R, Vomgerjpets FJG, Tsui JKC. Limb dystonia. In: Tsui JKC, Calne DB, eds. Handbook of Dystonia. New York, NY: Marcel Dekker, 1995:143–148.

76. Duchenne de Bologne GB. Spasme fonctionel et paralysies musculaires fonctionelles. In: L'Electrisation Localisee, vol I. Paris: Balliere, 1861:928–946.

77. Gowers WR. A Manual of Diseases of the Nervous System, vol. 2. London, UK: Churchill, 1888:656–674.

78. Naumann M, Reiners K. Long-latency reflexes of hand muscles in idiopathic focal dystonia and their modification by botulinum toxin. Brain. 1997;120:409–416.

79. Preibisch C, Berg D, Hofmann E, et al. Cerebral activation patterns in patients with writer's cramp: a functional magnetic resonance imaging study. J Neurol 2001;248:10–17.

80. Lenz FA, Byl NN. Reorganization in the cutaneous core of the human thalamic principal somatic sensory nucleus (ventral caudal) in patients with dystonia. J Neurophysiol 1999;11:3204–3212.

81. Elbert T, Candia V, Altenmuller F. Alternation of digital representation in somatosensory cortex in focal hand dystonia. Neuroreport 1998; 9:3571–3575.

82. Byl N, Merzenich M, Jenkins, W. A primate genesis model of focal dystonia and repetitive strain injury: I. Learning-induced de-differentiation of the representation of the hand in the primary somatosensory cortex in adult monkeys. Ann Neurol 1996;47:508–520.

83. Bara-Jiminez W, Catalan M, Hallett M. Abnormal somatosensory homunculus in dystonia of the hand. Ann Neurol 1998;44:828–831.

84. Deuschl G, Toro C, Matsumoto J, et al. Movement-related cortical potentials in writer's cramp. Ann Neurol 1995;38:861–868.

85. Ceballos-Baumann AO, Sheean G, Passingham RE, et al. Botulinum toxin does not reverse the cortical dysfunction association with writer's cramp. A PET study. Brain 1997;120:571–582.

86. Rosenbaum F, Jankovic J. Focal task-specific tremor and dystonia: categorization of occupational movement disorders. Neurology 1988;38:522–527.

87. DeLong MR, Crutcher MD, Gergopoulis AP. Primate globus pallidus and subthalamic nucleus: functional organization. J Neurophysiol 1985;53:530–543.

88. DeLong MR. Primate models of movement disorders of basal ganglia origin Trends Neurosci 1990;13:281–285.

89. Frasson E, Priori A, Bertolasi L, et al. Somatosensory disinhibition in dystonia. Mov Disord 2001;16:593–594.

90. Pujol J, Roset-Llobet J, Rosines-Cubells D, et al. Brain cortical activation during guitar-induced hand dystonia studied by functional MRI. Neuroimage 2000;12:257–267.

91. Tempel L, Perlmutter J. Abnormal cortical responses in patients with writer's cramp. Neurology 1993;43:2252–2257.

92. Bhatia KP, Marsden CD. The behavioral and motor consequences of focal lesions of the basal ganglia in man. Brain 1994;117:859–876.

93. Charness ME. Unique upper extremity disorders of musicians. In: Millender LH, Louis DS, Simmons BP, eds. Occupational Disorders of the Upper Extremity. New York, NY: Churchill Livingstone, 1992:117–151.

94. Hardy MA, Merritt WH. Psychological evaluation and pain assessment in patients with reflex sympathetic dystrophy. J Hand Ther 1988;1:155–164.

95. Jankovic J, Shale H. Dystonia in musicians. Semin Neurol 1989; 9:131–135.

96. Jankovic J. Can peripheral trauma induce dystonia and other movement disorders? Yes. Mov Disord 2001;16:7–11.

97. Katz R, Williams C. Focal dystonia following soft tissue injury: three

case reports with long term outcomes. Arch Phys Med Rehab 1990;71:345–349.

98. Jankovic J, Shale H. Dystonia in musicians. Seminars in Neurology 1989;9:131–135.

99. Leijinse J. Anatomical factors predisposing to focal dystonia in musicians' hand: principles, theoretical examples, clinical significance. J Biomechanics. 1996;30:659–669.

100. Quartarone A, Girlanda, P, Risitano G, et al. Focal hand dystonia in a patient with thoracic outlet syndrome. J Neurol Neurosurg Psychiatry 1998;65:272–274.

101. Weiner W. Can peripheral trauma induce dystonia? No. Mov Disord. 2001;16:13–22.

102. Wilson F, Wagner C, Homberg V, et al. Interaction of biomechanical and training factors in musicians with occupational cramps/focal dystonia. Neurology 1991;4:292–296.

103. Wilson F, Wagner C, Homberg V. Biomechanical abnormalities in musicians with occupational cramp/focal dystonia. J Hand Ther 1993;6:298–307.

104. Ridding M, Sheean G, Rothwell J, et al. Changes in the balance between motor cortical excitation and inhibition in focal, task specific dystonia. J Neurol Neurosurg Psychiatry 1995;59:493–498.

105. Odergren T, Iwasaki N, Borg J, et al. Impaired sensory motor integration during grasping in writer's cramp. Brain 1996;119:569–583.

106. Schott GD. The relationship of peripheral trauma and pain to dystonia. J Neurol Neurosurg Psychiatry 1985;48:698–701.

107. Schott GD. Induction of involuntary movements by peripheral trauma. An analogy with causalgia. Lancet 1986;2:712–715.

108. Frucht S, Fahn S, Fried B. Focal task-specific dystonia induced by peripheral trauma. Mov Disord 2000;15:329–335.

109. Topp K, Byl N. Repetitive strain injury-focal hand dystonia: anatomical analysis in owl monkeys. Mov Disord 1998;14:295–306.

110. Kolle B. Psychological approach to focal dystonia in musicians. In: Tubiana R, Amadio PC, eds. Medical Problems of the Instrumentalist Musician. London, UK: Martin Dunitz, 2000:363–368.

111. Frommer J. Idiopathic writing cramp as a psychosomatic disease: a qualitative analysis of three case reports. J Psychosom Med Psychoanal 1992;38:49–62.

112. Schulze A, Jacob HW, Guckler A. Psychosomatic determinants of writer's cramp. Psychother Psychosom Med Psychol 1992;42:201–205.

113. Windgassen K, Ludolph A. Psychiatric aspects of writer's cramp. Eur Arch Psychiatry Clin Neurosci 1991;241:170–176.

114. Bronfonbrener AG. Musicians with focal dystonia: a report of 58 cases seen during a ten-year period at a performing arts medicine clinic. Med Probl Perform Art 1995;10:121–127.

115. Grafman J, Cohen L, Hallett M. Is focal hand dystonia associated with psychopathology. Mov Disord 1991;6:29–35.

116. McKenzie AM, Nagajaran SR, Merzenich MM, et al. Somatosensory differences in somatosensory evoked responses using magnetic source imaging: patients with focal hand dystonia [Abstract]. New Orleans, LA: Society of Neuroscience; November 2000.

117. Sanger TD, Tarsy D, Pascual-Leone A. Abnormalities of spatial and temporal sensory discrimination in writer's cramp. Mov Disord 2001;16:94–99.

118. Tinassi M, Frasson E, Bertolasi L, et al. Temporal discrimination of somesthetic stimuli is impaired in dystonic patients. Neuroreport 1999;10:1547–1550.

119. Hallet M. Is dystonia a sensory disorder [Editorial]? Ann Neurol 1995;38:139–140.

120. Hallett M. Physiology of dystonia. Adv Neurol 1998;78:11–18.

121. Sanger TD, Pascual-Leone A, Tarsy D, et al. Nonlinear sensory cortex response to simultaneous tactile stimuli in writer's cramp. Mov Disord 2002;17:105–111.

122. Byl N, Merzenich M, Cheung S, et al. A primate model for studying focal dystonia and repetitive strain injury: effects on the primary somatosensory cortex. Phys Ther. 1996;727:39.

123. Byl N, Wilson F, Scott P, Oakes A. Sensory dysfunction associated with repetitive strain injuries of tendonitis and focal hand dystonia: a comparative study. J Ortho Sports Phys Ther 1996;23:234–244.

124. Xerri C, Merzenich MM, Jenkins W, et al. Representational plasticity in cortical area 3b paralleling tactual-motor skill acquisition in adult monkeys. Cerebral Cortex. 1999;9:264–276.

125. Groenewegen HJ, Berendse, HW, Wolters JG, et al. The anatomical relationship of the prefrontal cortex with the striatopallidal system, the thalamus and the amygdala: evidence for a parallel organization. Prog Brain Res 1990;85:95–116.

126. Sanger TD, Merzenich MM. Computational model of the role of sensory disorganization in focal task-specific dystonia. J Neurophysiol 2000;84:2458–2464.

127. Tubiana R. Incidence: classification of severity and results of therapy. In: Winspur I, Parry CBW, eds. The Musician's Hand. London, UK: Martin Dunitz Ltd., 2000:164-l67.

128. Wagner C. Determination of finger flexibility. Eur J Appl Physiol 1974;32:259–278.

129. Norkin CC, White DJ. Measurement of Joint Motion: A Guide to Goniometry, 2nd ed. Philadelphia PA: FA Davis Co; 1995.

130. Newmark J, Hochberg F. Isolated painless manual incoordination in musicians. J Neurol Neurosurg Psychiatry 1987;50:291–295.

131. Fry H. Overuse syndromes in musicians 100 years ago: an historical review. Med J Aust 1986;145:620–625.

132. Kendall FP, McCreary EK, Provance PG. Muscles: Testing and Function, 4th ed. Philadelphia: Lippincott, Williams & Wilkins, 1993.

133. Ayres J. Sensory Integration Praxis Test. Western Psychological Association. Los Angeles, CA; 1989.

134. McKenzie AA. A new test to measure stereognosis: key test [Abstract]. Annual Meeting: California Chapter of the APTA; Sacramento, CA, October 1997.

135. Byl N, Nagarajan SS, Newton N, et al. Effect of sensory discrimination training on structure and function in a musician with focal hand dystonia. Phys Ther Case Rep 2000;3:94–113.

136. Bohannon, RW. Stopwatch for measuring thumb movement time. Percept Mot Skills 1995;81:122–126.

137. Psychological Assessment Resources Inc. PAR Finger Tapper User's Guide. 1998.

138. Fung S, Byl N, Melnick M, et al. Functional outcomes: the development of a new instrument to monitor the effectiveness of physical therapy. Eur J Phys Med Rehabil 1997;7:31–41.

139. Mai N, Marguardt C. Treatment of writer's cramp: kinematic measures as assessment tools for planning and evaluating handwriting training procedures. In: Faure C, Keuss PJG, Lorette G, Vinter A, eds. Advances in Handwriting and Drawing. Paris, France: Europia, 1994:445–461.

140. Fahn S. Assessment of the primary dystonias. In: Munsat TL, ed. Quantification of Neurologic Deficits. Boston, MA: Butterworth, 1989:231–270.

141. Byl N, Nagarajan SS, McKenzie A. Effectiveness of sensory retraining: three case studies of patients with focal hand dystonia [Abstract]. Society for Neuroscience. November 4–9, 2000, New Orleans, LA.

142. Tubiana R, Chamagne P. Les affections professionnelles du member superieur chez les musicians. Bull Acad Natl Med 1993;177:203–216.

143. Von Reis G. Electromyographical studies in writer's cramp. Acta Med Scand 1954;149:253–260.

144. Hughes M, McLellan DL. Increased co-activation of the upper limb muscles in writer's cramp. J Neurol Neurosurg Psychiatry 1985;48:782–787.

145. Defendini, R, Fahn S. Magnetic resonance imaging of dystonic states. Adv Neurol 1988;50:265–275.

146. Gilman S, Junck L, Young A. Cerebral metabolic activity in idiopathic dystonia studied with positron emission tomography. Adv Neurol 1988;50:231–236.

147. Chase T, Tamminga C, Burrows H. Positron emission tomographic studies of regional cerebral glucose metabolism in idiopathic dystonia. Adv Neurol 1988;50:237–241.

148. Karbe H, Holfhof V, Rudolf J. Positron emission tomography demonstrates frontal cortex and basal ganglia hypometabolism in dystonia. Neurology 1992;42:1540–1544.

149. Byl N, McKenzie A. Treatment effectiveness of patients with a history of repetitive hand use and focal hand dystonia: a planned prospective follow up study. J Hand Ther 2000;13:289–301.

150. Mavroudais N, Caroyer J, Brunko E, et al. Abnormal motor evoked responses to transcranial magnetic stimulation in focal dystonia. Neurology 1995;45:1671–1677.

151. Gerloff C, Corwell, B, Chen R, et al. The role of the human motor cortex in the control of complex and simple finger movement sequences. Brain 1998;121:1695–709.

152. Tubiana R, Chamagne P. Occupational "cramps" of the upper limb. Ann Chir Main 1983;2:134–142.

153. Leversedge LA, Sylvester JD. Conditioning techniques in the treatment of writer's cramp. Lancet 1955;4:1147–1149.

154. Tecce JJ, Cattanachi L. Contingent negative variation. In: Niedermeyerie L, da Silva F, eds. Electroencephalography Related Fields. Baltimore, MA: Williams and Wilkins; 1994:887–910.

155. Tas N, Karatas GK, Sepici V. Hand orthosis as a writing aid in writer's cramp. Mov Disord. 2001;16:1185–1189.
156. Ranaawaya R, Lang A. Usefulness of a writing device in writer's cramp. Neurology 1989;39:149–150.
157. Koller WC, Vetere-Overfield B. Usefulness of a writing aid in writer's cramp. Neurology 1989;9:149–150.
158. Priori A, Pesenti A, Cappellari A, et al. Limb immobilization for the treatment of focal occupational dystonia. Neurology. 2001,56:405–409.
159. Berardelli A, Rothwell JC, Hallett M, et al. The pathophysiology of primary dystonia. Brain 1998;121:1105–1212.
160. Byrnes ML, Thickbroom GW, Wilson SA. The corticomotor representation of upper limb muscles in writers cramp and changes following botox injections. Brain 1998;232:977–988.
161. Liebert J, Tegenthoff M, Malin JP. Changes of cortical motor area size during immobilization. Electroenceph Clin Neurophys 1995;97:382–386.
162. Liepert J, Multner WHR, Bauder H, et al. Motor cortex plasticity during constraint-induced movement therapy in stroke patients. Neurosci Lett 1998;50:5–8.
163. Wolf SL, Lecraw DE, Barton L, et al. Forced use of hemiplegic upper extremities to reverse the effect of learned nonuse among chronic stroke and head-injured patients. Exp Neurol 1989;104:125–132.
164. Taub E, Crago JE, Uswatte G. Constraint-induced movement therapy: a new approach to treatment in physical medicine. Rehabil Psychol 1988;43:152–170.
165. Taub E, Miller NE, Novack TA, et al. Technique to improve motor deficit after stroke. Arch Phys Med Rehabil 1993;74:347–354.
166. Candia V, Elbert T, Altenmuller E, et al. A constraint-induced movement therapy for focal hand dystonia in musicians. Lancet 1999;353:42–43.
167. Candia V, Schafer T, Taub E, et al. Sensory motor returning: a behavioral treatment for focal hand dystonia of pianists and guitarists. Arch Phys Med Rehabil 2002;83:1342–1349
168. Blake DT, Hsiao SS, Johnson KO. Neural coding mechanisms in tactile pattern recognition: the relative contributions of slowly and rapidly adapting mechanoreceptors to perceived roughness. J Neurosci 1997;17:7680–7689.
169. Mountcastle VS, Henneman E. The representation of tactile sensibility in the thalamus of the monkey. J Comp Neurol 1952;97:409–440.
170. Zeuner KE, Bara-Jimenez W, Noguchi PS, et al. Sensory training for patients with focal hand dystonia. Ann Neurol 2002;51:593–598.
171. Ikeda A, Shibasaki H, Kaji R, et al. Abnormal sensorimotor integration in writer's cramp: study of contingent negative variation. Mov Disord 1999;17:683–690.
172. Porro CA, Francescato MP, Cettolo V, et al. Primary motor and sensory cortex activation during motor performance and motor imagery: a functional magnetic resonance imaging study. J Neurosci 1996;16:7688–7698.
173. Abbrazese G, Trompetto C, Schieppati M. The excitability of the human motor cortex increases during execution and mental imagination of sequential but not repetitive finger movements. Exp Brain Res 1996;111:476–472.
174. Decety J. Do imagined and executed actions share the same neural substrate? Brain Res Cogn Brain Res 1996;3:87–93.
175. DiGuisto EL, Bond N. Imagery and the autonomic nervous system: some methodological issues. Percept Mot Skills 1979;48:427–438.
176. Porter K, Foster J. The Mental Athlete. New York, NY: Ballantine Books, 1986.
177. Lafayette Instrument Company. Purdue Pegboard, Model 32020: Instructions and Normative Data.
178. Ramachandran VS, Rogers-Ramachandran D. Synaesthesia in phantom limbs induced with mirrors. Proc Soc London B 1996;263;377–386.
179. Yang TT, Gallen C, Schwartz B, et al. Sensory maps in the human brain. Nature 1994;368;592–593.
180. Topp KS, Byl N. Focal hand dystonia. Phys Ther Case Rep 1997;1:39–52.
181. Byl N, McKenzie A, Nagarajan SS. Differences in somatosensory hand organization: healthy flutist and flutist with focal hand dystonia. J Hand Ther 2000;13:302–309.
182. Byl N, Hamati D, Melnick M, et al. The sensory consequences of repetitive strain injury in musicians: focal dystonia of the hand. J Back Musculoskel Rehab 1996;7:27–39.

APPENDIX 5A. *Summary: Practical Guidelines for Sensory and Selective Sensory Motor Training*

I. **Goal: Restore the Somatosensory Representation of the Hand and Normal Fine Motor Control.**
 A. *Specific Sensory Activities*
  1. Active stimulation: active exploration of objects
   a. Nontarget sensory tasks
    i) Read braille (workbooks and regular books) and play card games using braille cards. Use one finger at a time.
    ii) Scan embossed letters through a windowed opening (4 mm to 8 mm, eyes closed)
    iii) Palpate plastic disks created with matched pairs of indented symbols of letters, figures/shapes.
    iv) Play games with eyes closed (Scrabble and dominoes).
    v) Put shapes into matched holes with eyes closed.
    vi) Place small party objects in a plastic bag and try to match objects with eyes closed.
    vii) Identify alphabet soup letters with exploration with target fingers.
    viii) Place small objects in large boxes of rice and beans; with eyes closed, bury hand in rice and find matching objects.
 B. *Target Sensory Tasks (without any tension in the hand)*
  1. Feel the instrument; do not use it or play it.
  2. Identify everything about the surface of the instrument, eyes closed (strings, fret, white keys, black keys).
  3. Place raised letters on the keys of the computer keyboard; palpate to determine if matched to underlying key.
  4. Explore target surface with each finger individually while keeping all other fingers relaxed.
 C. *Non-target Sensory Motor Tasks*
  1. Introduce a distinctive stimulus (e.g., sharp, dull, soft, design); subject must bend the metacarpal-phalangeal after the stimulus.
  2. Palpate different alphabet magnet letters (eyes closed) and spell words by placing letters on the refrigerator.
  3. Look at a picture on the wall, then close the eyes and feel for selected objects in a box that match the picture; with the unaffected side, feel the picture on the wall and with the affected digits place the objects appropriately on the picture where you remember they should go (like pin the tail on the donkey).
  4. Smoothly and efficiently remove small objects from wells of different sizes, progressing the task from easy to hard and slow to fast.
  5. Smoothly and efficiently, lightly hold a pen or pencil (just barely preventing it from dropping) and write using the proximal muscles of the shoulder and elbow; increase the difficulty and speed of what is being written.
  6. Working with puzzles with raised surfaces, put puzzles together with eyes closed.
  7. Eyes closed, feel pegs, lightly hold them, and efficiently place pegs into holes; progress difficulty by getting pegs of different sizes and increase speed.
  8. Forearms supinated, resting on the legs, hands relaxed, bend elbow and shoulder and take each finger to feel different parts of the body. Start slowly and then increase speed. Be accurate and only lightly feel area.
 D. *Target Sensory Motor Tasks*
  1. Close eyes and balance posture with gravity while holding and lightly exploring the feel of the instrument.
  2. Letting the hand be like a dead weight, use large, slow, free flowing circular movements of the shoulder to bring the hand to contact the playing surface of the instrument (e.g.,dropping the finger on the key of the piano, the string of the guitar, or the fret of the violin. Progressively decrease the range of proximal movement and increase the speed.
  3. With the hand as a dead weight, drop one finger at a time on the playing surface, creating a strong sound on the piano or a strong sound from the string of the guitar.
  4. With the weight of the hand relaxed on the playing surface, one finger at a time, initiate the pressure down on the key using the muscles inside the hand; then release the pressure down, but do not lift up.
  5. Begin sequencing movements of the digits on the instrument without tension, moving from muscles at the shoulder or elbow or inside hand.
  6. Begin to learn new music or type unfamiliar passages on the instrument.
  7. Put hand in shaving cream and begin making large circular movements, making the movements smaller and smaller and ultimately make the movements faster.
  8. Put Velcro on the pen and hold the pen between D2 and D3 and move the pen around between the fingers.
  9. With the pen between D2 and D3, practice placing the pen in the writing position.
  10. Holding the pen very lightly, practice making large circular movements from proximal shoulder and elbow and progress to making letters and writing sentences slowly increasing the speed.
II. **Passive Stimulation: Stimuli Delivered to the Skin**
 A. Place raised surfaces of different configurations on finger pads; subject has to identify (e.g. alphabet soup letters).
 B. Have a friend or family member write different numbers, letters, shapes and symbols on the involved fingers of the subject's affected hand (eyes closed).
  1. In the simple case, the subject must name the letter or word drawn.
  2. For complex designs, the subject must draw what he/she felt (angles, intersections, curves must be accurate)
  3. When the subject interprets the stimulus incorrectly, the friend will provide the stimulus again. If missed a second time, the friend will have the subject look at the design delivered, they have the subject close his/her eyes and deliver the stimulus again. This repetition and feedback is designed to increase the potential for learning.
III. **Selective Motor Training** (may need to stabilize an adjacent finger to prevent movement)
 A. Do simple tasks that are embedded in the target specific task.
 B. Do functional tasks (activities of daily living) using primarily the proximal shoulder and elbow muscles paired with using the muscles inside the hand for handling objects.

APPENDIX 5A. *Summary: Practical Guidelines for Sensory and Selective Sensory Motor Training (Continued)*

C. Forearms supinated, move one finger at a time using only the muscles inside the hand.
   1. Flex each individual finger and then all together at the metacarpal-phalangeal joint (increase speed).
   2. Alternate fingers.
   3. Straighten the interphalangeal joints with the metacarpal-phalangeal joints flexed.
   4. Pair finger movements (e.g., 2 and 4; 2 and 5).
D. Place forearms in pronation with no surface contact (forearm muscles must be quiet)
   1. Lift each individual finger by straightening interphalangeal joints (and not extending metacarpal-phalangeal joints).
   2. Lift digits in sequence by extending interphalangeal joints.
   3. Lift pairs of digits by extending interphalangeal joints.
E. Place forearms in pronation, with surface contact
   1. Lift each individual finger by straightening interphalangeal joints (and not extending metacarpal-phalangeal joints).
   2. Lift digits in sequence by extending interphalangeal joints.
   3. Lift pairs of digits by extending interphalangeal joints
F. Begin to do more complex fine motor tasks such as manipulating coins in the hand, manipulating the pen such as twirling with the fingers, weaving, beading, perhaps even juggling (as long as can do normally).
G. On the target instrument, eyes closed, perform flexion and extension movements of the digits including alternating movements, simulating a trill without lifting the digits.
   1. Balance posture with gravity.
   2. Keep forearm muscles quiet.
   3. Move from proximal metacarpal phalangeal joints.
   4. Move from muscles inside hand (intrinsic muscles).

IV. Biofeedback
A. Learning should be reinforced with biofeedback, visual and motor imaging, mental practice and mirror imagery.
B. Auditory and visual biofeedback should be integrated into the training program. Emphasis will be placed on retraining the most involved fingers.
   1. Patients should be given a biofeedback unit to take home for a month
   2. The biofeedback should be used help the patient learn to: (1) inhibit the co-contraction of agonists and antagonists (particularly the extrinsic finger extensors and flexors); (2) use the intrinsic muscles of the hand to initiate flexion at the metacarpal-phalangeal joint without recruiting the finger flexors; (3) abduct the fingers and extend the interphalangeal joints using the intrinsic muscles while keeping the extensor digitorum quiet; (4) release digit downward pressure without lifting and extending the finger with the extensor digitorum; (5) alternate and sequence adjacent digits by using the interossei and the lumbricals (on as well as off their instrument); and (6) complete common personal care and household activities, writing, keyboarding and the target specific task using the intrinsic muscles inside the hand and minimizing the use of the extrinsic muscles.
   3. A two-channel unit should be used. The patient will place one electrode on the flexor surface of the forearm and the second on the extensor surface. Each subject will also be shown how to use tape as a biofeedback mechanism. If the finger is curling excessively, tape on the extensor surface will be stretched, giving the subject earlier information about excessive flexion.

V. Mental Imagery, Visualization Techniques, Mental Rehearsal, and Mental Practice
A. Mental imagery, visualization, mental rehearsal and mental practice can reinforce learning.
B. Audio and audiovisual training tapes should be made for the subjects to use to develop the skills at imagery.
C. As soon as possible, the subject should be encouraged to image without the assistance of the tapes because self-imagery provides the most viable image. These tapes will initially focus on: (I) healing; (2) relaxation; (3) balancing the posture with gravity; (4) normalizing all hand functions in activities of daily living; (5) normalizing sensory processing (e.g., ability to discriminate all textures, letters, figures normally); (6) eliminating abnormal movements; (7) freely moving the upper limb using proximal shoulder and elbow joints; and (8) normalizing the target task (e.g., writing, computer, keyboard, instrument). Some of the tasks the subjects will be asked to image include: (1) lifting a glass; (2) using utensils; (3) brushing teeth; (4) cooking; (5) cleaning house; (6) picking up and manipulating small objects; (7) washing dishes; (8) writing; (9) using a keyboard; (10) picking up, retrieving and manipulating small objects; and (11) playing their musical instrument
D. The mental imagery must be reinforced with mental practice.
   1. The subjects will be asked to reflect back to the time when the hand was working normally.
   2. The subjects will constantly remind themselves how easy it was to do the task, how warm the hand felt, how each individual digit felt absolutely controlled, and how easy it was to control each digit separately and how coordinated the hand felt.
   3. The subjects will be asked to review the pleasure of performance in their job or on the target instrument including the satisfaction of the tone, accuracy, speed, and tension free movements as well as the confidence of knowing the hand position, the quality of the sensation, and the control of fine motor movement.

VI. Mirror Imagery
A. Mirror imagery can also be used to change the strategy for writing, keyboard techniques, handling objects and instrumental play.
B. Use mirrors as a type of virtual reality to restore the somatosensory function of the involved part.
C. The affected hand is placed out of view (e.g., behind the mirror).
D. The subject concentrates on the mirror image (e.g., the right hand looks like the left hand in the mirror).
E. The subjects try to replicate the mirror image with their affected side. The mirrors will be placed on a table surface, the keyboard or the target instrument.

APPENDIX 5B. *Example of Supervised Training Program: Two Hours (15 minute units of blocked time)*

1. Have the therapist draw designs on digits, increasing difficulty and give feedback on the target digits on the middle of the pads as well as ulnar and radial side of the digits to increase distinct representation
2. Retrieve small items from small well, timing the sequence and trying to get faster and faster (stopwatch). Also may retrieve small objects matched in pairs from a box of rice or noodles, again trying to increase time and accuracy.
3. Put small pegs in and out of holes, using pegs with different surfaces, trying to shorten the time to do the task and to do the task with minimum force and functional hand/finger/wrist positioning. Can also do this task with a metronome.
4. Work with grated surfaces (e.g., domes or threaded screws) on directionality (screws can be pasted on different surfaces in different orientations).
5. With eyes closed, play games such as dominos or Scrabble or solitaire with braille cards (give subject feedback) with the therapist who can give feedback about correctness.
6. Read letters and words in braille book (number one book). Read letters and words out loud to the therapist who can correct the patient.
7. Place unaffected hand in front of mirror (therapist's or patient's), affected hand behind mirror. Now create activities with both hands (e.g., write, keyboard work, pick up objects, manipulate and match objects, feel different surfaces). Therapist observes patient and gives feedback about correctness of the involved hand.
8. Use biofeedback to control co-contractions and spread of excitation. Start with electrodes and then use tape as feedback. First carry out sensory discrimination reading braille while keeping all of the muscles of the forearm quiet (move from the elbow and shoulder). Then progress to working on simple tasks where only the muscles inside the hand are used and the extrinsic muscles in the forearm are quiet. Then begin manipulating small objects in the hand and activities of daily living. Then work on trying to perform simple movements on the target task that can be done normally.
9. Progress to fine motor movements on tasks that can be done normally (such as manipulating small objects in tension). All movements must be normal before tasks are progressed in difficulty.

CHAPTER 5B

Practical Approaches to Managing Speech and Swallowing Dystonias

Celia F. Stewart

INTRODUCTION

Speech and swallowing disorders may result from dystonia. The speech disorder associated with dystonia is termed hyperkinetic dysarthria. This disorder may affect respiration, phonation, and articulation. Dysarthria may affect all of the phases of the swallow. We first review the speech disorders and then review the swallowing disorders associated with dystonia.

SPEECH DISORDERS

Individuals with dystonia may have breakdowns in their motor speech, making their speech difficult to understand. This difficulty may also lead to social isolation and dependency. To assist in clarifying the motor speech changes that accompany dystonia, the normal physiology of speech production must be identified.

Speech is a motor act that requires little concentration once it is learned. The energy source for speech is air. The diaphragm is the primary muscle of respiration[1] and air is inhaled and exhaled through the vocal tract. The diaphragm contracts and flattens; this enlarges the thoracic cavity by displacing the abdominal contents downward and expanding the thoracic volume. The external intercostals assist the diaphragm in increasing the size of the thoracic capacity. If these movements are not coordinated, the supply and control of air may be reduced. Lack of coordination occurs during inhalation when the abdominal muscles contract simultaneously with the diaphragm and push the abdominal contents upward.[2] This upward movement decreases the size of the thoracic cavity, which reduces the amount of air available for production of speech. Restriction of the air supply may lead to reduced loudness, illogical breath groups, limited pitch range, decreased intelligibility, and increased expiratory ef-

fort. Respiration for speech should be effortless and coordinated with phonation and resonation.

Adduction of the vocal folds in a stream of air produces phonation. During quiet respiration, the vocal folds are abducted to an intermediate position by the poster cricoarytenoid muscles. During optimal phonation, exhalation is initiated and the vocal folds are simultaneously stiffened and adducted to phonation neutral position. In this position, the vocal folds are adducted close enough to vibrate but do not touch.[3] The puff of air flowing through the narrow opening between the vocal folds generates a slight negative pressure and the vocal folds are sucked together. This medial movement of the membranous portion of the vocal folds closes the glottis and blocks the flow of air. Consequently, air pressure builds up below the vocal folds and eventually blows the vocal folds apart. The elastic qualities of the vocal folds and the suction created by the air moving between the vocal folds brings the vocal folds back to midline.[1,3] This oscillation or vibration of the vocal folds in the breath stream results in phonation. Throughout phonation, the vocal folds are stiffened and adducted by the thyroarytenoid, lateral cricoarytenoid, and interarytenoid muscles. When phonation stops, the posterior cricoarytenoid muscle abducts the vocal folds so that respiration may resume. Deviations from this pattern of movement may lead to strained voice production, as seen in patients with spasmodic dysphonia caused by laryngeal dystonia. Changes in the vibration pattern may result in altered voice quality, pitch, and loudness and decreased speech intelligibility.

The vocal tract is made up of the air passages above the level of the vocal folds. These air passages act as resonators and transform the sound from the glottis into meaningful speech. This is accomplished by changing shape, size, stiffness, and relative amount of constriction. Opening and closing the velopharyngeal port regulates nasality.[4] Vowels are produced by changing the size and shape of the vocal tract. Consonants are produced by constricting or blocking the flow of air through the vocal tract.[5] All movements must be coordinated with respiration and phonation. If these move-

Celia F. Stewart: Department of Speech-Language Pathology and Audiology, New York University, New York, New York.

Dr. Stewart has no commercial relationship with the funder.

ments are not coordinated, then breakdowns in speech production occur. Reduced precision of articulation leads to imprecise speech, decreased intelligibility, and effortful speech production.

Communication is a closed loop system. When individuals speak, others hear them and respond to their speech. In addition, individuals hear themselves speak and monitor their speech production. If speech production does not match the specific intention, then speech is modified. When speakers have a speech disorder, they may compensate for the impaired speech production by changing their respiration, phonation, and articulation. If this compensation is carried out in an effortful way, the compensation may be counterproductive and may worsen the symptoms (Allen EL, personal communication, 1989).

RESPIRATORY DYSTONIA

A rare dystonia is associated with breathing or respiratory dystonia. "(It) appears to be associated with spasmodic contractions in the upper airways or the diaphragm in most patients."[2] Respiratory dystonia is associated with generating increased expiratory effort to overcome the narrowing of the upper airway that is not coordinated with the movements of the diaphragm.[2] This rare form of dystonia may occur during quiet tidal breathing; however, it is more common during breathing for speech, and results in increased effort, irregular rate, and erratic depth of cycles. Dystonic respiratory movements usually increase with speech, oral panting, exercise, and stress. These movements decrease with quiet nasal respiration, sniffing, and breathing in the supine position, and are not present during sleep.[2,6,7]

SPASMODIC DYSPHONIA

Definition and Classification

Spasmodic dysphonia, the voice disorder associated with dystonia, may be one symptom of childhood-onset dystonia or it may be an isolated focal dystonia, which begins during adulthood.[8] Dystonic movements of the vocal folds are activated, in most patients, by connected speech. Unlike other voice disorders, the symptoms of spasmodic dysphonia usually disappear during nonlinguistic tasks. These tasks include sustaining vowels in falsetto, laughing, singing, coughing, clearing the throat, yawning, and sighing. In addition, the structure of the larynx is normal.[9] The predominant symptom of spasmodic dysphonia is increased effort when speaking. This effort may cause affected individuals to avoid speech by smiling and nodding.[9]

The three classifications of spasmodic dysphonia include: adductor, abductor, and mixed.[10]

Adductor Spasmodic Dysphonia

Adductor spasmodic dysphonia is most common form of the disorder and occurs in approximately 84% of individuals with spasmodic dysphonia.[8,11] Speakers with adductor spas-

modic dysphonia have increased expiratory effort or struggle during connected speech and a choked, rough, strained-strangled voice quality. Abrupt initiation and termination of voice results in intermittent aphonia, voice-breaks of varying lengths in vowels, staccato stutter-like phonatory blocks, and delayed phonation onset.[9,12–14] Vocal tremors or oscillatory movements imposed on top of the vibratory cycle occur frequently. These tremors or movements are characterized perceptually as a quavering voice quality that may make the patient sound old.[9,12,15] Individuals with adductor spasmodic dysphonia may speak with limited loudness, monopitch, monoloudness, altered inflection patterns, and intermittent bursts of loudness.[9,12–14,16] Some patients strain so severely to produce voice that nonspeech sounds, such as grunts and groans, are produced involuntarily.[12,13]

Abductor Spasmodic Dysphonia

Abductor spasmodic dysphonia has been called the antithesis of adductor spasmodic dysphonia.[17] Patients with abductor spasmodic dysphonia exhibit a whispering or breathy voice quality, interrupted by abrupt termination of voicing.[10,18,19] These abrupt voice terminations are triggered by voiceless consonants and result in strained, aphonic, whispered segments of speech,[10] and brief periods of silence between consonants and adjacent vowels.[17] These speakers frequently have vocal tremor, reduced overall speech intelligibility, difficulty while increasing the loudness of their voices, and may be misunderstood in noise.[10,17] During these times, patients are straining and pushing large quantities of air through their vocal tracts in an attempt to produce voice. As a result, patients may hyperventilate and feel dizzy or lightheaded.

Mixed Spasmodic Dysphonia

When patients present with a combination of adductor and abductor symptoms, they have mixed spasmodic dysphonia, the third classification of this disorder. Speakers with mixed spasmodic dysphonia have a mixture of strained-strangled, rough sounds, and breathy breaks.[8] The characteristics of the mixed type lie along a continuum; some patients have predominately adductor symptoms, while others have abductor-associated symptoms.

At times, individuals with spasmodic dysphonia overcompensate for their voice symptoms. This makes it difficult to determine if they have adductor or abductor spasmodic dysphonia.[18] For instance, speakers with adductor spasmodic dysphonia may consciously produce breathy or whispered voices to ease the strong adductor contractions of their vocal folds. The opposite compensation occurs when patients with abductor spasmodic dysphonia use increased effort to constrict the laryngeal area. This constriction then leads to an increase in expiratory drive as well as strained voices. Diagnosis of the appropriate type of spasmodic dysphonia may be difficult. This is, in part, because of these complex, compensatory techniques.

Treatment of Spasmodic Dysphonia

Some patients with spasmodic dysphonia may benefit from voice therapy, either in conjunction with botulinum toxin (BTX) injections or as a replacement for BTX injections.[20] Most patients do not require voice therapy after BTX therapy because their voice will sound normal or near normal after injection therapy.[11] As soon as dystonic symptoms are reduced by BTX therapy, affected individuals are able to coordinate the voice production subsystem with great efficiency. Some patients may have a suboptimal response to the BTX injections. These patients should be evaluated on an individual basis to determine why their voice production subsystems are not coordinated and why speech is produced in an effortful way. Clinicians must rely on their knowledge of the physiology of voice production mechanics and on physiologic empathy to identify the areas of breakdown.[8,21,22] It is not yet clear whether augmentation of the vocal folds with local collagen injections will improve voice quality in patients with abductor spasmodic dysphonia; however, this procedure has been found helpful in patients with hypophonia associated with parkinsonism.[23]

Treatment Techniques Used in Combination with BTX Therapy or Independent of BTX Therapy

Voice therapy for individuals with adductor, abductor, or mixed spasmodic dysphonia should focus on decreasing effort. This effort may result from the dystonia or from an individual's attempts to compensate for the dystonia (Allen EL, personal communication, 1989).[19] The strain may manifest itself as increased expiratory drive, effort at the level of the vocal folds, or lack of coordination between the expiratory drive, with the stiffness of the vocal folds (Allen EL, personal communication, 1989). If affected individuals have been speaking for many years with increased effort because of dystonia, they may no longer be aware of it. Patients may have learned to compensate for the dystonic muscle activity in an inappropriate way. Patients may increase the expiratory drive in an attempt to push through the increased muscle tightness in the larynx or the articulators. If patients have abductor spasmodic dysphonia, they may push too much air because of incomplete adduction. This compensation is counterproductive to speech production (Allen EL, personal communication, 1989). Therefore, the first step in therapy may be to make the patient aware of the counterproductive compensation and identify the extraneous muscle activity.

Patients may increase their awareness of the effort by consciously decreasing the effort levels and then by noticing the changes in their body. This contrast, between high and diminished efforts, may be elicited by having patients perform activities that will momentarily diminish the effort. These efforts include speaking on inhalation, producing a high-pitched sound in falsetto, singing glissando, and laughing.[9,12,13,24-26] These activities may act as a sensory trick and momentarily diminish the dystonic symptoms as well as the compensatory, counterproductive activities. When an activity is effective at diminishing effort, the speaking voice produced immediately following the sensory trick will also be diminished in effort. Helping patients to develop awareness of the different effort levels is the first step toward controlling the effort.

The next step toward controlling the effort is to diminish any remaining compensatory activities that are counterproductive. It is necessary to identify the location of the counterproductive compensation by observing the patients' posture, respiration, phonation, and articulation. The patients' attention is then drawn to the effort (Allen EL, personal communication, 1989). Control of expiratory drive may be enhanced by improving posture; letting go of extraneous muscle activity in the upper body; speaking briefly on inhalation; and taking a comfortable breath before speaking (Allen EL, personal communication, 1989).[19,27-29] Patients may need to focus on the respiratory cycle and ensure that they are exhaling a little air at the end of breath groups. Some patients do not need to focus specifically on respiration, as this will normalize when they decrease effort in their vocal folds.

When the center of counterproductive compensation is localized in the vocal folds, effort may be reduced by having patients resonate their voices in their facial mask, project their voices into the room, use shorter breath groups, and produce continuous phonation.[30]

These therapy procedures may help patients decrease extraneous movements and gain control over phonation. Some patients report having increased difficulty on specific consonants or vowels. These sounds should be identified and then patients with adductor spasmodic dysphonia can use h-initiated words. Those with abductor spasmodic dysphonia can use vowels, voiced continuants, or hum to decrease effort on those difficult sounds. These techniques are most effective when they are used consistently, in all speaking situations.

If the extraneous effort is localized in the articulators, it may be reduced by maintaining a freeway space between the upper and lower teeth, releasing the jaw, making lip flutters, speaking on inhalation, speaking into a word balloon, or feeling light contact of the articulators during speech. Some patients have sensory tricks such as holding a dowel in their mouth or putting their hand on the jaw while they speak. In addition, when laryngeal and respiratory symptoms are diminished, articulatory symptoms may improve.

One new voice therapy—speaking on inhalation—helps minimize the symptoms of spasmodic dysphonia for some patients.[28] Speaking on inhalation begins by having patients hum on inhalation so that they feel the back of their throats open when the hum is produced. The next step is to produce /i/ on inhalation, and then to count on inhaled air without straining. Patients then match the sound produced on inhalation with the sound produced on exhalation. Shulman[28] reports that some patients speak on inhalation all the time; however, some patients speak on inhalation only to facilitate speech on exhalation. Shulman[28] says that patients must work gradually to lengthen the time they speak on inhalation.

Some patients with adductor and abductor spasmodic dysphonia may shorten the side effects and lengthen the benefits received from the BTX injections by participating in short periods of voice therapy. If the breathiness after a BTX injection for adductor spasmodic dysphonia is severe or lasts for an extended period, voice therapy may be helpful.[20]

Before the BTX injection, patients with adductor spasmodic dysphonia use increased expiratory drive to vibrate the stiffened vocal folds. After the BTX injections, the vocal folds are weak and some patients do not decrease their expiratory drive. When the vocal folds are weakened, the excessive expiratory drive will blow the weak vocal folds out of the breath stream and they will not vibrate. In addition, the vocal folds may fatigue when they attempt to stiffen to resist the pressure from the strong airflow. Therefore, patients are advised to speak more quietly, reduce environmental noise, move closer to people when they speak, talk in a small group, and use a voice amplifier (on the telephone and in face-to-face communication). These suggestions may help patients maximize voicing.[19] In addition, effort may be reduced by shortening breath groups, minimizing extraneous muscle activity, optimizing posture, using laryngeal massage, or having patients yawn, laugh, sigh, and swallow.

Lundy et al.[31] and Nash and Ludlow[32] identified possible hyperfunction or involuntary contractions of supralaryngeal structures and palatal movements during speech. These studies indicate that compensatory movements may alleviate the strain during effortful speech. Murry and Woodson[20] used a combination of voice therapy and BTX injections to treat patients with SD. They found that those patients who received a period of voice therapy after BTX injection therapy had better voices for longer periods than those patients who received injections alone.

SWALLOWING DISORDERS

In patients with cervical dystonia, swallowing may be impaired because of the involvement of the muscles normally required for swallowing and as a complication of BTX injections. Using videofluoroscopy, one study demonstrated delayed initiation of swallow in all 12 patients with cervical dystonia.[33] Swallowing may be transiently compromised by BTX injections; however, permanent dysphagia may be an unfortunate consequence of a peripheral denervation procedure.

When treating patients who have dysphagia, the two major concerns are maintaining safety and sustaining adequate nutrition. There are four stages to the swallow. These include:

1. The oral preparatory phase is when food is placed in the mouth and masticated. This phase varies with different individuals; however, all people need to maintain both a labial and posterior seal to keep food in the mouth during mastication.
2. The oral phase begins when the tongue starts to move the bolus posteriorly and ends when the pharyngeal swallow is triggered.
3. The pharyngeal stage is triggered when the bolus passes the anterior faucial arches or the tongue base crosses the lower rim of the mandible. This phase is made up of a series of exquisitely timed movements, starting with elevation and retraction of the velum, elevation and anterior movement of the hyoid bone (which tucks the larynx under the tongue), closure of the laryngeal valve, and opening of the cricopharyngeal sphincter.[34] These movements are coordinated with tongue base and pharyngeal wall movements that generate pressure to propel the bolus safely into the esophagus.
4. The esophageal phase starts when the bolus enters the esophagus and ends when the food passes into the stomach.

Involuntary, irregular movements of the muscles may affect the first three phases of swallowing.[35] The esophageal phase is usually normal. The dystonic symptoms may worsen with volitional attempts to masticate food. Rapid, shallow, irregular breathing cycles may not be coordinated with swallowing.[35] The oral preparatory and oral phases of the swallow may be affected when an individual has a chin-elevated posture or by involuntary movements of the head or body. Lip closure may be intermittent due to involuntary oral movements and result in drooling, spillage of food out of the mouth, and increased difficulty swallowing because of an open-mouthed posture.[35] Tongue mobility may be reduced because of involuntary protruding, retracting, or lateralizing of the tongue. These movements may make it difficult to collect the food into a cohesive bolus and consequently, food may spill prematurely over the back of the tongue. Lingual movements may also be disorganized and result in slow oral transit times.

During the pharyngeal phase, swallowing may be altered by changes in respiration, reduced tongue movements, and inadequate laryngeal elevation. Involuntary inspirations may abduct the vocal cords during the swallow and cause food to spill into the airway. Involuntary pharyngeal wall contraction and posterior motion of the tongue may leave food residue in the vallecula and pyriform sinuses. This residue may increase with each swallow. In addition, incomplete or unsustained laryngeal elevation and closure may permit aspiration to occur from material that spills from the vallecula and pyriform sinuses.

Treatment of Swallowing Disorders

Traditional treatment strategies may be effective for patients with dystonia including modifying the size of the bolus, changing the viscosity of the food, using an effortful swallow, executing a chin-tuck procedure, using thermal stimulation, performing the Mendelssohn maneuver, doing the supraglotic swallow, and performing the super-supraglotic swallow. In addition, patients may benefit from relaxation techniques and eating in a quiet environment.

REFERENCES

1. Zemlin WR. Speech and Hearing Science: Anatomy and Physiology. 4th Ed. Englewood Cliffs, NJ: Prentice Hall; 1998.
2. Braun N, Abd A, Baer J, et al. Dyspnea in dystonia: a functional evaluation. Chest 1995;1309–1316.
3. Liebermann P. Direct comparison of subglottal and esophageal pressure during speech. J Acoust Soc Am 1968;48:1159–1164.
4. Bell-Berti F. An electromyographic study of velopharyngeal function in speech. J Speech Hear Res. 1976;19(2):225–40.
5. Borden GJ, Harris KS, Raphael LJ. Speech Science Primer: Physiology, Acoustics, and Perception of Speech. 3rd Ed. Baltimore, MD: Williams & Wilkins. 1994.
6. LeBlanche GR. Breathing Disorders of Individuals with Dystonia Musculorum Deformans [dissertation]. Chicago, IL: Northwestern University, Chicago; 1984.
7. Wilcox PG, Bassett A, Jones B, et al. Respiratory dyskinesia presenting as acute respiratory distress. Chest 1993;103:314–316.
8. Brin MF, Fahn S, Blitzer A, et al. Movement disorders of the larynx. In: Blitzer A, Brin MF, Fahn S, eds. Neurological Disorders of the Larynx. New York: Thieme, 1992:248–278.
9. Aronson AE, Brown JR, Litin EM, et al. Spastic dysphonia. I. Voice, neurologic, and psychiatric aspects. J Speech Hearing Disord 1968;33:203–218.
10. Aronson AE. Clinical Voice Disorders. New York: Thieme; 1985.
11. Blitzer A, Brin MF, Stewart CF. Botulinum toxin management of spasmodic dysphonia (laryngeal dystonia): a 12-year experience in more than 900 patients. Laryngoscope 1998;108:1435–1441.
12. Bloch CS, Hirano M, Gould WJ. Symptom improvement of spastic dysphonia in response to phonatory tasks. Ann Otol Rhinol Otolaryngol 1985;94:51–54.
13. Ludlow CL, Connor NP. Dynamic aspects of phonatory control in spasmodic dysphonia. J Speech Hear Res 1987;30:197–206.
14. Robe E, Brumlik J, Moore P. A study of spastic dysphonia. Laryngoscope 1960;70:219–245.
15. Finitzo T, Freeman F. Spasmodic dysphonia, whether and where: Results of seven years of research. J Speech Hear Res 1989;32:541–555.
16. Arnold GE. Vocal rehabilitation of paralytic dysphonia. Arch Otolaryngol 1962;76:358–368.
17. Zwitman DH. Bilateral cord dysfunctions: abductor type spastic dysphonia. J Speech Hear Disord 1979;44:373–378.
18. Brin MF, Blitzer A, Stewart C, et al. Treatment of spasmodic dysphonia (laryngeal dystonia) with local injections of botulinum toxin: review and technical aspects. In: Blitzer A, Brin MF, Fahn S, eds. Neurological Disorders of the Larynx. Thieme: New York, 1992:214–228.
19. Blitzer A, Stewart CF. Abductor spasmodic dysphonia. In: Stemple J, ed. Voice Therapy: Clinical Studies. 2nd Ed. Chicago: Mosby Year Book, 2000:467–478.
20. Murry T, Woodson GE. Combined modality treatment of adductor spasmodic dysphonia with Botulinum toxin and voice therapy. J Voice 1995;9:460–465.
21. Ludlow CL. Treatment of speech and voice disorders with botulinum toxin. JAMA 1990;264:2671–2676.
22. Ludlow CD, Naunton RF, Sedory SE, et al. Effects of botulinum toxin injections on speech in adductor spasmodic dysphonia. Neurology 1988;38:1220–1225.
23. Hill AN, Jankovic J, Vuong KD, et al. Treatment of hypophonia with collagen vocal fold augmentation in patients with parkinsonism. Mov Disord 2003;18:1190–1192
24. Izdebski K, Dedo HH. Selecting the side of recurrent laryngeal nerve section for spastic dysphonia. Otolaryngol Head Neck Surg 1981;89:423–426.
25. Robe E, Brumlik J, Moore P. A study of spastic dysphonia. Laryngoscope 1960;70:219–245.
26. Segre R. Spasmodic aphonia. Folia Phoniatr 1951;3:150–165.
27. Casper J. Confidential voice. In: Stemple JC, ed. Voice Therapy: Clinical Studies. Chicago: Mosby Year Book, 2000:128–139.
28. Shulman S. Symptom modification for abductor spasmodic dysphonia: inhalation phonation. In: Stemple JC. ed. Voice Therapy: Clinical Studies. Chicago: Mosby Year Book, 2000:479–486.
29. Stemple JC. Functional voice therapy for spasmodic dysphonia. In: Stemple JC, ed. Voice Therapy: Clinical Studies. Chicago: Mosby Year Book, 2000:434–437.
30. Lee L. Refocusing laryngeal tone. In: Stemple JC, ed. Voice Therapy: Clinical Studies. Chicago: Mosby Year Book, 2000:145–153.
31. Lundy DS, Lu FL, Casiano RR, et al. The effect of patient factors on response to outcomes to Botox treatment of spasmodic dysphonia. J Voice 1998;12:460–466.
32. Nash EA, Ludlow CL. Laryngeal muscle activity during speech breaks in adductor spasmodic dysphonia. Laryngoscope 1996;106:484–489.
33. Münchau A, Good CD, McGowan S, et al. Prospective study of swallowing function in patients with cervical dystonia undergoing selective peripheral denervation. J Neurol Neurosurg Psychiatry 2001;71:67–72.
34. Logemann JA. Evaluation and Treatment of Swallowing Disorders. Austin, TX: PRO-ED, 1998.
35. Bosma J, Geoffrey V, Thach B, et al. A pattern of medication induced persistent bulbar and cervical dystonia. Int J Orofacial Myology 1982;8:5–19.

CHAPTER 6

Pharmacologic Treatment of Generalized Dystonia

Stacy Horn and Cynthia L. Comella

TREATMENT OF GENERALIZED DYSTONIA

Generalized dystonia is a neurologic condition that results in sustained muscular contractions that typically cause twisting movements and abnormal postures.[1] The sustained contractures may be painful. The movements may be of variable speed and are often repetitive. Dystonia is typically worsened by activity.

Generalized forms of dystonia typically occur during childhood and most often start in one limb and then progress at a variable rate to involve the entire body.[2,3] Most patients with an onset of generalized dystonia before the age of 11 years experience initial symptoms in one leg. When the age of onset of generalized dystonia is greater than 20 years, the initial site of involvement is typically the arm.[3,4] When generalized dystonia becomes severe, the abnormal movements may occur during rest. Dystonia is typically aggravated by stress or fatigue and relieved by relaxation or sleep. Patients with dystonia may often employ sensory tricks, gestes antagoniste, which may be useful in relieving abnormal muscular contractions.[2,3]

The pharmacologic treatment of generalized dystonia may often be challenging; however, when pharmacotherapy is effective, it may result in dramatic changes in a patient's functional capacity. The treatment response to medications is variable; no specific features of the disease predict treatment response. The first decision regarding treatment is based on the exact type of generalized dystonia (i.e., primary or secondary generalized dystonia). The type of dystonia is determined through an extensive history that includes detailed information on past and present medications, birth and developmental history, and family history, as well as a detailed physical examination. The differential diagnosis and workup of generalized dystonia is discussed in detail in a separate chapter. Frequently used medications in the treatment of primary generalized dystonia are listed in Table 1.

MEDICATIONS

Dose Regulation and Drug Combinations

The choice of drug to initiate usually depends on the age of the patient, prior exposure to medications, other concurrent medications or medical problems, and the physician and patient bias. Levodopa therapy, as discussed below, is tried for all patients with young onset (age less than approximately 30 years), and those with onset in a limb. Drug dosage is initially low, gradually increased as tolerated, and adjusted to identify the most efficacious dose with a minimum of adverse effects (regulation of dose or optimization of dose). If the medication is of no benefit at a dose that causes adverse effects, then it is gradually tapered and discontinued. If a medication is documented as helpful, then it can be continued at the regulated dose and the next medication is added. When a medication is to be removed from a treatment program, the dose is tapered and only rarely abruptly discontinued.

Stacy Horn: Department of Neurological Sciences, Section of Movement Disorders, University of Pennsylvania, Philadelphia, Pennsylvania.

Cynthia L. Comella: Department of Neurological Sciences, Rush University, Chicago, Illinois.

Stacy Horn has no commercial relationship to disclose. Cynthia Comella has received research grants from Allergan Inc, Elan Biopharmaceuticals, and Ipgen Ltd.

TABLE 6-1. *Medications in the Treatment of Generalized Dystonia*

Medication	Typical therapeutic dosage
Levodopa	500–1,000 mg per day
Trihexyphenidyl	8–80 mg per day
Baclofen	25–120 mg per day
Clonazepam	1.5–12.0 mg per day
Tizanidine	Unclear
Tetrabenazine	25–75 mg per day

Levodopa

The treatment of primary generalized dystonia typically begins with a trial of levodopa. This trial is therapeutic as well as diagnostic in that this trial is used to identify a subset of patients with dopa-responsive dystonia (DRD). DRD is a form of generalized dystonia that is characterized by onset in childhood, diurnal variation, parkinsonism, gait disturbance, as well as dramatic and sustained response to levodopa, often in relatively low doses.[5,6] Patients with DRD frequently have a family history of dystonia. Recent findings have demonstrated a genetic heterogeneity with multiple loci and both autosomal dominant and recessive forms of the disease.[7–14] If DRD is left untreated, it may progress; however, patients have been reported to respond to levodopa therapy, even when treatment is delayed.[6] Patients with DRD have reduced striatal tyrosine-hydroxylase levels.[7] Patients with DRD respond to levodopa within days to a few months and many return to almost fully functional levels. The daily dosage of levodopa is 100–3,000 mg, with an average response to 500–1,000 mg/day.[6] Levodopa response is sustained without significant motor complications, which are observed in patients with idiopathic Parkinson's disease who are treated with levodopa.[6,15] This observation is frequently used to distinguish patients with DRD from those with an onset in childhood of juvenile Parkinson's disease (JPD). Patients with JPD, who frequently present with dystonia, develop motor fluctuations on therapy over time.

Because of the exquisite response in patients with DRD, it is important to administer a trial of levodopa in patients with primary dystonia. This medication is typically well tolerated, and in select cases, may cause dramatic and sustained improvement. If patients do not respond after 1 month of levodopa therapy, a second medication should be tried. The major side effects of levodopa include nausea, lightheadedness, sedation, confusion, or hallucinations.

Anticholinergic Medications

Anticholinergic medications are typically the next pharmacologic therapy for patients with primary dystonia. A number of clinical trials have evaluated the efficacy of anticholinergic medications in generalized dystonia.[3,16–19] These studies reported that high doses of anticholinergic medications may be required to produce clinical benefit; children can generally tolerate higher doses of these medications than adults. The side effects of anticholinergic medications may be central or peripheral in etiology. Central side effects may include sedation, forgetfulness, weight loss, or personality changes. Peripheral side effects may include blurred vision, dry mouth, or urinary retention. To reduce the incidence of side effects, anticholinergic medications are started at low doses and slowly increased. The major clinical studies that have evaluated the effectiveness of anticholinergic medications are discussed in the following paragraphs.

The most common anticholinergic medications include trihexyphenidyl and benztropine mesylate. Trihexyphenidyl works through direct inhibition of the parasympathetic nervous system. In addition, it has a relaxing effect on smooth musculature; this effect is exerted directly on the muscle tissue itself and indirectly through an inhibitory effect on the parasympathetic nervous system.[20] Trihexyphenidyl is available in 2-mg and 5-mg tablets and as a 2 mg per 5 mL elixir.[20] Benztropine, which has anticholinergic and antihistaminic effects, is available in 0.5-, 1.0-, and 2.0-mg tablets and also in an injectable form.[20]

Practitioners first began to try anticholinergic medications because of their efficacy in acute drug-induced dystonic reactions.[21] Fahn and Marsden were among the first investigators to describe, delineate, and further investigate the clinical response of dystonia to high doses of anticholinergics. In 1979, Fahn[16] reported the response of 35 patients to anticholinergic therapy. This study consisted of 14 children and 21 adults treated with a maximum dose of 40 mg/day of trihexyphenidyl. Fahn reported improvement in 10 children and four adults. Adults were less responsive due to their inability to tolerate high dosages of medication. In 1983, Fahn[17] published the results of an open-label, long-term trial involving 75 patients with dystonia of various etiologies; of these patients, 23 were children and 52 were adults. Patients were treated with an anticholinergic agent (i.e., trihexyphenidyl or ethopropazine) until clinical response was observed or intolerable side effects developed. The results of this study confirmed a difference in the response between adults and children. Children, who tolerate higher doses of anticholinergic medications than adults, tended to have a better clinical response with fewer side effects than adults. Adults experienced relatively less clinical improvement with significantly more side effects. Of the 23 children, 14 patients had a sustained and dramatic clinical response, with a median duration of 5 years. The average daily dose of trihexyphenidyl was 41 mg/day, with a dosage range of 8–80 mg/day. Of the 52 adults, 20 patients had sustained moderate to marked clinical improvement. Fewer than 50% of adult patients were treated for more than 2 years; most adult patients were treated for less than 1 year, with subsequent withdrawal because of intolerable adverse effects. The average daily dose of trihexyphenidyl was 24 mg/day. The average daily dose of ethopropazine was 350 mg/day. Fahn did not report any significant advantages of ethopropazine compared to trihexyphenidyl.

Marsden and colleagues[18] reproduced Fahn's results in a study that was published in 1984. In this open-label trial, 40 patients with dystonia (23 children and 17 adults) were treated with high doses of trihexyphenidyl. Fifty-two percent of the children received clinical benefit when treated with a median dose of 30 mg/day. Some children received up to 130 mg/day of trihexyphenidyl. Forty-one percent of adult patients gained clinical benefit on a median dose of 20 mg/day. Side effects were reported in 57% of children compared with 65% of adults.

In 1984, Nutt[22] performed a double-blind crossover study in nine patients with cranial dystonia. This study consisted of three arms: treatment with trihexyphenidyl at a maximum of 12 mg/day; a peripheral anticholinergic medication, tridihex-ethyl at a maximum dosage of 150 mg/day; and a placebo each for 6 weeks. Each phase of this study was abruptly ended after 6 weeks and the next arm of the study commenced. Patients were assessed at 3-week intervals. Assessment techniques included blink rate; presence of blepharospasm during 1 minute of task reading; clinical scoring of blepharospasm, dysarthria, facial, mandibular, and lingual involuntary movements; subjective scores; and blinded rating of videotapes.

Nine subjects completed all three phases of treatment, but four patients did not complete all 6 weeks of the titration. Six patients achieved the maximum dosage of trihexyphenidyl. One patient had an unequivocal clinical and subjective response to trihexyphenidyl treatment. The results of this small study suggest that a small subgroup of patients with cranial dystonia respond to anticholinergic therapy.

The results of a double-blind, crossover, prospective trial of high-dose trihexyphenidyl in 31 dystonic patients, who were under the age of 32 years, was published in 1986.[23] This study, which was conducted for 36 weeks, involved active treatment for 18 weeks and placebo treatment for 18 weeks. The maximum dose of trihexyphenidyl that was administered was 30 mg/day. Patients were videotaped and blindly rated. Seventy-one percent of patients experienced clinically significant improvement in their dystonia.

An open-label study published in 1986 examined the effects of high-dose anticholinergic therapy in adult patients.[19] Forty-four adults with various forms of dystonia were treated with anticholinergic medications; these patients started at low doses and were slowly increased to their maximum-tolerated dosage. Thirty-five patients with idiopathic dystonia, who received trihexyphenidyl therapy at average dosages of 21.5 mg/day, experienced moderate to marked improvement. Patients with symptomatic dystonia experienced only mild improvement on similar doses of anticholinergic medications. Younger patients, who had a shorter duration of dystonia and were able to tolerate higher dosages of medication, had the best overall response.

These studies assisted in the identification of anticholinergic therapy as a mainstay treatment for generalized dystonia and the collection of data from large, long-term retrospective studies. At Columbia University in New York, a retrospective study and chart review of 358 patients with dystonia was conducted; tardive and psychogenic dystonia were excluded.[24,25] Increasing trial doses of an anticholinergic agent were administered until clinical improvement or significant side effects were observed. Fifty-one percent of patients under the age of 20 experienced a good therapeutic response. This response was independent of the severity of dystonia and response rate was higher in those treated within 5 years of diagnosis. In patients with secondary dystonia, the response rate was 31%.

The large body of clinical data support the efficacy of anticholinergic therapy for generalized forms of dystonia. Children are more likely to have clinical improvement on an-

ticholinergic medications; however, they are also able to tolerate higher doses of anticholinergic medications. Adults may experience improvement in dystonia; however, side effects may be a limiting factor. In all patients, medication should be started at a low dose and slowly increased to clinical effect or when troublesome side effects are present. Trihexyphenidyl or benzhexol is typically started at 1–2 mg/day and increased by 1–2 mg every week on a three-times-per-day schedule until symptoms are improved or side effects occur.

Baclofen

Baclofen, a derivative of γ-aminobutyric acid (GABA), decreases the excitability of motor neurons and interneurons in the central nervous system (CNS); in addition, baclofen reduces spasticity in patients with spinal cord dysfunction and has also been used to treat dystonia.[26] Baclofen binds to the $GABA_B$ presynaptic receptor and inhibits calcium influx, thereby reducing the release of excitatory transmitters glutamate and aspartate. Baclofen is also reported to have CNS effects that may be relevant to its usefulness in dystonia. These CNS effects include:

- Promoting the accumulation of serotonin in the striatum;
- Decreasing firing of noradrenergic neurons in the locus ceruleus;
- Producing neuronal hyperpolarization in the substantia nigra pars compacta;
- Decreasing dopamine release in the striatum; and
- Increasing turnover of the inhibitory neurotransmitter glycine.[27–31]

Controlled studies in dystonia have not been conducted, however, baclofen is often used as a monotherapy or as polytherapy in patients with generalized dystonia. The major side effects of baclofen include confusion, lethargy, weakness, nausea, urinary frequency, or vomiting.

Baclofen therapy for generalized dystonia was reported only as case reports until the medication was studied in a retrospective trial of 108 patients with various forms of dystonia.[24,25] This study reported a 13% response rate in patients with generalized dystonia; the average dose was 82 mg/day. Therapeutic response was unrelated to gender or ethnic background; however, advanced age of onset was a factor for improved clinical response. Patients with a milder form of disease during the initiation of treatment tended to have a better clinical response. Duration of symptoms prior to institution of therapy did not affect response.

A second retrospective study was published in 1992.[32] This study focused attention on baclofen therapy in patients with idiopathic dystonia who were under the age of 21 years. A total of 80 patient charts were reviewed and 16 patients had received baclofen monotherapy or polytherapy. Fourteen patients had generalized dystonia. The mean age of onset of dystonia was 8.2 years; the mean treatment age was 13.9 years. Patients had an average disease duration of 5.7

years prior to the institution of baclofen. Seven patients had subjective clinical improvement with baclofen therapy. The average daily dose of baclofen in clinically responsive patients was 79 mg/day. Response to baclofen did not correlate with gender, age of onset, family history, or ethnic background. Patients with a shorter duration of symptoms tended to attain a better response. Five patients were followed for an extended amount of time (i.e., 3.8 years) and they continued to have good clinical responses to baclofen.

Another use of baclofen in patients with generalized dystonia has been intrathecal administration (ITB); this topic is discussed in this volume in those chapters that address its use in both children and adults. In brief, ITB therapy involves implantation of a pump in the abdomen; this pump delivers continuous specified doses of baclofen into the intrathecal space. In 1991,[32] case reports describing the efficacy of ITB for generalized dystonia began to appear. These initial case studies reported good clinical improvement of patients with medically refractive dystonia of various etiologies. In 1996, a retrospective study of 25 medication-refractory patients with severe segmental or generalized dystonia was conducted with ITB.[34] Of these 25 patients, 17 patients exhibited objective clinical evidence of spasticity in addition to their dystonia. Patients with refractory dystonia were given doses of ITB prior to implantation of the pump. Thirteen patients showed a favorable clinical response to ITB. These patients then underwent pump implantation. Of these patients, 10 were videotaped before and after the test doses. The videotapes were evaluated by two examiners who were blinded for the purposes of this study. The mean dystonia scores improved in 6 patients, however, the degree of improvement was not statistically significant. Of the 13 patients with an implanted pump, 11 patients were followed for a mean of 21 months. Continued subjective clinical response was reported by 6 of the 11 patients; 5 patients felt that the ITB had lost its effectiveness. Patients were also assessed using objective dystonia scores; 9 patients did not show an overall improvement on global scores or disability. Certain aspects of the dystonia, such as pain and muscle spasms, were helped with ITB. In long-term follow-up, complications were observed in 5 of the 13 patients.

An open-label study of 86 patients with generalized dystonia was conducted by Albright and colleagues.[35] Of these patients, 71% had dystonia associated with cerebral palsy. Patients were tested for response by either bolus or continuous infusion of baclofen. ITB pumps were subsequently implanted into 77 patients. The authors found a statistically significant improvement in dystonia scores over their previous baseline scores. The authors also reported a prolonged response over 29 months in 92% of patients. Side effects were reported in 26% of patients and surgical complications were reported in 38% of patients. Complications of ITB therapy include:

- Diminishing medication effects with continued need for escalating dosages of intrathecal baclofen;

- Cerebrospinal fluid leaks,
- Spinal headaches,
- Baclofen overdose with respiratory depression;
- Fibrosis at the catheter tip, and
- Skin erosion.

Although significant improvement with ITB has been reported in patients with generalized dystonia, patients who participated in these studies did not have primary generalized dystonia. These findings do not conclusively support the use of ITB for all patients with generalized dystonia.

Clonazepam

Clonazepam is another pharmacologic option for the treatment of generalized dystonia. This drug is a benzodiazepine that is centrally active and exerts it actions through inhibition of GABA. Clonazepam has been retrospectively studied and found to benefit patients with cervical dystonia and secondary dystonia.[24,25] In generalized dystonia, only 6% of 17 patients had a good clinical response. The average daily dosage of clonazepam was 3.7 mg/day; the typical treatment duration was 10 months. The age of onset of dystonia symptoms did not have an effect on response to clonazepam; however, patients treated within 5 years of onset tended to have a better clinical response. When clonazepam was compared to anticholinergic medications for the treatment of dystonia, anticholinergic medications were found to be significantly more effective with 50% of generalized dystonia patients improving with anticholinergic therapy. The major side effects of clonazepam include sedation and confusion. When discontinuing treatment, clonazepam should be gradually tapered; abrupt withdrawal could induce seizures.

Tizanidine

Tizanidine is a centrally acting, myotonolytic agent that works through agonistic activity at the noradrenergic α_2 receptors. This agonist activity causes both direct impairment of excitatory amino acid release from spinal interneurons and inhibition of facilitory ceruleospinal pathways.[36,37] Tizanidine has primarily been used to help control spasticity in pyramidal disease; however, it has been tried in patients with dystonia. In addition, tizanidine has been studied for its use in patients with cranial dystonia; an open-label, single-blind placebo study of 10 patients was completed.[38] This study included one patient with generalized dystonia. Patients were slowly optimized up to a total of 36 mg/day of tizanidine. Five patients dropped out of the study for various reasons. Of the remaining five patients, one patient experienced objective improvement in dystonia; one patient had subjective improvement. The results of this study were inconclusive. A large, double-blind placebo-controlled trial of patients with dystonia is required to determine the efficacy of this medication. Side effects of tizanidine include sedation, confusion, lightheadedness, weakness, nausea, insomnia, and hepatotoxicity.

Tetrabenazine

Tetrabenazine is a presynaptic monoamine-depleting agent. Multiple studies have investigated its effects in hyperkinetic movement disorders. This medication has not been approved for use in the United States, however, it is available in Europe and Canada. The major side effects of tetrabenazine include drowsiness, sialorrhea, insomnia, depression, akathisia, parkinsonism, and postural hypotension.[39,40]

In a double-blind, crossover placebo study published in 1982, tetrabenazine was studied in 19 patients with hyperkinetic movement disorders.[39] During this study, 12 patients with various forms of dystonia were treated. Patients received either placebo or escalating doses of tetrabenazine. The maximum dose of tetrabenazine was 200 mg/day for 6 weeks. Of the dystonia patients, nine patients had clinical improvement.

During 1988, Jankovic[40] completed a long-term retrospective study that evaluated the efficacy of tetrabenazine in hyperkinetic movement disorders. Patients who underwent treatment for hyperkinetic movement disorders ($n = 217$) were followed for an average of 18 months. Each patient was rated on a scale of 1 to 5 (1 = marked improvement, 4 = no response, 5 = worsening). The mean improvement in 19 patients with generalized dystonia was 2.8.

In a more recent retrospective study of 400 patients with various hyperkinetic movement disorders, response to tetrabenazine was monitored for an average of 28.9 months.[41] The patients were again rated on a scale of 1 to 5. In this group, 108 patients had idiopathic dystonia (41 with generalized dystonia). Sixty-three percent of all idiopathic dystonia patients had a marked clinical improvement and were maintained on doses of 25–75 mg/day. Side effects were reported by 81.8% of the 400 patients and were similar to those listed above.

These studies support the use of tetrabenazine in generalized dystonia, especially in patients who are refractory to other therapies. The major drawbacks of this therapy include expense and acquisition of tetrabenazine. It is important to monitor patients for side effects, especially depression.[39–41]

Marsden and colleagues[18] proposed triple therapy, known as the Marsden cocktail, comprising a dopamine depletor (reserpine/tetrabenazine [TBZ]), a dopamine-blocking agent, and in patients with severe dystonia, the addition of an anticholinergic. TBZ and the dopamine-blocking agent slow involuntary movements; the anticholinergic is used for its antidystonic effect as well as ameliorating some drug-induced parkinsonism. Depression is not an absolute contraindication to TBZ since if efficacious, reactive depression often improves.

Clinical experience has demonstrated that the addition of lithium may ameliorate the parkinsonian and depressive effects of TBZ, while enhancing the beneficial treatment effect on dystonia. Lithium attenuates the dopamine-depleting effects of reserpine and TBZ.[42] Lithium also inhibits the calcium-dependent release of dopamine and norepinephrine, but not serotonin; in addition, it also alters the reuptake and presynaptic storage of catecholamines, thereby inactivating the amines. When used alone, lithium does not have a significant beneficial effect in patients with dystonia.

Dopamine Agonists

Dopamine agonist therapy has been studied in patients with dystonia. Most published results are case reports. In 1988, a small study conducted in two phases was completed.[43] Twenty patients with cervical dystonia were initially enrolled in the first phase, which was a single-blind trial of the dopamine agonist lisuride. Treatment was initiated at 0.1 mg/day and slowly increased over 1 month to a maximum dosage of 4 mg/day. In this phase, three patients obtained substantial and sustained clinical improvement; seven patients obtained moderate to mild transient improvement that lasted for less than 1 month. The remainder of the patients had no change or worsening of symptoms. Nine patients went on to complete the second phase of the study. This phase was a double-blind, crossover study comparing lisuride to placebo. Each arm lasted for 5 to 7 days, with a 2-day washout period. The results of the double-blind phase mirrored the results of the single-blind phase. The major side effects of dopamine agonists include nausea, fatigue, lethargy, paranoia, hallucinations, edema, mood lability, and lightheadedness. Although the results of this study were promising, the long-term efficacy of dopamine agonist therapy for the treatment of primary generalized dystonia remains undetermined. A large, double-blind, placebo-controlled trial is needed to assess long-term safety and efficacy for the treat of generalized dystonia.

Clozapine

Clozapine is a dibenzodiazepine and an atypical neuroleptic medication with a relatively high affinity for D_1 and a low affinity for D_2 receptors. Clozapine has been studied for its use in refractory psychiatric disease and was found to improve tardive dystonia in some patients. Small-sized studies have investigated clozapine's effectiveness in dystonia. One study was a pilot study designed to determine efficacy.[44] Ten patients with moderate to severe idiopathic cervical dystonia were enrolled in this study. Clozapine was initially administered at 12.5 mg/day and increased by 12.5 mg to a maximum of 100 mg/day. Patients were assessed using standardized rating scales for dystonia; videotapes were blindly rated at conclusion of the study. Subjective improvement was reported in six patients at doses of 37 mg and 62 mg per day; eight patients reported improvement at 100 mg/day. An improvement in dystonia rating scale scores was seen in two patients taking 100 mg/day of clozapine; however, the degree of improvement was not statistically significant. This study did not definitively demonstrate clinical improvement of cervical dystonia with moderate doses of clozapine.

A second study of clozapine was an open-label trial in a total of five patients, four with generalized dystonia.[45] Clozapine was initiated at 12.5 mg/day; it was then increased by 250-mg increments to a maximum dosage of 900 mg/day. Patients were treated at their maximally tolerated dose for 2 weeks and then tapered off the medication. Patients reached statistical improvement (both subjectively and objectively) with clozapine treatment.

Side effects of clozapine are common and may, in some cases, be serious. These include lightheadedness, seizures, tachycardia, sedation, myoclonus, or leukopenia. Leukopenia has been associated with fatalities while taking clozapine and patients must have weekly white blood cell counts. A literature search failed to find any subsequent cases of leukopenia or mortality since mandatory monitoring has taken effect. Clozapine may be a beneficial medication in refractory patients; however, a large double-blind, placebo-controlled trial is needed to determine its efficacy.

STATUS DYSTONICUS

Treatment of status dystonicus or dystonic storms deserves special mention. Status dystonicus occurs when a patient with generalized dystonia has an acute worsening that may become life-threatening. Complications may be caused by metabolic derangement, hyperpyrexia, or respiratory complications. Marsden and colleagues[18] described treatment with a multidrug regimen including pimozide, trihexyphenidyl or benzhexol, and tetrabenazine. Marsden used this regimen in two patients with severe generalized dystonia and improvement was seen in one patient. In this treatment regimen, patients were tried on tetrabenazine and increased up to 75 mg/day. In addition, pimozide was added until symptom management or side effects. If necessary, benzhexol or trihexyphenidyl was then added at 6–30 mg/day. Manji and colleagues[46] published a series of 12 case studies of dystonia of various etiologies with acute worsening and their subsequent treatment responses. Two of these patients were diagnosed with primary torsion dystonia. Of these two patients, one responded to high-dosage anticholinergic therapy and the second responded to the medication regimen recommended by Marsden. Although only a few case reports exist in the literature supporting this treatment regimen, it may be helpful to control life-threatening situations when standard medication regimens fail.

CONCLUSION

Generalized idiopathic dystonia may be a severely limiting illness with a varied clinical response. Unfortunately, the pathophysiology of this disorder is not completely understood. As of this publication, physicians do not have a medication specifically designed to control the symptoms of generalized dystonia. Until this goal has been met, patients

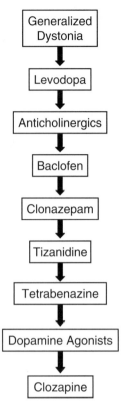

FIG. 1. Flow chart of medical therapies for generalized dystonia.

should be tried on the medications known to give the best clinical effect for generalized dystonia. A flow sheet for pharmacologic treatment of generalized dystonia may be found in Figure 1.

REFERENCES

1. Fahn S, Marsden CD, Calne DB. Classification and investigation of dystonia. In: Marsden CD, Fahn S, eds. Movement Disorders 2. London, UK: Butterworth; 1987:332–358.
2. Bressman SB. Dystonia update. *Clin Neuropharmacology.* 2000;23: 239–251.
3. Fahn S. Generalized dystonia: concept and treatment. Clin Neuropharmacol 1986;9(Suppl 2):S37–S48.
4. Marsden CD, Harrison MJG, Bundey S. Natural history of idiopathic torsion dystonia. Adv Neurol 1976;14:177–187.
5. Segawa M, Hosaka A, Miyagawa F, et al. Hereditary progressive dystonia with marked diurnal variation. Adv Neurol 1976;14:215–233.
6. Nygaard TG, Marsden CD, Duvoisin RC. Dopa-responsive dystonia. Adv Neurol 1988;50:377–384.
7. Rowland LP. Molecular basis of genetic heterogeneity: role of the clinical neurologist. J Child Neurol. 1998;13:122–132.
8. Gasser T. Idiopathic, myoclonic and dopa-responsive dystonia. Curr Opin Neurol 1997;10:357–362.
9. Ichinose H, Ohye T, Takahashi E, et al. Hereditary progressive dystonia with marked diurnal fluctuation caused by mutations in the GTP cyclohydrolase I gene. Nat Genet 1994;8:236–242.
10. Furukawa Y, Shimadzu M, Rajput AH, et al. GTP-cyclohydrolase I gene mutations in hereditary progressive and dopa-responsive dystonia. Ann Neurol 1996;39:609–617.
11. Lüdecke B, Dworniczak B, Bartholomé K. A point mutation in the tyrosine hydroxylase gene associated with Segawa's syndrome. Hum Genet 1995;95:123–125.

12. Van den Heuvel LPWJ, Luiten B, Smeitink JAM, et al. A common point mutation in the tyrosine hydroxylase gene in autosomal recessive l-dopa-responsive dystonia in the Dutch population. Hum Genet 1998;102:644–646.

13. Bräutigam C, Wevers RA, Jansen RJT, et al. Biochemical hallmarks of tyrosine hydroxylase deficiency. Clin Chem 1998;44:1897–1904.

14. Furukawa Y, Kish SJ. Dopa-responsive dystonia: recent advances and remaining issues to be addressed. Mov Disord 1999;14:709–715.

15. Nutt JG, Nygaard TG. Response to levodopa treatment in dopa-responsive dystonia. Arch Neurol 2001;58:905–910.

16. Fahn S. Treatment of dystonia with high-dosage anticholinergic medication. Neurology. 1979;29:605.

17. Fahn S. High dosage anticholinergic therapy in dystonia. Neurology. 1983;33:1255–1261.

18. Marsden CD, Marion MH, Quinn N. The treatment of severe dystonia in children and adults. J Neurol Neurosurg Psychiatry 1984;47:1166–1173.

19. Lang AE. High dose anticholinergic therapy in adult dystonia. Can J Neurol Sci 1986;13:42–46.

20. Trihexyphenidyl. In: Sifton DW, ed. Physicians' Desk Reference. Montvale NJ: Medical Economics, 2002:1855.

21. Ayd FJ. A survey of drug-induced extrapyramidal reactions. JAMA 1961;175:1054–1060.

22. Nutt JG, Hammerstad JP, de Garmo P, et al. Cranial dystonia: Double-blind crossover study of anticholinergics. Neurology 1984;34:215–217.

23. Burke RE, Fahn S, Marsden CD. Torsion dystonia: a double-blind, prospective trial of high-dosage trihexyphenidyl. Neurology. 1986;36:160–164.

24. Greene P, Shale H, Fahn S. Analysis of open-label trials in torsion dystonia using high dosages of anticholinergics and other drugs. Mov Disord 1988;3:46–60.

25. Greene P, Shale H, Fahn S. Experience with high dosages of anticholinergic and other drugs in the treatment of torsion dystonia. Adv Neurol 1988;50:547–556.

26. Davidoff RA. Antispasticity drugs: mechanism of action. Ann Neurol 1985;17:107–116.

27. Nishikawa T, Scatton B, Enomoto T, et al. Modulation of striatal serotonin metabolism by baclofen, a gamma-aminobutyric acid$_B$ receptor agonist. Tokai J Exp Clin Med 1989;14:375–380.

28. Guyenet PG, Aghajanian GK. Ach, substance P, and met encephalin in the locus coeruleus: pharmacological evidence for independent sites of action. Eur J Pharmacol 1979;53:319–328.

29. Seabrook GR, Howson W, Lacey MG. Electrophysiological characterization of potent agonists and antagonists at pre- and post-synaptic GABA$_B$ receptors on neurons in rat brain slices. Br J Pharmacol 1990;101:949–957.

30. Bowery NG, Hill DR, Hudson AL. Baclofen decreases neurotransmitter release in the mammalian CNS by an action at the novel GABA receptor. Nature 1980;283:92–94.

31. Potasher SJ. Baclofen: effects on amino acid release and metabolism in slices of guinea pig cerebral cortex. J Neurochem 1978;32:103–109.

32. Greene PE, Fahn S. Baclofen in the treatment of idiopathic dystonia in children. Mov Disord 1992;7:48–52.

33. Narayan RK, Loubster PG, Jankovic J, et al. Intrathecal baclofen for intractable axial dystonia. Neurology 1991;41:1141–1142.

34. Ford B, Green P, Louis ED, et al. Use of intrathecal baclofen in the treatment of patients with dystonia. Arch Neurol 1996;53:1241–1246.

35. Albright AL, Barry MJ, Shafron DH, et al. Intrathecal baclofen for generalized dystonia. Dev Med Child Neurol 2001;43:652–657.

36. Wagstaff AJ, Bryson HM. Tizanidine. A review of its pharmacology, clinical efficacy and tolerability in the management of spasticity associated with cerebral and spinal disorders. Drugs 1997;53(3):435–452.

37. Coward DM. Tizanidine: neuropharmacology and mechanism of action. Neurology 1994;44(11 Suppl 9):S6–S10.

38. Lang AE, Riley DE. Tizanidine in Cranial Dystonia. Clinical Neuropharmacology 1992;15(2):142–147.

39. Jankovic J. Treatment of hyperkinetic movement disorders with tetrabenazine: a double-blind crossover study. Ann Neurol 1982;11:41–47.

40. Jankovic J, Orman J. Tetrabenazine therapy of dystonia, chorea, tics and other dyskinesias. Neurology 1988;38:391–394.

41. Jankovic J, Beach J. Long-term effects of tetrabenazine in hyperkinetic movement disorders. Neurology 1997;48:358–362.

42. Reches A, Hassan MN, Jackson VR, Fahn S. Lithium attenuates dopamine depleting effects of reserpine and tetrabenazine but not that of alpha methyl-p-tyrosine. Life Sci 1983;33:157–160.

43. Teräväinen H, Calne S, Burton K, et al. Efficacy of dopamine agonists in dystonia. Adv Neurol 1988;50:571–577.

44. Burband P, Guehl D, Lagueny A, et al. A pilot trial of clozapine in the treatment of cervical dystonia. J Neurol 1998;245:329–331.

45. Karp BI, Goldstein SR, Chen R, et al. An open trial of clozapine for dystonia. Mov Disord 1999;14:652–657.

46. Manji H, Howard RS, Miller DH, et al. Status dystonicus: the syndrome and its management. Brain 1998;121:243–252.

CHAPTER 7A

Intrathecal Baclofen for Dystonia in Adults

Ruth H. Walker

INTRODUCTION

Medical therapy for dystonia remains suboptimal despite the use of oral medications with varying mechanisms of action. These medications include anticholinergic, γ-amino-butyric acid (GABA)-ergic, dopaminergic, and antidopaminergic agents. The benefits obtained with these medications are often limited by significant sedative effects.

With the development of intrathecal pump technology, direct delivery into the cerebrospinal fluid (CSF), of the GABA analogue baclofen (β-4-chlorophenyl-GABA) (Lioresal; intrathecal form manufactured by Medtronic, Minneapolis, MN) was explored, initially for spasticity,[1,2] and subsequently for severe dystonia.[3] This method enables the administration of baclofen directly into the CSF, achieving therapeutic effects with minimal sedation.[1] Clinical efficacy is seen at a plasma level of 100 times less than that necessary when given orally.[4]

After several initial positive reports, intrathecal baclofen (ITB) was administered to patients with dystonia of varying etiologies whose symptoms were not adequately controlled, or who developed intolerable side effects with maximal oral medical therapy. Some authors have reported positive results for children[5,6] and adults.[7] Other investigators report less success with ITB therapy, particularly in certain patients with specific types of symptomatic dystonia.[5,8] This chapter reviews the use of ITB and our own[9] and others' experience with ITB for dystonia in adults.

ITB FOR DYSTONIA: REVIEW OF SEVEN YEARS OF EXPERIENCE AT MOUNT SINAI MEDICAL CENTER

Between June 1993 and May 1998, 14 patients with dystonia had pumps implanted at the Movement Disorders Clinic.[9] Patients were considered for a trial dose of ITB if they had received extensive treatment for dystonia, including oral antidystonic and antispastic medications, without satisfactory control of symptoms or with unacceptable adverse effects. Patients underwent trial injections of ITB as described below. The highest dose administered during a trial was 200 μg.

Those patients who experienced a positive clinical response to trial injections of ITB proceeded to surgery and pump implantation. Exception to this practice was made in the case of a patient with severe generalized dystonia, on the premise that he might show benefit at higher ventricular CSF levels of baclofen than would be achieved with a single lumbar injection.[10] After pump placement, the dose of ITB was increased in increments of approximately 10% with each clinic visit, until the patient reported adequate improvement or dose-limiting adverse effects, or until a dose of 1,000 μg/day was achieved. Occasionally a higher dose was used when either the therapeutic effects appeared to wane because of tolerance or if additional benefit was sought. If adverse effects were reported, the dose was decreased until these symptoms resolved. The dose was then increased again in smaller increments to optimize the dose. After the highest tolerated dose had been determined, the dose was decreased in the same decrements to determine the lowest dose that produced maximal symptom reduction. Patients were videotaped prior to pump implantation and after dose optimization, and rated using the Burke-Fahn-Marsden Rating Scale (BFM)[11] by a rater blinded to the patient's treatment status.

Mean length of therapy with ITB was 41 months, with a range of 6–87 months. Mean dose for those patients who continued on ITB therapy was 658 μg/day, with a range of 90–1,300 μg/day. Frequently, worsening symptoms prompted dose increases.

Primary Dystonia

Fourteen patients with the *DYT1* mutation were screened with a trial dose of ITB. Nine of these patients proceeded to pump implantation (eight with generalized dystonia and one with idiopathic cranial segmental dystonia). A decrease in

Department of Neurology, Bronx Veterans Affairs Medical Center, Bronx, New York and Mount Sinai Medical Center, New York, New York.

The author has no commercial relationship to disclose.

BFM scores was seen in only three patients. Two of those patients whose scores decreased subsequently had the dose tapered and the pump removed without exacerbation of symptoms. Two patients reported subjective improvements that were not reflected in BFM scores. Three participants demonstrated a mild worsening of BFM scores with ITB treatment. Only one patient had reported benefit from oral baclofen; however, she did not respond to ITB.

Five patients had their pumps removed, subsequent either to complications or demonstration of lack of efficacy. One patient committed suicide. Three patients continued with ITB therapy.

Secondary Dystonia

Seven patients with symptomatic dystonia were screened with ITB. Five proceeded to pump implantation. Four patients had generalized dystonia, one case each because of perinatal hypoxia, presumed tardive dystonia, putaminal degeneration of unknown etiology,[12] and of unknown etiology associated with complex partial seizures. One patient had upper extremity tardive dystonia and akathisia.

The most significant effect was seen in the patient with upper extremity tardive dystonia, who had a dramatic improvement of his dystonia and akathisia, as reflected by the decrease in his BFM scores (22.5 to 1.5). Two patients reported subjective benefits that were not reflected in BFM scores.

One patient had her pump removed after complications and demonstration of lack of benefit. One patient died of cardiac causes unrelated to ITB. Three patients continued with ITB therapy.

USE OF ITB

The Intrathecal Pump

The intrathecal pump (SynchroMed EL infusion system; Medtronic) weighs 185 g, with a diameter of 70 mm and thickness of 27 mm. The exact site of implantation is individualized for each patient. The site depends upon body habitus; the location is usually the lateral lower abdomen (Fig. 1). The pump is inserted through a small incision into a subcutaneous pocket. Using a separate incision over the lumbar spine, the catheter is inserted into the lower thoracic intrathecal space and tunneled anteriorly to connect with the pump (Fig. 2). Optimal placement of the pump can help minimize physical stresses on the catheter.[13] The rate of infusion is programmed noninvasively by radiotelemetry with the programmer head held over the pump. The 20-mL reservoir containing the baclofen solution may be accessed for emptying or refilling through a port located in the center of the pump. Solutions are added or removed under sterile conditions using the specially designed refill kit containing a syringe, filter, tubing, template, and a needle that is used to pierce the skin and the membrane over the pump's refill port.

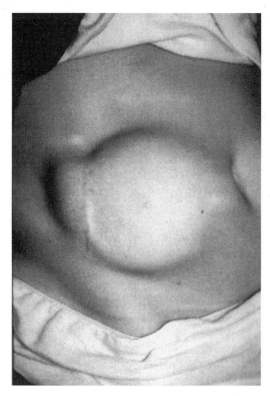

FIG. 1. Pump *in situ.*

The needle has its aperture on the side, similar to a sewing needle, thus, with each refill, it pierces the pump membrane without coring out a piece of the membrane, as would happen with a standard needle.

Three concentrations of baclofen are available; 50 μg/mL, 500 μg/mL, and 2000 μg/mL. The 50 μg/mL concentration is used for the trial dose and 500 μg/mL is used for initiation of therapy and maintenance at rates of less than approximately 300 μg/day. The frequency of refills may be every 3 to 4 weeks, up to every 3 months, depending on the infusion rate. The manufacturer recommends that the pump solution be changed at a minimum of every 3 months to avoid stasis of fluid in the pump and to minimize the potential for bacterial growth.

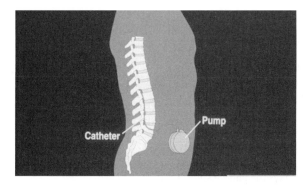

FIG. 2. Diagram of localization of pump and catheter.

Determining Response to ITB

Prior to the therapeutic trial, informed consent is obtained and the potential risks are fully discussed. The trial dose of ITB may range from 25–100 μg, depending on the patient's habitus and the etiology of dystonia.[4] Using a customary sterile lumbar puncture technique, an appropriate volume (typically 0.5–2 mL) of 50 μg/mL ITB is instilled into the lumbar intrathecal space. The patient is observed for 2–8 hours, with regular monitoring of symptoms and for signs of overdose. Peak effect is usually seen 30–60 minutes after injection. Ideally, the procedure should be repeated several times at intervals of not less than 24 hours, with some injections being either placebo or sham injections. Patients score their dystonia on a visual analogue scale and a dyskinesia rating scale,[14] and preferably should be rated by a blinded observer on videotape.[14] Day-to-day fluctuations of symptom severity may be a confounding factor and may necessitate repeat testing to confirm the reproducibility of the response. If there are no significant side effects and either no response or equivocal benefit, the trial may be repeated. In the next trial the dose is usually increased by 25 μg. If there is no benefit and there are significant side effects, the trial should not be repeated. If the patient has a positive response in terms of reduction in symptoms (regardless of whether it is quantitatively satisfactory, because dosage will be optimized during continuous infusion), pump implantation may be considered.

Although the manufacturers recommend using a dose not higher than 100 μg,[4] lack of response to a single bolus does not necessarily rule out a positive response to continuous ITB infusion because the drug may not reach effective concentrations within the neuraxis after a single lumbar puncture test dose.[10] Intrathecal infusion via an externalized catheter has been suggested as an option for screening patients, however, this procedure carries a risk of infection.[6] In view of the observation that patients with dystonia appear to require higher doses of ITB than those with spasticity,[9,15] the length of time required to reach a dose at which benefit may occur might expose the patient to a significant risk of meningitis.

Complications of trial dose administration can include sedation, ataxia, hypotension, nausea and vomiting, and treatment is supportive. Physostigmine may be used with some benefit, or removal of large volumes of CSF (see below).

Dose Titration

After initial placement, the pump is filled with the 500 μg/mL concentration of baclofen and programmed to deliver a total of twice the effective trial dose over 24 hours. If the patient showed a sustained response to the trial dose, this dose should be delivered over 24 hours.[4]

Thereafter, the rate is increased by 5–15%, with a time interval between increases of not less than 24 hours. For the first few days the patient should be carefully monitored in an inpatient setting, but subsequent adjustments can be performed in the outpatient clinic, and rate increases performed, for example, at weekly visits. Rate increases are stopped when the patient reports dose-limiting adverse effects, satisfactory control of symptoms, or a dose of 1,000 μg/day is achieved. After the maximum dose has been identified, a slow taper may be performed to determine the minimum effective dose. A dose of 1,000 μg/day is the maximum practical dose and necessitates pump refills every 4 weeks. In exceptional circumstances higher rates may be used, for example, if a patient who previously showed a good response has an exacerbation of symptoms resulting from disease progression or the development of tolerance. However, it should be noted that any sudden change in dose requirements may be indicative of a mechanical problem, such as a leaking or dislodged catheter.

The Medtronic intrathecal pump is designed to infuse its contents under a variety of programs. These include a continuous infusion or a complex dosing cycle, with different infusion rates at specific times of the day. For instance, when treating spasticity, patients may require a lower dose during the day, when increased lower extremity tone is needed in order to bear weight, and a higher infusion rate at night to treat painful nocturnal spasms. This complex dosing feature may also be used to increase the overall exposure to baclofen and avoid dose-limiting side effects during the day. For instance, a patient may receive 1,200 μg/day (50 μg/hr) with associated benefit but mild sedation. The pump could be reprogrammed to deliver 40 μg/hr for 16 hours and 70 μg/hr for 8 hours during sleep, when the sedative effects would be less troublesome.

Development of Tolerance

Lack of sustained clinical benefit, despite an apparently positive response to a test dose of ITB, may be explained by the development of tolerance, although as noted above, mechanical problems interfering with drug delivery need to be excluded. It may also be difficult to distinguish tolerance from an increase in symptom severity. In some cases, an increase in dose may be required to maintain benefit. Ford and coworkers[15] reported treating four patients with doses higher than 1,000 μg/day, with a maximal rate of 1,500 μg/day. We used a maximal dose of 1300 μg/day in one patient, although this was subsequently tapered to 1,000 μg/day. Some centers currently use an arbitrary practical maximal dose of 1,000 μg/day, necessitating a refill every four weeks. If higher drug concentrations become available, it may be possible to supersede this dose.

Progressive tolerance to ITB has been demonstrated in patients with spasticity,[16] and may be related to downregulation of $GABA_b$ receptors in the spinal cord, as demonstrated in a rat model.[17] A similar process may occur in dystonia. Drug holidays may be one mechanism of resensitizing receptors. Intrathecal fentanyl has been demonstrated to reduce spasticity in the presence of tolerance to baclofen[18]; however, this approach has not been reported in dystonia. Indeed, there may be a rationale for avoiding fentanyl and related agents in dystonia as they have been reported to cause dystonia.[19–22]

Disease Progression

Progression of disease may be a confounding factor when monitoring patient response and may mask a benefit from ITB. Longitudinal studies of dystonia symptoms have not been performed, but the disease is typically slowly progressive, although in occasional cases symptoms may remit. Symptoms may vary from day to day for idiopathic reasons, or in response to environmental stressors including psychological factors. Disease progression and the therapeutic effect of ITB may be assessed by slow, preferably double-blinded, tapering of ITB.[9] If the taper is performed too rapidly, there may be rebound exacerbation of symptoms as part of a withdrawal syndrome.[23]

Complications

Patients and treating physicians must be educated regarding the risks of ITB therapy because there is significant potential for morbidity and mortality related to baclofen withdrawal[24–29] or overdose.[30] During long-term infusion, patients should understand the importance of returning for regular pump refills. In particular, they should be educated regarding symptoms that may suggest infection, overdose, or withdrawal.

Signs of withdrawal include worsening dystonia, muscle spasm and rigidity, itching, and tachycardia, and may mimic sepsis or neuroleptic malignant syndrome.[24–29] Therapy is supportive and symptomatic. Oral baclofen may be given but is not always be helpful.[28] Intravenous benzodiazepines and general anesthesia may be required.

Signs of overdose include sedation, ataxia, hypotension, nausea, vomiting, and at high doses, respiratory depression, coma, and seizures, and treatment is supportive. Physostigmine (intravenous; 2 mg given over 2 minutes or intramuscular) has been used anecdotally,[31,32] and is recommended by the manufacturer for overdose[4] but may not always be efficacious.[33] It may also be beneficial to perform a lumbar puncture to remove large volumes of CSF.

Operator errors, such as inappropriate pump programming or refilling the reservoir with the wrong concentration of drug, may result in high morbidity or death.[24] A variety of equipment-related complications have been reported. These include infection, catheter fracture (Fig. 3), migration or kinking, pump or battery malfunction, and wound dehiscence.[9,23,34–38] Improvements in technology as well as education and experience of the patient and the health care provider may reduce the occurrence of these events in the future, although they continue to be a significant issue even after several years experience. Position-dependent leakage and microfractures of the catheter can pose a challenge to troubleshooting, even with the use of radio-opaque or radionuclide tracers.[39–41]

In the study by Walker et al.,[9] one patient with dystonia who was receiving ITB committed suicide. He had general-

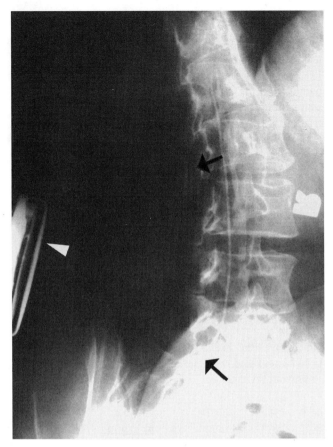

FIG. 3. Oblique lateral radiograph of lumbar spine showing fractured catheter, with broken ends indicated by arrows, and pump (arrowhead).

ized idiopathic dystonia and experienced a severe personal psychological trauma but was not noted to be depressed before this event. Another patient in our study who received ITB also committed suicide. He had progressive debility secondary to multiple sclerosis, which is associated with an increased risk of suicide. There was no evidence of depression related to ITB in other study patients, nor has this problem been reported in the literature, however, neuropsychiatric status was not specifically assessed. Because of our experience, we recommend that patients receiving ITB should be monitored for signs and symptoms of depression.

ITB may exacerbate hyperkinetic movements as reported in a case of secondary dystonia due to a metabolic disorder.[8] Oral baclofen has also been reported to cause dyskinesias in a patient with spinal spasticity.[42] In our series, we observed small increases in BFM scores in five patients receiving ITB that were not clinically significant.[9]

DISCUSSION

ITB for Dystonia

There are a number of reports of successful ITB therapy in selected cases, both pediatric and adult, with intractable dystonia from a variety of causes, including the *DYT1* mutation,[9] reflex sympathetic dystrophy,[43] parkinsonism,[15] pantothen-ate kinase-associated neurodegeneration (Hallervorden-Spatz disease),[5,32] chromosome 18p deletion,[44] stroke,[45] head injury,[46] cerebral palsy,[3,5,47] Friedreich's ataxia,[9] striatal necrosis,[48] and tardive dystonia.[9,49] The largest series of successful treatments were of patients with secondary dystonia who had a significant component of spasticity caused by head injury or stroke.[5,45,46] Albright and coworkers[5,6] (and this publication) have reported a number of successfully treated pediatric patients with dystonic cerebral palsy.

Two small series (13 patients[15] and 10 patients[50]) reported adults with primary or secondary dystonia who underwent pump implantation. (One patient from the former study[15] was included in our report.[9]) These studies confirm our findings of no consistent or predictable significant effect on dystonia symptoms with ITB. Some patients report a subjective benefit in the absence of an objective improvement. This may have been due either to a placebo effect or to insensitivity of the BFM rating scale to those domains that improved. It may be helpful for all patients receiving ITB to undergo dose optimization including blinded dose adjustments, to clarify if the patient is indeed deriving benefit from this therapy.

The underlying etiology of a patient's dystonia or their *DYT1* status was not predictive of the response to ITB. Patients with primary and secondary dystonia of varying etiologies responded or failed. The most striking improvement was in the patient with tardive dystonia,[9] as has been reported by others.[49]

There appears to have been more success in patients with dystonia in whom spasticity is also a significant component, for example, secondary to stroke,[45] head injury,[46] cerebral palsy,[3,5,47] and Friedreich's ataxia.[9] The presence of spasticity complicates objective assessment and may be difficult to distinguish from the dystonic component on clinical examination. However, dystonia in which spasticity is a significant feature may respond better to ITB, possibly because of a common mechanism in the spinal cord.

Site of Action of Baclofen in Dystonia

GABA$_b$ receptors, at which baclofen is known to act, are found throughout the mammalian central nervous system,[51] and are especially numerous in the basal ganglia. They are present both presynaptically and postsynaptically in the substantia nigra,[52,53] and have been shown to influence the activity of dopaminergic neurons.[54–57] Although the underlying pathophysiology of dystonia is not yet known, there is increasing evidence for dysfunction of substantia nigra dopaminergic neurons in humans with DYT1 dystonia,[58–60] making this a possible site of drug action.

Another potential site of therapeutic action of baclofen is at the level of cortical GABA$_b$ receptors. Cortical excitability, as demonstrated by transcranial magnetic stimulation, appears to be abnormally increased in dystonia[61,62] and may be reduced by ITB.[63]

Baclofen has been shown to have a presynaptic effect on descending pathways in the spinal cord, reducing excitatory neurotransmitter release.[64] It is likely that this is the site of therapeutic action in spasticity, and this mechanism may also play a role in patients in whom dystonia is combined with spasticity.

ITB for Other Neurologic Conditions

ITB is an accepted effective therapy for patients with spasticity of spinal and cerebral origins as a result of a variety of causes, including cerebral palsy, spinal cord injury, head injury, stroke, transverse myelitis, syringomyelia, spinal ischemia, hereditary spastic paraparesis, X-linked adrenoleukodystrophy, tropical paraplegia, amyotrophic lateral sclerosis, and multiple sclerosis. Significant benefit has been demonstrated as reductions in tone and spasticity,[37,65–67] quality of life, activities of daily living, level of function, and cost effectiveness.[65,67–72]

ITB has also been reported to be effective in a number of other neurological disorders, including stiff-person syndrome,[7,24,73–77] tetanus,[78–80] painful legs/moving toes,[7] Friedreich's ataxia,[9,37] noncortical myoclonus,[81,82] complex regional pain syndrome,[83] dysautonomia,[84] and Wilson's disease.[7]

SUMMARY

Clinical experience with ITB for adults with dystonia suggests that this therapy may be helpful for select patients who have unsatisfactory control of symptoms or intolerable side effects with maximal medical therapy. Unfortunately, it is not yet possible to determine in advance who will benefit from long-term infusion and who will not. Review of the literature suggests that ITB may be more helpful in patients with spasticity in addition to dystonia rather than dystonia alone.

Equipment-related complications are relatively common. These may be serious and limit therapy, and these complications may necessitate further invasive procedures. Development of tolerance may be a significant problem; some patients may be unable to achieve the apparent benefit they attained with the trial dose. Other complicating factors requiring further study are the difficulty in distinguishing the development of tolerance from progression of disease and the day-to-day fluctuations in symptoms.

For patients with dystonia who have failed maximal oral medical therapy, double-blinded intrathecal testing is recommended as the most objective method of determining initial responsiveness. Once ITB therapy has been established, dose optimization, which may include blinded dose reduction when practical, is suggested to determine sustained efficacy.

REFERENCES

1. Penn RD, Kroin JS. Intrathecal baclofen alleviates spinal cord spasticity. Lancet 1984;1:1078.

2. Dralle D, Muller H, Zierski J, Klug N. Intrathecal baclofen for spasticity. Lancet 1985;2:1003.
3. Narayan RK, Loubser PG, Jankovic J, et al. Intrathecal baclofen for intractable axial dystonia. Neurology 1991;41:1141–1142.
4. Lioresal Intrathecal [package insert]. Minneapolis, MN, Medtronic, Inc.; 2003.
5. Albright AL, Barry MJ, Fasick P, et al. Continuous intrathecal baclofen infusion for symptomatic generalized dystonia. Neurosurgery 1996;38:934–938; discussion 938–939.
6. Albright AL, Barry MJ, Shafton DH, et al. Intrathecal baclofen for generalized dystonia. Dev Med Child Neurol 2001;43:652–657.
7. Penn RD, Gianino JM, York MM. Intrathecal baclofen for motor disorders. Mov Disord 1995;10:675–677.
8. Silbert PL, Stewart-Wynne EG. Increased dystonia after intrathecal baclofen. Neurology 1992;42:1639–1640.
9. Walker RH, Danisi FO, Swope DM, et al. Intrathecal baclofen for dystonia: benefits and complications during six years experience. Mov Disord 2000;15:1242–1247.
10. Kroin JS, Ali A, York M, et al. The distribution of medication along the spinal canal after chronic intrathecal administration. Neurosurgery 1993;33:226–230.
11. Burke RE, Fahn S, Marsden CD, et al. Validity and reliability of a rating scale for the primary torsion dystonias. Neurology 1985;35:73–77.
12. Walker RH, Purohit DP, Good PF, et al. Severe generalized dystonia due to primary putaminal degeneration: case report and review of the literature. Mov Disord 2002;17:576–584.
13. Dickerman RD, Stevens QE, Schneider SJ. The role of surgical placement and pump orientation in intrathecal pump system failure: a technical report. Pediatr Neurosurg 2003;38:107–109.
14. van Hilten JJ, Hoff JI, Thang MC, et al. Clinimetric issues of screening for responsiveness to intrathecal baclofen in dystonia. J Neural Transm 1999;106:931–941.
15. Ford B, Greene P, Louis ED, et al. Use of intrathecal baclofen in the treatment of patients with dystonia. Arch Neurol 1996;53:1241–1246.
16. Akman MN, Loubser PG, Donovan WH, et al. Intrathecal baclofen: does tolerance occur? Paraplegia 1993;31:516–520.
17. Kroin JS, Bianchi GD, Penn RD. Intrathecal baclofen down-regulates GABA(B) receptors in the rat substantia-gelatinosa. J Neurosurg 1993;79:544–549.
18. Chabal C, Jacobson L, Schwid HA. An objective comparison of intrathecal lidocaine versus fentanyl for the treatment of lower extremity spasticity. Anesthesiology 1991;74:643–646.
19. Dehring DJ, Gupta B, Peruzzi WT. Postoperative opisthotonus and torticollis after fentanyl, enflurane, and nitrous oxide. Can J Anaesth 1991;38:919–925.
20. Khan ZH. Dystonic movements following thalamonal and alfentanil induction: a case report. Middle East J Anesthesiol 1998;14:281–286.
21. Stemp LI, Taswell C. Spastic torticollis during general anesthesia: case report and review of receptor mechanisms. Anesthesiology 1991;75:365–366.
22. Weinger MB, Swerdlow NR, Millar WL. Acute postoperative delirium and extrapyramidal signs in a previously healthy parturient. Anesth Analg 1988;67:291–295.
23. Siegfried RN, Jacobson L, Chabal C. Development of an acute withdrawal syndrome following the cessation of intrathecal baclofen in a patient with spasticity. Anesthesiology 1992;77:1048–1050.
24. Meinck HM, Tronnier V, Rieke K, et al. Intrathecal baclofen treatment for stiff-man syndrome: pump failure may be fatal. Neurology 1994;44:2209–2210.
25. Samson-Fang L, Gooch J, Norlin C. Intrathecal baclofen withdrawal simulating neuroepileptic malignant syndrome in a child with cerebral palsy. Dev Med Child Neurol 2000;42:561–565.
26. Alden TD, Lytle RA, Park TS, et al. Intrathecal baclofen withdrawal: a case report and review of the literature. Childs Nerv Syst 2002;18:522–525.
27. Kao LW, Amin Y, Kirk MA, et al. Intrathecal baclofen withdrawal mimicking sepsis. J Emerg Med 2003;24:423–427.
28. Greenberg MI, Hendrickson RG. Baclofen withdrawal following removal of an intrathecal baclofen pump despite oral baclofen replacement. J Toxicol Clin Toxicol 2003;41:83–85.
29. Coffey RJ, Edgar TS, Francisco GE, et al. Abrupt withdrawal from intrathecal baclofen: recognition and management of a potentially life-threatening syndrome. Arch Phys Med Rehabil 2002;83:735–741.
30. Anderson KJ, Farmer JP, Brown K. Reversible coma in children after improper baclofen pump insertion. Paediatr Anaesth 2002;12:454–460.
31. Muller-Schwefe G, Penn RD. Physostigmine in the treatment of intrathecal baclofen overdose. Report of three cases. J Neurosurg 1989;71:273–275.
32. Delhaas EM, Brouwers JR. Intrathecal baclofen overdose: report of 7 events in 5 patients and review of the literature. Int J Clin Pharmacol Ther Toxicol 1991;29:274–280.
33. Saltuari L, Baumgartner H, Kofler M, et al. Failure of physostigmine in treatment of acute severe intrathecal baclofen intoxication. N Engl J Med 1990;322:1533–1534.
34. Penn RD. Intrathecal baclofen for spasticity of spinal origin: seven years of experience. J Neurosurg 1992;77:236–240.
35. Teddy P, Jamous A, Gardner B, et al. Complications of intrathecal baclofen delivery. Br J Neurosurg 1992;6:115–118.
36. Coffey RJ, Cahill D, Steers W, et al. Intrathecal baclofen for intractable spasticity of spinal origin: results of a long-term multicenter study. J Neurosurg 1993;78:226–232.
37. Patterson VH, Watt M, Byrnes D, et al. Management of severe spasticity with intrathecal baclofen delivered by a manually operated pump. J Neurol Neurosurg Psychiatry 1994;57:582–585.
38. Gooch JL, Sandell TV. Botulinum toxin for spasticity and athetosis in children with cerebral palsy. Arch Phys Med Rehabil 1996;77:508–511.
39. Dickerman RD, Schneider SJ. Recurrent intrathecal baclofen pump catheter leakage: a surgical observation with recommendations. J Pediatr Surg 2002;37:E17.
40. Bardutzky J, Tronnier V, Schwab S, et al. Intrathecal baclofen for stiff-person syndrome: life-threatening intermittent catheter leakage. Neurology 2003;60:1976–1978.
41. Dawes WJ, Drake JM, Fehlings D. Microfracture of a baclofen pump catheter with intermittent under- and overdose. Pediatr Neurosurg 2003;39:144–148.
42. Ryan DM, Blumenthal FS. Baclofen-induced dyskinesia. Arch Phys Med Rehabil 1993;74:766–767.
43. van Hilten BJ, van de Beek WJ, Hoff JI, et al. Intrathecal baclofen for the treatment of dystonia in patients with reflex sympathetic dystrophy. N Engl J Med 2000;343:625–630.
44. Awaad Y, Munoz S, Nigro M. Progressive dystonia in a child with chromosome 18p deletion, treated with intrathecal baclofen. J Child Neurol 1999;14:75–77.
45. Meythaler JM, Guin-Renfroe S, Hadley MN. Continuously infused intrathecal baclofen for spastic/dystonic hemiplegia: a preliminary report. Am J Phys Med Rehabil 1999;78:247–254.
46. Meythaler JM, Guin-Renfroe S, Grabb P, et al. Long-term continuously infused intrathecal baclofen for spastic-dystonic hypertonia in traumatic brain injury: 1-year experience. Arch Phys Med Rehabil 1999;80:13–19.
47. Albright AL, Barry MJ, Painter MJ, et al. Infusion of intrathecal baclofen for generalized dystonia in cerebral palsy. J Neurosurg 1998;88:73–76.
48. Green C, Riley DE. Treatment of dystonia in striatal necrosis caused by Mycoplasma pneumoniae. Pediatr Neurol 2002;26:318–320.
49. Dressler D, Oeljeschlager RO, Ruther E. Severe tardive dystonia: treatment with continuous intrathecal baclofen administration. Mov Disord 1997;12:585–587.
50. Hou JG, Ondo W, Jankovic J. Intrathecal baclofen for dystonia. Mov Disord 2001;16:1201–1202.
51. Bowery NG, Hudson AL, Price GW. GABA A and GABA B receptor site distribution in the rat central nervous system. Neuroscience 1987;20:365–383.
52. Watts AE, Hicks GA, Henderson G. Putative pre- and postsynaptic ATP-sensitive potassium channels in the rat substantia nigra in vitro. J Neurosci 1995;15:3065–3074.
53. Lacey MG, Mercuri NB, North RA. On the potassium conductance increase activated by GABAB and dopamine D2 receptors in rat substantia nigra neurones. J Physiol (Lond) 1988;401:437–453.
54. Engberg G, Klingpetersen T, Nissbrandt H. GABA(B)-receptor activation alters the firing pattern of dopamine neurons in the rat substantia nigra. Synapse 1993;15:229–238.
55. Engberg G, Nissbrandt H. gamma-Hydroxybutyric acid (GHBA) induces pacemaker activity and inhibition of substantia nigra dopamine neurons by activating GABAB- receptors. Naunyn Schmiedebergs Arch Pharmacol 1993;348:491–497.
56. Tepper JM, Martin LP, Anderson DR. GABAA receptor-mediated inhibition of rat substantia nigra dopaminergic neurons by pars reticulata projection neurons. J Neurosci 1995;15:3092–3103.

57. Tepper JM, Paladini CA, Celada P. GABAergic control of the firing pattern of substantia nigra dopaminergic neurons. Adv Pharmacol 1998;42:694–699.

58. Augood SJ, Hollingsworth Z, Albers DS, et al. Dopamine transmission in DYT1 dystonia: a biochemical and autoradiographical study. Neurology 2002;59:445–448.

59. Rostasy K, Augood SJ, Hewett JW, et al. TorsinA protein and neuropathology in early onset generalized dystonia with GAG deletion. Neurobiol Dis 2003;12:11–24.

60. Perlmutter JS, Stambuk MK, Markham J, et al. Decreased [18F]spiperone binding in putamen in dystonia. Adv Neurol 1998;78:161–168.

61. Ikoma K, Samii A, Mercuri B, et al. Abnormal cortical motor excitability in dystonia. Neurology 1996;46:1371–1376.

62. Ridding MC, Sheean G, Rothwell JC, et al. Changes in the balance between motor cortical excitation and inhibition in focal, task specific dystonia. J Neurol Neurosurg Psychiatry 1995;59:493–498.

63. Siebner HR, Dressnandt J, Auer C, et al. Continuous intrathecal baclofen infusions induced a marked increase of the transcranially evoked silent period in a patient with generalized dystonia. Muscle Nerve 1998;21:1209–1212.

64. Bowery NG, Hill DR, Hudson AL, et al. Baclofen decreases neurotransmitter release in the mammalian CNS by an action at a novel GABA receptor. Nature 1980;283:92–94.

65. Penn RD, Savoy SM, Corcos DM. Intrathecal baclofen for severe spinal spasticity: a double-blind crossover study. N Engl J Med 1989;320:1517–1521.

66. Lazorthes Y, Sallerin-Caute B, Verdie JC, et al. Chronic intrathecal baclofen administration for control of severe spasticity. J Neurosurg 1990;72:393–402.

67. Hugenholtz H, Nelson RF, Dehoux E, et al. Intrathecal baclofen for intractable spinal spasticity: a double-blind cross-over comparison with placebo in 6 patients. Can J Neurol Sci 1992;19:188–195.

68. Meythaler JM, Steers WD, Tuel SM, et al. Continuous intrathecal baclofen in spinal cord spasticity. A prospective study. Am J Phys Med Rehabil 1992;71:321–327.

69. Becker WJ, Harris CJ, Long ML, et al. Long-term intrathecal baclofen therapy in patients with intractable spasticity. Can J Neurol Sci 1995;22:208–217.

70. Nance P, Schryvers O, Schmidt B, et al. Intrathecal baclofen therapy for adults with spinal spasticity: therapeutic efficacy and effect on hospital admissions. Can J Neurol Sci 1995;22:22–29.

71. Concalves J, Garcia-March G, Sanchez-Ledesma MJ, et al. Management of intractable spasticity of supraspinal origin by chronic cervical intrathecal infusion of baclofen. Stereotact Funct Neurosurg 1994;62:108–112.

72. Gianino JM, York MM, Paice JA, et al. Quality of life: effect of reduced spasticity from intrathecal baclofen. J Neurosci Nurs 1998;30:47–54.

73. Ford B, Fahn S. Intrathecal baclofen. Neurology 1994;44:1367–1368.

74. Penn RD, Mangieri EA. Stiff-man syndrome treated with intrathecal baclofen. Neurology 1993;43:2412.

75. Silbert PL, Matsumoto JY, Mcmanis PG, et al. Intrathecal baclofen therapy in stiff-man syndrome: a double-blind, placebo-controlled trial. Neurology 1995;45:1893–1897.

76. Stayer C, Tronnier V, Dressnandt J, et al. Intrathecal baclofen therapy for stiff-man syndrome and progressive encephalomyelopathy with rigidity and myoclonus. Neurology 1997;49:1591–1597.

77. Seitz RJ, Blank B, Kiwit JC, et al. Stiff-person syndrome with antiglutamic acid decarboxylase autoantibodies: complete remission of symptoms after intrathecal baclofen administration. J Neurol 1995;242:618–622.

78. Brock H, Moosbauer W, Gabriel C, et al. Treatment of severe tetanus by continuous intrathecal infusion of baclofen [letter]. J Neurol Neurosurg Psychiatry 1995;59:193–194.

79. Dressnandt J, Konstanzer A, Weinzierl FX, et al. Intrathecal baclofen in tetanus: four cases and a review of reported cases. Intensive Care Med 1997;23:896–902.

80. Engrand N, Guerot E, Rouamba A, et al. The efficacy of intrathecal baclofen in severe tetanus. Anesthesiology 1999;90:1773–1776.

81. Fouillet N, Wiart L, Arne P, et al. Propriospinal myoclonus in tetraplegic patients: clinical, electrophysiological and therapeutic aspects. Paraplegia 1995;33:678–681.

82. Olson WL, Morassutti DJ. Noncortical myoclonus: an experience with intrathecal baclofen. Neurology 2000;54(Suppl 3):A51.

83. Zuniga RE, Perera S, Abram SE. Intrathecal baclofen: a useful agent in the treatment of well-established complex regional pain syndrome. Reg Anesth Pain Med 2002;27:90–93.

84. Cuny E, Richer E, Castel JP. Dysautonomia syndrome in the acute recovery phase after traumatic brain injury: relief with intrathecal baclofen therapy. Brain Inj 2001;15:917–925.

CHAPTER 7B

Intrathecal Therapy for Dystonia in Children

A. Leland Albright

INTRODUCTION

Although dystonia in children and adolescents may affect only one or two body regions, it is more often generalized, affecting all or nearly all regions of the body. That generalized distribution may be because the most common causes of dystonia in children (e.g., cerebral palsy and head injury) affect large areas of the brain. Whether the dystonia is primary, secondary, or associated with a neurodegenerative condition, it often causes progressive disability, discomfort, and deformity.

Childhood dystonia is usually generalized, therefore, its treatment needs to have generalized effects similar to those observed with systemic medications. The commonly used oral medications for children and adolescents include baclofen (Lioresal, Novartis Pharmaceuticals Canada, Inc., Dorval, Quebec), trihexiphenidyl (Artane, Wyeth Pharmaceuticals, Collegeville, PA), clonazepam (Klonopin, Roche, Nutley, NJ), and l-dopa (Sinemet, Merck Sharp Dohme, Auckland, New Zealand). Those medications improve dystonia in 25–30% of individuals but improve it substantially in fewer, perhaps 5–10%. Oral medications are sometimes augmented with intramuscular botulinum toxin injections. Botulinum toxin therapy treats only the injected muscles in regions of the body; therefore, these injections are less beneficial in patients with generalized dystonia than they are in patients with focal dystonia.

After the administration of many oral medications, penetration of the drugs into the cerebrospinal fluid (CSF) is impeded by the blood-brain barrier. However, when medications are injected directly into the CSF, the resulting concentrations are many times higher (e.g., 100x) than after the administration of oral doses. Thus, intrathecal medications often produce substantially greater clinical effects, with fewer side effects than oral medications.

The treatment of dystonia with intrathecal medications is

Department of Pediatric Neurosurgery, Children's Hospital of Pittsburgh, Department of Neurosurgery, University of Pittsburgh School of Medicine, Pittsburgh, Pennsylvania.

The author is a consultant to Medtronic, Inc., Minneapolis, MN.

relatively new. The first case report was by Narayan et al. in 1991.[1] Narayan and coworkers treated an 18-year-old man with symptomatic generalized dystonia. This patient had been unresponsive to oral medications; however, a substantial improvement was observed with intrathecal baclofen (ITB). Since 1991, several authors have reported their experiences with ITB to treat dystonia, particularly generalized dystonia. There are a few reports of intrathecal morphine or clonidine to treat patients with dystonia. Ford et al.[2] treated two dystonic patients with intrathecal morphine; one patient later underwent a thalamotomy. Ford and his colleagues have treated several persons who became unresponsive to ITB. These patients were treated with mixtures of baclofen and morphine as well as with mixtures of baclofen and clonidine. No significant improvement was observed in any patient. Thus, the predominant intrathecal medication is baclofen. This is true in children as well as in adults.

PHARMACOLOGY OF BACLOFEN

Baclofen (β-4-chloro-phenyl-GABA) is a GABA agonist that acts primarily at $GABA_b$ receptors.[3] Oral baclofen is absorbed rapidly into the bloodstream, achieving plasma levels of 275 ng/mL. However, because of the blood-brain barrier, corresponding CSF levels are less than 12 ng/mL.[4] Intrathecal administration of 400 μg/day of baclofen results in CSF levels of approximately 400 ng/mL.[5] The half-life of intrathecal baclofen is approximately 4 hours.[6] Baclofen is cleared from the CSF by bulk flow at a rate of 30 mL/hr, which is approximately the CSF clearance rate.[7] After injection of baclofen into the lumbar CSF, baclofen concentrations decrease cephalad; concentrations at the craniovertebral level are approximately one-fourth those in the lumbar region.[8]

RATIONALE FOR ITB IN DYSTONIA

Baclofen is known to work at many sites in the central nervous system (CNS). It works in the superficial layers of the spinal cord by impeding the release of excitatory neurotransmitters such as glutamate.[9] In the brain, baclofen:

- Increases serotonin levels in the basal ganglia;
- Decreases dopamine release in the striatum;
- Inhibits noradrenergic neurons in the locus caeruleus;
- Hyperpolarizes neurons in the substantia nigra pars compacta; and
- Increases metabolism of the inhibitory neurotransmitter glycine.[10–14]

The mechanism by which baclofen affects dystonia is not known. It is probably related to baclofen's GABA-ergic activity at a cortical level, a spinal level, or both.

One hallmark of dystonia is simultaneous contraction of agonist and antagonist muscles. This may occur because of insufficient reciprocal inhibition at the brain stem and spinal cord levels. Baclofen might work at a spinal level to decrease the release of excitatory neurotransmitters, which cause simultaneous contractions. However, when ITB is given in bolus doses, spasticity improves. Bolus doses have considerably less of an effect on dystonia. Baclofen might also work at a cortical level, entering the intracranial subarachnoid space and migrating upward over the convexities. Once there, baclofen could inhibit the excessively stimulated premotor and supplementary cortex.

The current pathophysiologic model of dystonia proposes a lack of cortical inhibition. Continuous intrathecal infusion of baclofen does not improve dystonia within 2–4 hours, as it does in spasticity. Improvement is typically observed in 2–3 days, which is long enough for the medication to get up over the convexities. Dystonia also requires higher doses than in spasticity; these relatively higher doses would be needed to achieve therapeutic concentrations over the convexities. This also indicates that baclofen may be acting at a cortical level.

PATIENT SELECTION

Ideally, patients who might be candidates for ITB are evaluated in a multidisciplinary clinic by a team experienced in dystonia, spasticity, and other movement disorders. This team is knowledgeable about available treatment options; in this type of clinical setting, the treatment recommendations are from a group of experts rather than from an individual practitioner.

The general indication for ITB is severe, generalized dystonia that is unresponsive to oral medications. ITB has been used for individuals with hemidystonia or segmental dystonia; however, the primary indication for ITB is generalized dystonia. In this form of dystonia, symptoms, which are present more than 50% of the time, interfere with or prevent function.

The Barry-Albright Dystonia (BAD) scale grades dystonia in each of eight body regions including eyes, face, neck, trunk, and upper and lower extremities. The BAD scale rates dystonia on a 0–4 scale; scores of 3–4 are present when dystonia is present in at least three major body regions (e.g., extremities, trunk, and neck). The overall BAD score is usually between 15–20 in candidates for ITB therapy.[16,17]

More specific indications for ITB include increased comfort, enhanced function, and greater ease of positioning or care. ITB is particularly helpful for individuals who have both dystonia and spasticity. Before these patients are referred for ITB therapy, it is common for them to have undergone a spine fusion due to severe scoliosis. Spinal fusion is not a contraindication for ITB therapy; however, spinal fusion makes insertion of the intrathecal catheter more difficult.

During initial examination, most patients evaluated for ITB therapy by this author report that they had received multiple oral medications and were unresponsive to these drugs. The patients' dystonia is graded while they are on these medications. Because orally administered baclofen does not readily enter the CSF, response to oral baclofen does not predict response to intrathecal baclofen.

ITB is administered via an implanted pump that is connected to an intrathecal catheter (Fig. 1). The pump measures 70 by 27 mm, approximately the size of a hockey puck. The reservoir volume is 18 mL. A thinner pump (22 mm) has a 10-mL reservoir and is appropriate for smaller children who weigh less than 30–40 pounds. The limiting factor in ITB therapy is the patient's size, not patient age. I have placed a 10-mL pump into a 9-month-old infant.

An additional criterion for patient selection is reliability. Patients must return for periodic pump refills and dose ad-

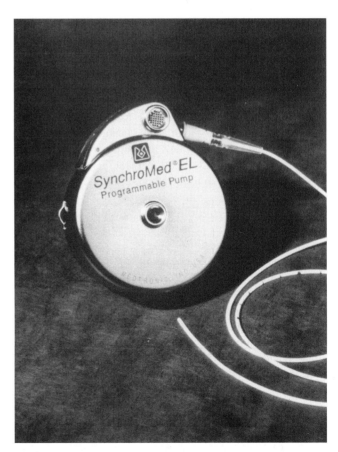

FIG. 1. SynchroMed EL programmable pump and one-piece intrathecal catheter (Medtronic, Inc., Minneapolis, MN).

justments. If pumps are not refilled in a timely manner, symptoms of baclofen withdrawal may occur; on occasion, these symptoms may be serious.

SCREENING TRIAL METHODS AND RESULTS

Before a pump is implanted for long-term ITB therapy, responsiveness to ITB is usually tested. Testing may be performed in two ways: bolus injections or continuous infusions. The goal of screening is to identify patients whose dystonia will be substantially improved by long-term ITB infusion. The endpoint in screening for dystonia is less clear than in screening spasticity. In subjects with spasticity of cerebral origin, a one-point decrease in mean Ashworth scores in the lower extremities is considered to be clinically significant.[18] There are no commonly accepted standards regarding objective criteria for a clinically significant response of dystonia to ITB. I consider a 25% decrease in the BAD score during two consecutive time intervals to be clinically significant. Other investigators use the traditional Fahn-Marsden scale and different criteria.[19] I use the BAD scale because most of his patients have secondary dystonia and often have impaired functional and cognitive abilities. For these patients, the BAD scale is probably more appropriate than the Fahn-Marsden scale.

The response of spasticity is tested with bolus injections of baclofen. Boluses of 50–100 µg are administered intrathecally and, within 2–4 hours, dramatic improvements are noted in lower extremity spasticity. Initially, testing of dystonia with ITB was also with bolus doses. Accounts in the medical literature reported that the response rate of dystonia to bolus injections was approximately 50%. This percentage is substantially lower than the 95% response rate of individuals with spasticity. It is also lower than the response of dystonia to continuous ITB infusion.[20] In 19 published cases, 79% of patients responded to baclofen infusion.[20] My colleagues and I often screen young patients (i.e., 3–6 years) and small patients (i.e., 30–50 pounds) with bolus doses of baclofen. These patients seem more likely to respond to bolus doses than older, larger children. We also screen patients diagnosed with mixed dystonia and spasticity; these patients are also screened with bolus injections. If their spasticity responds to the bolus dose and they are implanted with a pump, there is a strong likelihood that both the spasticity and dystonia will improve.

In the Spasticity and Movement Disorders program at the Children's Hospital of Pittsburgh, we typically screen dystonic patients via an implanted intrathecal catheter, which is inserted while in the operating room. The catheter enters the CSF at approximately L2–L3. If the dystonia is generalized, the catheter is then tunneled cephalad to the C1–C4 region. The distal end of the catheter is tunneled anteriorly, where it is connected to a subcutaneous infusion port (i.e., Bard port or Mediport). This port is implanted below the costal margin. After the incision is closed over the port, a Huber needle is inserted into the port and connected to an external mi-

croinfusion pump (i.e., Syringe-infusion Pump 2010, Medfusion, Duluth, GA). Baclofen infusion begins at a rate of 200 µg/day and increases by 50 µg every 8–12 hours until either the mean dystonia score decreases by 25%, unacceptable side effects occur, or the infusion rate is 900 µg/day without an improvement in the dystonia. While using this technique (when an external catheter and pump are used for the screening procedure), strict attention to sterile management of the apparatus is required to avoid infection.

After the screening trial is completed, the needle is withdrawn from the port, and the patient is discharged from the hospital for approximately 2 weeks, then returns for pump insertion. Approximately one-fourth of patients screened with continuous infusions experienced side effects during the screening trial. These side effects included headache, nausea, and drowsiness.

PUMP IMPLANTATION

Two commercially available pumps are available for intrathecal infusions. The SynchroMed pump (Medtronic, Inc. Minneapolis, MN) is an adjustable pump powered by a battery. This battery has a lifespan of 7–8 years. Its infusion rate may be adjusted using radiotelemetry via an external computer. By the year 2004, a smaller programmable pump with the same reservoir volume may be available.

The other available pump is a nonprogrammable, Freon gas-powered model (Infusaid). This pump runs indefinitely at a constant rate. Virtually all patients who receive ITB for dystonia require multiple dose adjustments; therefore, the programmable pump is used more commonly for these patients.

Pumps are surgically implanted while the patient is under general anesthesia. The operation lasts for approximately 1 hour. The pump is inserted anteriorly, usually below the right costal margin. In thin children and adults, pumps are placed in a subfascial pouch, just below fascia of the rectus abdominis and external oblique muscles, but above the corresponding muscles (Fig. 2). In individuals with 2 cm or more of subcutaneous tissue between the skin and abdominal fascia, the pump may be placed on the fascia. If patients have an intrathecal catheter in place from the screening trial, it is disconnected from the port and connected to the pump. If no catheter is in place, a single-piece catheter is inserted posteriorly at L2-L3 as described above and tunneled cephalad to the C1–C4 region. The distal end is then tunneled anteriorly and connected to the pump (Fig. 3). The catheter placement is higher than that for treating spastic quadriparesis (T2–T4) and appears to give greater improvement in dystonia in the upper extremities than catheters in the mid- or low-thoracic regions.[21]

POSTOPERATIVE MANAGEMENT

During the postoperative period, pumps are usually programmed to begin baclofen infusion at 200 µg/day. While patients are in the hospital, the dose is increased by approxi-

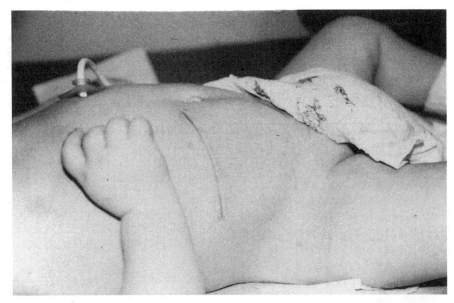

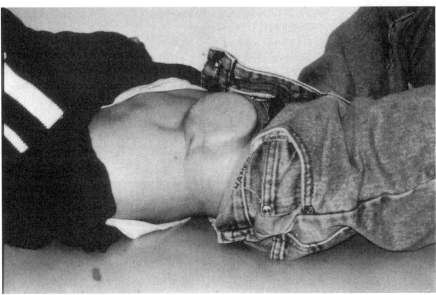

FIG. 2. Appearance of a pump placed above (top) and below (bottom) the abdominal fascia.

mately 50 μg each day; doses are increased until dystonia is appreciably improved. To diminish the risk of CSF leak, patients remain flat and on bed rest for 3–5 days. After patients are discharged, ITB doses are also adjusted when patients return for suture removal. Thereafter, at each refill, dystonia is reassessed and dose adjustments may be made. Most pumps have 18-mL reservoirs and must be refilled every 3 months. ITB doses for dystonia range from 200–2,000 μg/day. Doses of 500–1,000 μg/day are common and are higher than those used to treat spasticity. Doses are adjusted, with the primary goal of improvement of dystonia, and the secondary goal to improve function or facilitate care.

In my experience, in 69 patients diagnosed with generalized dystonia (70% associated with cerebral palsy) and screened by continuous infusion, 63 patients (91%) had clinically significant decreases in dystonia; 3 had equivocal responses; and 3 did not respond.[21] The mean baclofen dose at the time of response was 485 μg/day. Responses usually occurred after 2–3 days of infusion. Approximately 10% of individuals with severe, generalized dystonia lose their responsiveness to ITB over time; this lack of response usually occurs within the first year of therapy. The cause for unresponsiveness is not known. When response diminishes, it may sometimes be restored by changing the infusion mode from a continuous mode to intermittent bolus mode. In intermittent bolus mode, the pump delivers periodic boluses of 200–300 μg, every 6 hours. In addition, there is a low infusion rate during the intervals between boluses.

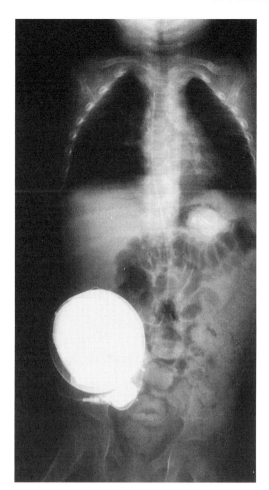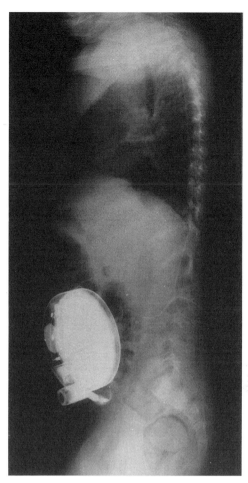

FIG. 3. Radiograph demonstrating the appearance of a pump and intrathecal catheter.

COMPLICATIONS OF TREATMENT WITH ITB

Approximately 25% of patients receiving long-term ITB infusion experience side effects. The most common side effect is constipation. In fewer than 10% of patients, with dose optimization, decreased neck or trunk control or drowsiness may occur. Treatment with ITB has complications, however, these complications are typically not related to the medication or the pump that infuses it. Complications occur in 30–40% of cases. The most common complications are infections, CSF leaks, and catheter malfunctions.

Infections within 1 month after pump/catheter implantation, usually associated *Staphylococcus aureus,* occur in 5–10% of patients. Most infections are treated by removal of the pump and catheter as well as the administration of intravenous antibiotics for 2 weeks. CSF leaks, which are often related to occult hydrocephalus, occur because CSF migrates out of the thecal sac; this leak occurs at the point where the catheter penetrates it. CSF migrates subcutaneously and accumulates in the lumbar region, around the pump, or both. Initially, CSF leaks are treated by bed rest and abdominal binders. If the leaks persist, they may be treated for 5 days with external lumbar catheters. Alternatively, CSF leaks may be surgically treated. During this surgery, the dura is sealed at the catheter entry point. Catheter problems include migration, kink, obstruction, and disconnection. These problems, which may be repaired in relatively minor operations, occur less frequently than in the past when two-piece catheters were used.

The relationship between ITB and seizures is not clear. There is no compelling evidence that ITB increases the frequency of seizures. In rare cases, a patient's seizures may seem worse when ITB therapy is initiated. However, for most patients, seizure frequency is unchanged.

The two potential medical complications of ITB therapy are baclofen withdrawal and baclofen overdose. The common symptoms of withdrawal include increased dystonia and itching. Less common symptoms include fever, agitation, seizures, and, in rare cases, psychosis. Whenever symptoms of withdrawal develop, it is recommended that patients immediately begin taking substantial doses of oral baclofen (e.g., 20 mg 3–4 times daily). These oral doses are continued until the cause of the problem is identified and treated. Baclofen overdose is usually secondary to programming the pump. Mild overdoses have been treated by physostigmine; however, mild overdoses probably do not need to be treated. Larger overdoses cause profound hypotension and respiratory depression. These overdoses are treated by artificial ventilation, stopping the pump, and performing a spinal tap to withdraw and barbitage CSF. Baclofen is not neurotoxic and infusion resumes after the excessive medication is metabolized (i.e., within 24–48 hours).

RESULTS OF ITB FOR DYSTONIA

After the first reports of the use of ITB for dystonia, several investigators used it to treat people with primary and secondary dystonia and confirmed its benefit in many patients. However, benefits occurred in a relatively smaller proportion of patients with dystonia than in treated patients with spasticity. In a 1998 summary of published cases, sustained improvement was reported in 28 of 38 cases (74%).[20] My colleagues and I have treated approximately 100 individuals who have generalized dystonia with ITB. Follow-up of 1 year or longer is available for 77 of these patients.[21] Prior to surgical pump implantation, the mean dystonia score on the BAD rating scale for this patient series was 18. Mean BAD scores after implantation were:

- 13 at 3 months;
- 10 at 6 months;
- 7 at 12 months; and
- 10 at 24 months.

All scores were significantly lower (P value of .003 or less) than at baseline. Mean dystonia scores of subjects with intrathecal catheters positioned at T4 or higher were significantly lower, and therefore better, than those whose catheters were positioned at T6 or lower.

Because the number of primary and secondary dystonia cases treated with ITB therapy is small, it is not possible to state with confidence whether the response of the two forms is similar. We tested two people who had been diagnosed with hemidystonia. These patients received an ITB screening trial. One of these patients improved. Children and adolescents with dystonia that is secondary to a neurodegenerative disorder, such as pantothenate kinase-associated neurodegeneration (Hallervorden-Spatz disease), do not seem to respond to ITB as well as those with secondary dystonia that is caused by a neurodegenerative disorder. However, the number of these patients treated thus far is small[21] and no definitive statement may be made.

The effects of ITB therapy on the functioning of patients with generalized dystonia are becoming clearer. We questioned patients whose dystonia had been treated with ITB therapy for 1 year or longer (i.e., a median of 26 months of ITB therapy). Eighty-six percent of these patients reported that quality of life and ease of care were improved. Speech improved in 33% and extremity function improved in 30–40% of these patients. Studies are underway to study the effect of ITB prospectively on speech and function in individuals with severe, generalized dystonia.

CONCLUSIONS

Generalized dystonia, particularly secondary dystonia, responds to long-term ITB infusion in 80–90% of individuals. ITB therapy is adjustable and reversible. Side effects and complications occur in approximately one-third of individuals and often require surgical correction; however, these may be treated without serious morbidity. ITB is probably the treatment of choice for individuals with severe generalized dystonia that does not respond adequately to treatment with oral medications.

REFERENCES

1. Narayan RK, Loubser PG, Jankovic J, et al. Intrathecal baclofen for intractable axial dystonia. Neurology 1991;41:1141–1142.
2. Ford B, Greene P, Louis ED, et al. Use of intrathecal baclofen in the treatment of patients with dystonia. Arch Neurol 1996;53:1241–1246.
3. Misgeld U, Bijak M, Jarolimek W. A physiological role for GABA$_b$ receptors and the effects of baclofen in the mammalian central nervous system. Prog Neurobiol 1995;46:423–462.
4. Knutsson E, Lindblom U, Martensson A. Plasma and cerebrospinal fluid levels of baclofen (Lioresal^R) at optimal therapeutic responses in spastic paresis. J Neurol Sci 1974;23:473–484.
5. Muller H, Zierski J, Dralle D, et al. Pharmacokinetics of intrathecal baclofen. In: Muller H, Zierski J, Penn R, eds. Local Spinal Therapy of Spasticity. Berlin: Springer 1988:155–214.
6. Penn RD, Kroin JS. Long-term intrathecal baclofen infusion for treatment of spasticity. J Neurosurg 1987;66:181–185.
7. Ochs G, Reimann I. Baclofen Intrathekal. Verla, Stuttgart: Thieme, 1995.
8. Kroin JS, Ali A, York M, et al. The distribution of medication along the spinal canal after chronic intrathecal administration. Neurosurgery 1993;33:226–230.
9. Davidoff RA. Antispasticity drugs: mechanisms of action. Ann Neurol 1985;17:107–116.
10. Nishikawa T, Scatton B, Enomoto T, et al. Modulation of striatal serotonin metabolism by baclofen, a gamma-aminobutyric acid$_b$ receptor agonist. Tokai J Exp Clin Med 1989;14:375–380.
11. Guyenet PG, Aghajanian GK. Ach, substance P, and metenkephalin in the locus coeruleus: pharmacological evidence for independent sites of action. Eur J Pharmacol 1979;53:319–328.
12. Seabrook GR, Howson W, Lacey MG. Electrophysiological characterization of potent agonists and antagonists at pre-and postsynaptic GABA$_b$ receptors on neurones in rat brain slices. Br J Pharmacol 1990;101:949–957.
13. Bowery NG, Hill DR, Hudson AL. Baclofen decreases neurotransmitter release in the mammalian CNS by an action at a novel GABA receptor. Nature 1980;283:92–94.
14. Potashner SJ. Baclofen: effects on amino acid release and metabolism in slices of guinea pig cerebral cortex. J Neurochem 1978;32:103–109.
15. Hallett M. The neurophysiology of dystonia. Arch Neurol 1998;55:601–603.
16. Albright AL. Intrathecal baclofen in cerebral palsy movement disorders. J Child Neurol 1996;11(Suppl 1):S29-S35.
17. Barry MJ, Van Swearingen JM, Albright AL. Reliability and responsiveness of the Barry-Albright dystonia scale. Dev Med Child Neurol 1999;41:404–411.
18. Albright AL, Barron WB, Fasick MP, Polinko P, Janosky J. Continuous intrathecal baclofen for spasticity of cerebral origin. JAMA 1993;270:2475–2477
19. Burke RE, Fahn S, Marsden CD, et al. Validity and reliability of a rating scale for the primary torsion dystonias. Neurology 1985;35:73–77.
20. Albright AL. Intrathecal baclofen for treatment of dystonia. In: Krauss JK, Jankovic J, Grossman RG, eds. Movement Disorders Surgery. Philadelphia: Lippincott, Williams and Wilkins, 2001:316–322.
21. Albright AL, Barry MJ, Shafron DH, Ferson SJ. Intrathecal baclofen for generalized dystonia. Dev Med Child Neurol 2001;43:652–657.

CHAPTER 8

Pharmacology of Botulinum Toxin Therapy

Mitchell F. Brin, Dirk Dressler, and K. Roger Aoki

INTRODUCTION

Since its first clinical use in the late 1970s,[6] botulinum toxin type A has become an important tool for the treatment of a variety of neurological and other disorders.[7] The therapeutic potential of botulinum toxin was first postulated in the early 19th century by Justinus Kerner, a German district physician who provided the first detailed clinical description of botulism and its association with faulty sausage production (Figure 1).[8–10] In the late 1800s and early 1900s, botulinum toxin was isolated and identified as the agent responsible for botulism.[11] With the advent of World War II, the enormous toxic potency of botulinum toxin was recognized by scientists, governments, and the military. Eventually, seven serotypes of botulinum neurotoxin were identified (A, B, C_1, D, E, F, G); however, most early studies focused on botulinum toxin type A as it was the first to be purified.[11] Military research produced a valuable stock of information about botulinum toxin type A and its mode of action. This groundwork provided a basis for subsequent therapeutic use.

Botulinum toxin is produced by *Clostridium botulinum*.[12] *C. botulinum* is an obligate anaerobic, rod-shaped, Gram-positive or Gram-negative (in older cultures) bacterium (Figures 2a and 2b).[13] The bacterium usually exists in a highly resistant spore form and is typically found in soil and water. Under appropriate pH values and strict anaerobic conditions, the spore form transforms into the vegetative form and produces botulinum toxin as an exotoxin. Botulinum toxin is

found throughout the world[14] and primarily affects animals, particularly sea birds living in wetland colonies.

The toxin most likely provides *C. botulinum* with territorial advantages over other bacteria. In humans, botulinum toxin poisoning may occur through ingestion of improperly preserved or stored food. Infant botulism follows ingestion of *C. botulinum* spores, often from soil or honey products. Due to poorly colonized intestinal flora which would normally compete with the botulinum bacteria, and lack of effective immune mechanisms, the spores germinate and synthesize botulinum toxin. Wound botulism occurs when *C. botulinum* colonizes infected wounds following injuries or surgery, or is injected during illegal drug use with contaminated needles.[15] The clinical picture of botulism is typically characterized by paresis usually affecting extraocular, pharyngeal, and esophageal muscles; ultimately, respiratory and limb

Mitchell F. Brin: Senior Vice President Development and Therapeutic Area Head BOTOX® & Neurology Allergan, LLC and Professor of Neurology University of California, Irvine, Irvine, California.

Dirk Dressler: Department of Neurology, Rostock University, Rostock, Germany.

K. Roger Aoki: Neurotoxin Research Program, Biological Sciences, Allergan, LLC Irvine, California.

Portions of this review were adapted from other reviews by the authors.[1–5]

Dr. Mitchell F. Brin and Dr. Roger Aoki are employees of Allergan, Inc.; Dr. Dirk Dressler has no commercial relationship to disclose.

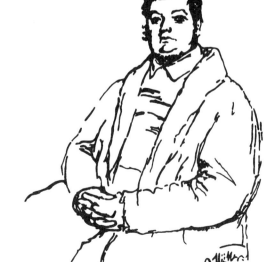

FIG. 8-1. Justinus Kerner (1786–1862). The German district physician and poet published the earliest systematic description of food botulism.[272]

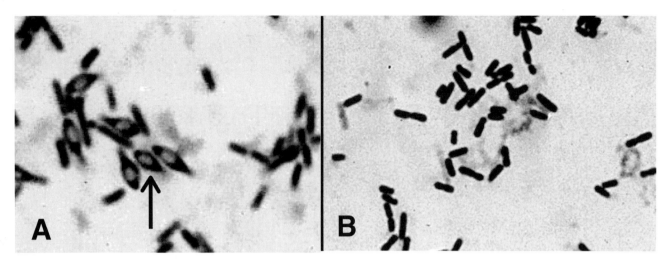

FIG. 8-2. *Clostridium botulinum* type F, Langeland strain. Brain heart culture medium. **A:** Spore form (arrow). 48 hours growth time. **B:** Vegetative form. 12 hours growth time. Figures courtesy of Ms. H King and Dr. HS Tranter, Public Health Laboratory Service, Centre for Applied Microbiology & Research, Salisbury, Wiltshire, UK.

muscles are affected. Symptoms of autonomic dysfunction may also occur, including dryness of mouth, conjunctival irritation, accommodation difficulties, bladder-voiding difficulties, heartburn, and constipation.[15,16]

NOMENCLATURE

Alan Scott, a US ophthalmologist, introduced botulinum toxin type A as a research chemodenervating agent for patients with the ocular disorder strabismus,[17] and called his manufactured research therapeutic "Oculinum."[18,19] The name oculinum reflected the strabismus use and was a combination linking "<u>ocul</u>" with "<u>lining</u>"-up-the-eye and the Latinate ending "<u>um</u>" (personal communication, Alan Scott). Dr. Scott used the toxin in 1980 for legs before treating blepharospasm in 1981, and treated the first 3 torticollis patients in 1983 (published by Tsui in 1984[20]), before treating a hemifacial spasm patient in 1984. At Columbia University, we began using the substance for blepharospasm and numerous non-ophthalmic neurologic disorders in 1984,[21] and coined the term "botox" to refer to botulinum toxin type A, which was the same product (Oculinum) manufactured by Dr. Scott.[22,23] We[24] and other clinicians[25] also used "BTX" or "BT."[26] Allergan, Inc (Irvine, CA) subsequently licensed Oculinum in 1989 and acquired the product in 1991 as "Oculinum Injectable." They changed the trade name to BOTOX®; this name was accepted by the FDA in 1992.

Dysport®, the finished product manufactured in the United Kingdom and originally distributed by Porton Products, now Ipsen Ltd. It was given its name, derived from Dystonia and Porton, on first licensure in the UK in 1991, and was discussed as such in 1993 and differentiated from BOTOX®.[27] Although the marketed finished products do not have the same properties, at times, in publications, one may discuss the neurotoxins without referring to brand names. Our basic science colleagues used BoNT, Botx, BoTX and BoTx as abbreviations[28] for the research raw material botulinum toxin, with BoNT/A referring to serotype A. "BTX" has been used for over 2 decades to refer to finished products, with BTX-A referring to serotype A. This nomenclature should not be confused with batrachotoxin ("poison dart frog" poison[29]) which has also been abbreviated as BTX. For the purpose of this review, BTX will be used to refer to both the raw material and finished product.

STRUCTURE

Botulinum toxin (BTX) in its native form contains a mixture of various proteins. The toxically and therapeutically active compound, botulinum neurotoxin, is a 150kD protein that demonstrates remarkable similarities to tetanus toxin, another clostridial toxin. To become biologically active, the 150kD protein must be nicked or cleaved into a light chain of 50kD and a heavy chain of 100kD. These chains are held together by a disulfide bond.[30,31]

The light chain of BTX type A (BTX-A) consists of 448 amino acids; the heavy chain comprises 848 amino acids.[30,31] The integrity of the disulfide bond is essential for BTX's biological activity. In addition to the 150kD BTX, BTX contains non-toxic proteins preventing gastric degradation after oral ingestion. The non-toxic protein + BTX complexes vary in size from 300kD to 900kD depending on specific BTX serotype and bacterial strain. These protein complexes contain hemagglutinin and non-toxic non-hemagglutinin (NTNH) proteins. Botulinum toxin type A is the only serotype forming a 900kD complex, which consists of hemagglutinin proteins of 600kD and a non-hemagglutinin protein of approximately 130 kD.[32] Serotype B, used in the commercial preparation is a 700 kD product.[33] Serotypes A, B, C₁, and hemagglutinin-positive D form 500kD and 300kD complexes; however, serotypes E, F, and hemagglutinin-negative D form only 300kD complexes.[34,35]

MODE OF ACTION: OVERVIEW

BTX inhibits cholinergic transmission at neuromuscular and autonomic postganglionic synapses, thereby reducing excessive muscular activity or likely glandular secretions. When BTX is injected into its target tissue (i.e., muscle or gland tissue), clinical effects are usually first observed after 2 to 5 days and reach their maximum therapeutic effect after 10 to 14 days. When injected into human skeletal muscles, most BTX-A effects resolve within 16 to 24 weeks. The duration of action seems to be shorter for BTX-B than for BTX-A,[36,37] and this is supported by the pre-clinical and clinical models cited below.[38] In a large clinical trial of the therapeutic use of BTX-A as BOTOX® for axillary hyperhidrosis, a glandular tissue, the overall mean duration of effect was 30.6 weeks (~7 months) and 28% of the patients completed the 16-month study after only 1 BTX-A treatment, reflecting over 1 year of benefit.[39]

The mode of action of BTX may be divided into extracellular and intracellular components. The heavy chain binds specifically to extracellular structures on cholinergic nerve terminals. These structures are termed acceptors rather than receptors because neither the acceptor protein nor any natural ligands have yet been identified. Bound BTX is internalized via endocytosis and the light chain is then transported across the vesicular membrane into the cytosol.[40]

The light chain of BTX is a zinc-dependent protease that cleaves one or more of the soluble NSF [N-ethylmaleimide-sensitive fusion] attachment protein receptor (SNARE), which transport the acetylcholine vesicle from the cytosol to the synaptic cleft. These proteins facilitate rapid vesicle fusion with neuronal plasma membrane and thus neurotransmitter exocytosis.[41] When this transport is interrupted, release of neurotransmitter from the neuromuscular or autonomic synapse is blocked and paresis or reduction of glandular secretion occurs. Different BTX serotypes cleave different SNARE proteins (Figure 3). BTX types A, C₁, and E cleave a synaptosomal associated protein of 25kD (SNAP-25), each at a unique site on this protein.[42–44] BTX types B, D, and F cleave vesicle-associated membrane protein (VAMP or synaptobrevin), each at a unique site.[45,46] BTX type C₁ cleaves syntaxin[47] (Table 1; Figure 4).

It was originally believed that the cholinergic blockade of the specific nerve terminal was permanent and that re-innervation of the target tissue was caused by axonal re-sprouting.[48,49] However, animal data with BTX-A has demonstrated that sprouting produces temporary re-innervation only during the early recovery phase. During the late recovery phase, the sprouts retract and the original terminal becomes functional once again.[50] After re-innervation is completed, the target tissue is fully functional.[51] There is no indication that post-botulinic re-innervation produces functionally substandard synapses.

Although traditionally called a neurotoxin because of its potential lethal effect on the organism as a whole by perturbing nervous system functioning, BTX-A is neither a cytotoxic agent nor an agent permanently altering nervous system function. It therefore can be viewed as a neuromodulator.

In addition to its effects on neuromuscular and autonomic efferent pathways, BTX-A most likely affects afferent pathways by blocking intrafusal fibers,[52–54] which is manifested in modification of sensory feedback to the central nervous system. Ludlow[55] and Zwirner et al.[56] proposed that reduced muscle activity and therefore feedback to the laryngeal motor neuron pools may be a primary mechanism of action of BTX-A. We[57] offered the possibility that toxin might have a direct effect on sensory afferents by blocking intrafusal fibers, resulting in decreased activation of muscle spindles. This would effectively change the sensory afferent system by reducing the Ia traffic.[57] Filippi et al.[52] supported this hypothesis by establishing that local injection of BTX-A directly reduces afferent Ia fiber traffic, and therefore exerts a modulatory effect on sensory feedback. This may also account for the clinical observation that injections of BTX-A have an effect on regional non-injected muscles, most striking in spastic limbs.[58]

Support for this mechanism derives from the cumulative work of Ryuji Kaji and colleagues.[59–64,64] He showed that the increase in severity of dystonic writer's cramp associated with enhancing Ia muscle spindle activity with the tonic vibration maneuver can be decreased by intramuscular injections of dilute lidocaine, which preferentially affects the afferent innervation of the muscle spindle. Both ethanol and lidocaine block sodium channels; however, ethanol blocks the channels for a longer duration than the anesthetic. Kaji has coined the term "muscle afferent block" or "MAB" for the treatment of lidocaine + ethanol, and has shown an effect in neck, jaw[63] and limb dystonia[59,60,60] and spasticity.[62,64,64] The benefit for each treatment only lasts a few weeks, and therefore is of limited use in most dystonic and spastic situations. However, this model of blocking Ia afferents supports the proposed mechanism of action with BTX-A on conditions associated with excessive muscle contraction.

It is notable that cranial dystonia is often associated with pain,[65,66] most commonly in cervical dystonia but also blepharospasm and occasionally troublesome limb and axial dystonia. Speculations about BTX-A's direct analgesic effects arose after it was noted that BTX-A treatment for dystonia and various other muscular hyperactivity syndromes alleviated not only motor symptoms but also pain.[67] The analgesic effects of BTX-A were first reported in 1985[20] in a pilot study of BTX-A treatment for cervical dystonia, characterized by abnormal, involuntary neck and shoulder muscle contractions and often resulting in significant, disabling musculoskeletal pain. Tsui et al. noted that the most marked benefit of BTX-A injections was pain relief in all 6 patients who reported severe neck pain due to muscle spasm.[20] In a small, double-blind, placebo-controlled extension of this pilot study, 16 patients treated with BTX-A experienced significantly reduced pain compared to placebo.[68] In subsequent open-label, prospective studies involving larger

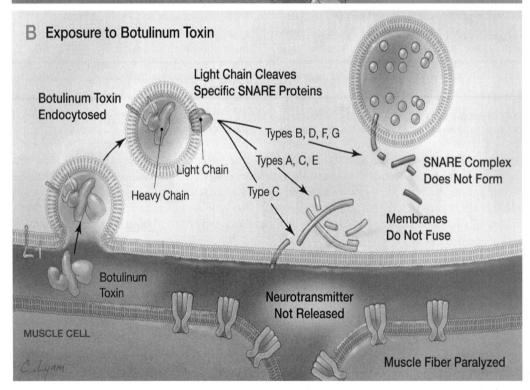

FIG. 8-3. Mechanism of Action of Botulinum Toxin. **A:** Release of acetylcholine at the neuromuscular junction is mediated by the assembly of a synaptic fusion complex that allows the membrane of the synaptic vesicle containing acetylcholine to fuse with the neuronal cell membrane. The synaptic fusion complex is a set of SNARE proteins, which include synaptobrevin, SNAP-25, and syntaxin. After membrane fusion, acetylcholine is released into the synaptic cleft and then bound by acceptors on the muscle cell. **B:** Botulinum toxin binds to the neuronal cell membrane at the nerve terminus and enters the neuron by endocytosis. The light chain of botulinum toxin cleaves specific sites on the SNARE proteins, preventing complete assembly of the synaptic fusion complex and thereby blocking acetylcholine release. Botulinum toxins types B, D, F, and G cleave synaptobrevin; types A, C, and E cleave SNAP-25; and type C cleaves syntaxin. Without acetylcholine release, the muscle is unable to contract. SNARE: soluble NSF-attachment protein receptor; NSF: N-ethylmaleimide-sensitive fusion protein; SNAP-25: synaptosomal-associated protein of 25 kd. (Reprinted from Arnon with permission of the publisher[273])

TABLE 8-1. *Putative Target Proteins of Botulinum Toxin (updated from Hunter)[264]*

Toxin type	Cellular substrate	Target cleavage site
BTX-A	SNAP-25[42,265]	Gln197-Arg198
BTX-B	VAMP/Synaptobrevin[45]	Gln76-Phe77
	Cellubrevin[266]	Unknown (likely similar to Synaptobrevin)*
BTX-C	Syntaxin 1A, 1B[47]	Lys253-Ala254
	SNAP-25[267]	Lys252-Ala253
BTX-D	VAMP/Synaptobrevin[46,265,268]	Lys59-Leu60
	Cellubrevin[46,268]	Ala67-Asp68
		Unknown (likely similar to Synaptobrevin)*
BTX-E	SNAP-25[42,265]	Arg180-Ile181
BTX-F	VAMP/Synaptobrevin[46,268,269]	Gln58-Lys59
	Cellubrevin[270]	Unknown (likely similar to Synaptobrevin)*
BTX-G	VAMP/Synaptobrevin[268]	Ala81-Ala82
TeTx	Synaptobrevin[270]	Gln76-Phe77
	Cellubrevin[271]	Unknown (likely similar to Synaptobrevin)*

*The differences in amino acid sequences between synaptobrevin and cellubrevin are at the C- and N-terminals; we speculate that the cleavage sites on cellubrevin are similar to those reported for synaptobrevin.
BTX-X, Botulinum toxin type X (X = serotype); TeTx, tetanus toxin.

numbers of patients, the authors reported pain relief in 74%–84% of cervical dystonia patients following BTX-A injections.[23,69,70,71,72] Additional double-blind, placebo-controlled studies confirmed the observed effects on pain of BTX-A in cervical dystonia patients.[73,74–76] These observations have been emphasized in subsequent reports.[77] Recently investigators[78] have noted that in some cases, the pain associated with cranial-cervical dystonia is either chronic muscle-tension-type headache or migraine headache, suggesting that headache is common in this population and BTX-A may be valuable in treating associated cranial pain.[79–81]

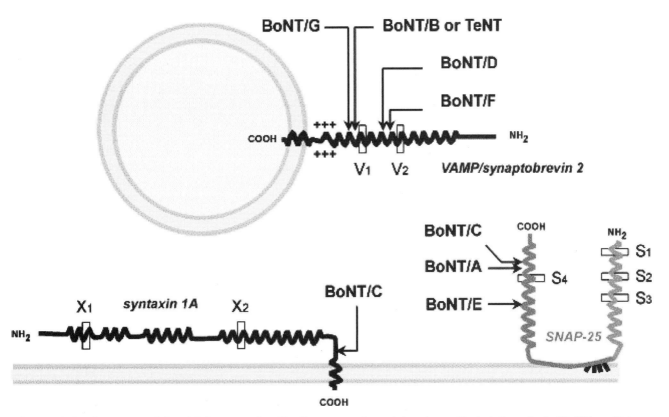

FIG. 8-4. Molecular targets of clostridial neurotoxins. The three synaptic proteins cleaved by botulinum toxin (BoNT) and tetanus toxin (TeNT) light chains are shown. The cleavage sites are indicated by arrows. The residues delimited by a box denote the sites that determine the binding specificity of the toxins light chains (also termed 'SNARE motif'). An additional binding site for the TeNT light chain on VAMP, rich in positive charges, is indicated. (Reprinted with permission from Humeau.[274])

In 1992, Memin et al. reported results from a pilot study conducted in Paris, France of BTX-A as treatment for spasticity following upper motor neuron lesion; five of 6 patients with pain experienced significant pain relief.[82] Also in 1992, Dengler et al. reported analgesic effects of BTX-A among 10 patients treated for spastic drop foot.[83] Later, a larger prospective study of patients with chronic limb spasticity due to various causes observed that 90% of 31 patients with painful flexor spasm or passive stretching experienced at least moderate pain relief and 26% experienced complete pain resolution after BTX-A injections.[84] Another prospective study in Thailand observed joint pain relief in 22 post-stroke spasticity patients.[85] Double-blind, placebo-controlled studies provided further support for the effect of BTX-A on pain relief in spasticity patients.[86,87]

Early in its use as a therapeutic agent, BTX-A was observed to provide pain relief in disorders other than dystonia and spasticity. Published case reports detail analgesic effects of BTX-A injections for muscle hypertrophy and myalgia associated with complex repetitive discharges[88] and for stiff-person syndrome.[89] In a prospective study of 60 achalasia patients, BTX-A improved chest pain associated with this disease of the esophagus.[90] Among 100 patients treated for anal fissure, 78% reported pain resolution within 3 days after initial injection.[91] Published reports of BTX-A for the relief of pain disorders,[77] includes pain associated with myofascial pain syndrome,[92-95] blepharospasm,[96] temporomandibular disorder and bruxism,[97-102] back pain,[103] painful myoclonus,[104] cervicogenic,[105] cluster,[106-108] tension type,[108-114,114] prostatic pain/sterile prostatitis,[115] and migraine headache.[108,116-120] For instance, in a double-blind, placebo-controlled study, cerebral palsy patients given BTX-A for postoperative pain following adductor-release surgery had significantly reduced pain scores, analgesic requirements, and hospital stays compared to placebo.[121] BTX-A has emerged as a promising option for patients suffering from chronic pain disorders.[77]

The association between BTX-A and pain relief was originally thought to relate only to its effect on muscle contraction. However, some studies of BTX-A for various conditions suggest that muscle relaxation may not directly coincide with pain relief, suggesting alternative mechanisms for analgesic effects of BTX-A. As noted above, there is experimental evidence that BTX-A affects afferent transmission,[52,54] which may be a factor in pain relief, and that BTX-A inhibits the release of substance P[122] and potentially other neuromodulators. Substance P is a neuropeptide that plays a role in pain perception, vasodilation, and neurogenic inflammation. Aoki has also shown experimentally that BTX-A relieves formalin-induced pain in laboratory animals.[123] This is an important observation in understanding the action of BTX-A on pain because formalin causes pain not through muscle tension, but by first directly stimulating nociceptors and then through local inflammation. It seems likely that the analgesic effects of BTX-A relate not only to its well-established effect at the neuromuscular juncture, but also to an effect on the nociceptor system.[4]

POTENCY MEASUREMENT

The potency of BTX is determined by *in vivo* mouse assays. One unit (U) of BTX has been defined as the amount of intraperitoneally administered BTX required to kill 50% (LD_{50}) of a group of 18g to 20g female Swiss Webster mice.[124-128] This unit is variously referred to as a mouse unit, or a mouse LD_{50} unit. Although the definition of a unit is internationally accepted, units of different serotypes[129] and of different therapeutic preparations of the same serotype[27,130-136] are not clinically equivalent. As a result of the biological properties of these products, there are no accepted methods of interconverting the units from one marketed neurotoxin to another.

Scott[137] injected BTX-A intramuscularly into 8 monkeys and determined the LD_{50} to be approximately 39 U/kg body weight. The lowest dose that caused systemic toxicity, 33 U/kg, was close to the fatal dose range of 38-42 U/kg; the LD_{50} dose was therefore close to the LD_{100} dose. This is different from mice, in which the LD_{90} is 2.2 times the LD_{50}. Herrero[138] showed that the LD_{50} for monkeys given BTX intravenously was 40 U/kg, similar to that found by Scott[137] for the intramuscular route of administration.

The lethal dose in humans is not known. Meyer and Eddie[139] reported a case of human botulism due to *Clostridium parabotulinum* type B in cheese and performed experiments to isolate and quantitate the exposure and potency of the orally ingested toxin (parabotulinum is an older terminology for botulinum). The[139,140] early estimates of the orally ingested lethal dose of botulinum toxin in humans are probably incorrect due to technical issues in quantitating the toxin, ability to identify multiple serotypes in samples and inaccurate assumptions. However, estimates from published data, including studies performed in primates, can be calculated. Lamanna[141] calculated that a dose of $\geq 10^5$ mouse LD_{50}/g food would be required to cause overt neurologic disease in humans. Based on calculations from monkey absorption studies, Smith suggests that the human lethal dose of ingested type A toxin is about 4 to 40 times the intravenous dose or 10^4 to 10^6 U.[142;143] Herrero[138] studied intravenous and intragastric administration of BTX-A in non-human primates and reported an intravenous LD_{50} of 40U/kg in rhesus monkeys, 66 U/kg in squirrel monkeys and an intragastric LD_{50} of 30,000U/kg in rhesus monkeys. Extrapolating Scott's[137] macaque monkey intramuscular data to a 70 kg human implies an intramuscular LD_{50} of nearly 3000 U. This makes accidental injection of a lethal dose highly unlikely. Although useful in select patients with pre-existing neurologic or neurodegenerative disease such as amyotrophic lateral sclerosis, myasthenia gravis or Lambert-Eaton syndrome,[144-153] troublesome side effects may occur at doses routinely used therapeutically, and well below the calculated LD_{50}, in such vulnerable patients.[154-159]

The different commercial preparations of botulinum toxin are distinct, and it is critical that treating physicians note which product is being utilized, particularly when treating patients in settings where multiple products and/or serotypes are available. In addition, when reading the scientific literature, the reader should be aware of which commercial product is described.

Differences in the potency labeling between different serotypes may be caused by different BTX susceptibilities of the mouse population used for testing. Differences between different preparations of the same serotype may also be due to differences in the test systems applied,[160] in addition to the properties of the neurotoxin complex, the formulation processes and assay conditions. Naturally, potency comparison is focused on BTX's therapeutic effect (i.e., its paretic or glandular blocking effect). However, therapeutic BTX preparations differ in more than their therapeutic effects. As described above, differences include the serotype used and the content, condition, and functioning of the BTX protein complexes, in addition to the excipients used in formulation. With this, differences in the rate of adverse events have been described[161–165] and differences in the risk of antibody formation may be assumed.[166]

Additionally, preclinical studies indicate that BOTOX® and Dysport® have different dose-response curves for muscle weakening efficacy (ED_{50}) and intramuscular lethal doses (LD_{50}).[5] Therefore, comparison between therapeutic BTX preparations based solely on their therapeutic effect may be misleading.[27] As a result, regulatory agencies now require the prescribing information for all therapeutic BTX preparations include statements indicating that units are neither equivalent nor convertible among different BTX products.

THERAPEUTIC PREPARATIONS

BTX for therapeutic use is commercially available as the type A preparations, BOTOX® and Dysport®, or the type B preparation, Myobloc™ (trade name in the US) or NeuroBloc® (trade name in Europe). All therapeutic BTX preparations are of natural origin and contain the neurotoxin core, non-toxic proteins, and formulation excipients. Content, condition, and functioning of the protein complexes and additives vary according to the particular formulation, molecular and complex characteristics, thus influencing their therapeutically relevant features. Each BTX serotype differs in its amino acid sequence and steric conformation.[167]

Specific Pharmacology: Botulinum Toxin Type A (BOTOX® and Dysport®)

BOTOX®, a BTX-A product manufactured by Allergan, Inc., Irvine CA, is the most widely used BTX product worldwide. BOTOX® has been studied since the late 1970s; it was approved for clinical use in 1989 and, until 1992, was distributed under the name Oculinum®. Each 100 U vial of BOTOX® contains: 5 ng of vacuum-dried 900kD BTX-A; 0.9 mg sodium chloride; and 0.5 mg serum albumin. The vial should be stored either in the refrigerator or at −5°C (according to the regional labeling) and reconstituted for use specifically with non-preserved normal saline. After reconstitution, the pH of the final solution will range from 5.5 to 7.0, depending upon the particular vial of sterile saline for injection. The preparation is unbuffered and will equilibrate with tissue pH quickly after injection. For microbiological reasons associated with the non-preserved diluent, the reconstituted product should be used within approximately 4 hours.

Dysport® is manufactured by Ipsen Ltd., Maidenhead, Berks, UK. This form of botulinum toxin type A was approved for clinical use in Europe in 1991. It is not approved in the US. Each 500 U vial of Dysport® contains: 12.5 ng of freeze-dried 500kD-900kD BTX-A,[168] 2.5 mg lactose, and 0.125 mg serum albumin. For storage and handling, Dysport® should be maintained at 4°C to 8°C. After reconstitution with normal saline, Dysport® has a pH value of approximately 7.0 and can be used for approximately 4 hours.

Both BOTOX® and Dysport® contain botulinum toxin type A (di-chain molecule as previously described) complexed with hemagglutinins (HA) and nontoxin-nonhemagglutinin (NTNH) proteins. The intraneuronal target for cleavage by BTX-A is the SNARE protein SNAP-25.

BTX-A is the only clostridial neurotoxin that is found in the largest complex of 900 kDa, also known as the LL form.[35,169] During fermentation, the bacteria produce the type A neurotoxin as a single chain polypeptide associated with various proteins to form complexes ranging in size from the LL form (~900 kD) to the L (~500 kDa) and M form (~300 kDa) as well as the free neurotoxin (150 kDa). During the later stages of fermentation, endogenous proteases nick the majority (> 95%) of single chain into the active di-chain form.[170] The bulk toxin for both BOTOX® (LL form) and Dysport® (LL and L forms) is purified from the other proteins in the fermentation broth. The bulk for BOTOX® and Dysport are purified by different methods and will have different physiochemical and clinical characteristics. Each product is formulated uniquely and packaged for commercial distribution. BOTOX® is vacuum dried whereas Dysport® is freeze dried. Both products require reconstitution with sterile saline for injection prior to use.

Despite the fact that the unit potencies of both products are determined with the mouse assay, there is no equivalence between a unit of BOTOX® and a unit of Dysport®. Reasons for the discrepancy include differences in assay procedures (especially the LD_{50} assay used to define the unit) for the two products[131,134,135,160,171,172] and different physiochemical properties due to the formulation, bulk toxin and/or final product manufacturing techniques. The diffusion and side effect profiles of the two products are distinct as well. Bigalke[173] demonstrated that Dysport® could attain a similar unit potency as BOTOX®, as determined by the mouse phrenic nerve hemidiaphragm preparation, by the addition of additional human serum albumin to the formulation of Dysport®. In a further clinical evaluation in the extensor digitorum brevis model, the authors demonstrated that the Dysport® formulation could be supplemented with additional human serum albumin to produce a similar effect to unmodified BOTOX®.[173,174]

TABLE 8-2. *Preclinical Comparison of the Local Murine Muscle Weakness and Systemic Safety of Intramuscular BOTOX® and Dysport®[5]*

	IM-ED$_{50}$ (U kg^{-1} body weight)	IM-LD$_{50}$ (U kg^{-1} body weight)	Safety margin IM-LD$_{50}$/IM-ED$_{50}$
BTX-A (BOTOX®) N=6	6.2 ± 0.6	81.4 ± 3.5	13.9 ± 1.7
BTX-A (Dysport®) N=6	22.9 ± 3.2*	160.8 ± 7.2*	7.6 ± 0.9*
BOTOX/Dysport ratio	1:3.7	1:1.98	1.8:1

*$P < .001$.

IM, intramuscular; ED$_{50}$, median effective dose; BTX-A, botulinum toxin type A.

The sensitivity of the Dysport® preparation to enhanced efficacy with additional albumin was also demonstrated with the Digit Abduction Score (DAS) assay[175], a murine preclinical model. This *in vivo* model was used to compare the efficacies of botulinum type A toxin preparations, BOTOX® and Dysport, for the induction of local muscle weakness. A direct dose-response evaluation was performed by using the clinically relevant vehicle, sterile saline (0.9% NaCl). The ability of mice to abduct their hind limb digits was scored with a five point score (0 – 4) system after a unilateral, intramuscular, hind limb injection. Treated mice were scored daily after a single intramuscular injection of the test article to determine onset of action and dose that produced peak efficacy; these data were used for identifying the IM-ED$_{50}$. A dose-related muscle weakness was observed in the DAS for BOTOX® and Dysport. Both products demonstrated onset of action by day 1 and a peak effect by day 3. Average ED$_{50}$ values ± s.e.m., n=3, for BOTOX®, and Dysport® were 4.7 ± 1 and 27 ± 5 units/kg, respectively. When nonspecific adsorption was blocked with the use of 0.5% bovine serum albumin (BSA) in saline, the ED$_{50}$ values were 3.4 ± 0.2 and 12.7 ± 5 units/kg for BOTOX® and Dysport, respectively. The apparent loss of Dysport® activity when reconstituted in saline was partially prevented with the addition of BSA. BOTOX® efficacy remained consistent regardless of the vehicle utilized. BOTOX® was approximately six-fold more potent than Dysport® when reconstituted with the clinically relevant vehicle, saline. BOTOX® and Dysport® are not interchangeable botulinum type A neurotoxin products.

Further preclinical comparison of BOTOX® and Dysport® in the murine digit abduction score assay supports the concept that a simple dose conversion between the two botulinum toxin type A complex-containing products is not possible.[5] A simple dose ratio requires parallel dose-response curves for the efficacy and safety doses. One method to illustrate this concept is to compare the dose required to inhibit a local muscle effect such as with the DAS assay with the dose, in the same system and injection location with a distal effect at higher doses. The local muscle effect is represented by the dose which elicits a 50% response (IM-ED$_{50}$ value). The IM-ED$_{50}$ comparison between BOTOX® and Dysport® demonstrated a ratio of 1 to 3.7 (Table 2) while the ratio comparing the systemic effect of the intramuscular dose (IM-LD$_{50}$ value) was 1 to ~2. The safety margins of the two products are clearly different demonstrating differing capacities of the products to remain within the injected murine muscles. Changes in the dose ratios between the products demonstrate the lack of parallel dose-response curves and thus demonstrate the inaccurate information conveyed by a simple dose ratio conversion between two BTX-A based products. However, interspecies differences in response make cross-species extrapolation of safety and efficacy data impossible, and leave the clinical relevance of these observations to be determined. Nevertheless, these pre-clinical data are consistent with the adverse event profile of the products in clinical trials (Table 3).

Botulinum toxin type A was also produced in Japan[176] for clinical research, and more recently in China,[177] but these are not manufactured under current Good Manufacturing Practice (cGMP) standards. The Chinese toxin is marketed under the name "BTX-A" and this should not be confused with either BOTOX® or Dysport®, both manufactured under internationally accepted cGMP standards.

TABLE 8-3. *Selected Adverse Effects Reported in Cervical Dystonia Studies*

	MYOBLOC™				Dysport®			BOTOX®			
Study no.	301[187]		302[36]		Poewe[225]			140[251,252]		503[253]	
Units	PBO	5,000	10,000	PBO	10,000	PBO	500	1,000	PBO	Mean 236.2*	Mean 156*	Mean 155**
Dysphagia (%)	3	11	22	5	28	10	29	39	4	7	8	15
Dry mouth (%)	3	14	24	3	44	5	18	33	0	1	0	1

140, Double-blind, placebo-controlled original BOTOX®. AE's for Dbl. Bld.
503, European crossover of original and current BOTOX®. AE's are for period I prior to the crossover.
*Original formulation.
**Current formulation.

Specific Pharmacology: Botulinum Toxin Type B (MyoBloc™/NeuroBloc®)

MyoBloc™/NeuroBloc® is the only marketed therapeutic BTX-B preparation. It is manufactured by Elan Biopharmaceuticals (Ireland) and was first approved for clinical use specifically for cervical dystonia during 2000. It is distributed in vials containing liquid solutions of 2,500 U, 5,000 U, or 10,000 U. Each vial of MyoBloc™/NeuroBloc® contains 10 ng, 50 ng, or 100 ng of 500–700kD BTX-B.[178] Its storage and handling temperature is 2°C to 8°C. After opening the vial, the time period of its use is not limited by product stability but by microbiological considerations. MyoBloc™/NeuroBloc® may cause discomfort when it is injected,[37,179,180] probably because of its low pH value.

BTX-B cleaves synaptobrevin/VAMP, which is one of the proteins in the complex responsible for docking and fusion/release of synaptic vesicle at the presynaptic membrane into the synaptic cleft. It is remarkable that synaptobrevin/VAMP knockout mice[181] continue to demonstrate SNARE function, suggesting that synaptobrevin may not be absolutely required for synaptic fusion. This observation is consistent with the above data suggesting a decreased effect of BTX-B in human[38,182] and preclinical[4,5] models.

The formulation of BTX-B is produced by fermentation of the Bean strain of *Clostridium botulinum* type B, and exists in noncovalent association with hemagglutinin and nonhemagglutinin proteins as a neurotoxin complex. The protein is synthesized as a single polypeptide of approximately 150 kDa, and nicked by proteases to form the heavy and light chains. The commercial preparation is an injectable solution that is clear and colorless-to-light yellow with a molecular weight of approximately 700 kDa. Each single-use vial that contain 5000 U of the product per milliliter includes 0.05% human serum albumin, sodium succinate, sodium chloride, sodium caprylate, sodium acetyltryptophanate, hydrochloric acid and water at a pH 5.6.[178,183,184] The method of calculating the LD_{50} in mice is specific to Elan Pharmaceuticals and is not available in the literature. Associated with the differences in specific details of their assay, such as the vehicle, dilution scheme, and laboratory protocols for various mouse LD_{50} assays, the Units of biological activity of Elan's product can not be compared to or converted into units of any other botulinum toxin or any toxin assessed with any other

specific assay method. The specific activity of Elan's product ranges between 70 and 130 U/ng.

Botulinum toxin type B, as manufactured Elan Pharmaceuticals, also had different dosing units, with the doses showing efficacy used in torticollis trials being between 2500 Units and 15,000 Units.[36,185–187]

In the pharmacodynamic studies performed in cynomolgus monkeys for registration,[184] it was concluded that a higher dose of MyoBloc™/NeuroBloc® than of BOTOX® was required to cause an equivalent degree of muscle weakness. In this species, a dose of 1440–2400 U/kg caused signs and symptoms of systemic botulism and 2400 U/kg was found to be lethal.

Sloop[182] carefully studied the extensor digitorum brevis (EDB) muscle in the foot and reported a dose-dependent decline in the compound muscle action potential (CMAP) amplitude, area, and mean rectified voltage (MRV) following a single IM injection of BOTOX® ranging from 1.25 U to 20 U, and a logarithmic dose response relationship. CMAP decrement was maximal by day 6, with a decrement of 68% on day 2, 92% on day 4, and 100% on day 6. This study showed a clear dose-dependent decrement in CMAP amplitude, area, and MRV recording from EDB. In a subsequent study,[38] Sloop and coworkers compared the effects of BOTOX® vs. MyoBloc™/NeuroBloc® in normal volunteers, and demonstrated that the muscle relaxing effect from MyoBloc™/NeuroBloc® was neither as complete nor as long lasting as that resulting from BOTOX®.

A preclinical comparison of MyoBloc™/NeuroBloc® with BOTOX® conducted with the DAS assay demonstrated that the two products have different efficacies and safety margins (Table 4). The BOTOX® results were described in the previous section. As in Sloop's studies, these preclinical results show a shorter duration of action from MyoBloc™/NeuroBloc®, and further demonstrate that the dose-response curves for MyoBloc™/NeuroBloc® and BOTOX® are not parallel, and a simple dose conversion value to convert units of one product into the units of the other product is not possible.

Lowe[37] recently compared the clinical efficacy and safety profile of BOTOX® and Myobloc® in glabellar lines. They observed the effects of the two preparations on patients with brow furrows assessing efficacy, duration of effect and adverse effects. Patients were injected with BTX-B in two different dose conversions against BTX-A to the corrugator-

TABLE 8-4. *Preclinical Comparison of the Local Murine Muscle Weakness and Systemic Safety of Intramuscular BOTOX® and MYOBLOC™/Neurobloc®* [249]

	IM-ED$_{50}$ (U/kg)	IM-LD$_{50}$ (U/kg)	Safety margin IM-LD$_{50}$/IM-ED$_{50}$
BTX-A (BOTOX®) N=6	6.2 ± 0.6	81.4 ± 3.5	13.9 ± 1.7
BTX-B (MYOBLOC™) N=6	20.8 ± 1.4*	104.6 ± 1.9*	5.4 ± 0.3*
BTX-A:BTX-B Ratio	1:3.4	1:1.3	2.6:1

*$P < .005$; IM, intramuscular; ED$_{50}$, median effective dose; BTX-A, botulinum toxin type A; BTX-B, botulinum toxin type B.

procerus complex. Some patients received 50 units of BTX-B (total of 1000 units) to 1 unit of BTX-A, while others received 100 units of BTX-B (total of 2000 units) to one unit of BTX-A. The patients treated with BTX-A received a total of 20 units. These patients were clinically assessed prior to treatment and 3 days, 1 week, 4 weeks, 12 weeks, and 16 weeks after treatment. It was notable that although the peak effect for both preparations (and both doses of BTX-B) were equivalent and both improved glabellar frown lines, duration of effect with BTX-A was at least 16 weeks. With 1000 units of BTX-B, dose duration was 6–8 weeks and with 2000 units of BTX-B, duration was 10–12 weeks. They observed that the Myobloc® treated group demonstrated a decrease in tearing and significantly increased pain on injection.[180]

Specific Pharmacology: Other Preparations

In addition to the commercially available therapeutic BTX preparations, other research preparations have been reported. BTX A preparations have been examined in Japan[188] and China.[177] In Germany, a preparation containing purified BTX-A neurotoxin (150kD), rather than the complexed BTX-A, is under development.[189] A different BTX-F preparations from Japan has been studied in patients with and without antibodies against BTX-A.[190–193] These preparations have not been approved for commercial use.

Immunogenicity

In clinical practice, the most common cause of "lack of benefit" is technical, including inadequate dosing, not injecting the muscles most involved in causing the unwanted posture, or difficulty with targeting the intended muscle. Therefore, the first consideration is whether the dose, injection site, and adjunctive therapies are appropriate. Additional considerations include a change in pattern of the underlying muscle contraction associated with the patient's condition, progression of the underlying disorder, changes in the patient's expectations or a mismatch in patient expectations vs. the potential results of therapy and the presence of a fixed contracture. Often, at the onset of therapy, the patient's condition is quite severe, and the improvement following the first treatment is substantial. Follow-up treatments are usually provided prior to the condition returning to its original baseline, and therefore the relief from subsequent treatments are not as dramatic as the first treatment. If a lack of therapeutic benefit continues with adjustment of dose and technique of administration (Table 5), the possibility of antibody-mediated resistance is considered (Figure 5).

When BTX-A was initially used for the treatment of strabismus, blepharospasm, and cervical dystonia, immunogenicity was not an issue.[194,195] It was believed that the amount of protein administered for those indications was too small to induce formation of neutralizing antibodies (C. Hatheway, personal communication, 1984). However, during the early 1990s, the first cases of BTX-A therapy failure were reported and antibody formation against Oculinum was demonstrated in patients with cervical dystonia.[196,197] Later antibody-induced therapy failure was also reported in a single patient treated with Dysport for blepharospasm.[198]

There is a paucity of data regarding the exact epidemiology of antibody-induced therapy failure. The common belief suggests that antibody-induced therapy failure had occurred in 5% to 10% of patients treated for cervical dystonia.[199]

With the advent of the current BOTOX® preparation that was introduced in November 1997, it was predicted that the frequency of antibody formation would decrease; this has been the experience of current users.[200,201] The authors had reported[202] on consecutive cervical dystonia patients treated with current BOTOX®, and found no evidence for immunoresistance. Recently, Jankovic reviewed his series of cervical dystonia patients treated with both the original BOTOX® (lot 79–11) and current BOTOX® and reported no patients had developed immunoresistance when treated exclusively with current BOTOX®.[201] After performing an analysis examining the influence of age and cumulative dose, they concluded that the low

TABLE 8-5: *Botulinum Toxin Therapy: Dose Modifiers*

Modifiers	Dose per muscle	
	Decrease dose if:	Increase dose if:
Patient weight	Low	High
Likely duration of therapy	Chronic	Acute
Muscle bulk	Very small	Very large
Number of body regions being treated simultaneously	Many	Few
Clinical muscle contractions or spasms	Mild	Severe
Concern for excessive muscle relaxation	High	Low
Previous results of therapy	Too much muscle relaxation	Inadequate muscle relaxation
Sternocleidomastoid, digastric or perilingual/pharyngeal injections	Bilateral injection	—
Prior denervation or nerve injury (hemifacial spasm, peripheral denervation surgery)	If present	—

From Brin.[250]

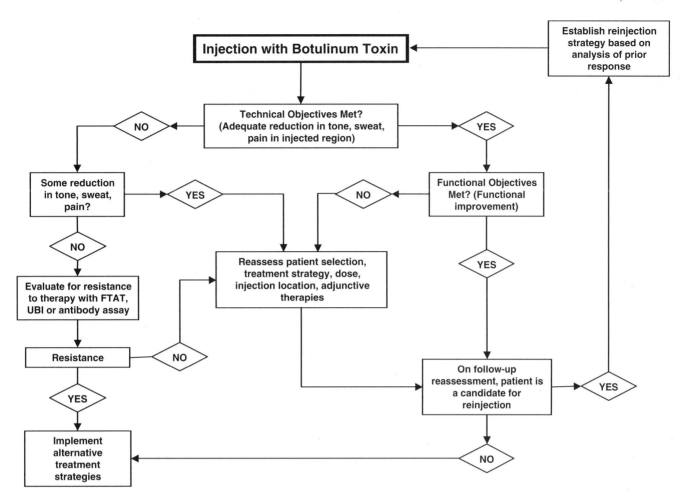

FIG. 5. Injection with botulinum toxin is individualized to the objectives of the patient in order to achieve optimum technical and functional outcomes. Occasionally a patient will not respond to BTX therapy. The first consideration is whether the dose, injection site, adjunctive therapies or patient selection are appropriate. If a lack of therapeutic benefit continues with adjustment of dose and technique of administration, the possibility of antibody-mediated resistance is considered. Functional resistance may be determined by the FTAT (Frontalis Type A Test) or UBI (Unilateral Brow Injection) (see text). If indicated, alternate treatment strategies could include introduction/modification of pharmacotherapy, surgical therapy, or an alternative serotype of botulinum toxin.

risk of antibody formation following current BOTOX® treatment is related to the lower protein exposure (Table 6). These observations have been confirmed in 326 patients with cervical dystonia treated for up to 9 treatments with a mean dose per treatment of 176 U and mean cumulative dose of 758 U.[203]

The formation of neutralizing antibodies is only one of many possible causes of BTX therapy failure.[204] As noted above, suboptimal response to BTX may be due to technical issues. Because these problems may be remedied, it is impor-

tant to consider them before concluding that neutralizing antibodies have developed (Figure 5). If the patient is still non-responsive after altering these variables, several methods are available for the detection of antibodies in the patient's serum.

In the mouse protection assay (MPA), a mouse population receives an injection of BTX that has been incubated with the test serum. If the proportion of mice dying during the test period is less than that of a control population, the test serum is presumed to contain antibodies that block BTX's biologi-

TABLE 8-6. *Protein Exposure with Currently Available Botulinum Toxin Preparations*

	BOTOX®[253]	Dysport®[131,254]	Neurobloc®/MYOBLOC™[183]
Units per nanogram (U/ng) in current formulation	20 U/ng	40 U/ng	100 U/ng
Nanogram (ng) protein per CD treatment	10 ng/200 U	18 ng/700 U	100 ng/10,000 U

CD, cervical dystonia.

cal action, referred to as neutralizing antibodies. The MPA is considered the gold standard for detection of neutralizing antibodies because, as a biologic assay, antibodies directed against non-toxic BTX proteins do not interfere with its result. Thus, the specificity of MPA is high.[205]

The mouse diaphragm assay (MDA) has been examined.[166,206] In this test, a preparation of a mouse hemidiaphragm with its attached phrenic nerve is placed in a device that measures the twitch force produced by repetitive electrical stimulation of the phrenic nerve. When BTX that has been incubated with a test serum containing BTX antibodies is applied, diaphragmatic paralysis occurs inversely proportional to the amount of BTX antibodies contained in the test serum. The MDA is able to produce quantitative results within a few hours. When the mouse diaphragm assay is applied, 38% of patients without complete therapy failure present with neutralizing antibodies suggesting that the mouse diaphragm assay may not be a clinically relevant assay.[206]

A recently introduced radioimmunoprecipitation assay (RIPA)[207] shows sensitivity and specificity similar to those of the mouse diaphragm assay.[208] The RIPA is quantitative and delivers results within a few hours. Further studies will be needed to confirm the utility of this test.

Rather than sending patients' serum for either type of assay, simple patient-based tests such as the frontalis type A antibody test (FTAT)[209,210] may be used for screening purposes. During this test, 15 U to 20 U of BOTOX® are injected into two sites of one corrugator muscle. If, after two weeks time, the patient can not furrow the injected side of their eye brow, they are "not resistant." If the corrugator can be activated properly, the patient is "resistant," indicating the presence of neutralizing antibodies. If the patient is not resistant, the opposite corrugator may be injected to maintain facial symmetry. A modification of this test is the "unilateral brow injection" (UBI) described by Hanna & Jankovic.[210] For this office-based assay, the physician injects one corrugator with 15–20 U of BOTOX® and examines the ability of the patient to furrow their brow at two weeks. Another patient-based test is the extensor digitorum brevis test,[211] also a qualitative test. Although the sensitivity of these tests are not adjusted to a control population, they have the advantage of being clinically relevant. The sternocleidomastoid test[206] is a quantitative patient-based test. It does not, however, have the simplicity or utility of the FTAT or UBI.[212]

Studies that have compared BTX-A-treated patient groups with or without antibody-induced therapy failure have identified several risk factors for antibody formation, including higher doses at each injection series and shorter intervals between injection series.[197,213] Higher doses and more frequent injections expose patients to more BTX protein. Reducing the amount of protein per treatment as well as the number of treatment cycles per year may help reduce the risk of antibody formation.[197,213,214] The various BTX products differ in the amount of BTX protein they contain per effective dose. In one retrospective study of clinical practice in Germany, mean doses of 187 U BOTOX® and 732 U of Dysport® were reported for the treatment of cervical dystonia.[161] Dividing these doses by the specific potencies of 20 U/ng for BOTOX® (pre 1997) and 40 U/ng for Dysport®, the resulting BTX protein exposure per treatment was 9.35 ng for BOTOX® and 18.3 ng for Dysport®. Based on these calculations, BOTOX® may be associated with a lower risk of antibody formation than Dysport®. As noted above, there have been no reports of resistance to therapy with the current formulation of BOTOX®.

A 10,000 U dose of NeuroBloc®/MyoBloc™ for the treatment of cervical dystonia, with a specific potency of 100 U/ng, contains approximately 100 ng of neurotoxin complex protein (Table 6). This would be expected to result in a higher risk of neutralizing antibody formation than the two BTX-A products. The only published antibody rates for NeuroBloc®/MyoBloc™ are found in the US Product Label and in the Summary Basis of Approval (SBA) available on the FDA website.[183] Using data from patients participating in studies 301, 302, 351, and 352, it appears that an ELISA assay was used to screen the samples for the MNA (a.k.a. MPA) and identify those patients who developed an antibody response. The ELISA assay has a high false-positive rate as the assay will identify antibodies to various epitopes in the toxin complex, in addition to those to the native toxin. The mouse neutralization assay (MNA), which is more specific, was then performed and the results were presented in the documents. A positive MNA was seen in 9.6% of patients at 12 months, 18.2% of patients by 18 months, and 22.6% of patients by 20 months. The regulatory reviewers stated that "these results indicate that there is substantial formation of antibodies in response to treatment with botulinum toxin type B, and that many patients will convert to having neutralizing antibodies within 2 years of beginning treatment . . . some analyses suggest that these responses may have an impact on the patient's decision to continue using the toxin."[183]

Neutralizing BTX antibodies are thought to persist for several years. Strategies to eliminate or inactivate them are difficult.[215] In some patients, the titer may drop over a period or years, and subsequent pre-treatment with mycophenolate[216] has been tried prior to another exposure as a method to avoid the precipitation of titer elevation (anamnestic response) with repeat treatment. In addition, plasmapheresis has been tried in an attempt to remove neutralizing antibodies.[217] Therefore, avoidance of BTX antibody formation is important. Antibody formation avoidance strategies include the use of the lowest effective BTX doses that produce a meaningful therapeutic effect and in most cases, and inter-injection intervals of at least 10 to 12 weeks.

SIDE EFFECTS AND SAFETY

Local side effects may occur as an extension of BTX's pharmacologic and therapeutic effects. For example, muscle relaxation—the desired therapeutic effect—affects both pathologic and physiologic muscle activities. BTX reduces physiologic muscle activity along with pathologic muscle activity. A reduction of physiologic muscle activity (i.e., muscle relaxation) may be compensated for by regional agonistic muscles; therefore, overall physiological function is usually not impaired by BTX therapy.

Local side effects may also include those associated with the procedure, such as pain, bleeding, and local soreness. Additional pharmacologic local effects are those that occur in tissue adjacent to the injection sites and are thought to be caused by diffusion of BTX limited to those adjacent tissues. The frequency of these local side effects is thought to be related to the characteristics of the surrounding tissue, the serotype and the formulation administered. Dysphagia is an established adverse event following treatment of cervical dystonia patients with all BTXs; this appears to be more pronounced with BTX-B (See Table 3). In cervical dystonia patients, there are reports of rare cases of dysphagia severe enough to warrant the insertion of a gastric feeding tube. There are also rare case reports in which subsequent to the finding of dysphagia a patient developed aspiration pneumonia and died.

Side effects may be termed systemic when they are symptomatic in body parts distant from the target tissue. BTX-A injected into a target muscle is rapidly bound to its acceptors on nerve terminals,[218] mitigating the potential for systemic side effects when usual therapeutic BTX-A doses are applied in patients with normal neuromuscular junctions. With therapeutic BTX-A doses in the order of only a few nanograms, physical analytic methods fail to detect systemic BTX-A. Single-fiber electromyography may reveal subtle alterations of neuromuscular transmission remote from the target muscles;[219–222] these findings have not been demonstrated as clinically relevant. Recently published radio-iodine studies with BOTOX® in rats at doses of ~210 U/kg, well beyond human therapeutic doses, have demonstrated that intact neurotoxin is localized to the injection region, and small soluble iodinated breakdown protein fragments may be found in remote sites.[223] This is consistent with the reduced potential for BTX-A systemic effects.

Results of several studies suggest that the rate of side effects differs between the two BTX-A preparations and may reflect the safety margin (Table 2). In a study of blepharospasm patients, Dysport® was associated with a higher rate of ptosis and a higher rate of adverse events overall than BOTOX®.[162] In a large retrospective study of patients with various types of dystonia,[161] Dysport® was also associated with more adverse events than BOTOX®. Additionally, in double-blind trials for the treatment of cervical dystonia, BOTOX® has been associated with a low rate of dry mouth (0.5%),[224] whereas Dysport® has been associated with a higher rate of dry mouth (18% to 33%),[225] and produces about three times more dysphagia than BOTOX® (Table 3).[163,164] Another study found much higher rates of dysphagia with Dysport® than BOTOX® (3% vs. 16%–17%, respectively).[165] However, some studies have not found adverse event differences.[226,227] Because the doses in these studies were pre-selected to conform to specific BOTOX®: Dysport® dose ratios (1:3 or

1:4), they may not represent the optimal doses for patients in a non-trial setting. Consequently, the adverse event rates obtained may not correspond to those in actual clinical practice given the general dose dependence of side effects with botulinum neurotoxins. The reasons for the reported increased rate of local side effects in most studies after injection therapy with Dysport® is not established; however, as suggested by preclinical results of the safety margin,[5] and as elaborated further by Aoki in subsequent studies,[228] these effects could be due to increased diffusion out of the muscle (Table 2).

As clinical experience with the first therapeutic BTX-B preparation (i.e., NeuroBloc®/MyoBloc™) accumulates, its unique side effect profile is beginning to emerge. It has a reportedly high incidence of dysphagia, dry mouth (see Table 3) and antigenicity (reviewed above). Although BTX-B affects neuromuscular cholinergic synapses,[36,187] its clinical effects on autonomic cholinergic synapses are considerably stronger,[229] as reflected by the adverse events reported.[230] It is unclear whether this reflects either a relatively higher affinity of BTX-B (as compared to BTX-A) for autonomic synapses or the observation that BTX-B doses for production of neuromuscular effects in humans are several fold higher than those of BTX-A, such that at therapeutic neuromuscular doses, autonomic synapses are stimulated by BTX-B. When BTX-B is used in therapeutic doses, systemic autonomic side effects including dryness of mouth, conjunctival irritation, accommodation difficulties, and heartburn are frequently observed.[164,230,231] Bladder dysfunction and fungal superinfection of exsiccotic mucosa may also occur.[230] These side effects seem to be more frequent with higher BTX-B doses than with lower doses.[230] With its high rate of systemic anticholinergic side effects, BTX-B may be less suitable for treatment of muscular indications than BTX-A, particularly when high doses are required. Whether BTX-B has advantages over BTX-A for treatment of autonomic indications remains to be determined. However, given its side effect profile, BTX-B should be used carefully in patients with pre-existing autonomic dysfunction, other anticholinergic treatment, or conditions in which anticholinergics are contraindicated.

The safe and effective use of BTX depends upon proper storage, selection of the dose, and proper reconstitution and administration techniques. Physicians providing therapy should read the product package insert carefully, and must understand the relevant anatomy of the area involved and any alterations to the anatomy due to prior surgical procedures.[232] An understanding of standard electromyographic techniques is also required in some situations.

Caution should be used when BTX treatment is used in the presence of inflammation at the proposed injection sites, and treatment is contraindicated in the presence of infection at the proposed injection sites, and in individuals with known hypersensitivity to any ingredient in the formulation. Treatment should be in an environment where ancillary medications (e.g., diphenhydramine, epinephrine) are available if needed.

Individuals with excessive weakness or atrophy in the target muscles or peripheral motor neuropathic diseases (e.g., amyotrophic lateral sclerosis, Machado-Joseph disease, or motor neuropathy) or neuromuscular junctional disorders (e.g., myasthenia gravis, Lambert-Eaton syndrome) should only receive BTX with caution. Patients with neuromuscular disorders may be at increased risk of clinically significant side effects including severe dysphagia from typical doses of BTX. Rare cases of administration of a botulinum toxin to patients with known or unrecognized neuromuscular disorders have reported that these patients may show extreme sensitivity to the typical clinical doses with a broader side effect profile.[156,157,233,234] In some of these cases, dysphagia has lasted several months and required placement of a gastric feeding tube. However, in motor neuron disease, treatment of sialorrhea has been carefully performed safely.[146]

Interactions with other drugs are rare. Reconstituting the botulinum toxin preparations with other drugs or liquids not listed on the product label is not advised, since the impact of the added ingredient (preserved saline, lidocaine, steroids, etc.) combined with the product remains unknown. In addition, there may be unknown interactions of the botulinum toxin with the other ingredients (active and inactive materials) found in any liquids beyond the approved non-preserved saline.

Aminoglycosides[235] may theoretically potentiate BTX's effects. In theory, since both BTX and aminoglycoside medications could exert action at the level of the neuromuscular junction, it was thought that clinically, the effects of BTX would be increased. However, there is no evidence in the published literature of increased clinically significant effects of therapeutically administered BTX-A in association with the use of aminoglycosides.

Historically, the concern that aminoglycosides could increase the effects of BTX was based upon theoretical speculation, and the clinical observation that patients with botulism worsened following the administration of aminoglycosides antibiotics.[236] In a study of 99 cases of infantile botulism, ventilatory assistance was required for 61% of infants receiving aminoglycosides after the onset of weakness compared to only 26% of those infants not receiving aminoglycosides. Indeed, the effects of aminoglycosides on patients with botulism had led to the suggestion that the administration of an aminoglycoside antibiotic may be a useful diagnostic tool in patients with suspected botulism;[237] the authors are not aware of any cases where this concept was instituted. Patients with botulism, however, do not have the same clinical characteristics as patients who have received therapeutic BTX-A. The quantity of therapeutic toxin is small and the area to be injected is carefully and precisely chosen by the physician to minimize any potential adverse events. This may be part of the reason why there are no reports of patients who receive both BTX-A and aminoglycosides developing any clinical problems.

There was only one case identified where BTX-A could have played a subclinical role in the patient's situation.[238] The patient underwent general anesthesia twice during treatment with botulinum toxin for a long history of blepharospasm. It was noted that the patient had a subclinical increased sensitivity to vecuronium, as demonstrated by the electrical stimulation used to monitor the patient. The authors postulated that potential remote effects of botulinum toxin produced subclinical denervation, similar to that postulated with single-fiber electromyography,[219–222] thus causing the patient to develop some non-clinically meaningful sensitivity to the effects of the vecuronium. Patients who receive vecuronium are already intubated and carefully monitored. However the anesthesiologist should be made aware when a patient has received BTX, as should be done with all medications preoperatively.[239]

There is a paucity of data regarding use during pregnancy for any commercially available serotype; teratogenicity has not been established.[240,241] The authors recommend against injecting patients who are pregnant or lactating.

Commercially GMP-produced BTX products contain albumin, a derivative of human blood. Based on effective donor screening and product manufacturing processes, it carries an extremely remote risk for transmission of viral diseases. A theoretical risk for transmission of Creutzfeldt-Jakob disease (CJD) also is considered extremely remote. No cases of transmission of viral diseases or CJD have ever been identified for BTX.

The incidence of some reported adverse events in clinical trials may be similar in a group receiving active treatment and placebo therapy. For instance, as outlined in the BOTOX® Cosmetic® package insert, the incidence of "headache" and "infection" is similar in the treated and placebo groups, as are some of the other adverse events (Table 14 in package insert[242]). In addition, some adverse events improve with optimizing individual therapy and/or experience. In the Allergan-sponsored clinical trials of BTX-A for the treatment of glabellar lines, blepharoptosis was reported for 2.1% (8/373) of subjects in the first treatment cycle and 1.2% (4/343) of subjects in the second treatment cycle; no patients who received placebo developed blepharoptosis.[242] Transient ptosis, though, has been reported in the literature in approximately 5% of patients undergoing treatment for the glabellar indication.

The long term safety of BTX-A has been demonstrated in controlled and observational studies spanning over 2 decades of research and over 14 years of marketed product in clinical application. These products have been used to treat millions of patients worldwide. Publications reviewing the long-term effects[39,243] are summarized in Table 7 for most presentations of dystonia, hemifacial spasm, stroke, and juvenile cerebral palsy.

Adverse events observed with BTX-A reflect its focal and reversible action. In most situations, adverse events are transient and can be mitigated through specific dose modifiers (Table 5), and optimization of therapy with experience with each individual patient. This is amplified by the experience noted above in the incidence of ptosis in the treatment of glabellar lines. Several long-term studies of dystonia patients have documented the safety of BTX-A for up to 10 years.[244,245]

TABLE 8-7. *Published Reports of Long Term Safety of BTX-A in Dystonia[243]*

Indication	Citation	N	Treatments	Results
HFS	Defazio, 2002[245]	65	10 years or more	AEs typically mild and well tolerated; declined from 1st to 10th year from 37% to 12% of patients
CD, HFS, BL, other	Hsuing, 2002[244]	235	At least 2 years; maximum 10 years	AEs reportedly minor and well tolerated; reported on 4.5% of treatments
OMD	Tan, 1999[255]	162	0.3 to 10 years; mean, 4.4 years	Local, transient AEs reported on 135 of 1213 visits (11.1%); dysphagia, dysarthria; AEs did not increase in frequency over time
SD	Blitzer, 1998[256]	901	12 years clinical experience; exact # of treatments NS	Mild breathiness 35% of patients, mild choking on fluids 15%, all other AEs <1% of patients
BL	Nussgens, 1995[257]	115	3 to 8 yrs	AEs were all local and transient and included ptosis, tearing, double vision, lid lag (all occurred in <5.4% of patients)
Focal hand dystonia	Karp et al., 1994[258]	53	37 at least 2 years	AEs were mild and transient and included mild weakness (21%), forearm atrophy (4%), and local pain (2%)
BL, MeS	Borodic, 1992[259]	11	Mean 11.3 injections over 3.5 years	No degenerative changes observed in orbicularis oculi muscles following repeated injections
Benign facial spasms	Ruusuvaara, 1990[260]	62	52–1 or 2 injections 20–3 to 5 injections	Mild/moderate ptosis 23%, diplopia 6.5%, facial paresis 6.5%
BL, HFS, MeS	Dutton, 1988[261]	290	175 > 2 injections 85 > 5 injections 30 > 10 injections	Local and transient AEs: dry eye, ptosis, photophobia, face weakness, lacrimation; sustained duration with repeated treatment
BL, HFS	Drummond, 2001[262]	39	39> 6 injections 17 > 12 injections 7 > 20 injections	No statistical or clinical change in duration with repeated treatment; adverse events not specified
Strabismus	Elston, 1985[263]	85	4 to 21 months	No local or systemic side effects

HFS, hemifacial spasm; CD, cervical dystonia; BL, blepharospasm; OMD, oromandibular spasm; SD, spasmodic dysphonia/ laryngeal dystonia; MeS, Meige's syndrome (segmental cranial dystonia); AEs, adverse events.

For instance, a study of 235 dystonia patients found that adverse events occurred on 4.5% of 2616 treatment cycles, and reportedly most were minor and well tolerated.[244] Another 10-year study found that the incidence of adverse events actually declined over this period, with 37% of 65 patients reporting an adverse event during the first year of treatment compared with only 12% of 65 patients during the tenth year of treatment.[245]

CONCLUDING COMMENT

The future of neuromodulator therapy is predicated on the quality of the translational interaction between basic science and clinical science.[67] It is the hope of the authors that continued research will further that interaction, and lead to greater understanding and appreciation of these unique molecules and remarkable therapies. There are very few medical specialties, which are not touched by botulinum toxin therapy—neurology, ophthalmology, gastroenterology, dermatology, otolaryngology, aesthetics, plastic surgery, urology and family practice. Botulinum toxin therapy can provide physicians and patients a therapeutic tool that delivers symptomatic relief for long periods, and positively impacts their quality of life.

REFERENCES

1. Brin MF. Botulinum toxin: new and expanded indications. Eur.J.Neurol. 1997;4:59–66.
2. Brin MF. Treatment of dystonia (Chapter: 26). In: Jankovic J, Tolosa E, eds. Parkinson's Disease and Movement Disorders. New York: Williams & Wilkins, 1998:553–578.
3. Brin MF. Botulinum toxin therapy: Basic science and overview of other therapeutic applications (Chapter: Blitzer A, Binder WJ, Boyd JB, Carruthers A, eds. Management of Facial Lines and Wrinkles. New York: Lippencott Williams & Wilkins, 2000:279–302.
4. Aoki KR. Pharmacology and immunology of botulinum toxin serotypes. J Neurol. 2001;248 Suppl 1:3–10.
5. Aoki KR. A comparison of the safety margins of botulinum neurotoxin serotypes A, B, and F in mice. Toxicon. 2001;39:1815–1820.
6. Scott AB. Botulinum toxin injection into extraocular muscles as an alternative to strabismus surgery. J.Pediatr.Ophthalmol.Strabismus 1980;17: 21–25.
7. Brin MF, Jankovic J. Other uses of botulinum toxin type A therapy (Chapter: Brin MF, Comella C, Jankovic J, eds. Dystonia Monograph. New York: Lippencott, 2003.
8. Kerner J. Das Fettgift und die Fettsaure und ihre Wirkungen auf den thierischen Organismus. Ein Beytrag zur Untersuchung des in verdorbenen Wursten giftig wirkenden Stoffes. Stuttgart, Tubingen:Cotta-Verlag, 1822.
9. Kerner J. Neue Beobachtungen uber die in Wurthemberg so haufig vorfallenden todlichen Vergiftungen durch den Genuss geraucherter Wurste. Tubingen:GF Osiander, 1820.
10. Kerner J. Vergiftung durch verdorbene Wurste. Tubinger Blatter f Naturwissensch u Arzneykunde 1817;3:1–25.
11. Schantz EJ, Johnson EA. Botulinum toxin: the story of its development for the treatment of human disease. Perspect.Biol.Med. 1997;40:317–327.

12. Hatheway CL. Bacterial sources of clostridial neurotoxins (Chapter: Simpson LL, ed. Botulinum neurotoxin and tetanus toxin. San Diego: Academic Press, Inc., 1989:3–24.

13. Nieman H. Molecular biology of clostridial neurotoxins (Chapter: Alouf J, Freer J, eds. Sourcebook of Bacterial Protein Toxins. New York: Academic Press, 1991:763–772.

14. Dolman CE. Botulism as a world problem (Chapter: Lewis KH, Cassel K Jr, eds. Botulism: Proceedings of a Symposium. Cincinnati: Public Health Service, 1964:5–30.

15. Shapiro RL, Hatheway C, Swerdlow DL. Botulism in the United States: a clinical and epidemiologic review. Ann.Intern.Med 1998;129:221–228.

16. Naumann M, Merz B, Bigalke H. Pure autonomic dysfunction in botulism type B. Archives of Pharmacology 2002;285:R31:89(Abstract)

17. Scott AB, Rosenbaum A, Collins CC. Pharmacologic weakening of extraocular muscles. Invest.Ophthalmol.Vis.Sci. 1973;12:924–927.

18. Therapeutics Committee. Oculinum: an ocular therapeutic use for a notorious toxin. Aust.N.Z.J.Ophthalmol. 1986;14:87–88.

19. Biglan AW, May M. Treatment of facial spasm with oculinum (C. botulinum toxin). J.Pediatr.Ophthalmol.Strabismus 1986;23:216–221.

20. Tsui JK, Eisen A, Mak E, Carruthers MJ, Scott A, Calne DB. A pilot study on the use of botulinum toxin in spasmodic torticollis. Can.J.Neurol.Sci. 1985;12:314–316.

21. Fahn S, List T, Moskowitz CB, Brin MF, Bressman S, Burke R, Scott A. Double-blind controlled study of botulinum toxin for blepharospasm. Neurology 1985;35 (Suppl 1):271(Abstract)

22. Blitzer A, Brin MF, Fahn S, Lange D, Lovelace RE. Botulinum toxin (BOTOX) for the treatment of "spastic dysphonia" as part of a trial of toxin injections for the treatment of other cranial dystonias [letter]. Laryngoscope 1986;96:1300–1301.

23. Brin MF, Fahn S, Moskowitz C, Friedman A, Shale HM, Greene PE, Blitzer A, List T, Lange D, Lovelace RE. Localized injections of botulinum toxin for the treatment of focal dystonia and hemifacial spasm. Mov.Disord. 1987;2:237–254.

24. Lange DJ, Warner C, Brin MF, List T, Fahn S, Lovelace R. Botulinum toxin therapy: Distant effects on neuromuscular transmission [abstract]. Muscle Nerve 1985;8:624(Abstract)

25. Sanders DB, Massey EW, Buckley EC. EMG monitoring of botulinum toxin in blepharospasm. Neurology 1985;35 (Suppl 1):272(Abstract)

26. Lorentz IT, Subramaniam SS, Yiannikas C. Treatment of idiopathic spasmodic torticollis with botulinum toxin A: a double-blind study on twenty-three patients. Mov.Disord. 1991;6:145–150.

27. Brin MF, Blitzer A. Botulinum Toxin—Dangerous Terminology Errors. J.R.Soc.Med. 1993;86:494

28. Samant HC, Gupta SK, Gupta OP. Palatal myoclonus. Ann.Otol.Rhinol.Laryngol. 1970;79:858–61.

29. Dart Frog Poison—http://chemweb.calpoly.edu/chem/bailey/377/PapersF2000/Caroline/. 2003.

30. DasGupta BR. The structure of botulinum neurotoxin (Chapter: Simpson LL, ed. Botulinum neurotoxin and tetanus toxin. New York: Academic Press, 1989:53–67.

31. Binz T, Kurazono H, Wille M, Frevert J, Wernars K, Niemann H. The complete sequence of botulinum neurotoxin type A and comparison with other clostridial neurotoxins. J.Biol.Chem. 1990;265:9153–8.

32. Sugii S, Sakaguchi G. Molecular construction of Clostridium botulinum type A toxins. Infect.Immun. 1975;12:1262–1270.

33. Hirtzer P, Chung J, Dias B, Kannan K, Patel N, Callaway J. Complex integrity of botulinum toxin type B (NeuroBloc Tm): implications for the incidence of secondary non-responders. Eur J Neurol 2000;7:113

34. Kondo H, Shimizu T, Kubonoya M, Izumi N, Takahashi M, Sakaguchi G. Titration of botulinum toxins for lethal toxicity by intravenous injection into mice. Jpn.J.Med.Sci.Biol. 1984;37:131–135.

35. Melling J, Hambleton P, Shone CC. Clostridium botulinum toxins: nature and preparation for clinical use. Eye. 1988;2:16–23.

36. Brin MF, Lew MF, Adler CH, Comella CL, Factor SA, Jankovic J, O'Brien C, Murray JJ, Wallace JD, Willmer-Hulme A, Koller M. Safety and efficacy of NeuroBloc (botulinum toxin type B) in type A-resistant cervical dystonia. Neurology 1999;53:1431–1438.

37. Lowe NJ, Yamauchi PS, Lask GP, Patnaik R, Moore D. Botulinum toxins types A and B for brow furrows: preliminary experiences with type B toxin dosing. J.Cosmet.Laser Ther. 2002;4:15–18.

38. Sloop RR, Cole BA, Escutin RO. Human response to botulinum toxin injection: type B compared with type A. Neurology 1997;49:189–194.

39. Naumann M, Lowe NJ, Kumar CR, Hamm H. Botulinum toxin type a is a safe and effective treatment for axillary hyperhidrosis over 16 months: a prospective study. Arch.Dermatol. 2003;139:731–736.

40. Pellizzari R, Rossetto O, Schiavo G, Montecucco C. Tetanus and botulinum neurotoxins: mechanism of action and therapeutic uses. Philos.Trans.R.Soc.Lond.B.Biol.Sci. 1999;354:259–268.

41. Martin TFJ. Stages of regulated exocytosis. Trends in Cell Biology 1997;7:271–276.

42. Schiavo G, Santucci A, DasGupta BR, Mehta PP, Jontes J, Benfenati F, Wilson MC, Montecucco C. Botulinum Neurotoxins Serotypes a and E Cleave Snap-25 at Distinct COOH-Terminal Peptide Bonds. FEBS Lett. 1993;335:99–103.

43. Binz T, Blasi J, Yamasaki S, Baumeister A, Link E, Sudhof TC, Jahn R, Niemann H. Proteolysis of SNAP-25 by Type-E and Type-A Botulinal Neurotoxins. J Biol Chem 1994;269:1617–1620.

44. Foran P, Lawrence GW, Shone CC, Foster KA, Dolly JO. Botulinum neurotoxin C1 cleaves both syntaxin and SNAP-25 in intact and permeabilized chromaffin cells: correlation with its blockade of catecholamine release. Biochemistry 1996;35:2630–2636.

45. Schiavo G, Benfenati F, Poulain B, Rossetto O, Polverino de Laureto P, DasGupta BR, Montecucco C. Tetanus and botulinum-B neurotoxins block neurotransmitter release by proteolytic cleavage of synaptobrevin. Nature. 1992;359:832–835.

46. Yamasaki S, Baumeister A, Blasi J, Link E, Cornille F, Roques B, Fykse EM, Sudhof TC, Jahn R, Niemann H, Binz T. Cleavage of Members of the Synaptobrevin/Vamp Family by Types D and F Botulinal Neurotoxins and Tetanus Toxin. J Biol Chem 1994;269:12764–12772.

47. Blasi J, Chapman ER, Yamasaki S, Binz T, Niemann H, Jahn R. Botulinum Neurotoxin-C1 Blocks Neurotransmitter Release by Means of Cleaving HPC-1/syntaxin. EMBO J 1993;12:4821–4828.

48. Duchen LW. Changes in the electron microscopic structure of slow and fast skeletal muscle fibres of the mouse after the local injection of botulinum toxin. J.Neurol.Sci. 1971;14:61–74.

49. Duchen LW. An electron microscopic study of the changes induced by botulinum toxin in the motor end-plates of slow and fast skeletal muscle fibres of the mouse. J.Neurol.Sci. 1971;14:47–60.

50. de Paiva A, Meunier FA, Molgo J, Aoki KR, Dolly JO. Functional repair of motor endplates after botulinum neurotoxin type A poisoning: biphasic switch of synaptic activity between nerve sprouts and their parent terminals. Proc.Natl.Acad.Sci.U.S.A 1999;96:3200–3205.

51. Borodic GE, Ferrante R, Pearce LB, Smith K. Histologic assessment of dose-related diffusion and muscle fiber response after therapeutic botulinum-A toxin injections. Mov.Disord. 1994;9:31–39.

52. Filippi GM, Errico P, Santarelli R, Bagolini B, Manni E. Botulinum-A Toxin Effects on Rat Jaw Muscle Spindles. Acta Oto-Laryngol. 1993; 113:400–404.

53. Dressler D, Eckert J, Kulowski B, Meyer BU. Somatosensory evoked potentials in writer's cramp: pathological findings reversed by botulinum toxin therapy. EEG Clin Neurophysiol 1995;94:59(Abstract)

54. Rosales RL, Arimura K, Takenaga S, Osame M. Extrafusal and intrafusal muscle effects in experimental botulinum toxin-a injection. Muscle Nerve 1996;19:488–496.

55. Ludlow CL, Hallett M, Sedory SE, Fujita M, Naunton RF. The pathophysiology of spasmodic dysphonia and its modification by botulinum toxin (Chapter: 24). In: Berardelli A, Benecke R, Manfredi M, Marsden CM, eds. Motor Disturbances II. New York: Academic Press, 1990: 273–288.

56. Zwirner P, Murry T, Swenson M, Wooodson G. Effects of botulinum toxin therapy in patients with adductor spasmodic dysphonia: acoustic, aerodynamic, and videoendoscopic findings. Laryngoscope 1992;102:400–406.

57. Brin MF, Blitzer A, Stewart C, Fahn S. Treatment of spasmodic dysphonia (laryngeal dystonia) with local injections of botulinum toxin: review and technical aspects (Chapter: 20). In: Blitzer A, Brin MF, Sasaki CT, Fahn S, Harris KS, eds. Neurological disorders of the larynx. New York: Thieme, 1992:214–228.

58. Borg-Stein J, Pine ZM, Miller JR, Brin MF. Botulinum toxin for the treatment of spasticity in multiple sclerosis. New observations. Am.J Phys.Med.Rehabil. 1993;72:364–368.

59. Kaji R, Rothwell JC, Katayama M, Ikeda T, Kubori T, Kohara N, Mezaki T, Shibasaki H, Kimura J. Tonic vibration reflex and muscle afferent block in writer's cramp. Ann.Neurol. 1995;38:155–162.

60. Kaji R, Kohara N, Katayama M, Kubori T, Mezaki T, Shibasaki H, Kimura J. Muscle afferent block by intramuscular injection of lidocaine for the treatment of writer's cramp. Muscle Nerve 1995;18:234–235.

61. Kaji R, Shibasaki H, Kimura J. Writer's cramp: a disorder of motor subroutine? [editorial; comment]. Ann.Neurol. 1995;38:837–838.

62. Kaji R, Mezaki T, Kubori T, Murase N, Kimura J. [Treatment of spasticity with botulinum toxin and muscle afferent block]. Rinsho Shinkeigaku 1996;36:1334–1335.

63. Yoshida K, Kaji R, Kubori T, Kohara N, Iizuka T, Kimura J. Muscle af-

ferent block for the treatment of oromandibular dystonia. Mov.Disord. 1998;13:699–705.

64. Mezaki T, Kaji R, Hirota N, Kohara N, Kimura J. Treatment of spasticity with muscle afferent block. Neurology 1999;53:1156–1157.

65. Chan J, Brin M, Fahn S. Idiopathic cervical dystonia: Clinical characteristics. Mov.Disord. 1991;6:119–126.

66. Jankovic J, Leder S, Warner D, Schwartz K. Cervical dystonia: Clinical findings and associated movement disorders. Neurology 1991;41:1088–1091.

67. Brin, M. F., Hallett, M., and Jankovic, J. (eds) Scientific and Therapeutic Aspects of Botulinum Toxin. New York:Lippencott Williams & Wilkins, 2002.

68. Tsui JK, Eisen A, Stoessl AJ, Calne S, Calne DB. Double-blind study of botulinum toxin in spasmodic torticollis. Lancet. 1986;2:245–247.

69. Tsui JK, Fross RD, Calne S, Calne DB. Local treatment of spasmodic torticollis with botulinum toxin. Can.J.Neurol.Sci. 1987;14:533–535.

70. Jankovic J, Schwartz K. Botulinum toxin injections for cervical dystonia. Neurology 1990;40:277–280.

71. Poewe W, Schelosky L, Kleedorfer B, Heinen F, Wagner M, Deuschl G. Treatment of spasmodic torticollis with local injections of botulinum toxin. One-year follow-up in 37 patients. J.Neurol. 1992;239:21–25.

72. Tsui JKC, Fross RD, Calne S, Calne DB. Local treatment of spasmodic torticollis with botulinum toxin. Can.J.Neurol.Sci. 1987;14:533–535.

73. Greene P, Kang U, Fahn S, Brin M, Moskowitz C, Flaster E. Double-blind, placebo-controlled trial of botulinum toxin injections for the treatment of spasmodic torticollis. Neurology 1990;40:1213–1218.

74. Blackie JD, Lees AJ. Botulinum toxin treatment in spasmodic torticollis. J.Neurol.Neurosurg.Psychiatry 1990;53:640–643.

75. Lorentz IT, Subramaniam SS, Yiannikas C. Treatment of idiopathic spasmodic torticollis with botulinum toxin A: a double-blind study on twenty-three patients. Mov Disord. 1991;6:145–150.

76. Lu CS, Chen RS, Tsai CH. Double-blind, placebo-controlled study of botulinum toxin injections in the treatment of cervical dystonia. J.Formos.Med.Assoc. 1995;94:189–192.

77. Brin MF, Binder WJ, Blitzer A, Schenrock L, Pogoda JM. Botulinum toxin type A for pain and headache (Chapter: Brin MF, Hallett M, Jankovic J, eds. Scientific and Therapeutic Aspects of Botulinum Toxin. New York: Lippencott Williams & Wilkins, 2002:233–250.

78. Galvez-Jimenez N, Lampuri C, Patino-Piecirilo R, Hargreave M. Dystonia and deadaches: the response to botulinum toxin (BTx) therapy. Mov.Disord. 2002;17:1141(Abstract)

79. Csala B, Deuschl G. [Craniocervical dystonia. Pragmatic general concept or nosologic entity?]. Nervenarzt. 1994;65:75–94.

80. Gobel H, Heinze A, Heinze-Kuhn K, Austermann K. Botulinum toxin A in the treatment of headache syndromes and pericranial pain syndromes. Pain. 2001;91:195–199.

81. Friedman J, Standaert DG. Dystonia and its disorders. Neurol.Clin. 2001; 19:681–705, vii.

82. Memin B, Pollack P, Hommel M, Perret J. Effects of botulinum toxin on spasticity. Rev.Neurol.(Paris) 1992;148:212–214.

83. Dengler R, Neyer U, Wohlfarth K, Bettig U, Janzik H. Local botulinum toxin in the treatment of spastic foot drop. J.Neurol. 1992;239:375–378.

84. Dunne JW, Heye N, Dunne SL. Treatment of chronic limb spasticity with botulinum toxin A. J.Neurol Neurosurg.Psychiatry 1995;58:232–235.

85. Viriyavejakul A, Vachalathiti R, Poungvarin N. Botulinum treatment for post-stroke spasticity: low dose regime. J Med Assoc.Thai. 1998;81:413–422.

86. Grazko MA, Polo KB, Jabbari B. Botulinum toxin A for spasticity, muscle spasms, and rigidity. Neurology 1995;45:712–717.

87. Hyman N, Barnes M, Bhakta B, Cozens A, Bakheit M, Kreczy-Kleedorfer B, Poewe W, Wissel J, Bain P, Glickman S, Sayer A, Richardson A, Dott C. Botulinum toxin (Dysport) treatment of hip adductor spasticity in multiple sclerosis: a prospective, randomised, double blind, placebo controlled, dose ranging study. J Neurol. Neurosurg.Psychiatry 2000;68:707–712.

88. Nix WA, Butler IJ, Roontga S, Gutmann L, Hopf HC. Persistent unilateral tibialis anterior muscle hypertrophy with complex repetitive discharges and myalgia: report of two unique cases and response to botulinum toxin. Neurology 1992;42:602–606.

89. Davis D, Jabbari B. Significant improvement of stiff-person syndrome after paraspinal injection of botulinum toxin A. Mov Disord. 1993; 8:371–373.

90. Fishman VM, Parkman HP, Schiano TD, Hills C, Dabezies MA, Cohen S, Fisher RS, Miller LS. Symptomatic improvement in achalasia after botulinum toxin injection of the lower esophageal sphincter. Am.J.Gastroenterol. 1996;91:1724–1730.

91. Jost WH. One hundred cases of anal fissure treated with botulin toxin: early and long-term results. Dis.Colon Rectum 1997;40:1029–1032.

92. Acquadro MA, Borodic GE. Treatment of myofascial pain with botulinum A toxin [letter]. Anesthesiology. 1994;80:705–706.

93. Diaz JH, Gould HJ. Management of post-thoracotomy pseudoangina and myofascial pain with botulinum toxin. Anesthesiology. 1999;91:877–879.

94. Cheshire WP, Abashian SW, Mann JD. Botulinum toxin in the treatment of myofascial pain syndrome. Pain. 1994;59:65–69.

95. Porta M. A comparative trial of botulinum toxin type A and methylprednisolone for the treatment of myofascial pain syndrome and pain from chronic muscle spasm. Pain. 2000;85:101–105.

96. Johnstone SJ, Adler CH. Headache and facial pain responsive to botulinum toxin: an unusual presentation of blepharospasm. Headache. 1998;38:366–368.

97. Girdler NM. Use of botulinum toxin to alleviate facial pain. Br. J. Hosp.Med. 1994;52:363

98. Van Zandijcke M, Marchau MM. Treatment of bruxism with botulinum toxin injections. J Neurol.Neurosurg.Psychiatry 1990;53:530

99. Ivanhoe CB, Lai JM, Francisco GE. Bruxism after brain injury: successful treatment with botulinum toxin-A. Arch.Phys.Med Rehabil. 1997;78:1272–1273.

100. Rijsdijk BA, van ES RJ, Zonneveld FW, Steenks MH, Koole R. [Botulinum toxin type A treatment of cosmetically disturbing masseteric hypertrophy]. Ned.Tijdschr.Geneeskd. 1998;142:529–532.

101. Tan EK, Jankovic J. Treating severe bruxism with botulinum toxin. J.Am.Dent.Assoc. 2000;131:211–216.

102. Freund B, Schwartz M, Symington JM. Botulinum toxin: new treatment for temporomandibular disorders. Br.J.Oral Maxillofac.Surg. 2000;38:466–471.

103. Foster L, Clapp L, Erickson M, Jabbari B. Botulinum toxin A and chronic low back pain: a randomized, double-blind study. Neurology 2001;56:1290–1293.

104. Polo KB, Jabbari B. Effectiveness of botulinum toxin type A against painful limb myoclonus of spinal cord origin. Mov.Disord. 1994; 9:233–235.

105. Freund BJ, Schwartz M. Treatment of chronic cervical-associated headache with botulinum toxin A: a pilot study. Headache. 2000;40:231–236.

106. Ginies PR, Fraimount JL, Siou DK, Chevallier J, Mann C, Colson P. Treatment of cluster headache by subcutaneous injection of botulinum toxin (abst) (Chapter: Jensen TS, ed. Progress in Pain Research and Management. 8th. ed. Seattle: IASP Press, 1996:501

107. Freund BJ, Schwartz M. The use of botulinum toxin A in the treatment of refractory cluster headache: case reports. Cephalalgia 2000; 20:329–330.

108. Smuts JA, Barnard PWA. Botulinum toxin type A in the treatment of headache syndromes: a clinical report of 79 patients. Cephalalgia 2000;20:332

109. Zwart JA, Bovim G, Sand T, Sjaastad O. Tension headache: botulinum toxin paralysis of temporal muscles. Headache. 1994;34: 458–462.

110. Relja M. Treatment of tension-type headache by local injection of botulinum toxin. Eur.J.Neurol. 1997;4 (suppl 2):S71–S74

111. Relja MA. Treatment of tension-type headache by local injection of botulinum toxin: 1-year followup. Cephalalgia 2000;20:336

112. Schulte-Mattler WJ, Wieser T, Zierz S. Treatment of tension-type headache with botulinum toxin: a pilot study. Eur.J Med Res. 1999; 4:183–186.

113. Porta M. A comparative trial of botulinum toxin type A and methylprednisolone for the treatment of tension-type headache. Curr. Rev. Pain 2000;4:31–35.

114. Carruthers A, Langtry JA, Carruthers J, Robinson G. Improvement of tension-type headache when treating wrinkles with botulinum toxin A injections. Headache. 1999;39:662–665.

115. Zermann D, Ishigooka M, Schubert J, Schmidt RA. Perisphincteric injection of botulinum toxin type A. A treatment option for patients with chronic prostatic pain? Eur.Urol. 2000;38:393–399.

116. Binder W, Brin MF, Blitzer A, Schenrock L, Diamond B. Botulinum toxin type A (BTX-A) for migraine: an open label assessment. Mov.Disord. 1998;13:241(Abstract)

117. Mauskop A, Basedo R. Botulinum toxin A is an effect prophylactic therapy of migraines. Cephalalgia 2000;20:422

118. Binder WJ, Brin MF, Blitzer A, Schoenrock LD, Pogoda JM. Botulinum toxin type A (BOTOX) for treatment of migraine headaches: An open-label study. Otolaryngol.Head Neck Surg. 2000;123: 669–676.

119. Silberstein S, Mathew N, Saper J, Jenkins S. Botulinum Toxin Type A as a Migraine Preventive Treatment. Headache. 2000;40:445–450.

120. Brin MF, Swope DM, Abassi S, O'Brien C, Pogoda JM. BOTOX for migraine: double-blind, placebo-controlled, region-specific evaluation. Cephalalgia 2000;20:421–422.(Abstract)

121. Barwood S, Baillieu C, Boyd R, Brereton K, Low J, Nattrass G, Graham HK. Analgesic effects of botulinum toxin A: a randomized, placebo-controlled clinical trial. Dev.Med Child Neurol. 2000;42: 116–121.

122. Ishikawa H, Mitsui Y, Yoshitomi T, Mashimo K, Aoki S, Mukuno K, Shimizu K. Presynaptic effects of botulinum toxin type A on the neuronally evoked response of albino and pigmented rabbit iris sphincter and dilator muscles. Jpn.J Ophthalmol 2000;44:106–109.

123. Cui M, Aoki KR. Botulinum toxin type A (BTX-A) reduces inflammatory pain in the rat formalin model. Cephalalgia 2000;20:414(Abstract)

124. Hatheway CL, Dang C. Immunogenicity of the neurotoxins of *Clostridium botulinum* (Chapter: 8). In: Jankovic J, Hallett M, eds. Therapy with Botulinum Toxin. New York: Marcel Dekker, 1994:93–107.

125. Schantz EJ, Kautter DA. Microbiological methods: Standardized assay for clostridium botulinum toxins. J.Association of Official Analytical Chemists 1977;61:96–99.

126. Schantz EJ. Purification and characterization of *C. botulinum* toxins (Chapter: Lewis KH, Cassel Jr. K, eds. Botulism. Washington D.C.: Public Health Service. U.S. Dept. of HEW, 1964:91–104.

127. Pearce LB, Borodic GE, First ER, Maccallum RD. Measurement of botulinum toxin activity: Evaluation of the lethality assay. Toxicol. Appl. Pharmacol. 1994;128:69–77.

128. Sellin LC, Thesleff S. Pre-and post-synaptic actions of botulinum toxin at the rat neuromuscular junction. J.Physiol. 1981;317:487–495.

129. Dressler D, Adib SF, Benecke R. Botulinum toxin type B for treatment of axillar hyperhidrosis. J.Neurol. 2002;249:1729–1732.

130. First ER, Pearce LB, Borodic GE. Dose Standardisation of Botulinum Toxin. Lancet. 1994;343:1035

131. Hambleton P, Pickett AM. Potency equivalence of botulinum toxin preparations. J.R.Soc.Med. 1994;87:719

132. Marion MH, Sheehy M, Sangla S, Soulayrol S. Dose standardisation of botulinum toxin. Journal of Neurology, Neurosurgery, and Psychiatry 1995;59:1:102

133. Marsden CD. Botulinum Toxin—Dangerous Terminology Errors—Reply. J.R.Soc.Med. 1993;86:494

134. Van den Bergh PY, Lison DF. Dose standardization of botulinum toxin. Adv.Neurol. 1998;78:231–235.

135. Wohlfarth K, Goschel H, Frevert J, Dengler R, Bigalke H. Botulinum A toxins: units versus units. Naunyn Schmiedebergs Arch.Pharmacol. 1997;355:335–340.

136. Dressler D, Rothwell JC, Marsden CD. Comparing biological potencies of Botox and Dysport with a mouse diaphragm model may mislead. J Neurol. 1998;245:332

137. Scott AB, Suzuki D. Systemic toxicity of botulinum toxin by intramuscular injection in the monkey. Mov.Disord. 1988;3:333–335.

138. Herrero BA, Ecklund AE, Street CS, Ford DF, King JK. Experimental botulism in monkeys — A clinical pathological study. Exp. Mol. Pathol. 1967;6:84–95.

139. Meyer KF, Eddie B. Perspectives concerning botulism. Z.Hyg. Infektionskr. 1951;133:255–263.

140. Lamanna C, Carr JC. The botulinal, tetanal, and enterostaphylococcal toxins: a review. Clin.Pharmacol.Ther. 1967;8:286–332.

141. Lamanna C, Hillowalla RA, Alling CC. Buccal exposure to botulinal toxin. J.Infect.Dis. 1967;117:327–331.

142. Smith LD. The action of the toxins (Chapter: 8). In: Botulism: The Organism, Its Toxins, The Disease. 1 ed. Springfield, IL: Charles C. Thomas, 1977:142–151.

143. Smith LD. The toxins of *Clostridium botulinum* (Chapter: 7). In: Botulism: The Organism, Its Toxins, The Disease. 1 ed. Springfield, IL: Charles C. Thomas, 1977:113–141.

144. Bentley CR, Dawson E, Lee JP. Active management in patients with ocular manifestations of myasthenia gravis. Eye. 2001;15:18–22.

145. Bushara KO. Sialorrhea in amyotrophic lateral sclerosis: a hypothesis of a new treatment—botulinum toxin A injections of the parotid glands. Med.Hypotheses 1997;48:337–339.

146. Giess R, Naumann M, Werner E, Riemann R, Beck M, Puls I, Reiners C, Toyka KV. Injections of botulinum toxin A into the salivary glands improve sialorrhoea in amyotrophic lateral sclerosis. J Neurol. Neurosurg. Psychiatry 2000;69:121–123.

147. Goncalves MR, Barbosa ER, Zambon AA, Marchiori PE. Treatment of cervical dystonia with botulinum toxin in a patient with myasthenia gravis. Arq Neuropsiquiatr. 1999;57:683–685.

148. Restivo DA, Lanza S, Marchese-Ragona R, Palmeri A. Improvement of masseter spasticity by botulinum toxin facilitates PEG placement in amyotrophic lateral sclerosis. Gastroenterology 2002;123:1749–1750.

149. Winterholler MG, Heckmann JG, Hecht M, Erbguth FJ. Recurrent trismus and stridor in an ALS patient: successful treatment with botulinum toxin. Neurology 2002;58:502–503.

150. Tan EK, Lo YL, Seah A, Auchus AP. Recurrent jaw dislocation after botulinum toxin treatment for sialorrhoea in amyotrophic lateral sclerosis. J Neurol.Sci. 2001;190:95–97.

151. Pal PK, Calne DB, Calne S, Tsui JK. Botulinum toxin A as treatment for drooling saliva in PD. Neurology 2000;54:244–247.

152. Friedman A, Potulska A. Botulinum toxin for treatment of parkinsonian sialorrhea. Neurol.Neurochir.Pol. 2001;35 Suppl 3:23–27.

153. Giladi N, Gurevich T, Shabtai H, Paleacu D, Simon ES. The effect of botulinum toxin injections to the calf muscles on freezing of gait in parkinsonism: a pilot study. J.Neurol. 2001;248:572–576.

154. Borodic G. Myasthenic crisis after botulinum toxin [letter]. Lancet. 1998;352:1832

155. Tarsy D, Borodic GE. Myasthenia gravis (MG) after botulinum toxin type A (BTX) for Meige syndrome (MGS). Mov.Disord. 2000;15 (Suppl 1):34(Abstract)

156. Emerson J. Botulinum Toxin for Spasmodic Torticollis in a Patient with Myasthenia Gravis. Mov.Disord. 1994;9:367

157. Mezaki T, Kaji R, Kohara N, Kimura J. Development of general weakness in a patient with amyotrophic lateral sclerosis after focal botulinum toxin injection. Neurology 1996;46:845–846.

158. Tarsy D, Bhattacharyya N, Borodic G. Myasthenia gravis after botulinum toxin A for Meige syndrome. Mov Disord. 2000;15:736–738.

159. Erbguth F, Claus D, Engelhardt A, Dressler D. Systemic effect of local botulinum toxin injections unmasks subclinical Lambert-Eaton myasthenic syndrome. J.Neurol.Neurosurg.Psychiat. 1993;56:1235–1236.

160. Mclellan K, Das RE, Ekong TA, Sesardic D. Therapeutic botulinum type A toxin: factors affecting potency. Toxicon. 1996;34:975–985.

161. Dodel RC, Kirchner A, Koehne-Volland R, Kunig G, Ceballos-Baumann A, Naumann M, Brashear A, Richter HP, Szucs TD, Oertel WH. Costs of treating dystonias and hemifacial spasm with botulinum toxin A. Pharmacoeconomics. 1997;12:695–706.

162. Nussgens Z, Roggenkamper P. Comparison of two botulinum-toxin preparations in the treatment of essential blepharospasm. Graefes. Arch. Clin. Exp. Ophthalmol. 1997;235:197–199.

163. Dressler D. Dysport produces intrinsically more swallowing problems than Botox: unexpected results from a conversion factor study in cervical dystonia. J.Neurol.Neurosurg.Psychiatry 2002;73:604

164. Dressler D, Benecke R. Autonomic side effects of botulinum toxin type B treatment of cervical dystonia and hyperhidrosis. Eur.Neurol. 2003; 49:34–38.

165. Ranoux D, Gury C, Fondarai J, Mas JL, Zuber M. Respective potencies of Botox and Dysport: a double blind, randomised, crossover study in cervical dystonia. J.Neurol.Neurosurg.Psychiatry 2002;72:459–462.

166. Goschel H, Wohlfarth K, Frevert J, Dengler R, Bigalke H. Botulinum A toxin therapy: neutralizing and nonneutralizing antibodies— therapeutic consequences. Exp.Neurol. 1997;147:96–102.

167. DasGupta BR. Structures of Botulinum Neurotoxin, Its Functional Domains, and Perspectives on the Crystalline Type A Toxin (Chapter: 2). In: Jankovic J, Hallett M, eds. Therapy with Botulinum Toxin. New York: Marcel Dekker, 1994:15–39.

168. Inoue K, Fujinaga Y, Watanabe T, Ohyama T, Takeshi K, Moriishi K, Nakajima H, Oguma K. Molecular composition of clostridium botulinum type a progenitor toxins. Infect.Immun. 1996;64:1589–1594.

169. Sakaguchi G, Kozaki S, Ohishi I. Structure and function of botulinum toxins (Chapter: Alouf JEF, ed. Bacterial Protein Toxins. London: Academic Press, 1984:433–443.

170. DasGupta BR, Sathyamoorthy V. Purification and amino acid composition of type A botulinum neurotoxin. Toxicon. 1984;22:415–424.

171. Pearce LB, Borodic GE, Johnson EA, First ER, MacCallum R. The median paralysis unit: a more pharmacologically relevant unit of biologic activity for botulinum toxin. Toxicon. 1995;33:217–227.

172. Krack P, Deuschl G, Benecke R, Ceballos-Baumann AO, Marion MH, Oertel WH, Poewe W. Dose standardization of botulinum toxin. Mov Disord. 1998;13:749–751.

173. Bigalke H, Wohlfarth K, Irmer A, Dengler R. Botulinum A toxin: Dysport improvement of biological availability. Exp.Neurol. 2001;168: 162–170.

174. Rollnik JD, Matzke M, Wohlfarth K, Dengler R, Bigalke H. Low-dose treatment of cervical dystonia, blepharospasm and facial hemispasm with albumin-diluted botulinum toxin type A under EMG guidance. An open label study. Eur.Neurol. 2000;43:9–12.

175. Peng K, Merlino G, Addeo J, Foster S, Spanoyannis A, Aoki KR. BOTOX® is six fold more potent than Dysport in the mouse digit abduction scoring assay. Mov.Disord. 1998;13 (Suppl 2):110(Abstract)

176. Nagamine T, Kaji R, Hamano T, Kimura J. [Treatment of focal dystonia with botulinum toxin]. Rinsho Shinkeigaku 1991;31:32–37.

177. Zhuang D, Yin-chin W. Treatment of blepharospasm, hemifacial spasm and strabismus with botulinum toxin. Chin.Med.J. 1992;105:476–480.

178. Setler P. The biochemistry of botulinum toxin type B. Neurology 2000;55:S22–S28

179. Dressler D, Benecke R. [Initial experiences with clinical use of botulinum toxin type B]. Nervenarzt. 2002;73:194–198.

180. Lowe NJ, Lask G, Yamauchi P. Efficacy and safety of botulinum toxins A and B for the reduction of glabellar rhytids in female subjects. J.Am.Acad.Dermatol. 2002;47:459(Abstract)

181. Schoch S, Deak F, Konigstorfer A, Mozhayeva M, Sara Y, Sudhof TC, Kavalali ET. SNARE function analyzed in synaptobrevin/VAMP knockout mice. Science. 2001;294:1117–1122.

182. Sloop RR, Escutin RO, Matus JA, Cole BA, Peterson GW. Dose-response curve of human extensor digitorum brevis muscle function to intramuscularly injected botulinum toxin type a. Neurology 1996;46:1382–1386.

183. United States Food and Drug Administration. Myobloc: Summary Basis of Approval Cervical Dystonia (http://www.fda.gov/cber/products/botelan120800.htm). 2002. Available from US Government through Freedom of Information.

184. Neurobloc European Public Assessment Report. 2002. European Agency for the Evaluation of Medicinal Products (http://www.eudra.org/human-docs/humans/epar/neurobloc/neuroblocM.htm).

185. Tsui JK, Hayward M, Mak EK, Schulzer M. Botulinum toxin type B in the treatment of cervical dystonia: a pilot study. Neurology 1995;45:2109–2110.

186. Lew MF, Adornato BT, Duane DD, Dykstra DD, Factor SA, Massey JM, Brin MF, Jankovic J, Rodnitzky RL, Singer C, Swenson MR, Tarsy D, Murray JJ, Koller M, Wallace JD. Botulinum toxin type B (BotB): A double-blind, placebo-controlled, safety and efficacy study in cervical dystonia. Neurology 1997;49:701–707.

187. Brashear A, Lew MF, Dykstra DD, Comella CL, Factor SA, Rodnitzky RL, Trosch R, Singer C, Brin MF, Murray JJ, Wallace JD, Willmer-Hulme A, Koller M. Safety and efficacy of NeuroBloc (botulinum toxin type B) in type A-responsive cervical dystonia. Neurology 1999;53:1439–1446.

188. Mezaki T, Kaji R, Hamano T, Nagamine T, Shibasaki H, Shimizu T, Kimura J. Optimisation of botulinum treatment for cervical and axial dystonias: Experience with a Japanese type A toxin. J.Neurol. Neurosurg. Psychiatry 1994;57:1535–1537.

189. Kohl A, Jost WH, Rosenwald D, Freudenberg B. Comparison of the effect of botulinum toxin type A (Botox®) with the highly-purified neurotoxin (NT 201) in the extensor digitorum brevis muscle test. Mov.Disord. 2000;15 (Suppl 3):165(Abstract)

190. Ludlow CL, Hallett M, Rhew K, Cole R, Shimizu T, Sakaguchi G, Bagley JA, Schulz GM, Yin SG, Koda J. Therapeutic use of type F botulinum toxin. N.Engl.J.Med. 1992;326:349–350.

191. Greene PE, Fahn S. Use of botulinum toxin type F injections to treat torticollis in patients with immunity to botulinum toxin type A. Mov Disord. 1993;8:479–483.

192. Greene PE, Fahn S. Response to botulinum toxin F in seronegative botulinum toxin A—resistant patients. Mov Disord. 1996;11:181–184.

193. Houser MK, Sheean GL, Lees AJ. Further studies using higher doses of botulinum toxin type F for torticollis resistant to botulinum toxin type A. J Neurol.Neurosurg.Psychiatry 1998;64:577–580.

194. Biglan AW, Gonnering R, Lockhart LB, Rabin B, Fuerste FH. Absence of antibody production in patients treated with botulinum A toxin. Am.J.Ophthalmol. 1986;101:232–235.

195. Gonnering RS. Negative antibody response to long-term treatment of facial spasm with botulinum toxin. Am.J.Ophthalmol. 1988;105:313–315.

196. Jankovic J, Schwartz KS. Clinical correlates of response to botulinum toxin injections. Arch.Neurol. 1991;48:1253–1256.

197. Jankovic J, Schwartz K. Response and immunoresistance to botulinum toxin injections. Neurology 1995;45:1743–1746.

198. Dressler D. Complete secondary botulinum toxin therapy failure in blepharospasm. J.Neurol. 2000;247:809–810.

199. Kessler KR, Skutta M, Benecke R. Long-term treatment of cervical dystonia with botulinum toxin A: efficacy, safety, and antibody frequency. German Dystonia Study Group. J.Neurol. 1999;246:265–274.

200. Jankovic J, Ahsan J, Vuong KDP. Comparison of immunogenicity of old versus current BOTOX in cervical dystonia. Naunyn Schmied. Arch. Pharmacol. 2002;365 (Suppl 2):R25(Abstract)

201. Jankovic J, Vuong KD, Ahsan J. Comparison of efficacy and immunogenicity of original versus current botulinum toxin in cervical dystonia. Neurology 2003;60:1186–1188.

206. Dressler D, Dirnberger G, Bhatia KP, Irmer A, Quinn NP, Bigalke H, Marsden CD. Botulinum toxin antibody testing: comparison between the mouse protection assay and the mouse lethality assay. Mov Disord. 2000;15:973–976.

207. Palace J, Nairne A, Hyman N, Doherty TV, Vincent A. A radioimmunoprecipitation assay for antibodies to botulinum A. Neurology 1998;50:1463-1466.

208. Dressler D, Dirnberger G. Botulinum toxin antibody testing: comparison between the immunoprecipitation assay and the mouse diaphragm assay. Eur.Neurol. 2001;45:257-260.

209. Hanna PA, Jankovic J, Vincent A. Comparison of mouse bioassay and immunoprecipitation assay for botulinum toxin antibodies [In Process Citation]. J.Neurol.Neurosurg.Psychiatry 1999;66:612-616.

210. Hanna PA, Jankovic J. Mouse bioassay versus Western blot assay for botulinum toxin antibodies: correlation with clinical response. Neurology 1998;50:1624-1629.

211. Kessler KR, Benecke R. The EBD test--a clinical test for the detection of antibodies to botulinum toxin type A. Mov Disord. 1997;12:95-99.

212. Dressler D, Schonle PW. Botulinum toxin to suppress hyperkinesias after hypoglossal-facial nerve anastomosis. Arch.Otorhinolaryngol. 1990;247:391

213. Greene P, Fahn S, Diamond B. Development of resistance to botulinum toxin type A in patients with torticollis. Mov Disord. 1994;9:213-217.

214. Borodic G, Johnson E, Goodnough M, Schantz E. Botulinum toxin therapy, immunologic resistance, and problems with available materials. Neurology 1996;46:26-29.

215. Dressler D, Bigalke H. Botulinum toxin antibody type A titres after cessation of botulinum toxin therapy. Mov Disord. 2002;17:170-173.

216. Duane DD, Monroe J, Morris RE. Mycophenolate in the prevention of recurrent neutralizing botulinum toxin A antibodies in cervical dystonia [letter]. Mov Disord. 2000;15:365-366.

217. Dressler D. Clinical presentation and management of antibody induced botulinum toxin therapy failure. Naunyn Schmiedebergs Arch.Pharmacol. 2002;365 (Suppl 2):R17(Abstract)

218. Takamizawa K, Iwamori M, Kozaki S, Sakaguchi G, Tanaka R, Takayama H, Nagai Y. TLC immunostaining characterization of Clostridium botulinum type A neurotoxin binding to gangliosides and free fatty acids. FEBS Lett. 1986;201:229-232.

219. Sanders DB, Massey EW, Buckley EG. Botulinum toxin for blepharospasm: single-fiber EMG studies. Neurology 1986;36:545-547.

220. Lange DJ, Brin MF, Warner CL, Fahn S, Lovelace RE. Distant effects of local injection of botulinum toxin. Muscle Nerve 1987;10:552-555.

221. Olney RK, Aminoff MJ, Gelb DJ, Lowenstein DH. Neuromuscular effects distant from the site of botulinum neurotoxin injection. Neurology 1988;38:1780-1783.

222. Girlanda P, Vita G, Nicolosi C, Milone S, Messina C. Botulinum toxin therapy: distant effects on neuromuscular transmission and autonomic nervous system. J Neurol.Neurosurg.Psychiatry 1992;55:844-845.

223. Tang-Liu DD, Aoki KR, Dolly JO, de Paiva A, Houchen TL, Chasseaud LF, Webber C. Intramuscular injection of 125I-botulinum neurotoxin-complex versus 125I-botulinum-free neurotoxin: time course of tissue distribution. Toxicon. 2003;42:461-460.

224. Hauser RA, Comella C, Brashear A, et al. A randomized, multicenter, double-blind, placebo-controlled study of original Botox (botulinum toxin type A) purified neurotoxin complex for the treatment of cervical dystonia. Mov.Disord. 2000;15:30-31.(Abstract)

225. Poewe W, Deuschl G, Nebe A, Feifel E, Wissel J, Benecke R, Kessler KR, Ceballos-Baumann AO, Ohly A, Oertel W, Kunig G. What is the optimal dose of botulinum toxin A in the treatment of cervical dystonia? Results of a double blind, placebo controlled, dose ranging study using Dysport. German Dystonia Study Group. J Neurol.Neurosurg.Psychiatry 1998;64:13–17.

226. Odergren T, Hjaltason H, Kaakkola S, Solders G, Hanko J, Fehling C, Marttila RJ, Lundh H, Gedin S, Westergren I, Richardson A, Dott C, Cohen H. A double blind, randomised, parallel group study to investigate the dose equivalence of Dysport and Botox in the treatment of cervical dystonia. J Neurol.Neurosurg.Psychiatry 1998;64:6–12.

227. Sampaio C, Ferreira JJ, Simoes F, Rosas MJ, Magalhaes M, Correia AP, Bastos-Lima A, Martins R, Castro-Caldas A. DYSBOT: a single-blind, randomized parallel study to determine whether any differences can be detected in the efficacy and tolerability of two formulations of botulinum

toxin type A--Dysport and Botox--assuming a ratio of 4:1. Mov Disord. 1997;12:1013-1018.

228. Aoki R, Francis J, Reynolds H, Leumer D. Comparison of the therapeutic windows of different botulinum neurotoxin preparations in an animal model. Neurology 2003;60 (suppl 1):A212-A213(Abstract)

229. Dressler D, Wittstock M, Benecke R. Botulinum toxin for treatment of jaw opening dystonia in Hallervorden-Spatz syndrome. Eur.Neurol. 2001;45:287-288.

230. Dressler D, Benecke B. Autonomic side effects of botulinum toxin type B therapy. Mov.Disord. 2002;(In Press)

231. Dressler D, Benecke R. Botulinum toxin typ B: moglichkeiten und grenzen der klinischen ansendung. Klin Neurophysiol 2001;32:240-243.

232. Brin MF, Anderson RL, Blitzer A, Carruthers A, Comella C, Consky E, Dubinsky R, Fahn S, Brueh BR, Hallett M, Jankovic J, Koman A, Kraft SP, Lang A, Ludlow C, Namerow NS, Rhew K, Simpson LL, Tsui J, Waters C, Woodson G. Training guidelines for the use of botulinum toxin for the treatment of neurologic disorders: Report of the Therapeutics and Technology Assessment Subcommittee of the American Academy of Neurology. Neurology 1994;44:2401-2403.

233. Borodic G. Myasthenic crisis after botulinum toxin. Lancet. 1998; 352:1832

234. Tuite PJ, Lang AE. Severe and prolonged dysphagia complicating botulinum toxin A injections for dystonia in Machado-Joseph disease. Neurology 1996;46:846

235. Santos JI, Swensen P, Glasgow LA. Potentiation of Clostridium botulinum toxin aminoglycoside antibiotics: clinical and laboratory observations. Pediatrics 1981;68:50-54.

236. Wilson R, Morris JG, Jr., Snyder JD, Feldman RA. Clinical characteristics of infant botulism in the United States: a study of the non-California cases. Pediatr.Infect.Dis. 1982;1:148-150.

237. Wang Y, Burr DH, Korthals GJ, Sugiyama H. Acute toxicity of aminoglycoside antibiotics as an aid in detecting botulism. Appl Environ Microbiol 1984;48:951-955.

238. Fiacchino F, Grandi L, Soliveri P, Carella F, Bricchi M. Sensitivity to vecuronium after botulinum toxin administration. J.Neurosurg.Anesthesiol. 1997;9:149-153.

239. Vidal-Marcos A, Sanz-Garcia M, Infante-Crespo B, Ruiz-Castro M, Rustarazo-Perez MT, Palma-Gamiz MA. [Botulinum toxin: clinical uses and anesthetic implications]. Rev.Esp.Anestesiol.Reanim. 1996;43:208-211.

240. Scott AB. Clostridial toxins as therapeutic agents (Chapter: 18). In: Simpson LL, ed. Botulinum neurotoxin and tetanus toxin. New York: Academic Press, 1989:399-412.

241. Moser E, Ligon KM, Singer C, Sethi KD. Botulinum toxin A (Botox) therapy during pregnancy (abstract). Neurology 1997;48:

242. Allergan, LLC. BOTOX® Cosmetic® US package insert for the indication of glabellar lines. 2002.

243. Naumann M, Moore AP. Long term safety of botulinum toxin type A. Mov.Disord. 2003;(In Press)

244. Hsiung GY, Das SK, Ranawaya R, Lafontaine AL, Suchowersky O. Long-term efficacy of botulinum toxin A in treatment of various movement disorders over a 10-year period. Mov Disord. 2002;17:1288-1293.

245. Defazio G, Abbruzzese G, Girlanda P, Vacca L, Curra A, De Salvia R, Marchese R, Raineri R, Roselli F, Livrea P, Berardelli A. Botulinum toxin A treatment for primary hemifacial spasm: a 10-year multicenter study. Arch.Neurol. 2002;59:418-420.

249. Aoki KR. Comparison of the duration of action and safety margins of botulinum toxin types A and B in mice. Ann.Neurol. 2001;50(3 Suppl): S32(Abstract)

250. Brin MF, The Spasticity Study Group. Dosing, administration, and a treatment algorithm for use of botulinum toxin A for adult-onset spasticity. Muscle Nerve 1997;20:S208-S220

251. Brashear A, Truong D, Charles D. A randomized double-blind, placebo-controlled study of intramuscular Botox for the treatment of cervical dystonia (CD). Mov.Disord. 1998;13 (Suppl 2):276(Abstract)

252. Hauser RA, Comella C, Brashear A. A randomized, multicenter, double-blind, placebo-controlled study of original Botox (botulinum toxin type A) purified neurotoxin complex for the treatment of cervical dystonia. Mov.Disord. 1999;15 (Suppl 2):30-31.(Abstract)

253. Naumann M, Yakovleff A, Durif F, Botox® Cervical Dystonia Prospective Study Group. A randomized, double-masked, crossover comparison of the efficacy and safety of botulinum toxin type A produced from the original bulk toxin source and current bulk toxin source for the treatment of cervical dystonia. J.Neurol. 2002;(In Press)

254. Quinn N, Hallett M. Dose standardisation of botulinum toxin [letter]. Lancet. 1989;1:964

255. Tan EK, Jankovic J. Botulinum toxin A in patients with oromandibular dystonia: long-term follow-up. Neurology 1999;53:2102-2107.

256. Hertzler JJ, Goldstein NP, Klass DW. Electroencephalogram in patients with palatal myoclonus. Electroencephalogr. Clin. Neurophysiol. 1970; 28:90

257. Nussgens Z, Roggenkamper P. Long-term treatment of blepharospasm with botulinum toxin type A. Ger J.Ophthalmol. 1995;4:363-367.

258. Karp BI, Cole RA, Cohen LG, Grill S, Lou JS, Hallett M. Long-Term Botulinum Toxin Treatment of Focal Hand Dystonia. Neurology 1994; 44:70-76.

259. Borodic GE, Ferrante R. Effects of repeated botulinum toxin injections on orbicularis oculi muscle. J.Clin.Neuroophthalmol. 1992;12:121-127.

260. Ruusuvaara P, Setala K. Long-term treatment of involuntary facial spasms using botulinum toxin. Acta Ophthalmol.(Copenh) 1990;68:331-338.

261. Dutton JJ, Buckley EG. Long-term results and complications of botulinum A toxin in the treatment of blepharospasm. Ophthalmology. 1988;95:1529-1534.

262. Drummond GT, Hinz BJ. Botulinum toxin for blepharospasm and hemifacial spasm: stability of duration of effect and dosage over time. Can. J. Ophthalmol. 2001;36:398-403.

263. Elston JS, Lee JP, Powell CM, et al. Treatment of strabismus in adults with botulinum toxin a. Br.J.Ophthalmol. 1985;69:718-724.

264. Huttner WB. Snappy exocytoxins. Nature. 1993;365:104-105.

265. Schiavo G, Rossetto O, Catsicas S, Delaureto PP, DasGupta BR, Benfenati F, Montecucco C. Identification of the Nerve Terminal Targets of Botulinum Neurotoxin Serotype-A, Serotype-D, and Serotype-E. J Biol Chem 1993;268:23784-23787.

266. Chen F, Foran P, Shone CC, Foster KA, Melling J, Dolly JO. Botulinum neurotoxin B inhibits insulin-stimulated glucose uptake into 3T3-L1 adipocytes and cleaves cellubrevin unlike type A toxin which failed to proteolyze the SNAP-23 present. Biochemistry 1997;36:5719–5728.

267. Williamson LC, Halpern JL, Montecucco C, Brown JE, Neale EA. Clostridial neurotoxins and substrate proteolysis in intact neurons: botulinum neurotoxin c acts on synaptosomal-associated protein of 25 kda. J Biol Chem. 1996;271:7694-7699.

268. Yamasaki S, Hu Y, Binz T, Kalkuhl A, Kurazono H, Tamura T, Jahn R, Kandel E, Niemann H. Synaptobrevin/vesicle-associated membrane protein (vamp) of aplysia californica: structure and proteolysis by tetanus toxin and botulinal neurotoxins type d and f. Proc Natl.Acad.Sci.U.S.A. 1994;91:4688-4692.

269. Schiavo G, Shone CC, Rossetto O, Alexander FCG, Montecucco C. Botulinum Neurotoxin Serotype-F Is a Zinc Endopeptidase Specific for VAMP/Synaptobrevin. J.Biol.Chem. 1993;268:11516-11519.

270. Grundemar L. [Sumatriptan and cardiac complaints. Careful cardiac anamnesis is needed prior to treatment]. Lakartidningen. 1994;91:1701-1702.

271. Breton S, Nsumu NN, Galli T, Sabolic I, Smith PJ, Brown D. Tetanus toxin-mediated cleavage of cellubrevin inhibits proton secretion in the male reproductive tract. Am.J.Physiol Renal Physiol 2000;278:F717-F725

272. Dressler, D. Botulinum Toxin Therapy. Stuttgart:Thieme-Verlag, 2000.

273. Arnon SS, Schechter R, Inglesby TV, Henderson DA, Bartlett JG, Ascher MS, Eitzen E, Fine AD, Hauer J, Layton M, Lillibridge S, Osterholm MT, O'Toole T, Parker G, Perl TM, Russell PK, Swerdlow DL, Tonat K. Botulinum toxin as a biological weapon: medical and public health management. JAMA. 2001;285:1059-1070.

274. Humeau Y, Doussau F, Grant NJ, Poulain B. How botulinum and tetanus neurotoxins block neurotransmitter release. Biochimie. 2000;82:427-446.

CHAPTER 9

Pharmacology of Phenol Injections

Jodi Frangiamore and Christopher O'Brien

INTRODUCTION

A nerve block, also referred to as chemodenervation, is defined as "the application of chemical agents to a nerve to impair, either temporarily or permanently, the conduction along the nerve."[1] Chemodenervation used in specific patient populations may be an extremely useful treatment for management of painful spasm, dystonia, or spasticity. The primary treatment goal is the reduction of focal muscle overactivity in a targeted muscle. There are currently two main products used for chemodenervation: phenol or botulinum toxin. This chapter focuses specifically on the current use of phenol, its history, pharmacology, and injection techniques.

The use of phenol (benzyl alcohol) dates back to ancient times; early Egyptians used the antiseptic derivatives of benzene for embalming. Phenol itself was first isolated in 1834 and its first medical use was as an antiseptic in 1867.[2] At a concentration of 0.2%, phenol is bacteriostatic; at concentrations greater than 1%, it is bacteriocidal.[3] During the early 1920s, phenol was unsuccessfully used in subcutaneous injections as a treatment for tetanus.[2]

EARLY THERAPEUTIC APPLICATIONS

One of the earliest attempts at localized neurolysis for blockade of sympathetic neuronal activity occurred in 1926 and was performed by Swetlow using alcohol. This investigator found that alcohol blocks were more effective in reducing sympathetic activity than procain hydrochloride; however, unacceptable complications ensued. For example, neuritis of the intercostal nerves was noted. Naturally, an agent was desired that would produce greater effects than procain hydrochloride, without the side effects of alcohol. Mandl[4] performed experiments on cats by exposing cervical ganglia and

then injecting 0.2 mL of 6% solution of phenol. Horner's syndrome readily developed and persisted for 14 days. Histologic results revealed complete necrosis of the injected nerves.

In 1925, Doppler studied the effect of phenol on blood vessels. He applied phenol to rabbit ovarian vessels and noted increased blood flow.[2,4,5] In 1949, Haxton was the first investigator to apply phenol to humans; he did so for the treatment of peripheral vascular disease. Haxton treated 220 subjects and reported favorable results, with fewer side effects than previously reported after alcohol injections.[4]

Haxton published a second paper[6] after he had injected up to 400 patients who had various diagnoses. These diseases included arteriosclerotic ischemia of the foot, intermittent claudication, erythrocyanosis, Raynaud's disease, acute thrombophlebitis, postphlebitic syndrome, and hyperhidrosis. He also began to use paravetebral injections with 10% solution of phenol in water. Haxton reported a complication rate of 20%. Adverse effects included neuritis and unwanted weakness. In one patient, these complications were permanent. Currently, these techniques are advocated only in rare cases because of the large percentage of complications.[2,5]

At about the same time, experiments injecting alcohol into the subarachnoid space were performed for the treatment of pain. By the late 1950s, phenol injections subsequently replaced alcohol injections. Brown, however, injected phenol into the subarachnoid of 55 patients with pain. He concluded that the procedure, as well as the results, was too unpredictable to be advocated.[2]

In 1955, Maher[7] first described intrathecal phenol injections. All of Maher's patients were affected by intractable pain resulting from cancer. This investigator described a technique during which he positioned patients with their painful side down. This was done in an attempt to block the specifically involved dorsal roots, using the hyperbaric properties of phenol compared to those of cerebrospinal fluid.[2,5,7,8] Maher also advocated the use of a phenol-glycerine mixture; he believed that this mixture would diffuse at a slower rate and localize most efficiently in the dorsal roots. Before phenol-glycerine injection, Maher would "protect" the distal roots below the desired

---

Jodi Frangiamore: Colorado Neurological Institute, Englewood, Colorado.

Christopher O'Brien: Prestwick Pharmaceuticals, Inc., Washington, DC.

113

level of block by injecting them with a heavy oil, X-ray contrast medium.[2,7] Overall, complications included transient ill effects such as headache, weakness, numbness, or sphincter problems. Approximately 1–33% of patients in this manner experienced such side effects. Permanent complications included urinary and fecal incontinence, limb weakness, or painful paresthesias. The death rate in the phenol-glycerine-treated patient population was 1–3%.[2,7,8–12] It is for this reason that intrathecal injections are not currently advocated.

In 1966, Nathan published on use of intrathecal phenol for the treatment of spasticity in patients with complete paraplegia. From that time forward, widespread use of phenol for spasticity caused by multiple sclerosis, cerebral palsy, stroke, and even Parkinson's disease has been reported.[8–12]

In 1966, Khalili and Benton[13] first described injections at the level of the peripheral nerve. By 1969, these investigators had performed 293 blocks in 120 patients. Khalili and Benton used 2–3% phenol in water and a sheath-insulated needle connected to a nerve stimulator. They reported a 10% rate of painful paresthesias following injection of mixed (sensorimotor) nerves. Spasticity improved for an average of 298 days.[2,5] This injection technique has increased safety and a lower percentage of side effects and has essentially replaced the use of intrathecal and epidural injections.[2,5,13] The primary use of phenol is for peripheral nerve injections; ongoing histologic studies and improved techniques have made this possible.

PHARMACOLOGY

The use of phenol for neurolysis is a localized treatment; therefore, standard pharmacologic discussions of absorption, distribution, metabolism, and excretion are not relevant. Thus, this chapter concentrates on the preparation and local physiologic effects of phenol.

Phenol or benzyl alcohol is the major oxidized metabolite of benzene.[1] As mentioned, it is bacteriostatic at a concentration of 0.2% and bactericidal at a concentration greater than 1%. The bactericidal effect is reduced at a low temperature and in an alkaline environment; therefore, this agent should be stored at room temperature. Phenol is available in an 89% solution and must be diluted to achieve the desired concentration.[14] It is water soluble at room temperature at a rate of 1:15, and is hyperbaric in comparison to cerebral spinal fluid.[14] If large quantities are injected or ingested, systemic distribution results in hepatic conjugation and 80% is excreted unchanged by the kidneys.[1,3,14]

The primary treatment effect is localized neuronal dysfunction caused by the denaturation of proteins. The extent of denaturation is a function of the phenol concentration as well as proximity to the injection site.

In a review of the literature, phenol concentrations used clinically have varied tremendously, from 0.2–10%.[1–13] The maximal safe dosage of phenol has not yet been established.[5] Felsenthal[3] reports the toxic dose as 8–15 g; however, there is no statement disclosing how this was concluded. The max-imum advisable dose within 24 hours is 1 g,[14] however, standard neurolytic therapy should not approach such a large quantity. Aqueous solutions of 3–5% are the most common for percutaneous blocks.[1,5] At concentrations of 2% or lower, phenol exhibits only local anesthetic properties when injected into the perineural space.[1] Phenol acts as a local anesthetic by blocking the influx of sodium ions, thereby preventing depolarization.[1,3,15–17] This agent appears to exhibit an immediate anesthetic effect, typically within 50 seconds and lasting up to 20 minutes.[3] The local anesthetic is directly proportional to the nerve size.[17] Phenol is not advocated for use as a local anesthetic as there are much more favorable and safer agents currently on the market.[2] Clearly, injection of phenol, or even normal saline, directly into a nerve may cause neuronal destruction that is independent of any pharmacologic effect. In most patients, direct neural injection is best avoided.

In solutions of relatively higher concentrations (i.e., >3%), phenol denatures protein. This action causes nerve destruction, denervation, muscle atrophy, and necrosis.[14] The extent of protein denaturation is dependent on the concentration of phenol and the proximity of the injection.[1] Reports suggest that at concentrations of greater than 5%, injury to the nerve is more severe than a crush injury.[16] Protein denaturation causes axonal demyelination and Wallerian degeneration, leading to muscle denervation.[16] As with other forms of denervation, positive sharp waves and fibrillation potentials emerge after 2–3 weeks. In electrophysiologic studies, axonal degeneration is evident within the injected nerve within 2 days of the phenol application.[1,16] The denervation is usually temporary, however, there have been rare cases of permanent denervation. The exact reason for permanent denervation remains unexplained.[5] It is possible that these cases reflect actual intraneural injection. The reported length of clinical effectiveness has varied tremendously. Based on EMG and non-EMG studies, estimates range from 2 days to permanent denervation.[1,2,4,5,9–11,13,15,16,18–20] The mean clinical effect was 308 days.[5] Wallerian regeneration of 1 mm/day occurs at similar rates after a crush injury.[14] Those patients who experience a permanent result may have a possible nerve infarction or vascular thrombosis in the nutrient vessels for the nerve. Full reinnervation may be slower than predicted because of resultant endoneural fibrosis.[14] Vascular thrombosis may impede nerve regeneration. In addition, spindle recovery may occur at a slower rate than with the neural elements.

In early studies, there was much debate whether phenol selectively destroyed neurons of different fiber diameters.[2,5,15,21,22] Thin gamma fibers were arguably more susceptible to phenol effects than larger alpha fibers. Subsequent studies disproved this hypothesis. Burkel and McPhee[21] published one such study in 1970. They surgically exposed sciatic nerves in rats and applied phenol, using one of two techniques. In one group, phenol was injected in such a manner that the entire solution remained inside the nerve. In the second group, phenol was dripped onto the surface of the nerve. The investigators then examined the nerve changes at various stages by electron microscopy. Burkel and McPhee[21] found that phenol did not bind to any specific cellular elements; rather, the agent spread diffusely. Phenol denatures protein in a nonselective fashion. The rats that were injected directly into the nerve demonstrated more complete nerve destruction and degeneration. The group exposed to phenol dripped onto the nerve demonstrated incomplete neural penetration and the axons in the center did not undergo Wallerian degeneration. All tissues close to the injection site were damaged, including blood vessels. After approximately 10 minutes, many of the blood vessels were completely occluded, causing decreased perfusion to the nerves. This was possibly a secondary cause of neural infarction. The overall consequence of these injections was Wallerian degeneration followed by nearly complete regeneration. Regeneration was noted by the increasing number of collagen fibers, which investigators hypothesized would make the nerves increasingly resistant with subsequent injections. The only observed difference in response of different fiber sizes was that the smaller diameter fibers degenerated and regenerated at a faster rate than larger diameter fibers.[21] This study was replicated in 1999, confirming that the largest variability in the completeness of the block was a function of the distance between phenol and the nerve.[18] These studies confirm that the accuracy of phenol placement is crucial for achievement of the best possible controlled denervation.

INJECTION TECHNIQUE

There are two main techniques advocated for peripheral injections of phenol: motor point blocks and motor nerve blocks. Both require precise knowledge of surface and gross anatomy and skill in using electrophysiologic methods.[14]

The technique of motor point blocks typically uses surface electrical stimulation to locate areas that contain many nerve fibers or motor end plates within the belly of the target muscle.[20,23] Multiple areas are located and then reference marks placed on the skin's surface. A Teflon-sheathed needle connected to a nerve stimulator is then inserted at the designated areas. The insulation ensures that stimulation occurs only at the needle tip, not along the entire shaft. Utilizing the technique of successive approximation, the tip position and stimulation intensity are manipulated until maximum contraction is produced with the lowest amplitude stimulation. Ideally, full fascicular contraction is produced with very low intensity stimulation (e.g., 0.25 mA). Aspiration is then performed to confirm that the needle is not within a blood vessel. The calculated amount of phenol solution is then injected. This procedure is repeated for all other motor points identified in this manner.[2,14,19,20,23,24]

For motor nerve blocks, the injector relies on anatomic knowledge and aims for a peripheral nerve. This is typically a motor nerve such as the musculocutaneous or obturator nerve. This technique also utilizes a Teflon-sheathed needle

connected to a nerve stimulator. Utilizing the technique of successive approximation, the tip position and stimulation intensity are manipulated until maximum contraction is produced with the lowest amplitude stimulation. Ideally, full target muscle contraction is produced with less than 1.0 mA stimulation intensity. If full contraction is produced only with high intensity, the needle position may not be adjacent to the nerve and should be repositioned. Aspiration is performed before injection to rule out intravascular injection.[23]

Each technique confers specific advantages and disadvantages. The motor point injections are technically more difficult to perform, require multiple injections, and take a larger volume of drug. In some patients, there is a graded or partial response with variable duration.[23] Experience has shown that motor nerve point blocks are associated with a lower risk of painful paresthesias. Most peripheral nerves contains both sensory and motor fibers while the small motor branches do not contain sensory fibers.[24,25] Motor nerve blocks inject a lower dose of phenol, with a more predictable and often complete blockade. However, the injector must have knowledge of the functional anatomy and be skilled at electrical stimulation technique to ensure avoidance of sensory nerves.[23]

With either technique, if the position of the needle elicits paresthesias, the needle should be repositioned before injection.[14] If high resistance to infusion is noted, the injection should not be forced. Such resistance may indicate that the needle is in a fixed space, such as a tendon or adjacent to bone. Slow injection rate is desirable to allow detection of any unwanted side effects.[14] Additives, such as epinephrine, increase the toxicity of the anesthetics when used in combination and typically are not recommended when performing phenol blocks.[14]

When injecting a nerve that is difficult to localize or injecting into an area with a higher risk of phenol effect on nontarget structures, adjunctive techniques may be advisable. These techniques include the use of ultrasound, as in the case of an iliopsoas injection.[26] To ensure precise injections, injectors may use an open technique, surgically exposing the nerve.[1,27] General anesthesia may be desirable when injecting young, apprehensive, or uncooperative patients or those in whom extreme spasticity interferes with positioning.[28]

Chemodenervation is performed only rarely as an isolated intervention. Optimal response often requires adjunctive therapy. Other interventions may be warranted including physical or occupational therapy, casting, bracing, posture and positioning, oral medications, local anesthetics, botulinum injections, surgeries, and implantable devices.[1,27]

POTENTIAL ADVERSE EFFECTS OF PHENOL

Before performing phenol injections, there must be an awareness of possible complications. Vigorous probing and multiple injections may cause trauma to the localized area and nerve. Therefore, it is advisable to utilize a small-gauge, beveled needle, which causes less nerve injury.[14] It is common for patients to feel postinjection soreness resulting from local tissue inflammation or necrosis. This may occur up to 24 hours after the injection.

If phenol is injected accidentally in a subcutaneous manner or if it remains in contact with the skin, necrosis may result. Chemical conjunctivitis may occur if phenol comes in contact with the eye. Standard flushing measures should be instituted.[14]

A compartment syndrome may develop after phenol injection. Tissue inflammation and venous thrombosis may cause a rise in compartment pressure, further compromising neurovascular status. Large injected volumes in a closed space may cause a reduction in perfusion, with resultant ischemia.

One common reported side effect after phenol injection is paresthesia or dysesthesia. The incidence of paresthesia ranges from 0–23%, with phenol concentrations of 2.0–5.0%.[14] Dysesthesias are usually reported within several days to 2 weeks postinjection. These sensations are commonly described as a burning sensation that is hypersensitive to tactile stimulation. The dysesthesias usually occur in a portion of the sensory distribution of the nerve that was blocked. Permanent sensory loss is rare; in most patients, sensory loss will resolve within 3 months.[1,14] This risk is highest with blockade of peripheral nerves that contain both motor and sensory fibers.[1,5,24] Some have argued the dysesthesias are not a side effect of a block but the result of an incomplete block. This argument has support as with reinjection the dysesthesias may often subside.[14] Infection is a rare complication as phenol is bacteriocidal.[3,14]

The most serious complication from phenol injections is the result of accidental vascular injection. One report described a patient who experienced arterial block, which followed an otherwise successful block of her brachioradialis and musculocutaneous nerves. Two days postinjection, the patient developed an arterial block that eventually required complete amputation of the limb.[20]

The cardiovascular and central nervous systems are particularly sensitive to systemic phenol. Cardiac dysrhythmias and venous thromboses have been reported after exposure to large amounts of phenol. One report describes a patient who ingested 70 mL of 42–52% phenol during a suicide attempt. She developed the symptoms noted above before respiratory arrest; she required intubation and mechanical ventilation. In less than 24 hours, the patient began to breathe independently, however, she experienced involuntary perioral movements and parkinsonism, including cogwheeling and resting tremor of both hands. By the 5th day, the involuntary movements and parkinsonism began to dissipate. By the 15th day, motor examination was normal and, on the 21st day, the patient was discharged.[29] It remains unclear which symptoms reflect hypoxia as opposed to the direct effects of phenol.

POTENTIAL ADVANTAGES OF PHENOL

Phenol has some advantages over other forms of chemodenervation such as botulinum toxin. It is low cost and easy to prepare and store.[1] When injected properly, effects are noted within 2–60 minutes. The average duration of effect lasts from 2 weeks to 6 months depending on the extent of neurolysis. Occasionally, longer duration or permanent effects are reported. The potential for immune-mediated resistance (antibody formation), a phenomenon sometimes noted after chemodenervation with botulinum toxin, seems extremely unlikely. The disadvantages of phenol injections include lack of selectivity, pain during the injection, vascular reactions, and tissue destruction effects.[23]

Phenol may offer some specific advantages in comparison to oral medications. Phenol is an accepted adjunctive treatment for spasticity, regardless of etiology.[23] At this time, experience with phenol for treatment of dystonia remains relatively limited. As a local therapy, phenol may have considerable effect in reducing local muscle contraction without associated systemic side effects. In contrast, oral spasticity or dystonia medications may be associated with more central side effects, such as dizziness, drowsiness, fatigue, diffuse muscle weakness, or and hepatotoxicity.[5]

Clinical observation suggests that phenol may have some effect beyond simple reduction in muscle contraction. Muscle tone is modulated by descending inhibitory pathways and peripheral afferents. Phenol may effectively alter spindle, gamma, or Ia activity. In this manner, phenol may indirectly reduce contractions. Specific physiologic effects in spasticity or dystonia have not yet been demonstrated, although some intriguing effects have been reported in patients with cervical dystonia who are resistant to botulinum toxin type A.[30]

CLINICAL APPLICATIONS

Spasticity

The use of phenol in motor control disorders has primarily been in the management of spasticity, therefore, a brief review serves as a point of reference when considering treating other motor control disorders. As a denervation agent, phenol seems most effective when the primary treatment goal is a reduction in focal muscle activity in a patient for whom less aggressive interventions have failed to produce improvement. This is not uncommon in the neurorehabilitation environment. Here, spasticity is defined as "a motor disorder characterized by a velocity-dependent increase in tonic stretch reflexes with exaggerated tendon jerks, resulting from hyperexcitability of the stretch reflex as one component of the upper motor neuron syndrome."[31,32] Thus it is a symptom rather than a diagnosis, and reflects brain or spinal cord injury that may be associated with a variety of disease states. These include stroke, multiple sclerosis, traumatic brain injury, and cerebral palsy.

If one therapeutic objective is reduction of contraction in a specific muscle or group of muscles, phenol denervation may be appropriate. If there is a partial contracture, one may be able to stretch soft tissues before full nerve regeneration occurs and muscle overactivity resumes, resulting in functional improvement well beyond the effects of the block.[14,18] These clinical scenarios are ones in which a large muscle is paired with a motor nerve that is easily accessible and unlikely to expose a sensory nerve to denervation. In large specialty rehabilitation centers, the most common phenol nerve blocks are performed for severe thigh adduction (i.e., the obturator nerve) or elbow flexion (i.e., the musculocutaneous nerve). In some centers, pediatric patients with multifocal spasticity receive phenol motor point blocks for knee flexion within the hamstring muscles. Specific expertise is required for many reasons, including for patient selection, injection technique, and management of potential complications. Although relatively low cost compared to botulinum toxin injections or some oral medications, the specific requirements noted above have limited the extent of phenol usage in the United States.[33–36]

Dystonia

The use of phenol for the treatment of dystonia is uncommon. Only a few attempts to help patients with cervical dystonia for whom botulinum toxin injections have failed have been reported.[30,37,38]

Three different techniques have been described.

1. A 5% phenol solution can produce an effective motor nerve block (accessory nerve branch), thereby reducing sternocleidomastoid muscle spasm. This method uses low volumes of fluid (e.g., 0.25 mL) delivered via Teflon-covered EMG needle and electrical stimulation. The primary risk is that of phenol coming into contact with nerve branches to the trapezius muscle or the auricular sensory nerve. Much more problematic is the potential effect of phenol on adjacent structures, such as the brachial plexus or carotid artery.
2. Motor point injections may be used to reduce focal contraction in cervical muscles as described by Massey.[37] No controlled clinical trials have been reported to date. This method uses larger volumes (1–2 mL per muscle) of phenol 5% solution. Pain on injection may be of moderate severity and excessive weakness may occur.
3. An alternative approach has been proposed.[38] In this setting, the primary treatment goal is the reduction of cervical muscle overactivity via alteration of muscle afferents. The short-term effect of intramuscular injection of local anesthetic agents may be prolonged with the addition small quantities of phenol. Selected overactive cervical muscles were injected with a solution of lidocaine and dilute phenol. During this open-label trial, patients apparently achieved 2 weeks of pain and spasm reduction with minimal side effects.[38]

As to the utility of the three methods described above, clarification of mechanism of action is required along with controlled clinical trials using standardized injection techniques.

REFERENCES

1. Gracies JM, Elovic E, McGuire J, et al. Traditional pharmacological treatments for spasticity Part I: local treatments. Muscle Nerve 1997;S6:61–91.
2. Wood, KM. The use of phenol as a neurolytic agent: a review. Pain 1978;5:205–209.
3. Felsenthal G. Pharmacology of phenol in peripheral nerve blocks: a review. Arch Phys Med Rehabil 1974;55:13–16.
4. Mandl F. Aqueous solution of phenol as a substitute for alcohol in sympathetic block. J Int Coll Surg 1950;13:566–568.
5. Botte M, Abrams A, Bodine-Fowler S. Treatment of acquired muscle spasticity using phenol peripheral nerve blocks. Orthopedics 1995;18:151–159.
6. Haxton, HA Paravertebral block with aqueous phenol in the treatment of vascular disease. Angiology 1953;4:268–280.
7. Maher RM. Further experiences with intrathecal and subdural phenol observations on two forms of pain. Lancet 1960;1:895–899.
8. Koppang K. Intrathecal phenol in the treatment of spastic conditions. Acta Neurol Scand 1962;38(Suppl 3):63–68.
9. Hansebout R, Cosgrove JB. Effects of intrathecal phenol in man. A histological study. Neurology 1966;16:277–282.
10. Baxter DW, Schacher U. Experimental studies on the morphological changes produced by intrathecal phenol. Can Med Assoc J 1962;86:1200–1205.
11. Sefanko S, Zebrowski S. Histological changes in the nerve roots and spinal cord after intrathecal administration of phenol for relief of spasticity. Pol Med J 1968;7:1204–1208.
12. Hughes J. Thrombosis of the posterior spinal arteries: a complication of an intrathecal injection of phenol. Neurology 1970;20:659–664.
12a. Nathan PW. Intrathecal phenol to relieve spasticity in paraplegia. Lancet 1959;2:1099–1102.
13. Khalili A, Benton J. A physiological approach to the evaluation and the management of spasticity with procaine and phenol nerve block. Clin Orthop 1966;47:97–104.
14. Lennard T. Physiatric Procedures in Clinical Practice. Philadelphia, PA: Hanley and Belfus, Inc., 1994.
15. Fusfeld R. Electromyographic findings after phenol block. Arch Phys Med Rehab 1968;49:217–219.
16. Bodine-Fowler S, Allsing S, Botte M. Time course of muscle atrophy and recovery following a phenol-induced nerve block. Muscle Nerve 1996;19:497–504.
17. Kirazli Y, On AY, Kismali B, et al. Comparison of phenol block and botulinus toxin type A in the treatment of spastic foot after stroke: a randomized, double-blind trial. Am J Phys Med Rehab 1998;77:510–515.
18. On AY, Kirazli Y, Kismali B, et al. Mechanisms of action of phenol block and botulinus toxin type A in relieving spasticity: electrophysiologic investigation and follow-up. Am J Phys Med Rehabil 1999;78:344–349.
19. Westerlund T, Vuorinen V, Kirvela O, et al. The endoneural response to neurolytic agents is highly dependent on the mode of application. Reg Anesth Pain Med 1999;24:294–302.
20. Gibson I. Phenol block in the treatment of spasticity. Gerontology 1987;33:327–330.
21. Burkel W, McPhee M. Effect of phenol injection into peripheral nerve of rat: electron microscope studies. Arch Phys Med Rehab 1970;51:391–397.
22. Brattstrom M, Moritz U, Svantesson G. Electromyographic studies of peripheral nerve block with phenol. Scand J Rehab Med 1970;2:17–22.
23. O'Brien CF. Injection techniques for botulinum toxin using electromyography and electrical stimulation. In: Mayer N, Simpson D, eds. The Role of Chemodenervation in Spasticity Management: A Self-Study Continuing Medical Educational Activity. WeMove February 2000. www.mdvu.org/classrooms/cme/spasticity_chemd/
24. Garland D, Lilling M, Keenan M. Percutaneous phenol blocks to motor points of spastic forearm muscles in head-injured adults. Arch Phys Med Rehabil 1984;65:243–245.
25. Botte M, Keenan M. Percutaneous phenol blocks of the pectoralis major muscle to treat spastic deformities. J Hand Surg 1988;13A:147–149.
26. Koyama H, Murakami K, Suzuki T, et al. Phenol block for hip flexor muscle spasticity under ultrasonic monitoring. Arch Phys Med Rehabil 1992;73:1040–1043.
27. Keenan MA. Management of the spastic upper extremity in the neurologically impaired adult. Clin Orthop 1988;233:116–124.
28. Griffith E, Melanpy CN. General anesthesia use in phenol intramuscu-

lar neurolysis in young children with spasticity. Arch Phys Med Rehabil 1977;58:154–156.

29. Kamijo Y, Soma K, Fukuda M, et al. Rabbit syndrome following phenol ingestion. J Toxicol Clin Toxicol 1999;37:4509–4511.

30. Massey JM. Treatment of spasmodic torticollis with intramuscular phenol injection. J Neurol Neurosurg Psychiatry 1995;58:258–259.

31. Young RR. Spasticity: a review. Neurology 1994;44:12–20.

32. Brown, P. Pathophysiology of spasticity. J Neurol Neurosurg Psychiatry 1994;57:773–777.

33. Gormley M, O'Brien C, Yablon S. Clinical overview of treatment decisions. Muscle Nerve 1997;S6:14–20.

34. Russman B, Tilton A, Gormley M. Cerebral palsy: a rational approach to a treatment protocol, and the role of botulinum toxin in treatment. Muscle Nerve 1997;6:S181-S193.

35. Pierson S. Outcome measures in spasticity management. Muscle Nerve 1997;6:S181-S193.

36. Herndon RM, ed. Handbook of Neurologic Rating Scales. New York: Demos Medical Publisher, 1997.

37. Ruiz PJ, Bernardos VS. Intramuscular phenol injection for severe cervical dystonia. J Neurol 2000;247:146–147.

38. Velickovic M, Benabou R, Brin MF. Cervical dystonia pathophysiology and treatment options. Drugs 2001;61:1921–1943.

CHAPTER 10

Role of Neurophysiology in the Treatment of Dystonia

M. Aramideh and J.W.M. Brans

INTRODUCTION

For many years, dystonia was considered a psychogenic disorder. Recognition of dystonia as an organic disorder and the availability of botulinum toxin treatment raised awareness about dystonia among medical professionals and the public. New cases are now more likely to be correctly diagnosed and appropriately treated.[1–5]

The diagnosis of dystonia is mainly based on patient's history and neurologic findings. Nonetheless, various electrodiagnostic tests have been applied as an extension of clinical evaluation. The first part of this chapter addresses the role of clinical neurophysiology in verifying the diagnosis and in elucidating the pathophysiology of dystonia. The second part focuses on the role of electromyography (EMG) in the treatment of dystonia.

NEUROPHYSIOLOGY AND DIAGNOSIS OF DYSTONIA

Confirmation of Diagnosis and Pathophysiology of Dystonia

During the last two decades, many neurophysiologic studies have been carried out in an attempt to distinguish dystonia from, in particular, voluntary movements and to confirm the clinical diagnosis of dystonia.[6–15]

Dystonic movements are usually distinguished from normal voluntary movements by coactivation of agonist and antagonist muscles, leading to abnormal movements or postures.[11,13,16] Dystonic movements may occur spontaneously or be precipitated by voluntary activity. At rest, mildly affected individuals may show no involuntary muscle activity.

M. Aramideh: Department of Neurology, Medical Center Alkmaar, Alkmaar, The Netherlands.

J.W.M. Brans: Department of Neurology, Medical Center Alkmaar, Alkmaar, The Netherlands.

The authors have no commercial relationship with the funder.

There are many electromyographic studies regarding dystonia; these studies analyze the types of involuntary motor activity and the frequency of dystonic discharges. EMG generally shows tonic, phasic, tremulous, or myoclonic discharges, and usually a combination of these abnormal discharges. There may be a crescendo phenomenon during buildup of tonic contraction. Frequency analysis may show a 4–7 Hz drive to the affected muscles.[14,17–20]

Antagonistic gestures or sensory trick maneuvers, which may reduce or abolish dystonic posturing, are well-known characteristics of dystonia. The effect of these maneuvers on dystonic movements may be investigated in detail, using various neurophysiologic techniques.[21–24] In a group of patients with blepharospasm, Gomez-Wong et al.[22] examined the effects induced by a sensory trick, consisting of finger contact with the face, on the electrically induced blink reflex and the blink reflex excitability recovery curve. In all subjects, during an average period of 10 minutes after the onset of finger-face contact, the area of R2 was significantly reduced and the amplitude of R1 was significantly enhanced in comparison to rest. However, there were no changes in the blink reflex excitability recovery curve.

In addition to electromyographic studies, there are many other neurophysiologic investigations used to assess underlying pathophysiology of dystonia as well as its differentiation from other movement disorders. These investigations include blink reflexes and blink reflex recovery curves, H-reflex reciprocal inhibition and recovery curve, evoked potentials, electroencephalographic (EEG) back-averaging, vestibular and oculomotor systems analyses, magnetic brain stimulation, and microstimulation during surgery.[6,7,12,16,25–44]

Neurophysiologic studies have emphasized the possible role of sensory feedback in the generation of dystonic movements.[45] The results of different neurophysiologic studies combined with clinical data, imaging, and pathologic studies, suggest that primary dystonia results from a functional disturbance of the basal ganglia. This disturbance may cause altered thalamic control of cortical motor planning and executive areas as well as abnormal regulation of brain stem and spinal cord inhibitory interneuronal mechanisms.[6,46]

Neurophysiology: Before and After Treatment

Neurophysiologic techniques may be applied to test a hypothesis about pathophysiology of dystonia. This may be done by showing possible alterations of a neurophysiologic test after treatment, whether or not combined with other data. For example, in a study on patients with cervical dystonia, Kanovsky et al.[30] found that the P22/N30 precentral component of the median nerve somatosensory evoked potential was higher before treatment. Moreover, Valls-Solé et al.[47] found no change in brain stem interneuronal excitability after botulinum treatment in patients with cervical dystonia. In a study in patients with dopa-responsive dystonia, Koelman et al.[48] showed normalization of soleus H-reflex excitability after L-dopa treatment.

Neurophysiology as a Therapy

Neurophysiologic techniques have been applied as a means of providing sensory feedback therapy (biofeedback) to patients with dystonia. By monitoring the affected muscles' activities with audiovisual displays, an attempt may be made to improve volitional control of the overactive muscle groups.[49–51] The mechanisms of improvement after EMG feedback therapy are poorly understood.

ELECTROMYOGRAPHY AND BOTULINUM TOXIN APPLICATION

There have been many studies emphasizing the use of EMG in detecting, selecting, and injecting the muscles involved in various dystonias.

Detection of Involved Muscles

Several studies have been performed in patients with cervical dystonia and writer's cramp. It has been shown that EMG may be used to accurately identify those muscles contributing to the dystonic posture.[19,52,53] Dystonic muscle activity is usually considered when an activity with an amplitude above a certain level is recorded and when its type is generally categorized into tonic, phasic or, tremulous activity.[20,54,55] Yet, studies of abnormal patterns of muscle activities have been largely restricted to more superficial muscles.

In a double-blind study using a needle EMG activity above 100 µV as the gold standard, Brans et al.[56] showed that physical examination has a low predictive value in the detection of involved muscles in patients with cervical dystonia. However, it remains unclear whether an activity above a certain level should be considered as dystonic activity. On the other hand, perhaps it is a compensatory activity to suppress dystonic activity of other muscles or it may be normal muscle activity. There is also unknown, relative variability of muscle activity among different individuals, or even within one individual at different times during longitudinal studies.

Selection of Most Active Muscle

EMG may be helpful to identify the most actively involved muscle—the muscle with discharges of the highest amplitude. It has been demonstrated that the most active muscle may change from one muscle to another after botulinum treatment.[57–59] Therefore, it has been postulated that EMG may be important to identify the "new" most active muscle, particularly in those patients responding less favorably to botulinum treatment or secondary nonresponders.[60] Yet, the double-blind randomized study of Brans et al.[56] showed an increased EMG activity in 20% of noninjected muscles after botulinum treatment and, surprisingly, in 27% of noninjected muscles after trihexyphenidyl treatment in patients with cervical dystonia. Brans et al.[56] also demonstrated that a switch from one most active muscle to another was equally distributed in both groups; therefore, this finding was not related to botulinum treatment but is probably a pathophysiologic phenomenon of cervical dystonia itself.

Botulinum Toxin Application Under Electromyographic Guidance

It is obvious that EMG may help to guide botulinum injections exactly into the desired muscles. EMG may be used to inject those muscles that cannot be identified easily, based on the clinical examination. Speelman and Brans[61] showed that without EMG guidance, 17–53% of the botulinum injections may be applied outside the selected muscles.[61] This observation also seems valid even for easily accessible muscles.

Borodic et al.[62] showed that after injection of botulinum toxin into the longissimus dorsi of mice, a botulinum toxin effect was apparent as far as 30 mm from the injection site. No effect was observed at 45 mm from the injection site.[62] However, the effect of higher amounts of toxin in actively contracting human muscles, as in patients with dystonia, is not known.

In the largest series of patients with cervical dystonia who were treated with botulinum toxin injections and received adequate follow-up, Jankovic et al.[63] did not use EMG. The results on treatment outcomes are comparable to those investigators who use EMG for botulinum toxin application.[63] Injection techniques vary considerably among different investigators; therefore, a precise and reliable comparison of clinical outcome is challenging. To determine the usefulness of EMG-guided botulinum toxin injections for the treatment of cervical dystonia, Comella et al.[52] carried out a randomized trial in 52 patients with cervical dystonia. The percentage of patients showing improvement did not differ significantly among those who received EMG-guided injections versus those who received non-EMG-assisted injections. However, the number of patients with marked improvement was greater in the EMG-assisted group. Those patients in the EMG-assisted group who had retrocollis, head tilt, and shoulder elevation had a relatively greater magnitude of benefit. There is still no evidence, based on results of a double-blind clinical study, to support the assumption that application of botulinum toxin injections under EMG guidance is superior to non-EMG-assisted application.

Lower Dosage Botulinum Toxin and Fewer Side Effects

It is clear that EMG enables the clinician to inject the toxin precisely within the muscle and, under ideal conditions, as close as possible to the neuromuscular junction. Results from several open studies suggest that the amount of toxin may be lower when the toxin is applied under EMG guidance.[64–66] Lower doses may reduce the risk of antibody production, the number and severity of side effects, and the cost of the treatment. However, some investigators believe that routine use of EMG is a more expensive approach. A double-blind randomized clinical trial to study outcomes of toxin injections with and without EMG guidance as well as with relative lower and higher doses is required to attempt to answer many important questions concerning the use of EMG and the optimal dose of botulinum toxin.

ELECTROMYOGRAPHY AND BOTULINUM TOXIN TREATMENT FAILURE

Subtypes of Dystonia and Predicting Treatment Outcome

EMG is an important and indispensable investigational technique to identify subgroups of patients with a certain type of dystonia who may respond less favorably to botulinum treatment. The results of EMG-guided injections may provide evidence to support the combination of botulinum toxin injections with other types of symptomatic treatments, the reduction or increase in the amount of injected toxin, or the prediction of treatment outcome. Tsui et al.,[67] using surface electrodes, defined two groups of patients with cervical dystonia. One group had an agonist-type dystonia, in which all involved muscles act together in the same direction. The other group had an antagonist-type of dystonia, in which the overactive muscles act in opposite directions. After botulinum toxin therapy, the number of patients responding favorably was relatively higher in the group with the agonist type of dystonia. Several studies investigated EMG activities in different portions of the orbicularis oculi muscles; in some studies, simultaneous EMG recordings were performed from the orbicularis oculi and the levator palpebrae in patients with blepharospasm. It appeared that the pretarsal portion of the orbicularis oculi is more often involved in dystonic activities. The magnitude of response increased after injection of botulinum toxin into that specific portion of the orbicularis oculi.[68] Aramideh et al.[69] also demonstrated that some patients with blepharospasm may also have a disturbed levator palpebrae activity, known as apraxia of eyelid opening, eyelid freezing, or involuntary levator inhibition.[17] Those patients with these combined types of activities responded less favorably to the treatment and required a ptosis crutch in addition to botulinum toxin injections. In another study, results showed that in this same clinical population, it is almost impossible to identify different subtypes of abnormal muscle activity based solely on clinical examination. Additional EMG investigation is required.[18,70]

Detection of Untreated Muscles

EMG studies may reveal that clinically unsuspected muscles may in fact be involved in dystonic movements. In 100 patients with cervical dystonia, Deuschl et al.[20] showed activity in muscles which were clinically unrecognized, particularly in patients with a rotational type of torticollis. However, as mentioned earlier, a certain background activity does not necessarily indicate dystonic activity and possible involvement remains uncertain.

Electromyography in Secondary Nonresponders

In patients who are possibly secondary nonresponders, the compound muscle action potentials from a particular muscle that has received a local injection of botulinum toxin may be investigated using surface electrodes. This procedure enables investigators to study the quantitative effect of botulinum toxin without the need for the patient's cooperation to contract the injected muscle. The extensor digitorum brevis is commonly used for this purpose.[71,72]

ELECTROMYOGRAPHY IN CLINICAL TRIALS

Objective Assessment of Effectiveness

Neurophysiologic techniques may be applied objectively to assess the effectiveness of treatment for dystonia. Quantitative analysis of EMG activities of certain muscles is possible with an optimal sensitivity and validity. Dressler and Rothwell[73] investigated the maximum voluntary EMG activity of the sternocleidomastoid muscle and its reduction in activity after botulinum toxin injections. This study was conducted on a group of patients with cervical dystonia. Dressler and Rothwell[73] demonstrated that EMG amplitude reductions could be applied with a precision of approximately 10%. This objective assessment (using the compound muscle action potential) may be valuable, particularly in blinded studies. It may reduce the chance of bias.

Studies on Different Botulinum Toxins and Dose Optimization

Quantitative EMG analysis of changes in muscle activity after botulinum toxin injections is an important method of objectively comparing the efficacy of different botulinum toxins.[74] The compound muscle action potential may be measured with reliability, before and after treatment. Dose-effect relationship may be monitored more precisely and the optimal dose required to induce sufficient paresis may be calculated for different toxin preparations. Single-fiber EMG studies may be carried out to investigate the remote effect of various toxins at different amounts and varying dilutions.[75–77]

TECHNIQUE OF ELECTROMYOGRAPHIC-GUIDED BOTULINUM TOXIN APPLICATION

The technique of botulinum toxin application varies considerably among investigators using EMG guidance. Some investigators use surface electrodes, which are not invasive, allowing only for recordings of superficial muscles. In addition, surface electrodes do not permit directed injections simultaneously with EMG recording. Wire electrodes are particularly useful to record EMG activity during movement of deeply located muscles; however, they do not permit targeted injection. Needle electrodes cause greater pain than other types of electrodes, tend to change position, and are suboptimal for simultaneous recording. Teflon-coated, hollow monopolar needle electrodes allow for targeted injections of botulinum into the selected muscles simultaneous with EMG monitoring. Standard EMG equipment and a clip to connect the EMG needle with EMG apparatus are also required. The same needle may be used for multiple injections in the same patient during a given session. The muscles selected for EMG-guided injections are likely to be involved in the abnormal movement or position, as determined by clinical evaluation, particularly the position of the head. When the electrode is inserted into the targeted muscle, the desired location of the needle may be determined by a full recruitment pattern, as demonstrated with voluntary activation of the muscle. The additional time for EMG-guided application of botulinum toxin is probably no more than 10 minutes.

CONCLUSION

Neurophysiology plays an important role in the diagnosis of dystonia as well as the investigation of its underlying pathophysiology. There is evidence in favor of the use of EMG guidance during application of botulinum toxin. Additional evidence should be based on future randomized, blinded studies. EMG is an indispensable tool in identifying the various subtypes of dystonia, which respond less favorably to treatment.

REFERENCES

1. Marsden CD, Fahn S. Dystonia 3. Summary and conclusions. Adv Neurol 1998;78:359–364.
2. Fahn S, Eldridge R. Definition of dystonia and classification of the dystonic states. Adv Neurol 1976;14:1–5.
3. Jankovic J. Etiology and differential diagnosis of blepharospasm and oromandibular dystonia. Adv Neurol 1988;49:103–116.
4. Marsden CD. Dystonia: the spectrum of the disease. Res Publ Assoc Res Nerv Ment Dis 1976;55:351–367.
5. Fahn S. Blepharospasm: a form of focal dystonia. Adv Neurol 1988;49:125–133.
6. Berardelli A, Rothwell JC, Day BL, et al. The pathophysiology of cranial dystonia. Adv Neurol 1988;50:525–535.
7. Aramideh M, Bour LJ, Koelman JH, et al. Abnormal eye movements in blepharospasm and involuntary levator palpebrae inhibition. Clinical and pathophysiological considerations. Brain 1994;117(Pt 6):1457–1474.
8. Cohen LG, Hallett M. Hand cramps: clinical features and electromyographic patterns in a focal dystonia. Neurology 1988;38:1005–1012.
9. Deuschl G, Goddemeier C. Spontaneous and reflex activity of facial muscles in dystonia, Parkinson's disease, and in normal subjects. J Neurol Neurosurg Psychiatry 1998;64:320–324.
10. Eekhof JL, Aramideh M, Bour LJ, et al. Blink reflex recovery curves in blepharospasm, torticollis spasmodica, and hemifacial spasm. Muscle Nerve 1996;19:10–15.
11. Hallett M. Analysis of abnormal voluntary and involuntary movements with surface electromyography. Adv Neurol 1983;39:907–914.
12. Hallett M. Physiology of dystonia. Adv Neurol 1998;78:11–18.
13. Hughes M, McLellan DL. Increased co-activation of the upper limb muscles in writer's cramp. J Neurol Neurosurg Psychiatry 1985;48:782–787.
14. Hallett M. Glossary of terms: EMG/EDX/clinical neurophysiology and the practice of medicine. Muscle Nerve 1992;15:1378–1382.
15. Kaji R, Ikeda A, Ikeda T, et al. Physiological study of cervical dystonia. Task-specific abnormality in contingent negative variation. Brain 1995;118(Pt 2):511–522.
16. Rothwell JC, Obeso JA, Day BL, et al. Pathophysiology of dystonias. Adv Neurol 1983;39:851–863.
17. Aramideh M, Ongerboer de Visser BW, Devriese PP, et al. Electromyographic features of levator palpebrae superioris and orbicularis oculi muscles in blepharospasm. Brain 1994;117(Pt 1):27–38.
18. Aramideh M, Ongerboer de Visser BW, Koelman JH, et al. Motor persistence of orbicularis oculi muscle in eyelid-opening disorders. Neurology 1995;45:897–902.
19. Dressler D. Electromyographic evaluation of cervical dystonia for planning of botulinum toxin therapy. Eur J Neurol 2000;7:713–718.
20. Deuschl G, Heinen F, Kleedorfer B, et al. Clinical and polymyographic investigation of spasmodic torticollis. J Neurol 1992;239:9–15.
21. Wissel J, Muller J, Ebersbach G, et al. Trick maneuvers in cervical dystonia: investigation of move. Mov Disord 1999;14:994–999.
22. Gomez-Wong E, Marti MJ, Cossu G, et al. The 'geste antagonistique' induces transient modulation of the blink reflex in human patients with blepharospasm. Neurosci Lett 1998;251:125–128.
23. Murase N, Kaji R, Shimazu H, et al. Abnormal premovement gating of somatosensory input in writer's cramp. Brain 2000;123(Pt 9):1813–1829.
24. Stejskal L. Counterpressure in torticollis. J Neurol Sci 1980;48:9–15.
25. Aramideh M, Eekhof JL, Bour LJ, et al. Electromyography and recovery of the blink reflex in involuntary eyelid closure: a comparative study. J Neurol Neurosurg Psychiatry 1995;58:692–698.
26. Blitzer A, Lovelace RE, Brin MF, et al. Electromyographic findings in focal laryngeal dystonia (spastic dysphonia). Ann Otol Rhinol Laryngol 1985;94(6 Pt 1):591–594.
27. Deuschl G, Toro C, Matsumoto J, et al. Movement-related cortical potentials in writer's cramp. Ann Neurol 1995;38:862–868.
28. Hallett M. The neurophysiology of dystonia. Arch Neurol 1998;55:601–603.
29. Kaji R, Rothwell JC, Katayama M, et al. Tonic vibration reflex and muscle afferent block in writer's cramp. Ann Neurol 1995;38:155–162.
30. Kanovsky P, Streitova H, Dufek J, et al. Change in lateralization of the P22/N30 cortical component of median nerve somatosensory evoked potentials in patients with cervical dystonia after successful treatment with botulinum toxin A. Mov Disord 1998;13:108–117.
31. Nakashima K, Rothwell JC, Thompson PD, et al. The blink reflex in patients with idiopathic torsion dystonia. Arch Neurol 1990;47:413–416.
32. Nakashima K, Thompson PD, Rothwell JC, et al. An exteroceptive reflex in the sternocleidomastoid muscle produced by electrical stimulation of the supraorbital nerve in normal subjects and patients with spasmodic torticollis. Neurology 1989;39:1354–1358.
33. van der Kamp W, Berardelli A, Rothwell JC, et al. Rapid elbow move-

ments in patients with torsion dystonia. J Neurol Neurosurg Psychiatry 1989;52:1043–1049.

34. van der Kamp W, Rothwell JC, Thompson PD, et al. The movement-related cortical potential is abnormal in patients with idiopathic torsion dystonia. Mov Disord 1995;10:630–633.

35. Koelman JH, Willemse RB, Bour LJ, et al. Soleus H-reflex tests in dystonia. Mov Disord 1995;10:44–50.

36. Koelman JH, Hilgevoord AA, Bour LJ, et al. Soleus H-reflex tests in causalgia-dystonia compared with dystonia and mimicked dystonic posture. Neurology 1999;53:2196–2198.

37. Stell R, Bronstein AM, Marsden CD. Vestibulo-ocular abnormalities in spasmodic torticollis before and after botulinum toxin injections. J Neurol Neurosurg Psychiatry 1989;52:57–62.

38. Colebatch JG, Di L, V, Quartarone A, et al. Click-evoked vestibulo-collic reflexes in torticollis. Mov Disord 1995;10:455–459.

39. Bronstein AM, Rudge P. Vestibular involvement in spasmodic torticollis. J Neurol Neurosurg Psychiatry 1986;49:290–295.

40. Lueck CJ, Tanyeri S, Crawford TJ, et al. Saccadic eye movements in essential blepharospasm. J Neurol 1990;237:226–229.

41. Bollen E, Van Exel E, van der Velde EA, et al. Saccadic eye movements in idiopathic blepharospasm. Mov Disord 1996;11:678–682.

42. Giladi N. The mechanism of action of botulinum toxin type A in focal dystonia is most probably through its dual effect on efferent (motor) and afferent pathways at the injected site. J Neurol Sci 1997; 152:132–135.

43. Greene PE, Bressman S. Exteroceptive and interoceptive stimuli in dystonia. Mov Disord 1998;13:549–551.

44. Pauletti G, Berardelli A, Cruccu G, et al. Blink reflex and the masseter inhibitory reflex in patients with dystonia. Mov Disord 1993;8: 495–500.

45. Hallett M. Is dystonia a sensory disorder? Ann Neurol 1995;38: 139–140.

46. Berardelli A, Rothwell JC, Hallett M, et al. The pathophysiology of primary dystonia. Brain 1998;121(Pt 7):1195–1212.

47. Valls-Sole J, Tolosa ES, Marti MJ, et al. Treatment with botulinum toxin injections does not change brainstem interneuronal excitability in patients with cervical dystonia. Clin Neuropharmacol 1994;17:229–235.

48. Koelman JH, Speelman JD, Hilgevoord AA, et al. Dopa-responsive dystonia and normalization of soleus H-reflex test results with treatment. Neurology 1995;45:281–285.

49. Jahanshahi M, Sartory G, Marsden CD. EMG biofeedback treatment of torticollis: a controlled outcome study. Biofeedback Self Regul 1991; 16:413–448.

50. O'Neill MA, Gwinn KA, Adler CH. Biofeedback for writer's cramp. Am J Occup Ther 1997;51:605–607.

51. Bird BL, Cataldo MF. Experimental analysis of EMG feedback in treating dystonia. Ann Neurol 1978;3:310–315.

52. Comella CL, Buchman AS, Tanner CM, et al. Botulinum toxin injection for spasmodic torticollis: increased magnitude of benefit with electromyographic assistance. Neurology 1992;42:878–882.

53. Finsterer J, Fuchs I, Mamoli B. Quantitative electromyography-guided botulinum toxin treatment of cervical dystonia. Clin Neuropharmacol 1997;20:42–48.

54. Wissel J, Kabus C, Wenzel R, et al. Botulinum toxin in writer's cramp: objective response evaluation in 31 patients. J Neurol Neurosurg Psychiatry 1996;61:172–175.

55. Poewe W, Wissel J. Use of botulinum toxin in the treatment of cervical dystonia. Baillieres Clin Neurol 1993;2:179–185.

56. Brans JW, Aramideh M, Koelman JH, et al. Electromyography in cervical dystonia: changes after botulinum and trihexyphenidyl. Neurology 1998;51:815–819.

57. Buchman AS, Comella CL, Stebbins GT, et al. Quantitative electromyographic analysis of changes in muscle activity following botulinum toxin therapy for cervical dystonia. Clin Neuropharmacol 1993;16:205–210.

58. Gelb DJ, Yoshimura DM, Olney RK, et al. Change in pattern of muscle activity following botulinum toxin injections for torticollis. Ann Neurol 1991;29:370–376.

59. Marin C, Marti MJ, Tolosa E, et al. Modification of muscle activity after BOTOX injections in spasmodic torticollis. Ann Neurol 1992;32:411–412.

60. Kanovsky P, Dufek J, Halackova H, et al. Change in the pattern of cervical dystonia might be the cause of benefit loss during botulinum toxin treatment. Eur J Neurol 2001;4:79–84.

61. Speelman JD, Brans JW. Cervical dystonia and botulinum treatment: is electromyographic guidance necessary? Mov Disord 1995;10:802.

62. Borodic GE, Joseph M, Fay L, et al. Botulinum A toxin for the treatment of spasmodic torticollis: dysphagia and regional toxin spread. Head Neck 1990;12:392–399.

63. Jankovic J, Schwartz K, Donovan DT. Botulinum toxin treatment of cranial-cervical dystonia, spasmodic dysphonia, other focal dystonias and hemifacial spasm. J Neurol Neurosurg Psychiatry 1990;53:633–639.

64. Rollnik JD, Matzke M, Wohlfarth K, et al. Low-dose treatment of cervical dystonia, blepharospasm and facial hemispasm with albumin-diluted botulinum toxin type A under EMG guidance. An open label study. Eur Neurol 2000;43:9–12.

65. Brans JW, de Boer IP, Aramideh M, et al. Botulinum toxin in cervical dystonia: low dosage with electromyographic guidance. J Neurol 1995;242:529–534.

66. Dubinsky RM, Gray CS, Vetere-Overfield B, et al. Electromyographic guidance of botulinum toxin treatment in cervical dystonia. Clin Neuropharmacol 1991;14:262–267.

67. Tsui JK, Eisen A, Calne DB. Botulinum toxin in spasmodic torticollis. Adv Neurol 1988;50:593–597.

68. Aramideh M, Ongerboer de Visser BW, Brans JW, et al. Pretarsal application of botulinum toxin for treatment of blepharospasm. J Neurol Neurosurg Psychiatry 1995;59:309–311.

69. Aramideh M, Ongerboer de Visser BW, Koelman JH, et al. Clinical and electromyographic features of levator palpebrae superioris muscle dysfunction in involuntary eyelid closure. Mov Disord 1994;9:395–402.

70. Aramideh M, Koelman JH, Speelman JD, et al. Eyelid movement disorders and electromyography. Lancet 2001;357:805–806.

71. Kessler KR, Benecke R. The EBD test: a clinical test for the detection of antibodies to botulinum toxin type A. Mov Disord 1997;12:95–99.

72. Adler M, Keller JE, Sheridan RE, et al. Persistence of botulinum neurotoxin A demonstrated by sequential administration of serotypes A and E in rat EDL muscle. Toxicon 2001;39:233–243.

73. Dressler D, Rothwell JC. Electromyographic quantification of the paralysing effect of botulinum toxin in the sternocleidomastoid muscle. Eur Neurol 2000;43:13–16.

74. Houser MK, Sheean GL, Lees AJ. Further studies using higher doses of botulinum toxin type F for torticollis resistant to botulinum toxin type A. J Neurol Neurosurg Psychiatry 1998;64:577–580.

75. Lange DJ, Rubin M, Greene PE, et al. Distant effects of locally injected botulinum toxin: a double-blind study of single fiber EMG changes. Muscle Nerve 1991;14:672–675.

76. Bhatia KP, Munchau A, Thompson PD, et al. Generalised muscular weakness after botulinum toxin injections for dystonia: a report of three cases. J Neurol Neurosurg Psychiatry 1999;67:90–93.

77. Girlanda P, Vita G, Nicolosi C, et al. Botulinum toxin therapy: distant effects on neuromuscular transmission and autonomic nervous system. J Neurol Neurosurg Psychiatry 1992;55:844–845.

CHAPTER 11

Surgical Therapies for Dystonia

William G. Ondo and Joachim K. Krauss

INTRODUCTION

Dystonia is defined as an involuntary, patterned muscle contraction that results in abnormal movements or postures. The diagnosis is based solely on clinical examination. Electromyographic co-contraction of agonist and antagonist muscles and other neurophysiologic features are characteristic, but not specific for the diagnosis of dystonia. Anatomic classifications categorize dystonia into generalized dystonia, affecting the entire body; hemidystonia, affecting one side of the body (usually caused by a structural lesion); segmental dystonia, affecting multiple, contiguous body parts; or focal dystonia, affecting one body part. The focal dystonias are usually named according to anatomy, such as ocular dystonia (blepharospasm), cervical dystonia (torticollis), and hand dystonia (writer's cramp).

Dystonic muscle activity is usually precipitated or exacerbated by planned, volitional muscle actions. Some focal dystonias that occur only with specific actions are termed task-specific. Any act requiring repetitive motions, such as writing, stenography, or playing musical instruments may evolve into a task-specific dystonia. Of these dystonias, writer's cramp is probably the most common.

As a rule, adult-onset dystonias usually remain localized to one part of the body. In contrast, dystonia that begins during childhood typically occurs in the limbs, and often spreads and becomes generalized. It is not clear whether this results from different pathophysiologies or whether it is a true age-dependent phenomenon.

Several other distinct forms of dystonia are classified separately. Tardive dystonia, seen after exposure to dopamine-blocking drugs, often results in neck and trunk extension, and may be severe.[1] Paroxysmal dyskinesias, which may oc-

cur in the setting of action (kinesiogenic) or rest (nonkinesiogenic), are predominately dystonic and may represent seizure activity within the basal ganglia.[2] Dopa-responsive dystonia, also known as DRD or Segawa's dystonia, results from several different enzymatic perturbations that impede the production of endogenous dopamine.[3,4] DRD responds dramatically to levodopa replacement therapy.

Dystonia may be primary or secondary. Many genetic or primary forms of dystonia have been linked; however, only *DYT1*, caused by a mutation in the gene on chromosome 9q34 that codes for the protein torsinA, can be diagnosed by commercially available DNA testing.[5,6] This specific condition is most commonly seen in people of Ashkenazi (Eastern European) Jewish origin; however, *DYT1* dystonia has been reported in various demographic regions. This form of dystonia usually presents during childhood with limb involvement, which then spreads to become generalized. The other genetic generalized dystonias have heterogeneous characteristics and demographics. Because most of these have only partial penetrance, the absence of a clear family history does not irrefutably preclude their existence.[7-11]

A variety of neurologic conditions such as static encephalopathies (dystonic cerebral palsy), Wilson's disease, Hallervorden-Spatz disease (more appropriately called neurodegeneration with brain iron accumulation type 1 or pantothenate kinase associated neurodegeneration), and Huntington's disease may include dystonia as part of their phenotype.[12,13] Any structural lesion within the basal ganglia, thalamus, or brain stem may also cause a secondary dystonia, especially in younger people.[14] Peripheral nerve injuries occasionally cause dystonia that tends to be painful and segmental.[15]

PATHOPHYSIOLOGY OF DYSTONIA

The exact pathophysiologic mechanisms resulting in either primary or secondary dystonia are unknown. Increasing evidence, however, suggests that altered signaling through the basal ganglia circuitry causes changes within the supplementary motor and sensorimotor cortices. In familial dystonia, the

William G. Ondo: Baylor College of Medicine, Department of Neurology, Houston, Texas.

Joachim K. Krauss: Department of Neurosurgery University Hospital, Klinikum Mannheim, Mannheim, Germany.

Dr. William Ondo is currently on the Speaker's Bureau for Allergan, Inc. Dr. Ondo has received study grants from Allergan in the past. He currently has no study grants from Allergan.

dopaminergic system is specifically implicated by positron emission tomography (PET) studies, which show a moderate reduction in putamen [^{18}F]dopa uptake.[16] Perlmutter et al.[17] reported reduced putaminal binding of [^{18}F]spiperone (a radioligand that is relatively specific for D2 receptors), and implicated the indirect basal ganglia pathway in the pathophysiology of dystonia. The indirect pathway may also play a key role in the production of levodopa-induced dyskinesias in patients with Parkinson's disease (PD)[18] and inhibit unwanted movement.[19]

According to current basal ganglia models, reduced dopaminergic input into the indirect and direct pathways results in increased globus pallidus internus (GPi) activity. In MPTP models of PD, microelectrode recordings of the GPi have consistently demonstrated increased GPi activity in the "off" state. The assumption is that patients with PD have increased GPi activity, although normal control data does not actually exist in humans. GPi recordings in patients with dystonia have been more variable. Overall, dystonia GPi firing rate is less than that seen in patients with PD in the "off"

state, and even less than that seen in normal non-human primates (Fig. 11-1). Importantly, however, the firing pattern is irregular and clumped.[20,21] Moreover, patients with dystonia show a higher number of GPi cells that respond to sensory stimulation and passive movement.[20,22] In these patients, this increased response to sensory input is also seen in the Vim thalamus.[20,23]

The authors' study data also shows that GPi firing in dystonia is much less than that seen in PD (24.5 ± 14.0 versus 84.7 ± 29.6 per minute, $P < .001$, Mann-Whitney rank sum test).[21] The dystonia firing pattern does seem irregular and clumped, and is similar to the pattern observed in PD patients who are experiencing dopaminergic-induced dyskinesia (Fig. 11-1). There is, however, no clear correlation between absolute GPi firing rate and surgical outcome. Furthermore, there are no statistical differences among the three classifications of dystonia: genetic, idiopathic (primary dystonia with no family history), or secondary (central nervous system [CNS] or peripheral lesion). The reliability of the single-cell recording data is somewhat limited; 11 of 16 surgeries

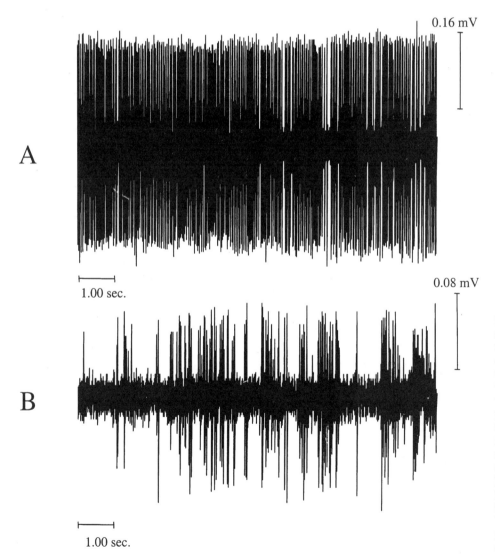

0.16 mV

A

1.00 sec.

0.08 mV

B

1.00 sec.

FIG. 11-1. Extracellular neuronal activity recorded in the GPi of patients with PD (**A**) and dystonia (**B**) using tungsten microelectrodes. Neuronal signals were filtered using a bandwidth of 300 Hz to 2–5 KHz, amplified and displayed with the Axon Instruments GS 3000 system (Axon Instruments, Foster City, CA). Neuronal activity was also stored for offline analysis of average firing rates, interspike intervals, and autocorrelation and cross-correlation histograms (DATAPAC 2000; Run Technologies, CA). GPi, globus pallidus internus; PD, Parkinson's disease.

required general anesthesia, which appears to slow the overall firing pattern. Nevertheless, the five patients with dystonia who did not require anesthesia still had a relatively slow, irregular firing pattern.

The GPi, which is the main basal ganglia outflow nucleus, functionally inhibits the VL/VA thalamus, which then stimulates the supplementary motor cortex (SMA). In PD, SMA activity is reduced, as predicted by this model, and may be increased by both dopaminergic treatment and pallidotomy.[24–28] In dystonia, however, the relationship between GPi output and cortical activity is less clear. Studies suggest that rostral SMA activity (i.e., rostral premotor and dorsolateral prefrontal cortex) is increased with limb movement in patients with primary and secondary dystonia.[16,29] Primary dystonia demonstrates decreased primary motor cortex activity, whereas dystonia that is secondary to basal ganglia lesions results in increased activity of the primary motor cortex.[16,29]

Kumar et al.[30] compared [^{15}O]H$_2$O PET images of a single patient with a primary but not clearly genetic dystonia. These comparisons were made before and after activation of bilateral GPi deep brain stimulators, which mimic the effects of lesioning. During joystick movements, activation of the GPi stimulators reduced PET activity bilaterally in the primary motor, lateral premotor, supplementary motor, anterior cingulate, and prefrontal areas. Reduced PET activity was observed ipsilaterally in the lentiform nucleus. No differences in activity were noted while the patient was at rest.

The thalamic conduit between the GPi and cortex is also clearly abnormal. Lenz and Byl[31] compared single-cell neuronal activity and microstimulation-evoked responses in the ventral caudal thalamus. They compared patients with dystonia to patients with essential tremor. The patients with dystonia showed a higher percentage of cells with multiple receptive fields (i.e., activity with innocuous cutaneous stimulation at different body parts). Furthermore, a higher percentage of cells had multiple projected fields. This sensory organization appears congruent to that seen in the cortex.

Therefore, GPi lesioning or high-frequency stimulation could possibly improve pathologic irregular GPi firing patterns in a manner that reduces cortical overactivity. Based on this theoretical rationale, as well as the observation that GPi lesioning improves dystonia and dyskinesia in PD, the GPi is now considered by many as the primary CNS target for the treatment of dystonia. Thalamic targeting for dystonia, however, has been long advocated and is still used successfully. Other traditionally used CNS targets, such as the cerebellum and spinal dorsal columns, have been largely abandoned.

HISTORY OF CENTRAL NERVOUS SYSTEM ABLATIVE SURGERY FOR DYSTONIA

During the 1940s, Meyers[32] was the first to lesion the basal ganglia to treat movement disorders. Spiegel et al.,[33] however, were the first to use a stereotactic frame for movement disorder surgery; Spiegel is therefore often credited as the

"father" of the field. As stereotactic techniques improved over the next two decades, basal ganglia surgery was performed for a variety of movement disorders, including dystonia. Cooper[34] first reported on a large series of patients using thalamotomy for dystonia and other movement disorders, including PD and athetosis. For many years, thalamotomy was clearly considered the surgical procedure of choice for patients with dystonia or PD. More recently, pallidal surgery has regained popularity for both PD and dystonia. This is largely because of improvements in understanding of the basal ganglia circuitry, coupled with improvements in surgical techniques, reducing the once unacceptable rates of visual field deficits and weakness.

GENERAL GUIDELINES FOR PATIENT SELECTION

Only a minority of patients with dystonia should be considered for CNS surgery. First, the dystonia must be severe enough to warrant surgery. Typically, patients with generalized or hemidystonia are candidates, as these patients are the most severely affected and most refractory to therapy. Reliable data regarding the treatment of most focal dystonias with CNS surgery are sparse, and most focal dystonias may be treated satisfactorily with botulinum toxin (BTX) injections and various medications. Nevertheless, severe refractory cases of cervical dystonia (CD) have been successfully treated with bilateral GPi targeting.[35–37]

Second, in all cases, patients being considered for surgery must have responded unsatisfactorily to more conventional and less invasive treatments. These include a variety of pharmacologic agents such as anticholinergics (e.g., trihexyphenidyl, benztropine, etc.), benzodiazepines (diazepam, clonazepam, etc.), baclofen, tizanidine, levodopa, and, in some patients, dantrolene. Other muscle relaxants including cyclobenzaprine, methocarbamol, carisoprodol, and metaxalone are also occasionally helpful. These medications are dose dependent. Therefore, in most patients, the dose should be augmented until adverse events become prohibitive. Furthermore, polytherapy with agents employing different mechanisms of action is usually superior to monotherapy. Again, adverse events eventually limit the dosing.

BTX is currently the mainstay of treatment for most focal dystonias, with or without adjunctive pharmacotherapy. BTX therapy is effective for discrete anatomic areas, especially in the face and neck. Involvement of larger anatomic areas, such as the legs, substantially increases the required dose of BTX. This may make its use problematic because:

1. The cost of therapy greatly increases with the large doses required for generalized dystonia;
2. Technically, large muscle injections are more variable; and
3. The development of neutralizing antibodies against the botulinum toxin correlates with higher and more frequent dosing.[38]

Other, less well-studied treatment alternatives include phenol injections, physiotherapy, and electrical stimulation.

Third, CNS dystonia procedures may be limited by the usual contraindications and restrictions of surgery and anesthesia. In contrast to patients with PD, who usually undergo similar procedures while awake, the severe muscle contractions seen in patients with dystonia often necessitate general anesthesia.

PALLIDOTOMY

The surgical procedures for pallidotomy vary depending on the center in which the surgery is performed. Specific surgical features that differ include: the stereotactic atlas and hardware; stereotactic imaging (magnetic resonance imaging [MRI] versus computed tomography [CT] versus ventriculography); techniques for macrostimulation lesion identification; and the use of and methods by which single-cell recording is performed to facilitate lesion placement. The following summarizes the techniques used by the authors at the Baylor College of Medicine and University of Mannheim.

1. After fixation of the stereotactic frame, stereotactic contiguous 1 mm axial scans are obtained via a helical CT scanner.
2. An initial target in the posteroventral GPi is chosen (20 mm lateral to the midline; 4 mm below the anterior commissure/posterior commissure (AC/PC) line; and 2 mm anterior to the midcommissural point).
3. Reformatting the images in axial, coronal, and sagittal planes and comparison with preoperative MRI is done to ensure accurate identification of the commissures and target.
4. A burr hole is made 7–9 cm above the orbital rim and 2 cm lateral to the midline.
5. Microelectrode trajectories are then planned at an angle of 35°–45° above the AC/PC line and parallel to the midsagittal line.
6. Microelectrodes, with an initial impedance measured between 0.5 and 1.2 megaohms, are used. The microelectrode is advanced via the guiding cannula. Single unit recordings are obtained from 20 mm above the tentative target to 5 mm below it.
7. The ventral border of the GPi is identified with the recording. In many patients, the optic tract is identified with microstimulation.
8. One to three trajectories are made in most patients. The microelectrode recording usually results in modifying the CT coordinates by up to 1–3 mm. This modification occurs most often in the vertical (Z) axis.
9. A 1.1-mm unipolar electrode with a 3-mm uninsulated tip is used for macrostimulation and lesion-making. The tip of the electrode is placed within 1 mm of the ventral border of the GPi, according to the mapping.
10. Macrostimulation is used to assess the threshold for the spread of current to the optic tract and internal capsule. This location is considered the final target in those pa-

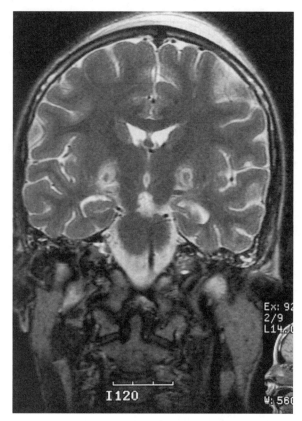

FIG. 11-2. Magnetic resonance imaging of a patient's status after simultaneous bilateral pallidotomy for generalized dystonia.

tients where no optic or capsular responses are elicited below 2 V. Otherwise, the electrode is withdrawn in 1.0-mm increments and the stimulation is repeated.
11. A radiofrequency lesion is made at 75°C for 60 seconds (Fig. 11-2).
12. The electrode is withdrawn 2 mm and a second similar lesion is made. During lesioning, the strength and mobility of the contralateral arm, speech, and visual fields are monitored.

Total operative time averages between 3 and 4 hours. The length of hospital stay averages approximately 3 days.

Efficacy of Pallidotomy: Baylor College of Medicine

Baylor College of Medicine has complete follow-up data on 16 patients, ages 5 to 56 years (mean, 21. ± 11.6), who have undergone GPi lesioning for generalized or hemidystonia (Table 11-1). Pallidotomy has not been performed on any patient with focal dystonia. Eleven of the 16 patients were children, under the age of 18 years. These 16 patients were taking a total of 39 different medications for dystonia at the time of surgery; 15 patients had received BTX injections during the previous year.

The pathogenesis of dystonia varied in this patient population. Six patients had a clear genetic dystonia, four of whom tested positively for *DYT1*. Five patients were thought to have idiopathic dystonia, but did not have a clear genetic

TABLE 11-1. *Characteristics of Sixteen Patients Undergoing Pallidotomy*

	Age at Surgery	Age at Onset	Initial Site of Dystonia	Current Site of Dystonia	Etiology	Surgical Site
1	15	3	Right leg	Generalized	Genetic[a]	Bilateral (s)
2	13	10	Right arm	Generalized	Genetic[a]	Bilateral (c)
3	14	7	Right arm	Generalized	Genetic[a]	Bilateral (c)
4	9	6	Right foot	Generalized right>left	Genetic[a]	Bilateral (s)
5	51	10	Right arm	Generalized	Genetic	Bilateral (c)
6	23	8	Right foot	Generalized	Genetic	Unilateral
7	16	10	Oral	Generalized	Idiopathic	Bilateral (c)
8	15	10	Right foot	Generalized	Idiopathic	Bilateral (c)
9	6	2	Bilateral legs	Generalized	Idiopathic	Bilateral (c)
10	7	6	Generalized	Generalized	Idiopathic	Bilateral (c)
11	47	5	Right leg	Generalized	Idiopathic	Unilateral
12	25	18	Left arm	Left hemidystonia	Focal Hypoxia	Unilateral
13	20	12	Right arm	Right hemidystonia	Peripheral trauma	Unilateral
14	56	46	Left arm	Generalized	Head trauma	Unilateral
15	18	13	Oral	Generalized	CNS bleed	Bilateral (c)
16	14	6	Generalized	Generalized	Global hypoxia	Bilateral (c)

[a]DYT1-positive
(c), concurrent; (s), staged; CNS, central nervous system.

history of dystonia. Five patients were thought to have secondary dystonia from peripheral trauma (1 patient), CNS trauma (1 patient), focal brain hypoxia (1 patient), global hypoxia (1 patient), and focal hemorrhage (1 patient). Patients were evaluated preoperatively and followed postoperatively at 3–6 months. In some patients, 2- and 3-year follow-up examinations were also available. In addition to general neurologic evaluation, patients underwent unblinded dystonia assessments with the Burke-Marsden-Fahn Dystonia Scale (BMFDS) and the Unified Dystonia Rating Scale (UDRS).[39,40] The UDRS is a detailed rating of dystonia amplitude (0–4) and duration (0–4) in 14 different areas of the body. An activity of daily living (ADL) scale based on the UDRS was also used. This scale included questions (each scored 0–5) regarding the patient's ability to write, eat, drink from a cup, and walk.

Eleven patients had bilateral procedures, which were staged in two patients and concurrent in nine patients. Overall, 14 of 16 patients demonstrated meaningful improvement (Table 11-2). One male patient, who had experienced global hypoxia secondary to drowning, failed to improve after simultaneous bilateral pallidotomy. This patient demonstrated a mixed movement disorder, consisting of generalized dystonia, chorea, and myoclonus. A second young

TABLE 11-2. *Individual Outcome Measures: Three-Month Follow-Up*

Patient	Pre-op UDRS scale	Post-op UDRS scale	Pre-op BMFDS	Post-op BMFDS	Pre-op ADL	Post-op ADL	# of pre-op meds	# of post-op meds
1	41	12	27	10	9	4	3	0
2	81	20	48	17	17	6	3	0
3	68	12	50	12	18	5	3	0
4	36	21	26	18	10	7	2	0
5	83	26	57	15	16	6	0	0
6	30	—	22	—	13	—	3	1
7	101	27	59	17	19	9	3	0
8	78	66	49	46	17	15	3	3
9	88	54	58	36	19	18	3	3
10	51	34	31	25	15	11	1	0
11	28	20	18	18	12	5	3	2
12	37	15	25	13	13	10	1	0
13	38	11	23	6	10	6	2	1
14	51	21	34	14	12	8	3	1
15	86	63	56	43	18	14	3	2
16	82	74	56	45	19	18	3	3
MEAN (S.D.)	63 (21)	32 (18)	41 (14)	22 (11)	15 (3)	9 (4)	1.8	1

UDRS, Unified Dystonia Rating Scale; BMFDS, Burke-Marsden-Fahn Dystonia Scale; ADL, Activities of Daily Living; meds, medications.

female, with an area of hemosiderin in the GPi and globus pallidus externus (GPe), experienced only mild improvement in one arm after a bilateral procedure; there was no other change in this patient's dystonia. Later, this patient responded well to an intrathecal baclofen pump.

The patients with genetic and primary dystonias (both *DYT1*-positive and *DYT1*-negative) consistently demonstrated marked benefits. Improvement in the idiopathic and secondary dystonias tended to be less dramatic and less consistent. Nevertheless, some patients with secondary dystonias experienced meaningful benefit.

It was difficult to compare the efficacy of unilateral versus concurrent bilateral procedures as this decision was clinically based upon the anatomic distribution of the dystonia. All patients with oromandibular and axial dystonia had bilateral procedures; therefore, it is difficult to know what improvement, if any, a unilateral pallidotomy would have had on their midline symptoms. The patients who underwent staged bilateral procedures experienced predominantly contralateral improvement after the first procedure, and further axial and bilateral improvement after the second procedure.

Improvement in different anatomic areas has been relatively consistent. The most dramatic benefit occurred in the hands and arms, which in many patients, returned to normal levels of function. Lower-extremity function and gait also consistently improved. However, midline structures did not respond as consistently, even with bilateral procedures. Over time, midline dystonia was also more likely to recrudesce.

The course of improvement is interesting and leads to considerable speculative debate. Normally, pallidotomy performed for PD immediately improves motor tone and dyskinesia. Motor tone in patients with dystonia may also improve almost immediately, but the actual action-induced dystonia does not usually begin to improve for 2–7 days. This improvement continues for up to 3 months. It is unknown whether this represents a relearning effect or some ongoing pathophysiologic change. Improvement has been generally maintained; however, there is some return of symptoms over time. Patients who initially responded remain much improved after a mean of 1.5 years of follow-up and several patients with longer follow-up periods remain improved after more than 3 years of postoperative evaluation.

Substantial complications related to surgery were limited to transient postoperative lethargy in one patient and mild unilateral weakness in another patient. In all patients except one, postoperative MRI demonstrated lesions that were confined within the GPi; the exception was the patient with transient weakness, in whom the lesion extended slightly into the internal capsule. There was no clear difference in adverse events between unilateral and bilateral procedures. The patient with postoperative lethargy had a bilateral procedure. No bulbar symptoms or cognitive compromise occurred in any patient.

Only four patients underwent extensive preoperative and postoperative neuropsychiatric testing. Three adults who were tested after a unilateral lesioning showed moderate im-

provement across a wide range of variables. These included verbal memory and language skills, areas that should not be affected by their improved motor function. A single child who was tested after a bilateral surgery showed no meaningful changes.

Based on long-term experience, the team at the Baylor Medical Center considers patients with dystonia to be ideal candidates for pallidotomy if they:

1. Have a primary genetic generalized dystonia;
2. Have no surgical contraindications;
3. Are refractory to other treatments, and
4. Have considerable disability referable to their limbs, rather than only midline structures.

It should be emphasized that patients who do not meet all of these criteria might still have a dramatic benefit from pallidotomy.

Efficacy of Pallidotomy: Literature Review

The authors' experiences with results of pallidotomy for dystonia have been generally consistent with results reported in other centers that perform pallidotomy for dystonia.[41–53] The delayed improvement has been consistently observed. However, most series are too small to assess factors that may otherwise predict response.

Iacono et al.[44] published an account of striking improvement after bilateral pallidotomies in a 17-year-old male with primary generalized dystonia, and subsequently reported mixed results in four additional patients.[45] Overall, two adults with craniocervical dystonia were noted as "markedly improved" by Iacono and colleagues. One of these patients underwent bilateral pallidotomies. The other patient, who had isolated cervical dystonia (CD), underwent a left pallidotomy. A 48-year-old patient with primary spasmodic dysphonia and left lower-extremity dystonia experienced moderate improvement in leg dystonia; however, there was no change in dysphonia after a right pallidotomy. A 24-year-old patient with secondary generalized dystonia, primarily appendicular in distribution, did not improve.

Vitek et al.[20,46] reported three patients who underwent unilateral pallidotomy. There was marked improvement in contralateral dystonic symptoms, with a significant reductions in the BMFDS of 72–80%. Comparison of preoperative and postoperative surface electromyographic (EMG) studies of overactive muscle groups revealed that during movement, there was decreased coactivation of agonist-antagonist muscle groups. A dramatic reduction in resting EMG activity after pallidotomy was also noted. One year after surgery, there was better residual improvement in appendicular signs. Axial symptoms might be better treated with bilateral pallidotomies. Vitek and colleagues (personal communication 2002) have also reported postpallidotomy results that were more favorable in patients with primary dystonia patients who tested positive for the *DYT1* gene.

Lozano and associates[42] reported remarkable improvement in an 8-year-old Ashkenazi male with familial (*DYT1*-negative) primary generalized dystonia following simultaneous bilateral pallidotomies. Improvement continued for 3 months after surgery.

Lin et al.[48] reported less favorable results in 18 patients who underwent bilateral pallidotomies. This difference could potentially be explained by the underlying condition, as all of their patients (*n* = 18) had secondary dystonia, including cerebral palsy (*n* = 8); hypoxic encephalopathy (*n* = 6), carbon monoxide poisoning (*n* = 2), and encephalitis (*n* = 2). Lin and colleages[48] also reported a delayed onset to maximal effect. Unlike other reports, they noted more axial improvement.

Pallidotomy may also improve symptomatic dystonia resulting from other neurodegenerative diseases. Cubo et al.[49] reported modest improvement following bilateral pallidotomy in a 13-year-old with Huntington's disease. The pallidal firing patterns were similar to those seen in idiopathic dystonia. The same center also reported modest improvement in a 10-year-old male with Hallervorden-Spatz disease and noted particular benefit in pain relief.[50] Paroxysmal dystonia is also reported to improve with pallidotomy.[51] Further reports of these and other diseases in which dystonia is a feature need to be evaluated before any recommendations are possible.

THALAMOTOMY

In most patients with dystonia, guidelines similar to those used for pallidotomy candidates govern the selection process for potential thalamotomy candidates. Patients must be severely incapacitated by their dystonic symptoms and refractory to medical managements. There are numerous potential surgical risks, and bilateral procedures carry the additional risk of dysarthria and other bulbar signs. The etiology of dystonia, either primary or secondary, must be clearly elucidated, if possible, as certain subgroups of dystonic patients may respond differently to thalamotomy and pallidotomy.

Surgical Techniques

In most medical centers, the surgical technique for thalamotomy in dystonic patients is similar to those techniques used in patients with PD.[54–58] However, the target has been more varied in dystonic patients. These targets include the VIM nucleus, ventrolateral thalamus, ventro-oralis internus nucleus, and centrum medianum. At the Baylor Medical Center, the target is located in the area designated, in the Hassler terminology, as the ventralis oralis (VOA/VOP).

General anesthesia is often required, especially in children who may not tolerate stereotactic procedures under local anesthesia. However, functional stereotactic procedures without patient feedback make target localization more difficult. The surgery usually provides a degree of immediate relaxation of the dystonic symptoms in patients who are awake; the surgery's full effect is not apparent until weeks or months after surgery. If an additional lesion is made, it is usually extended slightly anteriorly and medially.

Outcomes of Thalamotomy for Dystonia

The group at the Baylor College of Medicine reported on 17 patients with dystonia who underwent VOA/VOP thalamotomy.[54] Of these patients, 47% showed early moderate improvement that was sustained over time. Further improvement was noted in 12% of patients with time. Patients with secondary dystonia, who tended to do better than those with primary dystonia, experienced moderate to marked improvement in 50% of cases versus 43% of cases with primary dystonia. Similar to pallidotomy for dystonia, improvement with thalamotomy is often delayed and gradual. This is in contrast to the immediate effect that is seen when thalamotomy is used to treat patients with tremor. Comparison of the Baylor results with those of other centers is difficult because of differences in rating scales used for assessment, nuclei targeted during surgery, lengths of follow-up, and heterogeneous groups of patients being studied. Regardless, the Baylor results appear generally similar to those of other centers, with a moderate improvement seen overall.

Cooper[59,60] reported the first large series of thalamotomy for generalized dystonia. One hundred and four patients underwent unilateral surgery and 122 patients underwent bilateral surgery. The usual target was in the VIM, ventral caudal, and centromedian nuclei. The lesions were typically large and often repeated, if not effective. Overall, 69.7% of these patients experienced mild to moderate improvement. Cooper noted that, in many of his patients, there was deterioration in improvement over time. Axial and appendicular symptoms responded equally well. The mortality rate was 2%.

Kandel[61] performed 272 procedures on 188 patients with dystonia. The lesions were typically located in the VL nucleus; in some patients, lesions were added into the GPi and subthalamic nucleus. Overall, 54% of these patients showed substantial improvement and 22% showed good improvement in their dystonic symptoms. The reported mortality rate was 1.8% and the morbidity rate was 10%.

Tasker[51] reported thalamotomy results in 49 patients. Of these patients, 20 had primary dystonia and 29 had secondary dystonia. This investigator used physiologic guidance including microelectrode recording and stimulation to identify dystonic cells. The ideal target was the VIM nucleus, which is also the target for patients with tremor. Tasker noted that 68% of patients with secondary dystonia showed an improvement of more than 25%. Only 50% of primary dystonia patients showed similar improvement. Most improvement was seen in appendicular symptoms. Axial symptoms of gait, speech, and facial movement showed results that were more modest.

Krauss et al.[56] reported on the long-term results in patients with posttraumatic hemidystonia. All seven patients benefited from improvement of their dystonia during the early postoperative period. Five patients had transient side effects, consisting of hemiparesis in four patients. On long-term follow-up at a mean of 18 years postoperatively, hemidystonia was still improved in 4 patients; however, 3 patients had returned to baseline. Gross and associates[62] observed an immediate improvement in 51% of their patients; however, after 6 years, only 33% remained improved. The various other series reported similarly modest results overall.[63,64]

Surgical complications were documented in 35% of patients in the Baylor thalamotomy series. Confusion and contralateral hemiparesis were the most series problems; however, dysarthria and pseudobulbar palsy were also encountered. One patient (6%) experienced persistent neurologic deficits after a second procedure to enlarge the lesion. Other series report complication rates of 16–47%.[58–60] Additional complications that have been reported include dysphagia, gait disturbances, transient numbness, seizures, and death.

CENTRAL NERVOUS SYSTEM ABLATION CONCLUSIONS

Overall, thalamotomy moderately improves dystonia. Because of the relatively small number of patients undergoing thalamic lesioning, the varied methodologies, and inconsistent outcome assessments, no definitive recommendations about the surgical indications and ideal lesion placement may be made.

Experience with pallidotomy for dystonia, when compared to thalamotomy, suggests that patients may respond better to one or the other based on pathogenesis. Thalamotomy may be somewhat more efficacious in patients with secondary dystonia, as opposed to primary dystonia. Conversely, patients with primary dystonia, especially *DYT1*, probably respond more favorably to pallidotomy. These findings may suggest that pallidotomy is more appropriate for patients with primary dystonia and thalamotomy may be the potential procedure of choice in secondary dystonia.

DEEP BRAIN STIMULATION FOR DYSTONIA

High-frequency deep brain stimulation or DBS (Medtronic Activa System, Medtronic, Minneapolis, MN) is an accepted and widely used alternative to CNS lesioning in PD. Targets include: the VIM thalamus, which mostly improves tremor; the GPi, which mostly improves dyskinesia and rigidity; and the subthalamic nucleus (STN), which improves tremor, bradykinesia, and rigidity (Fig. 11-3). Physiologically, pulse frequencies of more than 50 Hz functionally inhibit local neuronal activity, thereby mimicking a lesion. The area of involvement is proportional to the square of the voltage.

DBS offers several potential benefits over traditional stereotactic ablative procedures. There may be less perioperative and postoperative morbidity with DBS, although this has only been formally assessed in essential tremor.[65] DBS

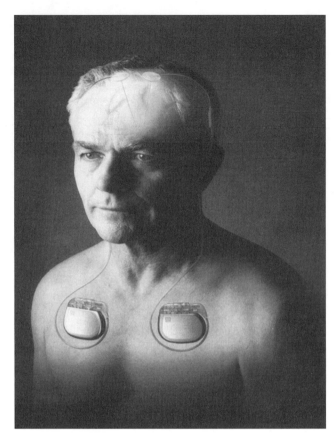

FIG. 11-3. Cartoon of the Activa deep brain stimulation system (Courtesy of Medtronic, Inc., Minneapolis, MN).

may be performed bilaterally without substantial morbidity. Most importantly, the device variables can be adjusted over time. Therefore, the functional size of the lesion, and to some extent, the actual placement can be changed by switching among different electrode contacts.

The Baylor College of Medicine team and other centers have noted partial long-term recrudescence after pallidotomy. This problem might be ameliorated by adjustments of the device parameters; however, long-term follow-up information on DBS is limited. The advantages of ablative procedures over DBS include a lower cost, less postoperative maintenance, less chance of infection, and proven long-term tolerability.

The surgical methods of DBS for the GPi and thalamus are similar, except for identification of the target site. Again, specific techniques may vary depending on the center where the surgery is performed.

The following summarizes the methods used by the authors' medical teams.

- A stereotactic head frame is secured to the patient's head after local anesthesia at the pin sites. CT-guided stereotaxis is used instead of MRI for the following reasons:
  1. Rapid scanning speed;
  2. Less patient discomfort;

3. Potentially greater accuracy;
4. Acceptance as the imaging technique for patients undergoing their second DBS implantation, because the device once implanted is a relative contraindication to MRI in some centers; and
5. Lower cost.

- The reconstructed CT images are used to find the AC/PC line.
- The target is chosen in relation to the midpoint of the intercommisure line. For GPi stimulation, the initial target is 20–22 mm lateral to and 4 mm below the AC/PC line, and 3 mm anterior to the AC/PC midpoint.
- For VIM/Vop stimulation, the initial target is 12–14 mm lateral and 1 mm below the AC/PC line, and 3–5 mm posterior to the AC/PC midpoint.
- A small scalp flap is elevated and a burr hole placed in the frontal bone 2–3 cm lateral of the midline and directly anterior to the coronal suture.
- The dura is opened and the cortical surface is viewed to avoid a sulcus.
- The stereotactic arc is secured to the frame using the coordinates determined from the stereotactic CT scan.
- A guiding cannula is inserted at the crown of the gyrus.
- The stylet is removed and microelectrode recording may be done as described above.
- After neurophysiologic identification of the DBS target, the electrode is placed into the cannula. The calculations are made such that the bottom contact is at the lower portion of the target.
- Intraoperative testing of the device is performed using a frequency of 130 Hz, a pulse width of 100 microseconds (μs), and a variety of electrode combinations and polarities to check for intrinsic and extrinsic effects.

In some patients, there is dramatic, immediate clinical improvement; in other patients, there is a less robust perioperative improvement. Therefore, clinical identification of the optimal site is sometimes less obvious than in PD. Minor adjustments in electrode placement may be made, depending on the effect of intraoperative test stimulation. Once the electrode is in an optimal location, it is secured to the skull with a burr-hole ring and cap. The electrode is then tunneled to a small incision placed behind the pinna of the ear. The wounds are closed in a manner such that the electrode may be retrieved, and the head frame is removed.

The pulse generators are implanted under general anesthesia. An incision is made beneath the clavicle, where a subcutaneous pocket is created for the pulse generator. A small incision is also made in the mastoid area and a subcutaneous tunneling device is used to create a tunnel for the extension wire down to the pulse generator. The Intrel II pulse generator (Medtronic) is small and subserves a single electrode, whereas the Kinetra pulse generator (Medtronic) is larger but can subserve two electrodes. The distal aspect of the electrode is retrieved and connected to the extension lead. With the pulse generator in place, the entire assembly is contained beneath the skin and all incisions are closed. Electrode placement is confirmed by CT. The stimulator is activated and programmed from 1–14 days after surgery.

The device allows for adjustment of four major parameters: voltage, pulse frequency, pulse width, and electrode montage (unipolar or bipolar among four discrete contacts on the electrode). The actual adjustments are made using a computer with a magnetic switch, which must be placed over the device located in the chest wall, therefore, adjustments are noninvasive. Investigators have proposed a variety of adjustment algorithms; however, the authors have found that the considerable variability among patients typically results in noteworthy improvisation on the part of the programmer. Typical final settings are approximately 1–6 V (voltage), 130–180 Hz (pulse frequency), and 180–300 μs (pulse width). Both bipolar and unipolar montages are used. Since the results of any individual adjustment may be delayed by minutes to hours, the process is often labor intensive and time consuming.

Pallidal Stimulation for Dystonia

Pallidal DBS has gained increasing importance in the treatment of patients with medically intractable dystonia over the past few years. Several studies with promising results have been published. Most studies, however, have reported only on relatively short follow-up periods, on single patients, or are retrospective. There are no controlled studies. Pallidal DBS has been shown to be beneficial in generalized dystonia, but also in focal and segmental dystonias.[35,37,66–81] The data available thus far are summarized (Table 11-3). DBS for cervical dystonia, which is the most frequent dystonia considered for surgery, is discussed later.

It has been suggested that the response of dystonia to pallidal DBS may depend on etiology, similar to the experience with pallidotomy. In general, patients with primary dystonia respond well, patients with secondary dystonia respond less well, and poorer results are expected in patients with secondary dystonia and structural lesions.[81] Nevertheless, in single instances of secondary dystonia with or without structural lesions remarkable benefit has been achieved with pallidal DBS. In light of the bilateral involvement of the basal ganglia circuitry in generalized and segmental dystonia, bilateral DBS should be preferred over unilateral surgery. Unilateral approaches are reserved, in general, for hemidystonia or focal dystonias. Adverse events, even with bilateral procedures, have been minimal and can be easily managed. Poor wound healing and hardware problems occur somewhat more frequently in dystonia patients than in patients with PD. There is some theoretical concern regarding the placement of a device into a child who is still growing. However, there are no reported cases of the electrode being displaced over time. Because of its novelty, it is unknown whether the

TABLE 11-3. *Pallidal Deep Brain Stimulation for Dystonia*

Author, year of publication	Patient(s), age	Dystonia, etiology	Distribution	Surgery	Reported outcome	Follow-up	Comments
Krauss, 1999	3, 42–53	Primary	Cervical	B	TWSTRS >50% imp of dystonia, pain + disability	6–15 m	—
Kumar, 1999	1, 49	Primary	Generalized	B	BFMDS 65% imp	18 m	Reduced PET activation of certain motor cortical areas during stim
Coubes, 1999	1, 8	Primary, DYT-1	Generalized	B	Excellent	30 m	—
Islekel, 1999	1, 42	Primary	Cervical	U	Marked imp	NA	—
Coubes, 2000	7, 8–27	Primary, DYT-1	Generalized	B	BFMDS 60–100% imp; mean 90%	1 yr (at least)	—
Angelini, 2000	1, 13	Secondary, CP (postvacc)	Generalized, choreoathetotic	B	Excellent	7 m	Life-threatening "dystonic storm" preoperatively
Tronnier, 2000	3	Primary (2), secondary, CP (1)	Generalized	B	Marked relief in primary, mild relief in secondary dystonia	6–18 m	—
Loher, 2000	1, 24	Secondary	Hemidystonia	U	Marked imp of dystonic posture, movements + pain	4 yr	After previous thalamotomy imp of tremor, but not of dystonia
Coubes, 2001	17, 8–26	Primary, DYT-1 (7)	Generalized	B	BFMDS mean 81% imp	3–36 m	Extended series
Andaluz, 2001	1, 61	Primary	Cervical + truncal	B	TWSTRS 50% imp	8 m	—
Kulisevsky, 2001	2, 35 + 65	Primary	Cervical	B	Mild imp of dystonia, but marked imp of pain	17–24 m	—
Brin, 2001	4, NA	Primary	Generalized (2), cervical (1), seg (1)	U	Mild imp (2), failure (2)	12 m	Wound healing problems in three patients, device removed in two
Gill, 2001	1, 11	Secondary, CP	Generalized, choreoathetotic	B	"Disappearance of hyperkinesia, modest imp of dystonia"	NA	—
Parkin, 2001	3, 23–67	Primary	Cervical	B	Marked imp of dystonia, pain + disability	2–6 m	—
Trottenberg, 2001	1, 70	Secondary, tardive	Segmental	B	BFMDS 73% imp	6 m	Patient had no effect with thalamic DBS
Muta, 2001	1, 61	Primary	Segmental axial and facial (Meige)	B	BFMDS 80% imp	NA	Prior bilateral thalamotomy without beneficial effect
Vercueil, 2001	8, 12–59	Primary (5), secondary (3)	Generalized (5), seg (2) hemidystonia (1),	B (7) U (1)	BFMDS > 50% mean imp	6–24 m	Thalamic DBS was not successful in three patients previously
Bereznai, 2002	6, 22–78	Primary, DYT-1 (1)	Generalized (1), seg (3), cervical (2)	B	BFMDS 73% mean imp, Tsui score 63% mean imp	3–12 m	—
Krauss, 2002	8, 28–53	Primary (6), secondary, CP (2)	Cervical (6), choreoathetotic (2)	B (7) U (1)	TWSTRS 63% imp of severity, 50% imp pain, 69% imp disability	12–30 m	Extended series of cervical dystonia, DBS adjunct to spinal surgery

B, bilateral; U, unilateral; TWSTRS, Toronto Western Spasmodic Torticollis Rating Scale; BFMDS, Burke-Marsden-Fahn Dystonia Scale; imp, improvement; stim, stimulation; m, month(s); yr, year(s); NA, not available; CP, cerebral palsy; seg, segmental; DBS, deep brain stimulation.

benefits of pallidal DBS persist over time. Long-term follow-up has become available only in few cases.

The most beneficial results in generalized dystonia were obtained in children with genetic *DYT-1*-positive dystonia. Coubes and colleagues[68] described a mean improvement of 90% in the BFMDS in seven patients (mean age at surgery, 14 years) at a follow-up of at least 1 year after surgery. Improvement was gradual within 3 months after bilateral implantation of pallidal electrodes. Six children managed to walk without assistance after surgery and became functionally normal. Pain rapidly resolved after surgery. Drugs were reduced in all patients resulting in improvement of alertness. All children could return to school. Substantial improvement of dystonia and related disability has also been achieved in adults with primary generalized dystonias. Bilateral DBS may also be beneficial in patients with segmental dystonia, and it may improve facial dystonia and blepharospasm in patients with a more generalized clinical picture of dystonia.[35,74,77,80]

It is unclear which patients with secondary dystonia are suited best for pallidal surgery. Some patients with choreoathetotic generalized dystonia secondary to cerebral palsy have been reported to benefit from bilateral pallidal DBS.[69,79] Published experience, however, has been limited to case studies. In our experience, 2 of 4 patients with choreoathetotic cerebral palsy were satisfied with the result of pallidal DBS at follow-up 2 years after surgery. Although, motor improvement on standard dystonia rating scales (the BFMDS and the UDRS scales) was modest, the gain in functional disabilities was rated highly useful by these severely disabled patients. Trottenberg and colleagues[74] reported a patient with tardive segmental dystonia who responded well to bilateral pallidal DBS, but who had been unresponsive to previous thalamic DBS.

Loher et al.[66] reported long-term follow-up on a patient who underwent pallidal stimulation for treatment of posttraumatic hemidystonia. The patient had developed left-sided, low-frequency tremor and hemidystonia after a severe head trauma sustained at 5 years of age. At 3 years postinjury, a thalamotomy was performed in the right hemisphere. The patient experienced relief of his tremor but not of the hemidystonia. At age 24, a monopolar electrode was placed in the right posteroventral GPi for long-term stimulation. Long-term pallidal stimulation resulted in marked improvement of dystonia-associated pain, phasic dystonic movements, and dystonic posture, which were accompanied by functional gain. Postoperative improvement was sustained at 4 years of follow-up. The Grenoble group achieved useful gains in three patients with generalized and multifocal dystonia who were poor responders to thalamic stimulation.[75]

Improvement of dystonia with pallidal stimulation may be delayed. Sometimes it may take even months until the full benefit is notable. In contrast, dystonia usually reoccurs within minutes when the pulse generators are switched off. Because dystonia often requires a wider pulse width and higher voltage settings than PD, depletion of the pulse gen-

erator batteries may occur within 2 years. It may occur more rapidly when the Intrel II pulse generator is used. The power consumption of the Intrel II is linear up to 3.6 V, but then rises abruptly because a second capacitor is activated. Because power consumption is linear with the Kinetra pulse generator (Kinetra, Golden, CO), it is more advantageous regarding battery life under such circumstances. Modifications in the techniques of stimulation should be explored. Battery life might be prolonged for example by cyclic stimulation modes.

Thalamic Stimulation for Dystonia

There are fewer published data reporting outcomes of thalamic DBS for the treatment of dystonia (Table 11-4).[74,75,82–86] Sellal and colleagues[83] were the first to report the effect of thalamic stimulation for treatment of hemidystonia. Unilateral stimulation in the somatosensory thalamus contralateral to the movement disorder resulted in excellent improvement of posttraumatic hemidystonia in a 16-year-old boy. The Grenoble group reported that thalamic stimulation did not improve mean BFMDS scores, but that nevertheless 6 of 12 patients achieved a good functional result.[75] Thalamic stimulation in the nucleus ventro-oralis anterior was reported to be successful in two patients who showed only a modest response to earlier pallidal stimulation.[82] Both of these patients had secondary dystonia. Improvement was noted to occur after a delay of months. A patient with severe postanoxic dystonia and bilateral necrosis of the basal ganglia underwent bilateral thalamic DBS and showed major improvement after 4 months of high-intensity DBS.[85] Previous pallidal stimulation was unsuccessful in this patient, although the stimulation period of only 6 weeks may have been too short to fully appreciate its effect. In a patient with essential myoclonic dystonia, thalamic DBS resulted in marked improvement of myoclonus scores but not of dystonia.[86]

The authors implanted a stimulator into the thalamus of a 30-year old woman with a 16-year history of right body hemidystonia, resulting from an abscess in her left putamen. Numerous medications had been ineffective and the patient had experienced only minimal response to BTX injections. The target site was more anterior to that used for tremor and was actually located in the Vop/Voa nucleus. The patient showed an immediate and dramatic improvement that persisted for 6 months. Conversely, Lozano et al. (personal communication 2002) reported only minimal improvement in two patients with hemidystonia caused by similar anatomic lesions.

We have reported our experience with long-term stimulation of the ventro-intermediate thalamus in a patient with dystonic paroxysmal nonkinesigenic dyskinesia.[84] This 37-year-old man had a 4-year history of severe and painful paroxysmal dystonia of the right arm. Long-term stimulation resulted in a decrease of the frequency, duration, and intensity of the paroxysmal movement disorder. These positive results have been maintained over the 4 years of follow-up.

TABLE 11-4. *Thalamic Deep Brain Stimulation for Dystonia*

Author, yr of publication	Patient(s), age	Dystonia, etiology	Distribution	Surgery	Reported outcome	Follow-up	Comments
Sellal, 1993	1 16	Secondary, head injury	Hemidystonia	U	Excellent, intermittent	8 m	Target nucleus: VPL, stim produced dysaesthesias poor wound healing: DBS removed
Loher, 2001	1 37	Secondary, after plexopathy	Paroxysmal nonkinesigenic	U	Marked decrease of frequency, intensity and duration of attacks	4 y	—
Trottenberg, 2001	1 60	Primary	Generalized myoclonic dystonia	B	Myoclonus score 80% imp, no imp of dystonia	24 m	—
Vercueil, 2001	12 18–25	Primary (4), secondary (8)	Generalized (9), seg (2), hemidystonia (1)	B (7) U (5)	Mean BFMDS unchanged, but good functional result in 6 patients	4 m–11 y	Pallidal stim in three patients later
Ghika, 2002	1 26	Secondary, postanoxic	Generalized	B	UDRS 50% imp	4 m	Patient committed suicide, previous pallidal stim was unsuccessful

B, bilateral; U, unilateral; BMFDS, Burke-Fahn-Marsden Dystonia Scale; imp, improvement; stim, stimulation; m, month(s); yr, year(s); VPL, ventroposterolateral thalamic nucleus; seg, segmental; UDRS, Unified Dystonia Rating Scale.

More data on thalamic DBS are required before recommendations on patient selection can be given. Thalamic DBS may be considered in particular in patients with secondary dystonia.

Multiple Central Nervous System Procedures

As discussed, pallidotomy and thalamotomy, as well as long-term stimulation of these target areas, may be efficient in different types of dystonia. The concurrent use of these on the same or opposite sides are two other possibilities that may improve efficacy and reduce adverse events. As detailed above, several patients were reported who underwent pallidal surgery after an unsatisfactory response to previous thalamic surgery. The Baylor experience included one patient with a secondary hemidystonia, after an acute ischemic injury (i.e., severed carotid artery). This patient underwent a thalamotomy,[87] with modest improvement. Some years later, the patient had a pallidotomy on the same side. The patient has done well after the second procedure. Another patient with a thalamotomy on one side and a pallidotomy on the other did well and did not experience any adverse events.

Pallidal Stimulation for Cervical Dystonia

CD is thought to arise from pathologic mechanisms within the basal ganglia circuitry. There is evidence in patients with CD that involvement is bilateral, regardless of the specific pattern. PET investigations of patients with CD have shown increased bilateral glucose metabolism in the lentiform nucleus. No substantial differences concerning the laterality, specific pattern, or severity of CD in individual patients was noted.[88] Bilateral basal ganglia involvement has also been suggested by a single-photon emission computed tomography (SPECT) study.[89] Striatal D2 receptor binding was substantially reduced in patients with CD compared to normal controls. However, with respect to the direction of head rotation, no noteworthy difference was found by intraindividual comparison of contralateral versus ipsilateral striatal epipride binding.

Bilateral rather than unilateral surgery is also supported by knowledge accumulated regarding the innervation of neck muscles. Earlier animal studies on ipsilateral versus contralateral control of the sternocleidomastoid (SCM) muscle yielded inconsistent results.[90] However, in a transcranial magnetic stimulation study of normal subjects, ipsilateral as well as contralateral SCM responses were evoked by stimulation of an area of cortex near the representation of the trunk.[91] The latency and waveforms of the motor-evoked potentials indicated a monosynaptic contralateral pathway and a disynaptic ipsilateral pathway. Another study showed that after amytal injection of the right internal carotid artery, fully cooperative patients were able to lift and turn their heads (on command) to the right and the left.[92] Ten of 14 patients had weakness of the right SCM compared to the left SCM. This finding suggests that most innervation of the SCM comes from the ipsilateral hemisphere.

Approximately 300 patients with CD were reported to have undergone functional stereotactic surgery in the 1960s and 1970s.[93] Historical reports are difficult to interpret; however, most patients apparently experienced mild to moderate benefit. The selection of the site and side on which to operate depended on the prevailing hypotheses and beliefs regarding the pathophysiology of CD. Hassler and Dieckmann[94,95] developed an elaborate theory on the correlates of specific types of CD in analogy to observations obtained from animal experiments. These researchers theorized that the target should be selected according to the phenotype of CD in the individual patient. Targets used by different surgeons included the ventral lateral nuclei of the thalamus (ventro-oralis anterior, ventro-oralis posterior, and ventro-oralis internus); the center median nucleus; the ventralis intermedius; the ventralis posteromedialis and posterolateralis; the pulvinar; Forel's fields H1 and H2; the zona incerta; the interstitial nucleus of Cajal; and the red nucleus.

The difficulties in choosing the appropriate side and site are exemplified by the contradictory recommendations of two historic authorities. While Cooper[96] recommended lesioning contralateral to the dystonic SCM muscle, Hassler and Dieckmann[94,95] stated that the ipsilateral side should be targeted. As early as 1977, Mundinger[97] reported his experience with thalamic stimulation for CD. However, the results were not published in the English literature and the study went unnoticed.

The authors have found that bilateral pallidal stimulation for CD may produce symptomatic and functional improvements, including marked relief of pain for up to 2.5 years of follow-up (Fig. 11-4).[36,98] Several other groups have also published their experience with pallidal DBS for CD (Table 11-3).[35,37,81,99-101] One year or greater follow-up is available

in five patients with complex CD who had tonic postures and phasic head movements. During the early postoperative period, these patients experienced immediate relief; however, the full benefit of long-term DBS could only be appreciated over the following few months, with adjustment of the stimulation settings. Phasic components improved early; however, dystonic postures improved later. During follow-up, anticholinergic medication was tapered off in all patients.

The gradual postoperative improvement of CD was reflected by evaluation with the modified Toronto-Western Spasmodic Torticollis Rating Scale (TWSTRS). All subscores were improved substantially by 3 months after surgery: the severity score improved by 38%, the disability score by 54%, and the pain score by 38%. At the last follow-up, all scores were further improved. The severity score had improved by 63%, the disability score by 69%, and the pain score by 50% compared to preoperative scores. The difference in the subscores at the last follow-up compared to the 3 month follow-up was significant for the severity and functional disability subscores, but not for the pain subscore. One patient was completely pain-free at the last follow-up; all other patients still complained of residual neck pain or tension. The first patient in this series experienced several exacerbations of CD during late follow-up (i.e., after 18 months). Two such episodes were caused by unilateral electrode fractures and two to battery depletion. Each time, CD worsened within a few hours. After replacement of the nonfunctioning hardware, clinical improvement occurred with much less delay than before. No patient experienced a permanent complication as a result of the surgical procedures or long-term DBS. During adjustment of the stimulation settings, some patients experienced a feeling of perioral tightness. This feeling was sometimes associated with mild dysphagia and difficulty speaking, but these associated problems could be eliminated by decreasing the voltage of the stimulation. Pallidal DBS also improved severe cervical choreoathetotic dyskinesias in

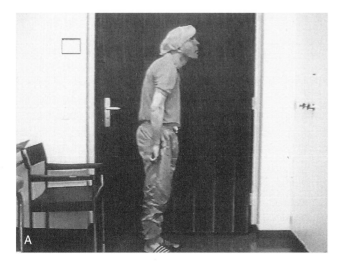 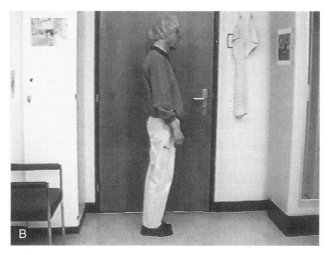

FIG. 11-4. Video stills of a 47-year-old man with complex cervical dystonia (CD), characterized mainly by sagittal shift and retrocollis. (**A**) presurgical and (**B**) 9 months after bilateral pallidal stimulation.

patients with cervical myelopathy undergoing spinal surgery and spinal stabilization.[36]

The authors' positive experience with long-term pallidal stimulation for complex CD corresponds well with the limited experience reported by other centers. Parkin and colleagues[37] reported on bilateral pallidal DBS in three patients. A 36-year-old woman with her head turned and tilted to the right had marked relief of associated neck ache and tremor. Within 1 month, her neck posture improved and, after 6 months, the head turn was reduced from 70° to 10°; head tilt was reduced from 30° to 15°. In a 67-year-old woman with head tremor and right head rotation, pallidal DBS resulted in reduction of the head turning from 60° to 10°. DBS settings were symmetric with large pulse widths (90–210 μs) and high amplitudes (at a mean of 4 V) at a frequency of 130 Hz. The Toronto group has also reported marked improvement upon bilateral pallidal stimulation in two patients with CD.[81] Islekel et al.[99] treated a 42-year-old woman with head rotation to the right; they used unilateral pallidal DBS contralateral to the head turning. The left SCM became flaccid on intraoperative test stimulation of the right pallidum at 100 Hz. The patient was said to become symptom-free after a week of test stimulation.

Indications

The indications for long-term bilateral pallidal stimulation for CD remain to be further elaborated. This technique is useful in patients with complex CD because they are poor candidates for peripheral procedures. Such patients include those with continuous phasic movements; marked dystonic head tremor or myoclonus; sagittal and lateral translations; and anterocollis with involvement of deep cervical muscles.[102,103]

Long-term bilateral pallidal stimulation may also become an alternative in patients with more complex forms of CD (e.g., those with shoulder elevation). Furthermore, a single operation might produce the same or greater benefit than serial procedures; as shown later, peripheral surgery may require serial procedures in some patients. The cost of chronic stimulation for patients with CD is relatively high. This is due, in particular, to shorter battery life and the younger age of the patients compared to those with other movement disorders.

Technical Aspects

The basic principles and rationales for pallidal stimulation for patients with CD and cervical dyskinesias are the same as those described above for generalized dystonia.[104] The authors prefer simultaneous bilateral surgery under local anesthesia. The amplitudes needed to achieve clinical benefit are higher, as compared to patients with pallidal stimulation for PD. The voltage in bipolar stimulation mode averaged 3.8 V; in a single instance, it was as high as 4.5 V. In addition, there

was a narrow therapeutic window for the intensity of stimulation. Multiple postoperative visits for stimulation programming were required. Over several months, the threshold for evoking unwanted effects increased; this allowed for a gradual increase of the intensity. The authors documented three occurrences of lead fracture, two of them in one patient. Because patients with other movement disorders often complained of discomfort when the connectors of the DBS system were placed behind and above the ear, the authors placed the connectors in the subcutaneous tissue of the neck in the first patients of this series. The increased tension from the dystonic posturing probably contributed to the lead fracture. Therefore, connectors are now routinely placed again behind the ears.

SPINAL PROCEDURES

Intrathecal Baclofen Pump

Patients with severe generalized dystonia may benefit from continuous intrathecal administration of baclofen via subcutaneously implanted programmable pumps.[105–114] Sustained improvement of dystonia has been reported in approximately 70% of patients with baclofen pumps. Those patients who experience severe concomitant spasticity are probably the most suitable candidates for this type of treatment. Patients are usually screened to determine if they are appropriate candidates for continuous intrathecal administration with bolus test injections of baclofen via lumbar punctures or infusions via intrathecal catheters. Nevertheless, some patients with relatively mild improvement on test injection have meaningfully benefited from baclofen pumps. Complications of treatment include catheter-related problems, infections, acute baclofen withdrawal, and baclofen overdosing, which can result in excessive weakness.

At the Parkinson's Disease Center of Baylor College of Medicine, investigators implanted 10 patients with baclofen pumps (2 males and 8 females, with a mean age of 43.2 [range, 21–66]). These patients had severe segmental or generalized dystonia and did not respond satisfactorily to oral medications and botulinum toxin injections. The Baylor patients were described as follows:

- Three patients had peripherally induced dystonia;
- Two patients had idiopathic dystonia;
- Two patients experienced brain injury;
- Two had static encephalopathy; and
- One had an unknown neurodegenerative disorder.

The anatomic distribution of the dystonia varied among patients. Three patients experienced segmental dystonia involving the neck, arms, or abdominal muscles. Seven other patients had generalized dystonia. The average duration of dystonia before implantation was 11.0 years (range, 1.7–35.0 years). All patients received test doses of bolus intrathecal baclofen before implantation. Two patients had a relatively poor initial response to the test dose; however, they still received implantations for continuous infusion. Neurologic assessments were conducted immediately after the implantations, 1 month postimplantation, and approximately every 3 months thereafter.

The average duration of follow-up was 4.7 years (range, 0.7–11.1). One patient had the pump explanted after 22 months. Initially, five patients markedly improved; two patients moderately improved; two patients mildly improved; and one patient experienced no improvement. Both patients who failed to respond to the initial test of intrathecal baclofen improved on continuous infusion with pump. In four patients, the level of improvement lessened over time, although they remained improved over their preoperative state.

All 10 patients continued oral medications and eight patients continued to receive BTX injections. In the authors' experience, patients with secondary, spastic dystonia involving primarily the legs and trunk may be the best candidates for continuous intrathecal baclofen infusion. Side effects were usually mild and improved with reduction of dose. Side effects included seven patients with nausea; two patients with paresthesia/numbness of the lower limbs; two patients with bladder urgency; and one patient with blurred vision. Only two patients needed revisions of the pump. All others experienced uninterrupted functioning of the equipment.

Long-Term Spinal Cord Stimulation

Over the past few years, long-term epidural cervical spine dorsal column stimulation (DCS) for the treatment of patients with CD has been largely abandoned. During this technique, quadripolar electrodes were placed longitudinally in the epidural space at C2–C4. The hypothetical rationale for this procedure's mechanism was based on a modified concept of the gate control theory. This theory suggested that altered sensory input might modify motor functioning. Stimulation frequencies were often in the range between 500–700 Hz.

Beneficial responses were described in several series.[115,116] Waltz[116] reported moderate to marked improvement in 69 of 90 patients (76%) with CD. Conversely, in a series of 25 patients, Fahn[117] reported almost complete lack of benefit on follow-up. Four patients experienced transient, mild benefit; one patient received benefits from long-lasting improvement. In a subsequent double-blind study of a series of 10 patients with CD, Goetz and colleagues[118] found no objective improvement.

PERIPHERAL SURGERY FOR CERVICAL DYSTONIA

Peripheral surgery for patients with CD is considered mainly in those patients who are primary or secondary nonresponders to botulinum toxin injections.[119–123] Patients with a long history of CD might not respond to BTX injections because of fibrosis or contractures of dystonic muscles or abnormal

ossifications. However, these patients might be appropriate candidates for selective myectomies. The goals of the surgery are to improve the dystonic posture or provide relief of local pain via peripheral denervation.[123,124] In general, this surgical treatment is reserved for those patients who experience functional disability as a result of their dystonic movement disorder. To reduce drug dosages, surgical treatment may be used as an adjunct to conservative treatment.

All patients with CD who are being considered for peripheral surgery should have preoperative CT or MRI scans of the head and cervical spine. In certain exceptional cases, CD and segmental craniocervical dyskinesia are related to mass lesions within the posterior fossa.[125,126] In general, these tumors are extra-axial tumors, such as meningiomas or schwannomas. Dystonia may improve after tumor resection, and, within 1 year, it may completely remit. Extension and flexion radiographs of the cervical spine should be obtained in patients with severe neck pain or radicular pain. Radiographic results assist in planning treatment of coexistent spinal instability or radicular compression. Patients should not have had BTX injections for at least 3–4 months before surgery.

History of Peripheral Surgery for Cervical Dystonia

Surgical treatment of patients with CD has a long and comprehensive history.[93,127,128] As early as 1641, the German surgeon Minnius sectioned the SCM muscle in a patient with CD. In 1834, Bujalski is credited for performing the first denervation of cervical muscles by ligation of the spinal accessory nerve.[127] Surgical treatment of patients with CD became more popular in the late nineteenth and early twentieth centuries. Initially, intradural procedures involved sectioning of the posterior cervical roots. Thereafter, attention shifted to the anterior roots. In the 1920s, McKenzie[129] developed intradural sectioning of the anterior upper cervical roots, in combination with sectioning of the intradural spinal accessory nerve. The procedure was refined by Dandy[130] and Hamby and Schiffer.[131,132] Intradural sectioning of the spinal accessory nerve aimed at sectioning only the fibers leading to the SCM muscle, while leaving the innervation of the trapezius intact. Later, the operating microscope was added as a technical aid to the procedure.

Extradural approaches, including posterior ramisectomy and peripheral nerve sectioning, were developed and popularized by Bertrand[133,134] in the 1970s. Bertrand emphasized the more selective nature of these procedures and lower frequency of side effects. Over the past few years, in many centers worldwide, extradural denervations have replaced intradural sectioning. Iontophoresis, which involves suppression of labyrinthine activity, never gained widespread acceptence.[135] During the 1980s, microvascular decompression (MVD) of the spinal accessory nerve was added to the armamentarium of surgical treatment options.[136,137] Several studies reported on its efficacy; however, this procedure never became widely accepted. Its lack of acceptance was due mainly to its conceptual difficulties with regard to the pathophysiology of CD.

General Methods

In all patients, it is essential to identify the culpable muscles correctly. These are best identified by a scrupulous physical examination, while patients allow and oppose the dystonic posture. Such passive movements may induce dystonic tremor, which may also be useful in identifying the most involved muscles. In some patients, hypertrophy of dystonic muscles may be prominent; however, compensatory muscles may also be hypertrophic. Temporary blocks with local anesthetics injected into different muscles may be useful in determining the contribution of a single muscle to the overall dystonic activity. To further differentiate the involvement of various muscles in patients with complex CD, serial injections into various muscles may be performed at different times. EMG guidance may be useful to elucidate the dystonic pattern.[123,138,139] Four-channel EMG should routinely include recording of the SCM, trapezius, splenius, and semispinalis muscles. In individual patients, recordings of the levator scapulae, scalene, longissimus colli, and paraspinal erector trunci muscles should also be performed. Activity in different muscles is compared while at rest and during head maneuvers.

Myotomy and Myectomy

There are limited data on the long-term benefits of myotomy and myectomy for CD. Most surgeons have used myotomies and myectomies as an adjunct to other surgical procedures. There are few instances in which patients have been operated on exclusively with myectomy.[140–142] Some reviews have stated that myectomies offer only little benefit; in the past few years, myectomies were abandoned by several surgeons. However, poor selection of candidates may have contributed to unsatisfactory results. Patients with complex CD will not achieve any benefit from unilateral sectioning of single muscles. The authors have rarely performed myotomies and myectomies as a first step in patients with rotational CD. More frequently, these surgeries were performed as an adjunct to selective denervation, or for treatment of dystonic activity in muscles that cannot be otherwise denervated.[123,141] The posterior neck muscles are adequately denervated by posterior ramisectomies; however, dystonic activity in the scalene muscles, levator scapulae, and omohyoid is difficult to control by selective denervation. In such patients, selective myotomies or myectomies are useful.

The simplest choice of surgical treatment for patients with CD is sectioning of the SCM muscle on the side that is opposite to the direction of the chin rotation. Sectioning of the SCM is appropriate for a few, well-selected patients; namely, those patients with torticollis who present with marked dystonic activity in the SCM and minimal dystonia in the contralateral posterior neck muscles. This procedure is usually combined with selective denervation of the peripheral branches of the spinal accessory nerve to the SCM.

Denervation procedures are not performed in patients who present with painful dystonic activity of the trapezius muscle that results in elevation and anteversion of the shoulder or contributes to ipsilateral head tilt as this would prohibit the ability to elevate the arm above the horizontal. These patients may benefit from partial myotomy/myectomy of the upper portion of the trapezius muscle, using an asleep-awake-asleep operative technique.[143]

Chen[140] has published the largest series on myotomies/myectomies for the treatment of patients with CD. In these series, myotomies/myectomies were combined with selective peripheral denervations in certain patterns of CD. Treatment plans included selective resections of dystonic muscles for various patterns of CD, including torticollis, laterocollis, anterocollis, and retrocollis. Excellent or marked improvement was described in 83% of the 60 patients in this series. In addition, no complications were reported. In a series of 15 patients with retrocollis, bilateral partial resections of the upper part of the trapezius muscles, splenius, semispinalis capitis, and semispinalis cervicis muscles were performed.[141] The outcomes during the postoperative follow-up period of 3–10 years were reported as excellent or markedly improved in 87% of patients. Persistent side effects were not present in these patients. In contrast, the long-term results of nonselective SCM sectioning in another series of 11 patients were less favorable.[142] At a mean follow-up of 4 years, a good or fair outcome was reported in 45% of patients. When used as an adjunct to other surgeries, it is difficult to appreciate the contribution of selective myotomy/myectomy. Nevertheless, additional improvement was achieved in the authors' patients who underwent selective sectioning of specific muscles as described above.[123] All three patients who underwent partial myectomies of the trapezius muscle benefitted. They experienced local pain relief and improvement of the dystonic posture of the shoulder.[143]

Technical Aspects

- The surgeon outlines the contours of the dystonic muscles to be sectioned. This is done with a marker on the patient's skin while the patient is awake. The choice of the positioning depends mainly on the topography of the muscles that are to be sectioned.
- Short-acting muscle relaxants are administered only for induction of general anesthesia.
- Skin incisions are made over the belly of the involved muscles. During dissection of the subcutaneous tissue care is taken to preserve sensory nerve branches.
- A bipolar-stimulation forceps is useful to identify fine motor nerve branches and elicit contractions in the corresponding muscles. This allows for indentification of brachial plexus branches when performing myectomies of the scalene muscles.

- The belly of the muscle is cut transversly, either with a monopolar electrode or sharply with scissors, until the posterior sleeve of the muscle fascia is reached.
- Then, in most patients, the proximal and distal stumps are cut, resecting approximately 3 cm of the muscle along its longitudinal axis.
- The gap is filled with a piece of spongostan, which can be soaked in a local anesthetic such as bupivacaine.
- Postoperatively, patients are placed on antiphlogistic medications.

Intradural Anterior Rhizotomy and Sectioning of the Spinal Accessory Nerve

Several variations of intradural anterior rhizotomy and sectioning of the spinal accessory nerve have been developed over the years (Fig. 11-5).[129–132,144–149] The typical procedure includes bilateral intradural sectioning of the C1–C3 anterior roots and the caudal rootlets of the spinal accessory nerves. Restricted and selective sectioning is advisable to avoid postoperative side effects. For example, in a patient with rotational CD, unilateral anterior rhizotomy combined with contralateral spinal accessory nerve sectioning may be sufficient. In patients with retrocollis, sectioning of the spinal accessory nerves would not be useful. Denervation, if performed bilaterally using this approach, is limited below the anterior roots of C3. The C4 root may be sectioned on one side; however, this may endanger the functioning of the diaphragm. Thus, this intradural approach cannot control dystonic activity that is mediated via the C4–C6 roots.

The reported results and complication rates of different series are highly variable. Most studies claim useful postoperative improvement in 60–90% of patients.[132,144,145,147,149] However, it not always clear if symptomatic amelioration of the abnormal postures or movements translated to overall improvement in functional disability, especially given the relatively high number of side effects. In the series by Friedman et al.,[147] the head returned to a neutral position in 59% of the postoperative patients. The likelihood of the head returning to a normal position during the postoperative phase was inversely related to the duration of CD. Some studies reported only very modest results after anterior intradural rhizotomy.[150] Hernesniemi and Keränen[142] reported that no patients reported a good outcome, based on their self assessments for the surgical result, disability, and working capacity.

Complications of the standard bilateral, intradural denervation are frequent and may become persistent and disabling. Mortality with the standard procedure usually is less than 1%. However, in some series, mortality was as high as 12%.[144] Side effects include dysphagia, neck weakness, cerebrospinal fluid fistulas, and infection. Neck weakness or instability is estimated to occur in approximately 40% of patients who have undergone bilateral rhizotomy.[145] Transient dysphagia may occur in approximately 30% of patients. Ra-

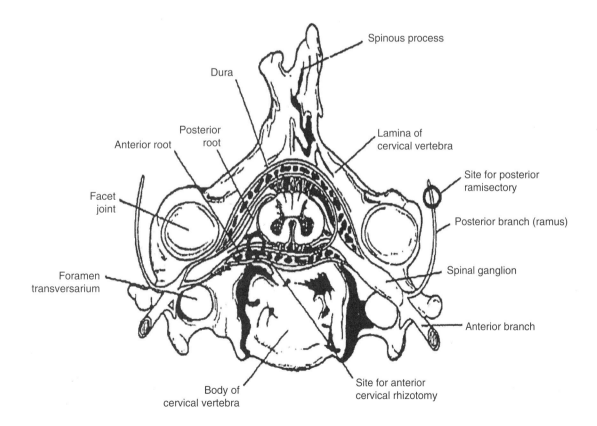

FIG. 11-5. Cartoon showing the lesioning sites for rhizotomy and ramisectomy surgeries.

diologic swallowing abnormalities were described in up to 95% of postoperative patients; frequently, this represented an aggravation of preexisting pharyngeal dysfunction.[151] In rare patients, bilateral infarctions of the medulla oblongata with bilateral Wallenberg's syndrome or ischemia of the upper spinal cord with tetraparesis were reported.[152,153]

Technical Aspects

- Intracranial sectioning of nerve roots is performed with the patient sitting or in the prone position, with the head fixed in a Mayfield head holder.
- The posterior neck muscles are divided within the ligamentum nuchae in the dorsal midline.
- A small suboccipital craniotomy, widening the posterior rim of the foramen magnum and laminectomies of the three upper cervical vertebrae, is performed.
- After opening of the dura, the upper spinal cord, the medulla oblongata, the cerebellar tonsils, the upper cranial nerve roots, the spinal accessory nerves and blood vessels of the cervicomedullary junction and the upper cervical medulla are visualized with the operating microscope. The anterior nerve roots are ventral to the dentate ligament.
- Each rootlet is stimulated with a bipolar nerve stimulator and then divided.
- Arterial blood vessels that accompany the nerve roots should be spared.
- If sectioning is carried out down to the C4 root (unilaterally), it is advisable to monitor muscular activity of the diaphragm.
- When sectioning of the spinal accessory is performed, the nerve usually is cut at the C1 level, where it crosses the upper margin of the dentate ligament.
- Bipolar stimulation may be used to further delineate the nerve rootlets of the spinal accessory nerve, which supply the SCM, trapezius, and pharyngeal muscles.
- Evoked muscle contractions may be monitored with surface electrodes.
- When present, anastomotic branches between the C1 roots and spinal accessory nerves should be divided.
- In rare patients, a more prominent anastomosis, the McKenzie branch, may be found. When the McKenzie branch is present, this branch should also be sectioned.

Posterior Ramisectomy and Selective Peripheral Denervation

Extradural sectioning of the posterior, primary divisions of the cervical nerve roots is also known as ramisectomy (Fig. 11-5). Bertrand[133] coined the term selective peripheral denervation, meaning the combination of sectioning the peripheral branch of the spinal accessory nerve to the SCM muscle, combined with posterior ramisectomy from C1–C6. In contrast to anterior rhizotomy, during a posterior ramisectomy, there is no need for laminectomy and opening of the dura. At the C1 and C2 levels, either extradural rhizotomies

or ganglionectomies or posterior ramisectomies may be performed. Taira and colleagues[154] have extended the concept of selective peripheral denervation to include other muscles. They described techniques to denervate the anterior C3 and C4 branches to the levator scapulae muscle as well as the ansa cervicalis and descending branch of the hypoglossal nerve to the omohyoid muscle.

Beneficial results with posterior ramisectomy and selective peripheral denervation are reported in 70–90% of patients in surgical series. Few persistent side effects have been noted.[103,133,134,155,156] In contrast, in a retrospective study that investigated the long-term outcome after selective extradural denervation, benefit was less robust at a mean of 5 years.[157] Long-term improvement was reported in approximately one-third of patients, with a 30% reduction in dystonia.

In an update on their series of 112 patients, Braun and Richter[158] reported that 14% of patients achieved complete relief of symptoms; 33% of patients demonstrated marked improvement; 24% of patients experienced moderate improvement, and 31% had only minimal or no improvement. In this series, the outcome was correlated with the initial response to botulinum toxin injections. Overall, 83% of patients who were secondary non-responders to botulinum toxin injections were satisfied with outcomes after surgery; however, only 50% of primary nonresponders considered the postoperative result as beneficial. Patients with more widespread dystonia (e.g., involving the extremities and trunk) demonstrated less improvement. Chawda et al.[159] found that patients with CD who experience moderate or severe degenerative spondylosis were less responsive to selective peripheral denervation, as compared to patients with zero or minimal degenerative changes.

The risk for complications with selective peripheral denervation is low. No instances of head or neck instability have been reported. Immediately after the operation, most patients have a variable sensory deficit in the distribution of the greater occipital nerve. Usually, this is well tolerated and patients only rarely complain about numbness. This sensory deficit usually improves within months. Rarely, patients experience prolonged local pain. Instances of inadvertent sectioning of the trapezius branch of the spinal accessory nerve have been described.[158] Extensive denervation procedures in one operative session should be avoided to reduce the risk of dysphagia.

Technical Aspects

- The operation is performed under general anesthesia.
- Patients are positioned in a half-sitting position or prone, with the head fixed in a Mayfield head holder.
- Positioning depends mainly on the muscles to be denervated. When only the posterior rami are to be approached (e.g., in patients with retrocollis), the authors prefer the prone position because it reduces the possibility of certain intraoperative adverse events such as air embolism.
- When the SCM on one side and posterior neck muscles on

the contralateral side are to be denervated (e.g., in patient with torticollis) a sitting or half-sitting position is preferred.

- When sitting or half-sitting positions are used, it is useful to monitor for air embolism using precordial Doppler ultrasound or transesophageal Doppler, coupled with online registration of end-expiratory partial carbon dioxide pressure.
- Only short-acting muscle relaxants are given for induction of anaesthesia.
- Muscle relaxants are not given during the procedure so that stimulation of nerve branches will elicit responses of the neck muscles.

For denervation of the SCM muscle:

- A 5-cm skin incision is made at its posterior margin.
- The branch to the trapezius muscle of the spinal accessory nerve is first identified in the lateral neck triangle.
- Great care should be taken not to injure the greater auricular nerve which crosses the operative field to avoid postoperative cutaneous sensory deficits.
- When the main trunk of the spinal accessory nerve is identified, the branches to the SCM muscle are stimulated with a bipolar forceps.
- These branches are sectioned and the stumps are resected as far as possible to avoid regeneration of the nerve fibers.
- Small nerve fibers to the SCM muscle may branch off from the trapezius branch of the spinal accessory nerve. These branches should be sectioned as well.
- When the underside of the SCM muscle is elevated, further branches supplying the caudal portion of the muscle may be detected and denervated.
- The authors always close the wound by an intracutaneous suture to obtain a good cosmetic result.

The denervation of the posterior rami to the neck muscles is performed via an extra incision.

- This extra incision runs in the midline of the neck, from the external occipital protuberance to the spinous process of C6.
- Unilateral or bilateral ramisectomies are performed, depending on the pattern of CD.
- After reaching the spinal processes from C1–C6, the posterior neck muscles can be laterally mobilized by subperiostal dissection. The authors prefer the technical variant described by Braun and Richter,[155,158] creating a cleavage plane between the semispinalis capitis and the semispinalis cervicis muscles. The inferior oblique capitis muscle is detached from its origin at the spinous process of C2.
- The procedure then proceeds further laterally to the articular facets.
- The posterior branches are identified in the cleavage plane that has been created at the point where they emerge lateral to the facet joints.
- Strong muscle contractions of the posterior neck muscles are evoked by bipolar stimulation.
- It is important to also identify smaller nerve branches to

the multifidus muscle, the semispinalis muscles, and the splenius muscle. The nerve branches are cut and resected as far as possible to avoid their regeneration. The operation microscope may be helpful to identify and section the branches.

- The C3 and C4 posterior rami are usually identified with ease; however, the C5 and C6 rami may be smaller and harder to identify. The C2 ganglion is located between the archs of C1 and C2 and the ventral and dorsal rami can be identified.
- At this point, the greater occipital nerve can be sectioned. The authors prefer performing a C2 ganglionectomy.
- The most difficult branch to find is the posterior branch of C1 or the suboccipital nerve. It is located approximately 2 cm lateral to the midline between the vertebral artery and the posterior arch of the atlas in the sulcus of the vertebral artery. Venous bleeding may occur from the venous plexus of the vertebral artery.
- Finally, any remaining tiny nerve branches are sought and sectioned. Bertrand advised to carefully avoid overdistraction of the neck muscles because the motor response could be reduced upon intraoperative stimulation.

Microvascular Decompression of the Spinal Accessory Nerve

MVD of the spinal accessory nerve for treatment of patients with CD is based upon the same rationale as when the procedure is used to treat cranial neuropathies, such as hemifacial spasm.[136] Proponents of MVD suggest the existence of two pathogenetically different types of CD: CD of "central origin" and "spasmodic torticollis of 11th nerve origin."[136,160] In other cranial neuropathies such as hemifacial spasm or trigeminal neuralgia, clinical symptoms are thought to be related to contact of small blood vessels with the vulnerable root. This contact results either in ectopic excitation and ephaptic transmission, or nuclear hyperexcitability.[161] The transition zone between central (i.e., oligodendroglia) and peripheral (i.e., Schwann glia) myelination is regarded as an area particularly vulnerable to compression. In one study, the average extension of glial spread into the facial nerve has been found to measure 2.5 mm. In another study, glial spread was slightly shorter; however, this segment has been described to be less than 0.1 mm in the spinal accessory nerve.[162]

Thus, it is difficult to understand how MVD of the spinal accessory nerve should work. Furthermore, with decompression for hemifacial spasm and trigeminal neuralgia, the benefit is apparent immediately after the operation. The improvement after MVD in patients with CD is delayed. It is even more difficult to understand how CD can be improved by MVD when muscles other than the SCM are involved in dystonic activity.

Technically, studies that report on the benefits of MVD for patients with CD involve sectioned rootlets of the spinal accessory nerve, the spinal accessory nerve proper, anastomoses between the accessory nerve roots and the posterior C1 and C2 roots, lysis of "cross-sectional adhesions" and "hypertrophied dentate ligaments" and division of the posterior C1 and C2 roots.[163–165]

The offending arteries usually were described as loops of the posterior inferior cerebellar artery and the vertebral artery, and, in rare patients, the posterior spinal arteries. Freckmann and associates[164,166] performed MVD of the spinal accessory nerve in 33 patients. Remarkably, they thought that postoperative improvement in their patients was not related to vascular decompression but to lysis from anastomoses and "adhesions" of the spinal accessory nerve related to "pathogenic factors in the afferent part of head control." In another series of 22 patients, who underwent "microneural decompression" of the spinal accessory nerve, a compressive vessel was thought to be responsible for CD in only 6 patients.[163] In a few studies, as in the series reported by Jho and Jannetta,[136] no nerve sections performed.[167]

Outcome data of MVD for treatment of patients with CD is limited. The assignment of postoperative benefits to MVD was of particular concern. This was done although, in most cases, multiple "adhesiolyses" and nerve sectionings were performed that might have contributed to postoperative benefit. The suggestion is that MVD is more successful in patients with rotational torticollis than in other forms of CD. In the series of Freckmann and colleagues,[164] 5 of 33 patients (15%) were reported with excellent results, 10 patients (30%) with good results, and 12 patients (36%) with less improvement. Postoperative death of 1 patient was reported caused by "medullary symptoms with severe respiratory insufficiency." Surgical morbidity included cerebrospinal fluid leaks, meningitis, and stroke. In one series, the frequency of complications was as high as 27%. At long-term follow-up of between 5 and 10 years, Jho and Jannetta[136] claimed a cure for CD in 65% of their patients (13/20 patients); substantial improvement in 4 patients (20%); moderate improvement in 1 patient (5%); and minimal improvement in 2 patients. The majority of these patients showed gradual improvement over 2 years. However, patients in the "cured" group were said to continue to "have some subtle tendency to move their necks to the prior abnormal position when they relaxed their head in the neutral position."

Peripheral Surgery for Cervical Dystonia: Conclusions

Various surgical alternatives for the treatment of CD are available. At this time, the recommendation is for selective targeting of dystonic activity, which may involve staged procedures and combination of different techniques. Peripheral denervation and posterior ramisectomies are clearly less invasive than intradural procedures and appear to have similar, if not better, postoperative benefit with lower complication rates. Myotomies and myectomies are useful adjuncts to other surgical procedures. A problem with peripheral surgery is that, in some patients with CD, dystonic muscle activity may recruit muscles other than those that were initially involved. Carefully conducted prospective studies with adequate assessment of postoperative outcome are urgently needed.

PERIPHERAL SURGERY FOR GENERALIZED DYSTONIA

Peripheral denervation of appendicular muscles may be performed to treat severe spasticity. In particular, soleus neurotomy is a useful treatment option for the spastic equinus foot.[168] Decq and colleagues[169] reported application of the concept of peripheral denervation to treat foot dystonia as part of generalized dystonia. A series of 11 patients included 1 patient with equinus deformity, 2 patients with varus deformity, 4 patients with toe deformities, 2 patients with mixed varus and toes deformity, and 2 patients with mixed equinovarus and toes deformity. Preoperative selection of the muscles to be denervated was performed with local anesthetic blocks. Peripheral denervation involved sectioning of the soleus nerve in 3 patients, the tibial nerve in 6 patients, and the flexor hallucis and digitorum longus nerves in 8 patients. All patients experienced symptomatic and functional improvements at a mean follow-up of 16 months.

CONCLUSIONS

A variety of surgical techniques may benefit some patients with both focal and generalized dystonias. In most cases, surgery is reserved for medically refractory patients; however, as techniques improve, the threshold for surgery will continue to lower. More detailed, better-controlled, comparative data are needed to identify the optimal surgical candidates.

ACKNOWLEDGMENTS

The authors wish to acknowledge the invaluable assistance of Robert Grossman M.D., Joseph Jankovic M.D., Manjit Sanghera Ph.D., and Mike Almaguer, R.N.

REFERENCES

1. Burke R, Fahn S, Jankovic J, et al. Tardive dystonia: late onset and persistent dystonia caused by antipsychotic drugs. Neurology 1982;32:1335–1346.
2. Demirkiran M, Jankovic J. Paroxysmal dyskinesia: clinical features and classification. Ann Neurol 1995;38:571–579.
3. Ichinose H, Ohye T, Takahashi E, et al. Hereditary progressive dystonia with marked diurnal fluctuation caused by mutations in the GTP cyclohydrolase I gene. Nat Genet 1994;8:236–242.
4. Furukawa Y, Shimadzu M, Rajput A, et al. GTP-cyclohydrolase I gene mutations in hereditary progressive and dopa-responsive dystonia. Ann Neurol 1996;39:609–617.
5. Ozelius LJ, Hewett JW, Page CE, et al. The early-onset torsion dystonia gene (DYT1) encodes an ATP-binding protein. Nat Genet 1997;17:40–48.
6. Augood SJ, Penney JB Jr, Friberg IK, et al. Expression of the early-onset torsion dystonia gene (DYT1) in human brain. Ann Neurol 1998;43:669–673.
7. Warner TT, Jarman P. The molecular genetics of the dystonias. J Neurol Neurosurg Psychiatry 1998;64:427–429.
8. Almasy L, Bressman SB, Raymond D, et al. Idiopathic torsion dysto-

nia linked to chromosome 8 in two Mennonite families. Ann Neurol 1997;42:670–673.

9. Leube B, Hendgen T, Kessler KR, et al. Evidence for *DYT7* being a common cause of cervical dystonia (torticollis) in Central Europe. Am J Med Genet 1997;74:529–532.

10. Quinn NP. Essential myoclonus and myoclonic dystonia. Mov Disord 1996;11:119–124.

11. Waters CH, Takahashi H, Wilhelmsen KC, et al. Phenotypic expression of X-linked dystonia-parkinsonism (Lubag) in two women. Neurology 1993;43:1555–1558.

12. Scott B, Jankovic J. Delayed onset progressive movement disorders. Neurology 1996;46:68–74.

13. Jankovic J, Fahn S. Dystonic disorders. In: Jankovic J, Tolosa E, eds. Parkinson's Disease and Movement Disorders. 4th ed. Philadelphia: Lippincott, Williams & Wilkins, 2002:513–552.

14. Marsden CD, Obeso JA, Zarranz JJ, et al. The anatomic basis of symptomatic hemidystonia. Brain 1985;108:463–483.

15. Jankovic J. Can peripheral trauma induce dystonia and other movement disorders? Yes! Mov Disord 2001;16:7–12.

16. Playford E, Fletcher N, Sawle G, et al. Striatal [18F]dopa uptake in familial idiopathic dystonia. Brain 1993;116:1191–1199.

17. Perlmutter JS, Stambuk MK, Markham KT, et al. Decreased [^{18}F]spiperone binding in idiopathic focal dystonia. J Neurosci 1997;17:843–850.

18. Papa SM, Chase T. Levodopa induced dyskinesias improved by a glutamate antagonist in parkinsonian monkeys. Ann Neurol 1996;39:574–578.

19. Mink JW, Thach WT. Basal ganglia intrinsic circuits and their role in behavior. Curr Opin Neurobiol 1993;3:950–957.

20. Vitek JL, Zhang J, Evatt M, et al. Gpi pallidotomy for dystonia: clinical outcome and neuronal activity. Adv Neurol 1998;78:211–219.

21. Sanghera MK, Grossman RG, Kalhorn CG, Hamilton WJ, Ondo WG, Jankovic J.Basal ganglia neuronal discharge in primary and secondary dystonia in patients undergoing pallidotomy. Neurosurgery 2003;52:1358–1370

22. Mandir AS, Lenz FA. Rationales for pallidal surgery: what are the mechanisms? In: Krauss J, Grossman RG, Jankovic J, eds. Pallidal Surgery for Treatment of Parkinson's Disease and Movement Disorders. Philadelphia: Lippincott-Raven, 1998:55–66.

23. Ikoma K, Samii A, Mercuri B, et al. Abnormal cortical motor excitability in dystonia. Neurology 1996;46:1371–1376.

24. Eidelberg D, Moeller JR, Ishikawa T, et al. Regional metabolic correlations of surgical outcome following unilateral pallidotomy for Parkinson's disease. Ann Neurol 1996;39:450–459.

25. Samuel M, Ceballos-Baumann AO, Turjanski N, et al. Pallidotomy in Parkinson's disease increases supplementary motor area and prefrontal activity during performance of volitional movements. An H$_2$^{15}O PET study. Brain 1997;120:1301–1313.

26. Rascol O, Sabatini U, Chollet F, et al. Supplementary and primary sensory motor area activity in Parkinson's disease. Regional cerebral blood flow changes during finger movements and the effects of apomorphine. Arch Neurol 1992;49:144–148.

27. Jenkins IH, Fernandez W, Playford ED, et al. Impaired activation of the supplementary motor area in Parkinson's disease is reversed when akinesia is treated with apomorphine. Ann Neurol 1992;32:749–757.

28. Grafton AT, Waters C, Sutton J, et al. Pallidotomy increases activity of the motor association cortex in Parkinson's disease: a positron emission tomographic study. Ann Neurol 1995;37:776–783.

29. Ceballos-Baumann AO. Overactivity of primary and association motor areas in secondary hemi-dystonia (SHD) due to thalamic or basal ganglia lesions: a PET study. Mov Disord 1994;9 (Suppl 1):238.

30. Kumar R, Dagher A, Hutchison W, et al. Globus pallidus deep brain stimulation for generalized dystonia: clinical and PET investigation. Neurology 1999;53:871874.

31. Lenz FA, Byl NN. Reorganization in the cutaneous core of the human thalamic principal somatic sensory nucleus (ventral caudal) in patients with dystonia. J Neurophys 1999;82:3204–3212.

32. Meyers R. Surgical experiments in the therapy of certain extrapyramidal diseases: a current evaluation. Acta Pychiatr Neurol 1951;67:1–42.

33. Spiegel EA, Wycis HT, Marks M, et al. Stereotaxis apparatus for operations on the human brain. Science 1947;106:349–350.

34. Cooper IS. An investigation of Neurosurgical alleviation of parkinsonism, chorea, athetosis, and dystonia. Ann Intern Med 1956;5:381–392.

35. Bereznai B, Steude U, Seelos K, et al. Chronic high-frequency globus pallidus internus stimulation in different types of dystonia: a clinical, video, and MRI report of six patients presenting with segmental, cervical, and generalized dystonia. Mov Disord 2002;17:138–144.

36. Krauss JK, Loher TJ, Pohle T, et al. Pallidal deep brain stimulation in patients with cervical dystonia and sever cervical dyskinesias with cervical myelopathy. J Neurol Neurosurg Psychiatry 2002;72:249–256.

37. Parkin S, Aziz T, Gregory R, et al. Bilateral internal globus pallidus stimulation for the treatment of spasmodic torticollis. Mov Disord 2001;16:489–493.

38. Jankovic J, Schwartz K. Response and immunoresistance to botulinum toxin injections. Neurology. 1995;44:1743–1746.

39. Burke RE, Fahn S, Marsden CD, et al. Validity and reliability of a rating scale for the primary torsion dystonias. Neurology 1985;35:73–77.

40. Comella C, Leurgans S, Chimura T, et al. The unified rating scale: initial concurrent validity testing with other dystonia scales. Neurology 1999;(Suppl 2):A292.

41. Tasker RR: Surgical treatment of the dystonias. In: Gildenberg P, Tasker RR, eds. Textbook of Stereotactic and Functional Neurosurgery. New York: McGraw-Hill, 1996:1015–1032.

42. Lozano AM, Kumar R, Gross RE, et al. Globus pallidus internus pallidotomy for generalized dystonia. Mov Disord 1997;12:865–870.

43. Lin JJ, Lin SZ, Lin GY, Chang DC, Lee CC. Application of bilateral sequential pallidotomy to treat a patient with generalized dystonia. Eur Neurol 1998;40:108–110.

44. Iacono R, Kuniyoshi S, Lonser R, et al. Simultaneous bilateral pallidoansotomy for idiopathic dystonia musculorum deformans. Pediatr Neurol 1996;14:145–148.

45. Iacono R, Kuniyoshi SM, Lonser RR, et al. Experience with stereotactics for dystonia: case examples. Adv Neurol 1998;78:221–226.

46. Vitek J, Evatt M, Zhang JU, et al. Pallidotomy and deep brain stimulation as a treatment for dystonia. Neurology 1999;52(Suppl 2):A294.

47. Kumar R, Lozano AM, Hutchison WD, et al. Pallidal procedures for the treatment of refractory dystonia. Mov Disord 1997;12:865–870.

48. Lin JJ, Lin GY, Shih SZ, et al. Pallidotomy and generalized dystonia. Mov Disord 1999;14:1057–1059.

49. Cubo E, Shannon KM, Penn DR, et al, Internal globus pallidotomy in dystonia secondary to Huntington's disease. Mov Disord 2000;15:1248–1251.

50. Justesen CR, Penn RD, Kroin JS, et al. Stereotactic pallidotomy in a child with Hallervorden-Spatz disease. J Neurosurg 1999;90:551–554.

51. Bhatia KP, Marsden CD, Thomas DG. Posteroventral pallidotomy can ameliorate attacks of paroxysmal dystonia induced by exercise. J Neurol Neurosurg Psychiatry 1998;65:604–605.

52. Sa D, Teive H, Grande C, et al. Bilateral simultaneous pallidotomy for generalized dystonia. Neurology. 1999;52(Suppl 2):A521.

53. Ford B, Winfield L, Frucht S, et al. Treatment of severe generalized dystonia using stereotactic pallidotomy. Neurology 2000;54(Suppl 3):A219.

54. Cardoso F, Jankovic J, Grossman RG, et al. Outcome after stereotactic thalamotomy for dystonia and hemiballismus. Neurosurgery1995;36:501–597.

55. Tasker RR, Doorly T, Yamashiro K. Thalamotomy in generalized dystonia. In: Fahn S, Marsden CD, Calne DB, eds. Dystonia 2: Advances in Neurology. New York, NY: Raven Press, 1988:615–631.

56. Krauss J, Mohadjer M, Braus D, et al. Dystonia following head trauma: a report of nine patients and review of the literature. Mov Disord 1992;7:263–272.

57. Tasker RR, Lenz F, Yamashiro K, et al. Microelectrode techniques in localization of stereotactic targets. Neurol Res 1987;9:105–112.

58. Tasker RR, Organ LW, Hawrylyshyn P, eds. The Thalamus and Midbrain of Man: A Physiological Atlas Using Electrical Stimulation. Springfield, IL: Charles C. Thomas; 1982.

59. Cooper IS. Twenty-year follow-up study of the neurosurgical treatment of dystonia musculorum deformans. In: Eldridge R, Fahn S, eds. Dystonia: Advances in Neurology. New York, NY: Raven Press, 1976:423–452.

60. Cooper IS, ed. Involuntary Movement Disorders. New York: Harper & Row; 1969:160–292.

61. Kandel EI. Functional and Stereotactic Neurosurgery. Watts G, trans; Walker AE, trans-ed. New York: Plenum Press; 1989.

62. Gros C, Frerebeau PH, Perez-Dominguez E, et al. Long-term results of stereotaxic surgery for infantile dystonia and dyskinesia. Neurochirurgia (Stuttg) 1996;19:171–178.

63. Andrew J, Fowler CJ, Harrison MJD. Stereotaxic thalamotomy in 55 cases of dystonia. Brain 1983;106:981–1000.

64. Laitinen LV. Short-term results of stereotaxic treatment for infantile cerebral palsy. Confin Neurol 1965;26:258–263.

65. Schuurman PR, Bosch DA, Bossuyt PM, et al. A comparison of continuous thalamic stimulation and thalamotomy for suppression of severe tremor. N Engl J Med 2000;342:461–468.

66. Loher TJ, Hasdemir MG, Burgunder JM, et al. Long-term follow-up study of chronic globus pallidus internus stimulation for posttraumatic hemidystonia. J Neurosurg 2000;92:457–460.

67. Vayssiere N, Hemm S, Zanca M, et al. Magnetic resonance imaging stereotactic target localization for deep brain stimulation in dystonic children. J Neurosurg 2000;93:784–790.

68. Coubes P, Roubertie A, Vayssiere N, et al. Treatment of DYT-1 generalized dystonia by stimulation of the internal globus pallidus. Lancet. 2000;355:2220–2221.

69. Angelini L, Nardocci N, Estienne M, et al. Life-threatening dystonia-dyskinesias in a child: successful treatment with bilateral pallidal stimulation. Mov Disord 2000;15:1010–1012

70. Brin MF, Germano I, Danisi FO, et al. Deep brain stimulation (DBS) of pallidum in intractable dystonia [Abstract]. Mov Disord 1998; 13:274.

71. Caputo E, Krack P, Tamma F, et al. Dystonic tremor treated by unilateral pallidal deep brain stimulation after secondary failure of thalamic stimulation [Abstract]. Mov Disord 1998;13:135.

72. Kulisevsky J, Gironell A, Molet J, et al. Bilateral pallidal stimulation for intractable pain in idiopathic dystonia [Abstract]. Mov Disord 1998;13:99.

73. Tronnier VM, Fogel W. Pallidal stimulation for generalized dystonia. Report of three cases. J Neurosurg 2000;92:453–456.

74. Trottenberg T, Paul G, Meissner W, et al. Pallidal and thalamic neurostimulation in severe tardive dystonia. J Neurol Neurosurg Psychiatry 2001;70:557–559.

75. Vercueil L, Pollak P, Fraix V, et al. Deep brain stimulation in the treatment of severe dystonia. J Neurol 2001;248:695–700.

76. Krack P, Vercueil L. Review of the functional surgical treatment of dystonia. Eur J Neurol 2001;8:389–399.

77. Muta D, Goto S, Nishikawa S, et al. Bilateral pallidal stimulation for idiopathic segmental axial dystonia advanced from Meige syndrome refractory to bilateral thalamotomy. Mov Disord 2001;16:774–778.

78. Pahapill P, Lozano A, Lang A. Pallidal stimulation for treatment of Parkinson's disease. In: Krauss J, Jankovic J, Grossman R, eds. Surgery for Parkinson's Disease and Movement Disorders. Philadelphia: Lippincott Williams & Wilkins, 2001:170–187.

79. Gill S, Curran A, Tripp J, Melarickas L, et al. Hyperkinetic movement disorder in an 11-year-old child treated with bilateral pallidal stimulators. Dev Med Child Neurol 2001;43:350–353.

80. Andaluz N, Taha JM, Dalvi A. Bilateral pallidal deep brain stimulation for cervical and truncal dystonia. Neurology 2001;57:557–558.

81. Alkhani A, Khan F, Lang AE, et al. The response to pallidal surgery for dystonia is dependent on the etiology [Abstract]. Neurosurgery 2000;47:504.

82. Villemure JG, Vingerhoets F, Temperli P, et al. Dystonia: pallidal or thalamic target [Abstract]. Acta Neurochir 2000;142:1194.

83. Sellal F, Hirsch E, Barth P, et al. A case of symptomatic hemidystonia improved by ventroposterolateral thalamic electrostimulation. Mov Disord 1993;8:515–518.

84. Loher TJ, Krauss JK, Burgunder JM, et al. Chronic stimulation of the ventrointermediate thalamus is effective for treatment of peripherally-induced dystonic paroxysmal nonkinesigenic dyskinesia. Neurology 2001;56:268–270.

85. Ghika J, Villemure JG, Miklossy J, et al. Postanoxic generalized dystonia improved by bilateral Voa thalamic deep brain stimulation. Neurology 2002;58:311–313.

86. Kupsch A, Trottenberg T, Meissner W, et al. Neurostimulation of the ventral intermediate thalamic nucleus alleviates hereditary essential myoclonus. J Neurol Neurosurg Psychiatry 1999;67:415–416.

87. Krauss J, Jankovic J. Hemidystonia secondary to carotid artery gunshot injury. Childs Nerv Syst 1997;13:285–288.

88. Magyar-Lehmann S, Antonini A, Roelcke U, et al. Cerebral glucose metabolism in patients with spasmodic torticollis. Mov Disord 1997;12:704–708.

89. Naumann M, Pirker W, Reiners K, et al. Imaging of the pre- and post-synaptic side of striatal dopaminergic synapses in idiopathic cervical dystonia: a SPECT study using ^{123}I epidepride and ^{123}I beta-CIT. Mov Disord 1998;13:319–323.

90. Kavaklis O, Shima F, Kato M, et al. Ipsilateral pallidal control on the sternocleidomastoid muscle in cats: relationship to the side of thalamotomy for torticollis. Neurosurgery 1992;30:724–730.

91. Thompson ML, Thickbroom GW, Mastaglia FL. Corticomotor representation of the sternocleidomastoid muscle. Brain 1997;120:245–255.

92. DeToledo JC, Dow R. Sternomastoid function during hemispheric suppression by amytal: insights into the inputs to the spinal accessory nerve nucleus. Mov Disord 1998;13:809–812.

93. Krauss JK, Pohle T. Historical review of functional stereotactic neurosurgery for treatment of cervical dystonia [Abstract]. Mov Disord 1998;13–S2:134.

94. Hassler R, Dieckmann G. Die stereotaktische Behandlung des Torticollis aufgrund tierexperimenteller Erfahrungen über die richtungsbestimmten Bewegungen. Nervenarzt 1970;41:473–478.

95. Hassler R, Dieckmann G. Stereotactic treatment of different kinds of spasmodic torticollis. Confin Neurol 1970;32:135–143.

96. Cooper IS. Effects of thalamic lesions upon torticollis. N Engl J Med 1964;270:967–972.

97. Mundinger F. New stereotactic treatment of spasmodic torticollis with a brain stimulation system [in German]. Med Klin 1977;72:1982–1986.

98. Krauss JK, Pohle T, Weber S, et al. Bilateral deep brain stimulation of the globus pallidus internus for treatment of cervical dystonia. Lancet 1999;354:837–838.

99. Islekel S, Zilelei M, Cakmur R, et al. Pallidal stimulation: an effective method in the treatment of spasmodic torticollis [Abstract]. Mov Disord 2000;15(Suppl 3):162.

100. Kavaklis O, Shima F, Kato M, et al. Ipsilateral pallidal control on the sternocleidomastoid muscle in cats: relationship to the side of thalamotomy for torticollis. Neurosurgery 1992;30:724–730.

101. Tasker RR. Overview of the surgical treatment of spasmodic torticollis. In: Gildenberg PL, Tasker RR. Textbook of Stereotactic and Functional Neurosurgery. New York: McGraw-Hill, 1998:1053–1058.

102. Krauss JK, Grossman RG. Operative techniques for pallidal surgery. In: Krauss JK, Grossman RG, Jankovic J, eds. Pallidal Surgery for the Treatment of Parkinson's Disease and Movement Disorders. Philadelphia: Lippincott-Raven, 1998:121–133.

103. Bertrand CM, Lenz FA. Surgical treatment of dystonias. In: Tsui JKC, Calne DB, eds. Handbook of Dystonia. New York: Marcel Dekker, 1995:329–345.

104. Krauss JK, King DE, Grossman RG. Alignment correction algorithm for transformation of stereotactic atlas coordinates into frame coordinates in image-guided functional neurosurgery. Neurosurgery. 1998;42:806–812.

105. Albright AL. Intrathecal baclofen for treatment of dystonia. In: Krauss JK, Jankovic J, Grossman RG, eds. Surgery for Parkinson's Disease and Movement Disorders. Philadelphia: Lippincott, Williams and Wilkins, 2001:316–322.

106. Albright AL, Barry MJ, Fasick P, et al. Continuous intrathecal baclofen infusion for symptomatic generalized dystonia. Neurosurgery. 1996;38:934–938.

107. Albright AL, Barry MJ, Painter MJ, et al. Infusion of intrathecal baclofen for generalized dystonia in cerebral palsy. J Neurosurg 1998;88:73–76.

108. Ford B, Greene P, Louis ED, et al. Use of intrathecal baclofen in the treatment of patients with dystonia. Arch Neurol 1996;53:1241–1246.

109. Ford B, Greene PE, Louis ED, et al. Intrathecal baclofen in the treatment of dystonia. Adv Neurol 1998;78:199–210.

110. Narayan RK, Loubser PG, Jankovic J, et al. Intrathecal baclofen for intractable axial dystonia. Neurology 1991;41:1141–1142.

111. van Hilten BJ, van de Beek WJT, Hoff JI, et al. Intrathecal baclofen for the treatment of dystonia in patients with reflex sympathetic dystrophy. N Engl J Med 2000;343:625–630.

112. Grande MA, Chacon J, Trujillo A, et al. Intrathecal perfusion pump with baclofen in generalized dystonia. Rev Neurol 2000;30:138–140.

113. Walker RH, Danisi FO, Swope DM, et al. Intrathecal baclofen for dystonia: benefits and complications during six years of experience. Mov Disord 2000;15:1242–1247.

114. Hou G, Ondo WG, Jankovic J. Continuous intrathecal baclofen infusion in dystonia [Letter]. Mov Disord 2001;16:1201–1202.

115. Gildenberg PL. Treatment of spasmodic torticollis by dorsal column stimulation. Appl Neurophysiol 1978;41:113–121.

116. Waltz JM. Chronic stimulation for motor disorders. In: Gildenberg

PL, Tasker RR, eds. Textbook of Stereotactic and Functional Neurosurgery. New York: McGraw-Hill, 1998:1087–1099.

117. Fahn S. Lack of benefit from cervical cord stimulation for dystonia. N Engl J Med 1985;313:1229.

118. Goetz CG, Penn RD, Tanner CM. Efficacy of cervical cord stimulation in dystonia. Adv Neurol 1988;50:645–649.

119. Brin MF, Jankovic J, Comella C, et al. Treatment of dystonia using botulinum toxin. In: Kurlan R, ed. Treatment of Movement Disorders. Philadelphia: Lippincott, 1995:183–246.

120. Hanna PA, Jankovic J. Mouse bioassay versus Western blot assay for botulinum toxin antibodies: correlation with clinical response. Neurology 1998;50:1624–1629.

121. Jankovic J, Brin MF. Therapeutic uses of botulinum toxin. N Engl J Med 1991;324:1186–1194.

122. Jankovic J, Schwartz K. Botulinum toxin injections for cervical dystonia. Neurology 1990;40:277–280.

123. Krauss JK, Toups EG, Jankovic J, et al. Symptomatic and functional outcome of surgical treatment of cervical dystonia. J Neurol Neurosurg Psychiatry 1997;63:642–648.

124. Weigel R, Rittmann M, Krauss JK. Spontaneous cranio-cervical osseous fusion caused by cervical dystonia. J Neurosurg 2001;95:115–118.

125. Krauss JK, Seeger W, Jankovic J. Cervical dystonia associated with tumors of the posterior fossa. Mov Disord 1997;12:443–447.

126. Pohle T, Burgunder JM, Krauss JK. Petroclival meningioma as a cause of ipsilateral cervicofacial dyskinesias. J Neurol Neurosurg Psychiatry 2000;68:113–114.

127. Iskandar BJ, Nashold BS Jr. History of functional neurosurgery. Neurosurg Clin North Am 1995;6:1–25.

128. Putnam TJ, Herz E, Glaser GH. Spasmodic torticollis. Arch Neurol Psychiatry 1949;61:240–247.

129. McKenzie KG. Intermeningeal division of the spinal accessory and roots of the upper cervical nerves for the treatment of spasmodic torticollis. Surg Gynecol Obstet 1924;39:5–10.

130. Dandy WE. An operation for the treatment of spasmodic torticollis. Arch Surg 1930;20:1021–1032.

131. Hamby WB, Schiffer S. Spasmodic torticollis: results after cervical rhizotomy in 80 cases. Clin Neurosurg 1970;17:28–37.

132. Hamby WB, Schiffer S. Spasmodic torticollis: results after surgical rhizotomy in 50 cases. J Neurosurg 1969;31:323–326.

133. Bertrand CM. Selective peripheral denervation for spasmodic torticollis: surgical technique, results, and observations in 260 cases. Surg Neurol 1993;40:96–103.

134. Bertrand CM. Surgical management of spasmodic torticollis and adult-onset dystonia. In: Schmidek HH, Sweet WH, eds. Operative Neurosurgical Techniques. 3rd ed. Philadelphia: Saunders, 1995: 1649–1659.

135. Svien HJ, Cody DT. Treatment of spasmodic torticollis by suppression of labyrinthine activity: report of a case. Mayo Clin Proc 1969; 44:825–827.

136. Jho HD, Jannetta PJ. Microvascular decompression for spasmodic torticollis. Acta Neurochir 1995;134:21–26.

137. Pagni CA, Naddeo M, Faccani G. Spasmodic torticollis due to neurovascular compression of the 11th nerve. J Neurosurg 1985;63: 789–791.

138. Comella CL, Buchman AS, Tanner CM, et al. Botulinum toxin injection for spasmodic torticollis: increased magnitude of benefit with electromyographic assistance. Neurology 1992;42:878–882.

139. Russo LS Jr, Arce C. Simultaneous four-channel electromyography as an adjunct to selective denervation in the treatment of spasmodic torticollis [Abstract]. Ann Neurol 1990;28:266.

140. Chen X. Selective resection and denervation of cervical muscles in the treatment of spasmodic torticollis: results in 60 cases. Neurosurgery 1981;8:680–688.

141. Chen XK, Ji SX, Zhu H, Ma AB. Operative treatment of bilateral retrocollis. Acta Neurochir 1991;113:180–183.

142. Hernesniemi J, Keränen T. Long-term outcome after surgery for spasmodic torticollis. Acta Neurochir 1990;103:128–130.

143. Krauss JK, Koller R, Burgunder JM. Partial myotomy/myectomy of the trapezius muscle with an asleep-awake-asleep anesthetic technique for treatment of cervical dystonia. J Neurosurg 1999;91: 889–991.

144. Arseni C, Maretsis M. The surgical treatment of spasmodic torticollis. Neurochirurgia 1971;14:177–180.

145. Colbassani HJ Jr, Wood JH. Management of spasmodic torticollis. Surg Neurol 1986;25:153–158.

146. Fabinyi G, Dutton J. The surgical treatment of spasmodic torticollis. Aust NZ J Surg 1980;50:155–157.

147. Friedman AH, Nashold BS Jr, Sharp R, et al. Treatment of spasmodic torticollis with intradural selective rhizotomies. J Neurosurg 1993; 78:46–53.

148. Gauthier S, Perot P, Bertrand G. Role of surgical anterior rhizotomies in the management of spasmodic torticollis. Adv Neurol 1988;50: 633–635.

149. Speelman JD, van Manen J, Jacz K, et al. The Foerster-Dandy operation for the treatment of spasmodic torticollis. Acta Neurochir Suppl (Wien) 1987;39:85–87.

150. Meares R. Natural history of spasmodic torticollis, and effect of surgery. Lancet 1971;2:149–150.

151. Horner J, Riski JE, Ovelmen-Levitt J, et al. Swallowing in torticollis before and after rhizotomy. Dysphagia 1992;7:117–125.

152. Scoville WB. Motor tics of the head and neck: surgical approaches and their complications. Acta Neurochir. 1978;45:338.

153. Sweet WH. What should the neurosurgeon do when faced with a malpractice suit? Clin Neurosurg 1975;23:112–124.

154. Taira T, Mitsuyama T, Okami N, et al. Selective peripheral denervation for spasmodic torticollis involving the levator scapulae muscle [in Japanese]. No Shinkei Geka. 1999;27:25–31.

155. Braun V, Richter HP. Selective peripheral denervation for the treatment of spasmodic torticollis. Neurosurgery 1994;35:58–62.

156. Davis DH, Ahlskog JE, Litchy WJ, et al. Selective peripheral denervation for torticollis: preliminary results. Mayo Clin Proc 1991;66: 365–371.

157. Ford B, Louis ED, Greene P, et al. Outcome of selective ramisectomy for botulinum toxin resistant torticollis. J Neurol Neurosurg Psychiatry 1998;65:472–478.

158. Braun V, Richter HP. Selective peripheral denervation and posterior ramisectomy in cervical dystonia. In: Krauss JK, Jankovic J, Grossman RG, eds. Surgery for Parkinson's Disease and Movement Disorders. Philadelphia: Lippincott, Williams and Wilkens, 2001:335–342.

159. Chawda SJ, Munchau A, Johnson D, et al. Pattern of premature degenerative changes of the cervical spine in patients with spasmodic torticollis and the impact on the outcome of selective peripheral denervation. J Neurol Neurosurg Psychiatry 2001;68:465–471.

160. Shima F, Fukui M, Kitamura K, Kuromatsu C, Okamura T. Diagnosis and surgical treatment of spasmodic torticollis of 11th nerve. Neurosurgery 1988;22:358–363.

161. Nielsen VK. Electrophysiology of the facial nerve in hemifacial spasm: ectopic/ephaptic excitation. Muscle Nerve 1985;187:161–164.

162. Lang J. Über Bau, Länge und Gefässbeziehungen der zentralen und peripheren Strecken der intrazisternalen Hirnnerven. Zbl Neurochir 1982;43:217–255.

163. Aksik I. Microneural decompression operations in the treatment of some forms of cranial rhizopathy. Acta Neurochir 1993;125:64–74.

164. Freckmann N, Hagenah R, Herrmann HD, et al. Treatment of neurogenic torticollis by microvascular lysis of the accessory nerve roots B indication, techniques and first results. Acta Neurochir 1981;59: 167–175.

165. Shima F, Fukui M, Matsubara T, Kitamura K. Spasmodic torticollis caused by vascular compression of the spinal accessory root. Surg Neurol 1986;26:431–434.

166. Freckmann N, Hagenah R, Herrmann HD, et al. Bilateral microsurgical lysis of the spinal accessory nerve roots for treatment of spasmodic torticollis. Acta Neurochir 1986;83:47–53.

167. Alafaci C, Salpietro FM, Montemagno G, et al. Spasmodic torticollis due to neurovascular compression of the spinal accessory nerve by the anteroinferior cerebellar artery: case report. Neurosurgery 2000;47: 768–771.

168. Decq P, Filipetti P, Cubillos A, et al. Soleus neurotomy for treatment of the spastic equinus foot. Neurosurgery 2000;47:1154–1160.

169. Decq P, Ochiai T, Filipetti P, et al. Peripheral neurectomies in the treatment of dystonic foot [Abstract]. Acta Neurochir. 2000;142: 1195.

PART III

Individual Dystonias: Management Considerations

CHAPTER 12

Blepharospasm and Hemifacial Spasm

Joseph King Ching Tsui

INTRODUCTION

Blepharospasm and hemifacial spasm are frequently discussed together because of their many similarities in symptoms and signs. However, they are two distinct neurologic entities. Blepharospasm refers to involuntary eyelid closure of central origin, and is a form of focal dystonia. Hemifacial spasm is caused by irritation of the facial nerve at its exit zone. In this chapter, these two distinct conditions are discussed.

BLEPHAROSPASM

Blepharospasm manifests as involuntary eyelid closure, usually bilateral, though it may sometimes be unilateral at onset. Contractions of the orbicularis oculi are the hallmark of the condition; however, other facial musculature is frequently involved. When lower facial and jaw muscles are also active, the combination of essential blepharospasm and orofacial or oromandibular dystonia is sometimes known as Meige's syndrome.[1] Marsden proposed the name Brueghel's syndrome, based on one of this artist's painting of a woman with facial grimacing suggestive of cranial dystonia.[2] Essential blepharospasm is a common form of focal dystonia, second in prevalence to cervical dystonia (CD) and writer's cramp. The incidence of essential blepharospasm has been reported to be 5 per million per year; oromandibular dystonia is said to affect 3 per million per year.[3] These figures are viewed as a gross underestimation because of inadequate ascertainment.

Etiology

The term blepharospasm should be used in the context of a syndrome. Essential blepharospasm refers to those patients whose condition has no obvious underlying cause, is a focal dystonia, or is part of the manifestations of generalized dystonia. Secondary blepharospasm may result from a variety of conditions including neuroleptic drugs, midbrain lesions, encephalitides, parkinsonism, and Wilson's disease. Genetic linkage to chromosome 18p (designated *DYT7*) has been described in a German family with adult-onset craniocervical dystonia[4]; however, the majority of cases are sporadic with no linkage to this region. Approximately 35% of patients presenting with essential blepharospasm may have dystonia that spreads to become segmental.[5] Although patients with parkinsonism may have associated blepharospasm, those patients presenting with essential blepharospasm are not prone to develop parkinsonian syndromes.[6]

In the past, essential blepharospasm was considered by some researchers to be of psychogenic origin, however, the body of evidence over the last three decades supports the organic nature of this condition. In patients with essential blepharospasm, electrophysiologic studies have shown shortened silent periods of the facial muscles.[7] This suggests hyperexcitability of cortical neurons or a lack of inhibition of those neurons that supply the facial muscles. Physiologic studies showed that reciprocal inhibition in forearm muscles was reduced in patients with essential blepharospasm.[8] Positron emission tomography (PET) studies with fluorodeoxyglucose (FDG) detect abnormal metabolism in the cerebellum and pons regions while patients are awake. PET studies also demonstrate abnormal metabolism in the superior medial frontal region while patients are asleep.[9] Overactivity of the striatum has also been reported.[10] These findings support the suggestion that the abnormal eyelid movements associated with blepharospasm are of central origin.

Clinical Features and Diagnosis

The onset of blepharospasm is typically insidious. Initially, blinking may increase in response to bright light, accompanied by a sensation of eye irritation. Dry eyes and tearing are common complaints. Many patients seek advice from an ophthalmologist who confirms no specific local eye pathology. The symptoms may progress slowly and the eyes may

Joseph King Ching Tsui: Pacific Parkinson's Research Centre, University of British Columbia, Vancouver, British Columbia.

The author has no commercial relationship to disclose.

involuntarily shut for periods of time; these episodes of eye closure may sometimes affect the patient's daily activities, such as driving, reading, or watching television. Symptoms are typically aggravated by stress and may improve after sleep. In extreme cases, persistent closing of the eyes might qualify the patient to register as being legally blind. Some patients describe "tricks" that may help to abort prolonged periods of eye closure. These tricks include gently touching the lateral canthus, rubbing the eyelids, or talking.

Blepharospasm may be difficult to distinguish from tics or eyelid-opening apraxia. Tics are usually suppressible and may be associated with other stereotypic abnormal movements. Eye closure is brief and frequent, and in most cases suppressible by voluntary effort for short periods of time. Tics seldom produce prolonged periods of complete eye closure. Patients describe an internal urge to shut the eyes.

Eyelid-opening apraxia is related to lack of contractions of the levator palpebrae superioris.[11] This condition may occur in isolation and be associated with patients who present with parkinsonism. Patients are not able to open their eyes after closing them; compensatory contractions of the frontalis muscles are frequent phenomena. Eyelid-opening apraxia is also characterized by the lack of contractions of the orbicularia oculi's periorbital fibers, as well as other lower facial muscles.

In contrast to typical blepharospasm, hemifacial spasm, as its name implies, is a unilateral condition. Twitches on one side of the face are obvious and complete closure of the eye is usually accompanied by pulling of the lower face and mouth toward the ear.

The differential diagnosis of blepharospasm also includes ptosis in myasthenic syndromes or ocular myopathy, which is characterized by absence of spasms of periorbital muscles. In case of doubt, Tensilon test (Hoffman-LaRoche, Nutley, NJ) or electromyography (EMG) may be performed to rule out these possibilities.

There are no laboratory tests or imaging techniques that confirm the diagnosis of essential blepharospasm. Diagnosis is based on careful history taking and a complete neurological examination. Exclusion of secondary causes of involuntary eye closure is crucial.

Treatment of Blepharospasm

Pharmacologic agents

As with other forms of dystonia, many oral medications have been used to treat blepharospasm. In general, these medications have not been efficacious. Side effects are frequent, and in many cases, dose limiting. Because the etiology remains unknown, various drugs that work in antagonism have been reported to benefit individual patients. Some examples are anticholinergic drugs (e.g., trihexyphenidyl, benztropine); cholinergic drugs (e.g., choline, deanol); dopaminergic agents (e.g., levodopa and dopamine agonists); and anti-dopaminergic drugs (e.g., haloperidol, tetrabenazine). Other categories of medication that have been used to treat ble-

pharospasm include GABAergic drugs (e.g., baclofen), benzodiazepines (e.g., lorazepam, clonazepam, diazepam), and anticonvulsants (e.g., carbamazepine).

Anticholinergic drugs have been the mainstay of therapy for idiopathic torsion dystonia. Before beneficial effects are obtained, these drugs have to be administered at relatively high dose levels; therefore, they are better tolerated in children than in adults. For trihexyphenidyl, side effects such as dry mouth and blurred vision are common. Frequently, doses up to 40 mg/day or higher may be required; at such high doses, dose-limiting side effects may include forgetfulness, mental confusion, and abnormal behaviors. In the older population, (in men) prostate problems, acute urinary retention, and precipitation of latent glaucoma are cautions to be observed. Baclofen is a drug that has been reported to benefit patients with blepharospasm.[12] As with anticholinergic drugs, at higher doses, the adverse effects of oral baclofen may overshadow the beneficial effects. In general, botulinum toxin injections have replaced oral medications as the treatment of choice in essential blepharospasm and other focal dystonias.

Surgical Treatments

The goal of surgical treatment is to stop contractions of the orbicularis oculi. Cessation of these contractions may be achieved through myectomy,[13] facial nerve avulsion, or differential sectioning of the facial nerve.[14] The rate of recurrence is high after these procedures; permanent damage to muscular or nervous tissues is undesirable. These procedures are reserved for those who do not respond to botulinum toxin injections.

Botulinum Toxin Injections

Stemming from other ophthalmologic applications, botulinum toxin (BTX) injections are utilized in the management of blepharospasm,[15] and are the treatment of choice for blepharospasm. This method of therapy is discussed below.

HEMIFACIAL SPASM

Hemifacial spasm is characterized by spasms of muscles on one side of the face. In most patients, the symptoms are unilateral, however, bilateral facial spasms have been reported.[16] In rare cases, hemifacial spasm may be associated with trigeminal neuralgia or glossopharyngeal neuralgia.[17]

Etiology

Irritation of the facial nerve at its root exit zone causes muscles supplied by this nerve to contract involuntarily. Physiologic evidence of ephaptic conduction has been reported and accounts for spontaneous facial movements.[18] All facial muscles innervated by the facial nerve may be involved. The source of irritation is most commonly a loop of blood vessel, typically a branch from the posterior inferior cerebellar artery. However, other arterial branches (e.g., anterior inferior cerebellar, acoustic, or internal auditory) may be responsible; it is less common for a vein to be responsible for irritation to the facial nerve. Hemifacial spasm is relatively more common in individuals of Asian descent. In a Korean series, the offending blood vessels, which were found during surgery, were reported in the anterior inferior cerebellar artery (43%); posterior inferior cerebellar artery (36.4%); vertebral artery (1.4%); multiple blood vessels (19%); and in a vein (0.2%).[19] Recovery from Bell's palsy may sometimes be associated with facial twitches that are indistinguishable from classic cases of hemifacial spasm; however, in those with Bell's palsy there may be associated facial weakness and synkinetic movements.

Clinical Features and Diagnosis

It is typical for patients with hemifacial spasm to complain of an insidious onset of twitching on one side of the face, at the outer angle of the lower eyelid. At first, the symptoms are intermittent and not bothersome. Slow progression involving the lower face and the upper eyelid usually ensues, and, in severe cases, the eye may become closed, with the face pulled toward the ear; this may continue for a period of time. Occasionally, clicking inside the ear may be noted; this is usually caused by spasms of the stapedius muscle, which is attached to the eardrum. The symptoms become worse when the patient is anxious. As the irritation is just outside the central nervous system, symptoms persist during sleep. The mechanical nature of this condition is illustrated by the fact that some patients report attenuation or aggravation of the symptoms according to varying postures of the head in bed. Some patient may be able to find a head position that reduces the twitching at bedtime, thus facilitating sleep.

The diagnosis of hemifacial spasm is based on the clinical history and neurologic examination. A history of slowly progressive unilateral facial twitches that spread, over a period of several years, from the outer corner of the lower lid is highly suggestive of hemifacial spasm. During the course of examination, facial spasms may be observed. Apart from a slight facial asymmetry, which is common in this condition (even while patients are at rest), there should be no facial motor weakness. Careful examination of the trigeminal and auditory nerves, as well as of the cerebellar system, should be performed to rule out a compressive or destructive lesion at the cerebellopontine angle. Atypical features would include facial muscle weakness, twitching starting from the lower face, impairment of facial sensation, hearing loss, cerebellar signs, other long tract signs, and rapid progression of symptoms. If unsure, a computed tomography (CT) scan or magnetic resonance imaging (MRI) should be performed. These tests may or may not demonstrate the offending vessel, however, they can assist in precluding the presence of a structural cerebellopontine angle lesion. These lesions include a tumor, vascular malformation, aneurysm, or arachnoid cyst.

Recent use of magnetic resonance angiography may improve the yield.[20]

Treatment

Oral Medications

Carbamazepine is the classic and most commonly used drug used to treat patients with hemifacial spasm. Before the availability of BTX-A injections, this drug was the only consistently effective drug for symptomatic relief. Side effects, which include dizziness, vertigo, and gastrointestinal upset, may necessitate discontinuation of therapy. In many patients, the drug appears to lose its effectiveness after a variable period of time. Phenytoin is another anticonvulsant that may reduce facial twitches in some patients. Gabapentin has been reported to be effective in controlling symptoms in five patients; doses ranged from 900 mg/day up to 1,600 mg/day.[21] More extensive studies have to be carried out to evaluate this drug.

Surgical Treatments

Unilateral periorbital myectomy was reported to be effective and safe for the treatment of individuals with hemifacial spasm. This procedure offered an option for patients who did not want to undertake a neurosurgical operation.[22] Its popularity has declined significantly after the introduction of treatment with BTX injections. During a periorbital myectomy, the orbicularis oculi and other facial muscles may be selectively denervated; this may be combined with musculocutaneous resection.[23] Recurrence is common and, with the availability of BTX injections, this operation has become obsolete. Facial nerve block with phenol is a procedure that is seldom performed.[24]

In most cases, when successfully performed, microvascular decompression offers a cure for the condition. This procedure, which was introduced in 1975, is also known as the Janetta procedure.[25] Recurrence, which may occur within 2 years after a successful surgery, may occur in up to 10% of patients.[26] In another series of 703 patients who were followed for 10 years, 84% had excellent results; 7% improved partially; and 9% had recurrent symptoms. Complications included deafness (2.6%), facial weakness (0.9%), brain stem infarction (0.3%), and death (0.1%).[27]

Botulinum Toxin Injections

In one series of 158 patients with hemifacial spasm, 110 patients received BTX-A injections and 25 patients were treated with microvascular decompression.[28] For those patients receiving BTX-A injections, 95% had marked to moderate improvement without significant adverse reactions. In the group of patients treated surgically, 7 had permanent complications related to the surgery. Because hemifacial spasm is a benign condition by itself, it would be reasonable to select BTX-A injections as the treatment of choice. First reported in 1984,[29] this treatment has become most popular because of its simplicity in application, effectiveness, and safety.

BOTULINUM TOXIN INJECTIONS

BTX-A was the first serotype of botulinum toxin used therapeutically in the treatment of diseases. Investigated with three other neuromuscular toxins, Scott et al.[30] published a report in 1973 regarding the efficacy and safety of BTX-A in producing reversible weakness in the lateral rectus of a monkey. This weakness occurred without significant systemic or local toxic effects in 1973.[30] In 1990, the National Institutes of Health[31] published a consensus statement that included a recommendation on the use of BTX-A in the treatment of blepharospasm and hemifacial spasm. Benefit usually begins 1–3 days after treatment, but occasionally a latent period of 2–3 weeks may be encountered. Typically, effects peak in 2 weeks and excellent results are maintained for 6–8 weeks. By the end of 12–16 weeks, most patients require repeat injections. The technique of injections is similar for hemifacial spasm and blepharospasm; the only difference is in the selection of facial muscles for treatment.

Two distinct serotypes of BTX are available commercially: types A and B. BOTOX (Allergan, Inc., Irvine, CA) and Dysport (Ipsen, Inc. Maidenhead, Berks, United Kingdom) are botulinum toxin type A. Myobloc™ (Elan Biopharmaceuticals, Inc., Dublin, Ireland) is botulinum toxin type B. Botulinum toxin type F is not commercially available; it has been shown to be effective in the treatment of dystonia, but its duration of effectiveness is too short to be of practical importance for the treatment of blepharospasm.[32] It may be considered an alternative to those resistant to the currently available forms of BTX.

BOTOX is supplied in dry powdered form; each vial of BOTOX contains 100 mouse units (MU, median lethal dose [LD_{50}], biologic unit) or 5 ng of protein. The powder must be reconstituted with normal saline that is free of preservatives. The shelf life of BOTOX may be significantly longer than several hours after its reconstitution; however, it is recommended the unused portion of the vial should be discarded at the end of the day because of sterilization precautions. It is estimated that 1 MU of BOTOX is probably equivalent to 4–5 MU of Dysport, and to approximately 50–70 MU of Myobloc. It is notable that there are no studies to support a fixed conversion dilution ratio among the marketed products. The following sections describe the use of BOTOX.

Preparation and Syringes

Tuberculin syringes with removable needles are best to use for injection of botulinum toxin. These syringes are graduated with 0.01-mL marks, with 100 graduations. The required quantity of normal saline is drawn up into the syringe, and using the supplied needle, the cork of the vial is pierced. A vacuum sucks in the contents of the syringe. It is helpful to direct the needle toward the side of the bottle to avoid mechanical impact to the toxin at the bottom of the vial. Bubbles on the surface of the vial's contents quickly disappear when the syringe is temporarily disconnected from the needle. The syringe is then reconnected to the needle and the desired amount of BTX-A drawn up into the syringe. It is important to change the needle to a 30-gauge for performance of the injections.

Dilution and Volume

Different centers use different dilution factors when reconstituting BOTOX. The more common dilution factor is 100 MU/mL (i.e., the addition of 1 mL to a vial of 100 MU). This dilution factor carries the convenience of taking each graduation of the tuberculin syringe to be 1 MU. However, the accuracy of delivering small doses like 1 MU may be compromised. When small doses are used for facial muscles, some injectors may prefer to add 2 mL or 4 mL to a vial of 100 MU. The dilution factor that is chosen should be the one that is most comfortable to work with, based upon the physician's experience and the individual technical needs of the patient. In some clinics that handle injections on different parts of the body, it may be advantageous to use a uniform concentration to avoid confusion or mixing up of the shared vials.

Injection Technique

As a rule, it is ideal to inject BTX-A directly into the target muscle. However, after repeated treatment, most facial muscles undergo atrophy and become very thin. Under these circumstances, subcutaneous injections may suffice. Most facial muscles are located over bone; therefore, diffusion of BTX-A is directed along the tissue planes of the muscles. The use of EMG is unnecessary for facial muscles that are commonly injected. An oblique needle approach is used to ensure injections into superficial layers. A general principle is to direct the needle away from possible injury to important structures, such as the globe of the eye.

Muscles Selection, Dose, and Sites of Injection

Most abnormal facial movements may be easily observed during the course of examination. The selection of muscles is seldom a problem during the first visit. The orbicularis oculi is the most common muscle to be injected, followed by risorius and depressor anguli oris. After injecting the orbicularis oculi, it may be expected that, in some cases, diffusion of BTX into the lower face may benefit patients with hemifacial spasm. It is advisable that, in mild cases, only the upper face is to be treated initially in order to avoid excessive lower facial weakness.

- The orbicularis oculi may be divided into two parts. The periorbital fibers are similar to a flat, wide section of rubber band around the eye. Contractions of this portion of the orbicularis oculi cause the eye to squint shut. The pretarsal fibers span transversely across the upper eyelid. This part of the muscle closes the eye in a fashion that mimics ptosis. Perpendicular to these fibers run the levator palpebrae superioris, which stops short of the edge of the lid by approximately 7.5 mm. In most cases of hemifacial spasm, only the periorbital fibers need to be injected; however, in most patients with blepharospasm, the pretarsal fibers are treated as well. There are variants of blepharospasm with only the pretarsal fibers involved; the same technique may be used to treat eyelid-opening apraxia.[33] For the best results, injections have to be distributed around the periorbital fibers about the orbital rim. However, the middle portion of the upper lid has to be avoided to prevent ptosis caused by diffusion into the levator palpebrae superioris. The medial portion of the lower lid should also be omitted because of its proximity to the drainage area of the tear duct. There is also the possibility of diffusion into the inferior rectus muscle, thus leading to diplopia. Pretarsal injections may be performed in two to three sites by creating blebs of BTX just above the lashes of the upper lid. When administered in this manner, there is very little chance of producing ptosis.
- The risorius is located along an imaginary line drawn from the tragus of the ear to the angle of the mouth. Bilateral, simultaneous contractions of these muscles produce a wide grin. A usual site of injection is the midpoint of the muscle's length. The needle should be tangential to the surface of the skin. For this muscle, subcutaneous injection may be advantageous to avoid diffusion into the underlying buccinator muscle, which would cause the patient to bite the inside of the cheek when eating. Bilateral injections into this muscle are indicated in some patients with blepharospasm who also have lower facial involvement. In those patients with hemifacial spasm, it may be necessary to inject the unaffected risorius to maintain facial symmetry.
- The depressor anguli oris is a triangular piece of muscle attached from the angle of the mouth, spanning down to the lower edge of the mandible. It depresses the angle of the mouth. Bilateral contraction gives rise to a "sad" look. Although not always involved in hemifacial spasm, if the risorius and levator labii superiores are injected, unopposed action of these muscles causes excessive droopiness of the angle of the mouth. When these muscles are injected, care should be taken to avoid the facial artery.
- The zygomatic major pulls the angle of the mouth toward the prominence of the zygoma. The levator labii superioris is located just medial to the zygomatic major. In some patients with hemifacial spasm, these two muscles may cause irritating twitches, which may be more annoying than other facial muscle twitches. Droopiness of the

mouth's angle occurs when these muscles are injected with BTX; most patients tolerate twitching better than droopiness. Therefore, these muscles are less frequently treated.
- The frontalis muscle raises the eyebrow. It attaches to the eyebrow anteriorly and spans through an aponeurosis in the scalp, over the hemicranium to an occipital component over the occipital bone (i.e., occipitofrontalis). Injections of BTX into the forehead just over the eyebrow effectively reduce twitching in this muscle. Uncommonly, the occipital component may be involved in hemifacial spasm and injections into this part of the muscle may be required.
- The platysma is a thin and superficial piece of muscle spanning from the lower edge of the mandible to cover the anterior part of the neck. In some patients, two or three strands of this muscle may be prominent. In patients with hemifacial spasm, direct injections into these strands improve the unsightly "gooseneck" appearance.
- The orbicularis oris is the most difficult muscle to treat. It is a sphincter around the mouth and is linked to many other muscles, thus pulling it in different directions. Injections into any part of this muscle affect the other attached muscles, producing an unpredictably, abnormally shaped mouth. Eversion of certain parts of the lips is common; in some cases, drooling of saliva or leakage of food may occur. Patients should be warned of these problems before attempting to treat pursing of the lips in orofacial dystonia associated with blepharospasm.

The doses used for the above muscles vary according to different centers. Table 12-1 is a list of suggested starting doses.

As repeated treatments are performed, these doses should be modified; doses may be reduced if excessive weakness occurs. In general, the doses required for hemifacial spasm are less than those required for blepharospasm; frequently, the initial results are more dramatic for hemifacial spasm. However, after a series of injections for hemifacial spasm, the face becomes asymmetric. The eyebrow may not lift as high as the noninjected side; the eye may not shut as well; and grinning is wider on the noninjected side. Many patients request injections on the unaffected side to improve facial symmetry.

TABLE 12-1. *Starting Doses*

Muscles	Mouse units of BOTOX
Orbicularis oculi, periorbital	2.5 to 5 per site, × 4
Orbicularis oculi, pretarsal	1 to 2 per site, × 2–3
Risorius	2.5 to 5
Depressor anguli oris	5 to 7.5
Levator labii superiores	2.5 to 5
Zygomatic major	1.25 to 5
Frontalis	5 to 10 per site, × 2
Platysma	2.5 to 5 per strand

Adverse Effects

Side effects of BTX-A therapy are usually minor and transient; no significant systemic toxic effects have been reported with facial injections of BTX. Spontaneous resolution is the rule. Most adverse effects are associated with local trauma related to the injections and to excessive weakness in the injected muscles or neighboring muscles, which may be affected by diffusion of BTX-A.

- Ecchymoses are common and inevitable. These may be reduced by using smaller gauged needles and by choosing a smaller injection volume. In patients taking aspirin, local pressure for a longer period may be needed after each injection.
- Ptosis is related to diffusion of BTX-A into the levator palpebrae superiores and may be avoided by not injecting the middle portion of the upper eyelid (while performing periorbital injections). When pretarsal injections are performed, the needle should be kept as close as possible to the lashes of the upper lid.
- Diplopia is caused by diffusion of BTX into the extraocular muscles. The inferior rectus muscle on the floor of the orbit is particularly susceptible, especially during injections into the medial portion of the lower lid. Occasionally, when the upper lid crosses the pupil and interferes with binocular visual fusion, ptosis may cause diplopia. In this situation, elevation of the upper eyelid resolves the diplopia.
- In some patients, tearing problems may occur, either as dry eyes or as excessive tearing. Dry eyes may be related to the effect of BTX-A on the lachrymal gland, which is innervated by cholinergic fibers. Excessive weakness of the orbicularis oculi may result in failing to shut the eye during sleep. Exposure of the eye leads to tearing or dry eyes. If left unattended, conjunctivitis may be a complication. Patients should be informed of this possibility and advised to wear an eye patch during sleep.
- An occasional patient may report blurring of vision, presumably due to slowing of pupillary reaction following BTX-A injections. This is rather uncommon in clinical practice with BTX-A.
- Droopiness of the angle of mouth is common after injections into the risorius, levator labii superiores, and zygomatic major. Injecting the depressor anguli oris may partially counteract this undesirable effect.
- Most patients with hemifacial spasm are pleased with the initial results when annoying twitching is significantly reduced. However, after a series of injections, most patients complain of facial asymmetry, particularly of asymmetric smile and eyebrows. In these cases, the unaffected side needs to be injected, according to patient wishes.
- Biting the inside of the cheek may occur if injections into the risorius are performed too deep into the tissue.
- Dysphagia may occur when injecting the platysma and may be avoided by dose or technical modifications of future injections.

- Depigmentation around the orbit has been reported in African Americans treated with BTX injections; however, this has not been observed in another series of patients.[34]

Resistance to Treatment

Primary treatment failure is uncommon, however, in some patients, it may be difficult to reduce abnormal facial movements without inducing significant facial weakness. In such cases, a satisfactory response cannot be achieved and adjunctive pharmacotherapy and/or surgical treatment may be considered.

Antibodies to BTX-A are not observed in patients receiving facial injections; this is true after both short-term[35] and long-term[36] treatment. Antibody formation is apparently related to frequency of treatment as well as dosage of BTX-A. It is advisable to enforce a treatment interval of no less than 9 weeks. The practice of administering booster doses every 2 to 3 weeks should not be done.

OTHER TREATMENTS

Chemical Myectomy

Injections of doxorubicin induce local destruction of muscle fibers. These injections have been employed in treating blepharospasm and hemifacial spasm. In one series, patients were treated with this method at 10-plus weekly intervals, until symptoms were controlled. Nine of 18 patients with blepharospasm and 6 of 9 patients with hemifacial spasm reported complete relief of symptoms for 1–6 years.[37] However, some patients required supplementary BTX-A injections; a few patients required surgical correction in their eyelids. Local skin inflammation may necessitate discontinuation of treatment with doxorubicin injections.

Supportive Treatment

In some cases, occupational and rehabilitation therapies are important to supplement medical treatment. In some patients, secondary depression may necessitate psychiatric consultations or psychological counseling. Stress aggravates symptoms of blepharospasm and hemifacial spasm; therefore, stress management techniques form an important part in the overall management of patients with these conditions. Patient support groups may provide additional, detailed information regarding coping with the challenges of day-to-day activities.

REFERENCES

1. Meige H. Les convulsions de la face. Une forme clinique de convulsion faciale, bilaterale et mediane. Rev Neurol 1910;21:427–433.
2. Marsden CD. Blepharospasm-oromandibular dystonia syndrome (Brueghel's syndrome): a variant of adult-onset torsion dystonia? J Neurol Neurosurg Psychiatry 1976;59:1204–1209.
3. Nutt JG, Muenter MD, Melton LJ III, et al. Epidemiology of dystonia

in Rochester, Minnesota. In: Fahn S, Marsden CD, Calne DB, eds. Advances in Neurology. Volume 50: Dystonia 2. New York: Raven Press, 1988;361–365.

4. Leube B, Hendgen T, Kessler KR, et al. Sporadic focal dystonia in Northwest Germany: molecular basis on chromosome 18p. Ann Neurol 1997;42:111–114.

5. Defazio G, Berardelli A, Abbruzzese G, et al. Risk factors for spread of primary adult onset blepharospasm: a multicenter investigation of the Italian movement disorders study group. J Neurol Neurosurg Psychiatry 1999;67:613–619.

6. Soonawala N, Bhatia KP, Yeung JH, et al. Idiopathic blepharospasm does not lead to a parkinsonian syndrome: results of a questionnaire-based follow-up study. J Neurol 999;246:283–286.

7. Curra A, Romaniello A, Berardelli A, et al. Shortened cortical silent period in facial muscles of patients with cranial dystonia. Neurology 2000;11;54:130–135.

8. Panizza M, Lelli S, Nilsson J, Hallett M. H-reflex recovery curve and reciprocal inhibition of H-reflex in different kinds of dystonia. Neurology 1990;40:824–848.

9. Hutchinson M, Nakamura T, Moeller JR, et al. The metabolic topography of essential blepharospasm: a focal dystonia with general implications. Neurology 2000;12;55:673–677.

10. Esmaeli-Gutstein B, Nahmias C, Thompson M, et al. Positron emission tomography in patients with benign essential blepharospasm. Ophthal Plast Reconstr Surg 1999;15:23–27.

11. Lepore FE, Duvoisin RC. "Apraxia" of eyelid opening: an involuntary levator inhibition. Neurology 1985;35:423–427.

12. Fahn S, Hening WA, Bressman S, et al. Long-term usefulness of baclofen in the treatment of essential blepharospasm. Adv Ophthal Plastic Reconstr Surg 1985;4:219–226.

13. McCord CD, Shore JW, Putnam JR. Treatment of essential blepharospasm: II. A modification of exposure of the muscle stripping technique. Arch Ophthalmol 1984;102:269–273.

14. Callahan A. Blepharospasm with resection of part of orbicularis nerve supply. Arch Ophthalmol 1963;70:508–511.

15. Scott AB, Kennedy RA, Stubbs HA. Botulinum A toxin injection as a treatment for blepharospasm. Arch Ophthalmol 1985;103:347–350.

16. Tan EK, Jankovic J. Bilateral hemifacial spasm: a report of five cases and a literature review. Mov Disord 1999;14:345–359.

17. Kobata H, Kondo A, Iwasaki K, et al. Combined hyperactive dysfunction syndrome of the cranial nerves: trigeminal neuralgia, hemifacial spasm, and glossopharyngeal neuralgia: 11-year experience and review. Neurosurgery 1998;43:1351–1361; discussion, 1361–1362.

18. Nielsen VK. Pathophysiology of hemifacial spasm: I. Ephaptic transmission and ectopic excitation. Neurology 1984;34:418–426.

19. Chung SS, Chang JW, Kim SH, et al. Microvascular decompression of the facial nerve for the treatment of hemifacial spasm: preoperative magnetic resonance imaging related to clinical outcomes. Acta Neurochir (Wien) 2000;142:901–7.

20. Ho SL, Cheng PW, Wong WC, et al. A case-controlled MRI/MRA study of neurovascular contact in hemifacial spasm. Neurology 1999;10;53:2132–2139.

21. Bandini F, Mazzella L. Gabapentin as treatment for hemifacial spasm. Eur Neurol 1999;42:49–51.

22. Garland PE, Patrinely JR, Anderson RL. Hemifacial spasm. Results of unilateral myectomy. Ophthalmology 1987;94:288–294.

23. Spector GJ. Selective facial neurectomy for spastic disorders of the facial nerve. Otolaryngol Head Neck Surg 1985;93:168–173.

24. Elmqvist D, Toremalm NG, Elner A, et al. Hemifacial spasm: electrophysiological findings and the therapeutic effect of facial nerve block. Muscle Nerve 1982;5:S89–94.

25. Jannetta PJ. The cause of hemifacial spasm: definitive microsurgical treatment at the brainstem in 31 patients. Trans Am Acad Ophthalmol Otolaryngol 1975;80(3 Pt 1):319–322.

26. Payner TD, Tew JM Jr. Recurrence of hemifacial spasm after microvascular decompression. Neurosurgery 1996;38:686–390.

27. Barker FG II, Jannetta PJ, Bissonette DJ, et al. Microvascular decompression for hemifacial spasm. J Neurosurg 1995;82:201–210.

28. Wang A, Jankovic J. Hemifacial spasm: clinical findings and treatment. Muscle Nerve 1998;21:1740–1747.

29. Frueh BR, Felt DP, Wojno TH, et al. Treatment of blepharospasm with botulinum toxin. A preliminary report. Arch Ophthalmol 1984;102: 1464–1468.

30. Scott AB, Rosenbaum A, Collins CC. Pharmacologic weakening of extraocular muscles. Invest Ophthalmol 1973;12:924–927.

31. National Institutes of Health: Consensus Statement on the Use of Botulinum Toxin. 1990;8:1–20.

32. Mezaki T, Kaji R, Kohara N, et al. Comparison of therapeutic efficacies of type A and F botulinum toxins for blepharospasm: a double-blind, controlled study. Neurology 1995;45(3 Pt 1):506–508.

33. Aramideh M, Ongerboer de Visser BW, et al. Pretarsal application of botulinum toxin for treatment of blepharospasm. J Neurol Neurosurg Psychiatry 1995;59:309–311.

34. Roehm PC, Perry JD, Girkin CA, et al. Prevalence of periocular depigmentation after repeated botulinum toxin A injections in African American patients. J Neuroophthalmol 1999;19:7–9.

35. Biglan AW, Gonnering R, Lockhart LB, et al. Absence of antibody production in patients treated with botulinum A toxin. Am J Ophthalmol 1986;101:232–235.

36. Song KH. Botulinum toxin type A injection for the treatment of frown lines. Ann Pharmacother 1998;32:1365–1367.

37. Wirtschafter JD, McLoon LK. Long-term efficacy of local doxorubicin chemomyectomy in patients with blepharospasm and hemifacial spasm. Ophthalmology 1998;105:342–346.

CHAPTER 13

Treatment of Cervical Dystonia

Joseph Jankovic

DIAGNOSIS AND EVALUATION OF CERVICAL DYSTONIA

Cervical dystonia (CD) is a focal dystonia affecting the neck that produces patterned, repetitive, and clonic (spasmodic) or tonic (sustained) muscle contractions resulting in abnormal movements and postures of the head and neck. The term spasmodic torticollis is used commonly to describe this form of dystonia.[1] However, because it is not always spasmodic (jerky) and does not always consist of torticollis (head turning), the term cervical dystonia is preferred as a generic descriptor of dystonic movements or postures involving the neck. In addition to neck turning (torticollis), CD may produce neck flexion (anterocollis), extension (retrocollis), and head tilt (laterocollis), as well as lateral or sagittal shift. In approximately one-third of all patients, CD progresses to involve contiguous body parts, including the facial and oromandibular regions, shoulder, and arms.[2] The prevalence of all forms of focal dystonia has been estimated to be 12.9 per 100,000;[3] CD is the most common form of dystonia in patients referred to movement disorder clinics.[4,5]

Two studies conducted in separate movement disorders clinics reviewed the clinical characteristics of patients with CD and noted remarkably similar results. Three hundred patients were studied at Baylor College of Medicine, Houston, Texas;[5] 61% of these patients were women, with mean age at symptom onset of 41.8 years. Two hundred sixty-six patients were studied at the Neurologic Institute (NI), New York, New York ($n = 266$); 65% of these patients were women, with mean age at symptom onset of 41.3 years.[4] In the Baylor group, torticollis was present in 82%; laterocollis

in 42%; retrocollis in 29%; and anterocollis in 25%. However, the majority of patients (66%) had a combination of these abnormal postures. Scoliosis was present in 39% of these patients. In the NI group, 83% of the patients had "constant" head deviation and 17% had only "intermittent" deviation. CD was accompanied by local pain in 68% of patients in the Baylor group and 75% of the NI patients.

Oscillatory movements of the head, noted in 60% of the patients with CD studied at Baylor, are typically produced either by repetitive dystonic contractions of neck muscles (dystonic tremor) or by essential-type tremor involving the head. In most patients, these two types of tremor may be identified clinically. Their differentiation may be aided by the use of electromyography (EMG).[6,7] Essential-type tremor typically has a relatively high frequency of greater than 7 Hz (with peaks at 9 Hz and 11 Hz) compared to the frequency of dystonic tremor at 3–7 Hz (with a peak at 5 Hz).

Dystonic tremor, an actual component of the dystonia, is somewhat more irregular; it is most obvious when the patient voluntarily attempts to move in the direction opposite to the force of the dystonia. Thus, if the patient has torticollis to the right but attempts to maintain a primary position, then lateral oscillation of the head (dystonic tremor) might be seen as the patient attempts to look straight ahead. However, when the patient stops resisting the dystonic pulling of the neck, the dystonic tremor ceases (a null point). In contrast, patients with coexistent essential-type tremor tend to continue to exhibit the head oscillation, regardless of the direction of the force of the dystonia. Using this clinical differentiation, head tremor has been identified in 60% of all patients with CD. This head tremor was categorized as dystonic in 38%; essential in 30%; and a combination dystonic-essential in 8% of patients.[5] Deuschl et al.[6] provided support for this clinical differentiation by using EMG polygraphic recordings.

In the Baylor patients with CD and a low-frequency tremor that was thought to be dystonic in origin, EMG tremor activity ceased when the patients used a geste antagonistique (sensory trick) to stop the movement. This phenomenon was not observed in patients with essential-type tremor. In some patients, head tremor may precede the onset

Joseph Jankovic: Professor of Neurology, Director of Parkinson's Disease Center, and Movement Disorders Clinic, Department of Neurology, Baylor College of Medicine, Houston, Texas.

Portions of this review were adapted from other reviews by the author, including: Jankovic J, Fahn S, Dystonic Disorders, In: Jankovic, J, Tolosa E eds. Parkinson's Disease and Movement Disorders. 3rd ed. Baltimore: Williams and Wilkins, 1998.

The author wishes to disclose research grant funding from Allergan, Inc., Elan Biopharmaceuticals, and Ipsen.

of dystonia symptoms and be the initial manifestation of focal dystonia (dystonic tremor).[8]

In addition to head tremor, CD is also associated with hand tremor. This tremor is phenomenologically similar to typical essential tremor.[9] Postural tremor involving the hands was noted in 27% of the Baylor group and in 23% of the NI group.[4] In another study involving 220 patients with CD, postural tremor was present in 21% of patients and apparent before the onset of cervical dystonia symptoms.[10] Further physiologic and genetic studies are needed to explore the relationship between typical essential tremor and postural tremor associated with dystonia.

In most patients with CD, there is no identifiable cause. Such idiopathic CD is usually a manifestation of primary dystonia that, in some patients, is clearly of genetic origin. A comprehensive discussion of the genetics of dystonia is beyond the scope of this chapter.

A gene mutation or a locus has been identified in several families with CD. *DYT1* dystonia is caused by a single GAG deletion mutation in the TOR1A (*DYT1*) gene on chromosome 9. This form of dystonia is associated with childhood onset of generalized dystonia (including CD), predominantly involving the limbs.[11] In addition to *DYT1* dystonia, several other genetic forms of primary torsion dystonia have been identified and designated as *DYT6* and *DYT13*. A gene locus in the 8p21-q22 region has been identified in a large German-American Mennonite family with cranial-cervical and limb dystonia.[12] This dystonia, designated as *DYT6* in the 8p21-q22 region, is clinically similar to *DYT1,* however, the involvement is more generalized and includes the head and neck. Another genetic dystonia, designated *DYT13* and mapped to chromosome 1p36.13–36.22 in an Italian family, is manifested by cranial-cervical or upper limb dystonia, both of which are a common presentation of adult-onset dystonia.[13] These findings highlight the importance of identifying the specific gene mutation involved, and studying gene abnormalities in many patients with dystonia. Such studies may help to determine the frequency of specific genetic causes in a general patient population with dystonia and, in particular, in those with cranial dystonia and CD.

Of the nongenetic causes of CD, trauma and drugs are probably the most common. Eleven percent of the Baylor patients[5] had "significant" neck injury less than 1 year before the onset of CD symptoms. Nine percent of the NI group[4] reported trauma in the period 3 months before the onset of neck dystonia. The topic of a cause-and-effect relationship between peripheral injury and dystonia, including CD, has stimulated lively discussions and debates. These discussions continue as the pathophysiologic mechanisms of posttraumatic dystonia are not well understood and because of related psychological and legal issues.[14,15]

Cervical dystonia can also develop after exposure to neuroleptic drugs (tardive dystonia).[16,17] Tardive dystonia accounted for up to 6% of the patients within the Baylor series; however, the frequency of this cause of dystonia has been gradually declining. This decline is the result of introduction

of atypical neuroleptics, which have a lower risk of tardive dyskinesia, including tardive dystonia, when compared to the traditional neuroleptics.

In addition to dystonia, there are many other causes of abnormal head position or torticollis (pseudodystonia). When a secondary cause is suspected, neuroimaging studies, including head and cervical magnetic resonance imaging (MRI), should be considered (Table 13-1).[18] In addition, tests designed to exclude potentially treatable causes, such as Wilson's disease, should be performed, particularly in patients with young-onset CD and in atypical cases.

The course of CD may vary from one individual to another, but most patients report deterioration during the first 5 years. After that time, the symptoms tend to stabilize.[19,20] Although some series have reported that up to 23% of patients with spasmodic torticollis achieve spontaneous and lasting remissions,[21,22] a remission rate of 10% is probably more accurate.[4] Remission, if it occurs, is most frequently noted during the first 3 years after the onset of symptoms. Remission is more likely in patients with spasmodic or "jerky" dystonia than in patients with constant neck deviation. However, in most patients, cervical dystonia is a lifelong disorder. In about 20% of patients, dystonia progresses to segmental or generalized dystonia.

To hold their head in a primary position, most patients learn certain maneuvers to relax the neck muscles. These sensory tricks or gestes antagonistique are often not sufficient to overcome the disability.[23] The mechanism of sensory tricks is unknown. Naumann et al.[24] conducted a study using $H_2^{15}O$ positron emission tomography (PET) on patients with CD. These investigators found that keeping the head in primary position (while using a sensory trick) decreased motor corti-

TABLE 13-1. *Causes of Abnormal Neck Postures*

1. Cervical dystonia
2. Atlanto-axial dislocation
3. Cervical fracture
4. Degenerative disc disease
5. Osteomyelitis
6. Klippel-Feil syndrome
7. Congenital torticollis associated with absence or fibrosis of cervical muscles
8. Postradiation fibrosis
9. Posttraumatic acute stiff neck
10. Infectious or postinfectious pharyngitis
11. Painful lymphadenopathy, adenitis
12. Posterior fossa tumor
13. Arnold-Chiari syndrome
14. Syringomyelia
15. Spinal cord tumor
16. Bobble-head doll syndrome (with third ventricle cyst)
17. Nystagmus
18. Sandifer's syndrome
19. Extraocular muscle palsies, strabismus
20. Head thrusts with oculomotor apraxia
21. Hemianopia
22. Spasmus nutans
23. Focal seizures

cal activation to the side that is contralateral to which the head tends to turn. Decreased activation was also noted in the anterior part of the supplementary motor cortex. In addition, the sensory trick was associated with increased activation of the parietal cortex, ipsilateral to the direction of dystonic head rotation. Despite sensory tricks, most patients cannot control the neck pulling. Because of this neck pulling and constant head movement, patients have difficulties with reading, writing, driving, and other activities of daily living.

TREATMENT OF CERVICAL DYSTONIA

Before discussing pharmacologic therapy, chemodenervation, and surgery, it is important to highlight the role of physical therapy in the treatment of CD. Stretching and range-of-motion exercises are recommended to help prevent contractures and other complications of chronically sustained abnormal neck postures. Muscle relaxation techniques and sensory feedback therapy, while not necessarily providing a dramatic relief, serve as useful ancillary treatments.[23] Finally, in some patients, specially constructed cervical braces may be useful to enable them to maintain a desired position and serve as a substitute for the sensory trick.

Pharmacotherapy

Pharmacotherapy may be useful in some patients with CD; however, in most patients with CD, medications may be ineffective, partially effective, or complicated by undesirable side effects.[25] In one study, 39% of patients with CD improved with anticholinergic drugs (e.g. trihexyphenidyl, ethopropazine, etc.).[26] Although anticholinergics are probably the most effective drugs in the treatment of dystonia, their benefits are often limited by the development of undesirable side effects. These effects may include nausea, dry mouth, forgetfulness and cognitive changes, drowsiness, blurred vision, glaucoma, and urinary retention.

Other drugs that occasionally ameliorate symptoms of CD include baclofen, carbamazepine, and tetrabenazine.[27] Muscle relaxants, such as diazepam, lorazepam, cyclobenzaprine, or tizanidine, may also provide benefit in some patients; however, these have never been systematically evaluated in CD. In some patients, oral and intrathecal baclofen may be helpful.[28,29]

Chemodenervation

Clearly, the most important advance in the treatment of CD has been the introduction of chemodenervation by local injection of botulinum toxin (BTX).[30] It is hardly necessary to emphasize that to optimize the response to BTX therapy, the dosage and the site of injection must be individualized. While dose guidelines are available, the clinician must rely on a careful assessment of the patient as well as previous experience to select the most appropriate muscles and doses. The most important determinants of a favorable response to BTX treatments are a proper selection of the involved muscles and an appropriate dosage.[31] This may be accomplished by a careful evaluation of the patient.

Patients should be examined while sitting, standing, walking, and writing; this examination is conducted with their eyes open and then with their eyes closed. This allows for a full and uncompensated expression of the abnormal movement and posture. During this examination:

- The head is passively moved to determine the full range of motion and whether there is an associated contracture;
- The neck muscles are carefully palpated to assess the intensity of contraction and determine the muscle mass and degree of hypertrophy, and
- The neck is carefully examined to identify points of tenderness.

It is important to document the findings, including with the use of video recordings, and attempt to quantify the severity of the dystonia and its response to treatment. This may be done by utilizing clinical rating scales, such as the Toronto Western Spasmodic Torticollis Rating Scale (TWSTRS)[32,33] and the Unified Dystonia Rating Scale (UDRS).[34]

The efficacy and safety of BTX in the treatment of CD has been demonstrated in several controlled and open trials.[35–42] As of 2003, there are three preparations available commercially for clinical use. BOTOX (Allergan, Inc., Irvine, CA) and MYOBLOC (Elan Biopharmaceuticals, Inc., Dublin, Ireland,) or Neurobloc are available in the United States and Europe; Dysport (Ipsen, Maidenhead, Berk, United Kingdom) is chiefly used in Europe. Double-blind, placebo-controlled studies demonstrated relatively modest improvement.[36] However, open-label studies generally report a more dramatic effect, partly because of greater flexibility in selecting the proper dosage and site of injection allowed in open-label trials as compared to controlled studies.[43] For example, in an open trial of 303 patients with medically intractable CD, the author noted a substantial improvement in both function and control of head-neck movement in 92% of patients treated with BOTOX.[37] Furthermore, 93% of patients had marked relief from their neck pain. The average latency between injection and the onset of improvement (and muscle atrophy) was 1 week; the average duration of maximum improvement was 3.5 months. In most patients, however, the beneficial effects lasted an additional 6 weeks. On average, the injections were repeated every 4–6 months. Only 14% of these patients failed to improve after one or more visits; 6% of these patients consistently failed after repeated attempts. Botulinum toxin type A (BTX-A) was compared to oral trihexyphenidyl in a prospective, randomized, double-blind trial involving 64 patients with CD. In this comparison, the response to the toxin was substantially superior to that observed with trihexyphenidyl.[44] In this regard, changes in scores on the TWSTRS disability subscale substantially favored the toxin.

Improvements similar to those obtained with BTX-A (BOTOX or Dysport) have been obtained in patients treated for CD with botulinum toxin type B (BTX-B; Myobloc or Neurobloc).[40,41,45,46] In a double-blind, controlled trial of 122 patients with CD treated with BTX-B (MYOBLOC or Neurobloc), the author observed a dose-response effect, particularly at doses of 10,000 units.[45] Using the TWSTRS, 77% of the patients were found to respond at week 4. Other studies have subsequently confirmed the efficacy of BTX-B,[40] even in patients who are resistant to BTX-A.[41] In a 16-week, randomized, multicenter, double-blind, placebo-controlled trial of BTX-B, 109 patients who previously responded well to BTX-A were randomized to one of three treatment groups: placebo; 5,000 units; and 10,000 units. These doses were administered into two to four cervical muscles.[40] At week 4, the total TWSTRS score compared to baseline improved by 4.3 for the placebo group, 9.3 for the 5,000-unit group ($P = .01$), and 11.7 for the 10,000-unit treatment group ($P = .0004$). Improved TWSTRS scores were accompanied by noteworthy improvements in pain, disability, and severity. The estimated median time until the total TWSTRS score returned to baseline was 63 days for the placebo group, 114 days for the 5,000-unit group, and 111 days for the 10,000-unit treatment group. The most frequent side effects included dysphagia and dry mouth.

An identical design was used in another study of BTX-B in CD with one exception: the patients were resistant to BTX-A as determined by the F-TAT (evaluation of muscle paralysis after unilateral frontalis injection).[41] Seventy-seven patients were randomly assigned to receive placebo or 10,000 units of BTX-B. At week 4, the total TWSTRS scores improved by 2 (placebo) and 11 (10,000 units with $P = .0001$). There was also significant improvement in secondary and tertiary outcome measures including global assessments and pain visual analogue scores as well as other measures of pain, disability, and severity. The estimated duration of effect, based on Kaplan-Meier survival analysis, was 112 days (12–16 weeks). Subsequent studies have suggested that dosages as high as 45,000 units of MYOBLOC or Neurobloc may be needed to achieve optimal response.

Botulinum toxin type F (BTX-F) has also undergone clinical testing. In a retrospective study of 18 BTX-A-resistant patients treated with BTX-F for at least 1 year, Chen et al.[47] reported that all patients initially improved, however, 4 patients became resistant to BTX-F. This resistance correlated with a higher dose per visit and a higher cumulative dose. Furthermore, the duration of benefit with BTX-F, although longer than initially reported,[48] was still relatively short at 7.9 weeks. For this and other reasons, it is questionable whether BTX-F will ever become commercially available.

In addition to a robust effect on involuntary muscle spasms and abnormal head position, patients with CD also experience marked relief of their pain following BTX injection. This symptomatic improvement is also frequently associated with substantial reduction of depression[19] and leads to a meaningful improvement in overall function.

BTX treatment is rarely associated with serious complications. When adverse effects occur, they are usually temporary and resolve in a few days. Complications, such as dysphagia and neck weakness, are usually related to regional spread of the toxin's biologic activity. Systemic side effects, such as generalized weakness and malaise, rarely occur. These rare effects may possibly occur as a result of blood distribution or, less likely, a retrograde axonal transport to the spinal motor neurons.[49] The mechanism of brachial plexopathy, rarely reported after BTX treatment for CD, is unknown.[50,51] Most complications resolve spontaneously, usually within 2 weeks.

Dysphagia, the most feared side effect of BTX injections, is rarely disabling. This side effect can usually be managed by instructing the patient to change the diet to soft food. An injection into both sternocleidomastoid (SCM) or scalenus muscles is most frequently associated with dysphagia.[38,52,53] One study showed that dosages as small as 20 units (administered as a single injection into the SCM muscle) completely eliminated muscle activity and could produce neck weakness and dysphagia.[54]

While BTX-A and BTX-B cause similar side effects, particularly dysphagia and neck weakness, BTX-B (MYOBLOC or Neurobloc) appears to cause more local pain at the time of injection. This pain is perhaps because of its acidic pH. BTX-B is also associated with a higher frequency of dry mouth. The comparison between pharmacology, clinical effects, safety, and immunogenicity is beyond the scope of this chapter, but the reader is referred to other reviews related to this topic.[55]

There have been only a few long-term studies of BTX treatment in CD,[56] however, the collective experience suggests that most patients continue to benefit, unless they develop immunoresistance associated with blocking antibodies.[14,57,58] Brashear et al.[59] showed that two-thirds of patients receiving BTX reported that the injections continue to provide satisfactory relief. Measuring paralysis 2 weeks after injection in the extensor digitorum brevis (EDB), Sloop et al.[60] found that patients with CD who continued to respond clinically to BTX-A demonstrated the same degree of muscle paralysis in the EDB as did naïve subjects (who were never treated with BTX).

EMG may be helpful in some patients with obese necks or those in whom the involved muscles are difficult to identify by palpation.[31,61–64] Some investigators have reported that EMG-assisted injections enhance clinical response by facilitating the accuracy of injection.[39,61,65] One study attempted to determine the usefulness of EMG-assisted BTX injections.[65] The study found that the percentage of patients showing any degree of improvement after BTX therapy was similar, whether the injections were EMG-assisted or non-EMG-assisted. The investigators also noted "a significantly greater magnitude of improvement" in patients treated with the EMG-assisted method. In addition, "a significantly greater number of patients with marked benefit" were in the group randomly assigned to the EMG-assisted method of treatment. Because most patients (70–79%) had previously been treated with BTX, some patients may have been experiencing residual effects from a previous injection; thus, interpretation of the results is difficult. Furthermore, the patients who were treated without EMG assistance received a

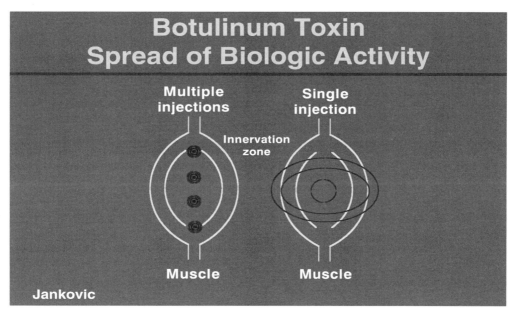

FIG. 13-1. Diagram showing the difference of injecting one single bolus (right) and distributing the total dose into four separate injections into the target muscle, thus containing the spread of the biologic activity within the target muscle.

higher dose, indicating more severe dystonia; thus, this may possibly explain the lesser degree of observed improvement.

Because of the additional discomfort, time, and expense required for EMG-assisted BTX injections, the routine use of EMG-guided technique seems impractical, and the consensus among most BTX injectors is that, in most patients, EMG guidance is not needed. This technique should be reserved for those patients who have had minimal or no benefit from previous clinically guided injections or those in whom the affected muscles are difficult to palpate. In those whose muscles are not palpable, EMG guidance may be used as an extension of the clinical examination.

In addition to the role of EMG, there are other controversies related to injection techniques. These controversies include whether the total dose per muscle should be injected as a single bolus injection or whether it should be distributed into several small injections. Figure 13-1 illustrates why the use of several injections seems to be a more rational approach.

There is considerable variation among different investigators regarding injection techniques; number of injections used per muscle; doses; combinations of muscles injected; and the use of EMG guidance. In most patients, examination of abnormal head position, coupled with muscle palpation and localization of pain or tenderness, facilitates the correct selection of involved muscles. Guidelines for doses of BTX into muscles usually involved in the production of certain abnormal postures are available (Figs. 13-2, 13-3; Tables 13-2, and 13-3). Because each patient is different, an indi-

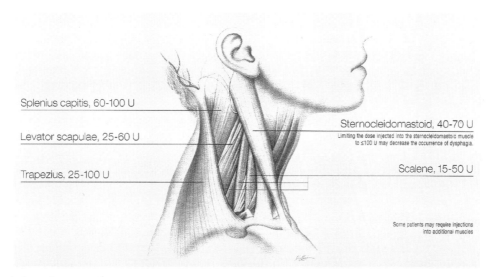

FIG. 13-2. Lateral view of the neck exposing the most frequently injected muscles and the average doses of BOTOX (Allergan, Inc., Irvine, CA) used.

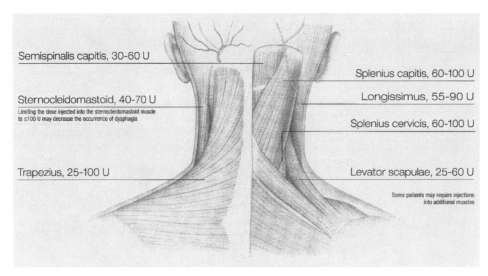

FIG. 13–3. Posterior view of the neck exposing the most frequently injected muscles and the average doses of BOTOX (Allergan, Inc., Irvine, CA) used.

vidualized approach is extremely important, and there are many exceptions to the suggested guidelines.

Although most patients obtain satisfactory relief of their CD with BTX treatment, some clinical features seem to be predictive of the degree of response. For example, patients with long-duration dystonia before their initial injection were found to respond less favorably than those who were treated relatively early in the course of their disease; prolonged dystonia may have produced fixed contractures in these patients.[38] Fortunately, with the advent of BTX therapy, dystonia-related contractures are now quite rare.

Surgery

Before the advent of BTX therapy, surgical denervation procedures had been used extensively to treat patients with CD. Surgery is now a rare but still useful therapeutic option. This is particularly true in those patients who fail to respond to repeated BTX injections; failure occurs because of secondary unresponsiveness, due to development of immunoresistance. Forty of the 300 patients (13%) followed at Baylor Medical Center eventually required surgery, consisting of selective cervical rhizotomy, with or without myotomy.[5] While 10% of patients noted worsening of symptoms after the surgery, 38% experienced either a noticeable improvement in their ability to control head position or a reduction in their pain.

When performed by an experienced neurosurgeon, selective peripheral denervation has been of benefit in as many as 76% of patients. This procedure may be useful in those who are resistant to botulinum toxin treatment.[66–68] The effects of 70 intradural or extradural denervation procedures were reported in 46 patients who had severe CD and no longer responded to BTX.[67] During follow-up, with a mean duration of 6.5 years, 21 of the patients (46%) reported excellent or marked improvement, as assessed on a global outcome scale. There was no difference in outcome distribution when patients who still responded to BTX were compared to the BTX nonresponders. Using a modified TWSTRS scale, statistically significant improvements were found, not only in the severity of dystonia but also in occupational and domestic work as well as in various activities of daily living.

The results of this study are comparable with those of Ford et al.[68] who reported an open-label, retrospective study of a selective denervation for severe CD. Sixteen patients who were refractory to injections with BTX-A were included in this retrospective study. Using functional capacity scales, the investigators concluded that 6 patients (37.5%) had a moderate or complete return of normal neck function. Some improvement was noted in 12 of 14 patients (85.7%), as demonstrated by the TWSTRS dystonia rating scale. The assessment was applied to blinded ratings of videotaped examinations; however, surgery failed to return these patients

TABLE 13-2. *Cervical Muscles Frequently Involved in Abnormal Head Positions in Cervical Dystonia**

Torticollis (rotatocollis)	Ipsilateral splenius, contralateral sternocleidomastoid
Laterocollis	Ipsilateral sternocleidomastoid, splenius capitis, scalene complex, levator scapulae, postvertebrals
Shoulder elevation	Ipsilateral trapezius, levator scapulae
Retrocollis	Bilateral splenius capitis, upper trapezius, deep postvertebrals
Anterocollis	Bilateral sternocleidomastoid, scalene complex, submental complex

* Cervical dystonia generally involves a combination of head positions.

TABLE 13-3. *Cervical Muscles Frequently Injected with Botulinum Toxin*

Muscle	Origin	Insertion	Action
Sternocleidomastoid	Manubrium of the sternum and medial 1/3 of the clavicle	Mastoid process	Contralateral rotation; anterior flexion
Trapezius	Medial end of superior nuchal line, external occipital protuberance, ligamentum nuchae and spines C7–T12	Scapula, acromion process, and lateral third of the clavicle	Elevation of the scapula and shoulder, extension of the neck
Splenius capitis	Lower half of the ligamentum nuchae and spines of C7–T5	Mastoid process	Ipsilateral rotation; extension of the neck
Levator scapulae	Transverse processes of C1–C4	Superior angle of the scapulae	Elevate the scapulae and shoulder
Scalene complex	Transverse processes of C1–C7	Superior surface of the first rib between subclavian groove and rib tubercle	Ipsilateral turn with flexion of the head [anterocollis]
Deep postvertebrals: 1. Longissimus capitis 2. Semispinalis capitis	1. Transverse process lower cervical, upper thoracic vertebrae 2. Lower cervical and upper thoracic vertebrae	1. Mastoid process lateral to splenius insertion 2. Medial part of occiput	1 and 2: ipsilateral tilt, extension of the neck

to their occupations. Based on the reported experience, surgical treatment, which is tailored to a specific pattern of dystonic activity in an individual patient, may be a valuable alternative in the long-term management of CD in patients who fail to obtain satisfactory relief from pharmacologic treatment or botulinum toxin injections.[69]

In addition to peripheral surgery, patients with severe generalized dystonia that includes CD may benefit from stereotactic surgery.[70–72] These surgeries include thalamotomy; pallidotomy; and high-frequency deep brain stimulation (DBS) of the globus pallidus interna (GPi). In a series of patients with generalized dystonia, investigators at the Baylor Center observed marked improvement following surgery. In some patients, dystonia-related disability changed from dependent functioning to completely independent functioning.[34] Several reports have documented meaningful benefits of bilateral GPi DBS in ameliorating CD associated pain and motor symptoms.[73–75] An ablative lesion or high-frequency stimulation of the GPi may produce dystonia, as well as improve dystonia. This suggests that the pattern of discharge in the basal ganglia, rather than the actual location or frequency of discharge, is pathophysiologically relevant to dystonia.[76]

REFERENCES

1. Jankovic J, Fahn S. Dystonic disorders. In: Jankovic J, Tolosa E, eds. Parkinson's Disease and Movement Disorders. 4th ed. Philadelphia: Lippincott Williams and Wilkins, 2002:331–357.
2. Tan EK, Jankovic J. Botulinum toxin A in patients with oromandibular dystonia: long-term follow-up. Neurology 1999;53:2102–2105.
3. Duffey P, Butler AG, Hawthorne MR, et al. The epidemiology of primary dystonia in the north of England. Adv Neurol 1998;78:121–125.
4. Chan J, Brin M, Fahn S. Idiopathic cervical dystonia: clinical characteristics. Mov Disord 1991;6:119–126
5. Jankovic J, Leder S, Warner D, et al. Cervical dystonia: clinical findings and associated movement disorders. Neurology 1991;41:1088–1091.
6. Deuschl G, Heinen F, Kleedorfer B, et al. Clinical and polymyographic investigation of spasmodic torticollis. J Neurol 1992;239:9–15.
7. Deuschl G, Krack P, Lauk M, et al. Clinical electrophysiology of tremor. J Clin Neurophysiol 1996;13:110–122.
8. Jedynak CP, Bonnet AM, Agid Y. Tremor and idiopathic dystonia. Mov Disord 1991;6:230–236.
9. Jankovic J. Essential tremor: a heterogenous disorder. Mov Disord 2002;17:638–644.
10. Rondot P, Marchand MP, Dellatolas G. Spasmodic torticollis—review of 220 patients. Can J Neurol Sci 1991;18:143–151.
11. Bressman SB, Sabatti C, Raymond D, et al. The DYT1 phenotype and guidelines for diagnostic testing. Neurology 2000;54:1746–1752.
12. Almasy L, Bressman SB, Raymond D, et al. Idiopathic torsion dystonia linked to chromosome 8 in two Mennonite families. Ann Neurol 1997;42:670–673.
13. Valente EM, Bentivoglio AR, Cassetta E, et al. DYT13, a novel primary torsion dystonia locus, maps to chromosome 1p36.13–36.32 in an Italian family with cranial-cervical or upper limb onset. Ann Neurol 2001;49:362–366.
14. Jankovic J. Can peripheral trauma induce dystonia and other movement disorders? Yes! Mov Disord 2001;16:7–112.
15. Weiner WJ. Can peripheral trauma induce dystonia? No! Mov Disord 2001;16:13–22.
16. Adityanjee, Yeken AA, Jampala VC, et al. The current status of tardive dystonia. Biol Psychiatry 1999;45:715–730.
17. Van Harten NP, Kahn RS. Tardive dystonia. Schizophrenia Bull 1999;25:741–748.
18. Suchowersky O, Calne DB. Non-dystonic causes of torticollis. Adv Neurol 1988;50:501–508.
19. Jahanshahi M, Marion MH, Marsden CD. Natural history of adult-onset idiopathic torticollis. Arch Neurol 1990;47:548–552.
20. Lowenstein DH, Aminoff MJ. The clinical course of spasmodic torticollis. Neurology 1998;38:530–532.
21. Jayne D, Lees AJ, Stern GM. Remission in spasmodic torticollis. J Neurol Neurosurg Psychiatry 1984; 47:1236–1237.
22. Friedman A, Fahn S. Spontaneous remissions in spasmodic torticollis. Neurology 1986;36:398–400.
23. Jahanshahi M. Factors the ameliorate or aggravate spasmodic torticollis. J Neurol Neurosurg Psychiatry 2000;68:227–229.
24. Naumann M, Magyar-Lehmann S, Reiners K, et al. Sensory tricks in cervical dystonia: perceptual dysbalance of parietal cortex modulates frontal motor programming. Ann Neurol 2000;47:322–328.
25. Jankovic J. Dystonia: Medical therapy and botulinum toxin. Adv Neurol 2004;94:275–286.
26. Greene P, Shale H, Fahn S. Analysis of open-label trials in torsion dystonia using high dosages of anticholinergics and other drugs. Mov Disord 1988;3:46–60.
27. Jankovic J, Beach J. Long-term effects of tetrabenazine in hyperkinetic movement disorders. Neurology 1997;48:358–362.

28. Ford B, Greene PE, Louis ED, et al. Intrathecal baclofen in the treatment of dystonia. Adv Neurol 1998;78:199–210.

29. Hou JG, Ondo W, Jankovic J. Intrathecal baclofen for dystonia: benefits and complications during six years of experience. Mov Disord 2001;16:1201–1202.

30. Jankovic J. Treatment of cervical dystonia with botulinum toxin. Mov Disord In press, 2004.

31. Jankovic J. Needle EMG guidance is rarely required. Muscle Nerve 2001;24:1568–1570.

32. Comella CL, Stebbins GT, Goetz CG, et al. Teaching tape for the motor section of the Toronto Western Spasmodic Torticollis Scale. Mov Disord 1997;12:570–575.

33. Consky ES, Lang AE. Clinical assessments of patients with cervical dystonia. In: Jankovic J, Hallett M, eds. Therapy with Botulinum Toxin. New York: Marcel Dekker, Inc., 1994:211–237.

34. Ondo WG, Desaloms M, Jankovic J, et al. Surgical pallidotomy for the treatment of generalized dystonia. Mov Disord 1998;13:693–698.

35. Blackie JD, Lees AJ. Botulinum toxin treatment in spasmodic torticollis. J Neurol Neurosurg Psychiatry 1990;53:640–643

36. Greene P, Kang U, Fahn S, et al. Double-blind, placebo-controlled trial of botulinum toxin injections for the treatment of spasmodic torticollis. Neurology 1990;40:12131218.

37. Jankovic J, Schwartz K. Botulinum toxin injections for cervical dystonia. Neurology 1990; 40:277–280.

38. Jankovic J, Schwartz KS. Clinical correlates of response to botulinum toxin injections. Arch Neurol 1991;48:1253–1256.

39. Poewe W, Schelosky L, Kleedorfer B, et al. Treatment of spasmodic torticollis with local injections of botulinum toxin. One-year follow-up in 37 patients. J Neurol. 1992;239:21–25.

40. Brashear A, Lew MF, Dykstra DD, et al. Safety and efficacy of Neurobloc™ (botulinum toxin type B) in type A responsive cervical dystonia. Neurology 1999;53:1439–1446.

41. Brin MF, Lew MF, Adler CH, et al. Safety and efficacy of NeuroBloc™ (botulinum toxin type B) in type A-resistant cervical dystonia. Neurology 1999;53:1431–1438.

42. Lorentz IT, Subramaniam SS, Yiannikas C. Treatment of idiopathic spasmodic torticollis with botulinum toxin A: a double-blind study on twenty-three patients. Mov Disord 1991;6:145–150.

43. Koller W, Vetere Overfield B, Gray C, Dubinsky R. Failure of fixed-dose, fixed muscle injection of botulinum toxin in torticollis. Clin Neuropharm 1990;13:355–358.

44. Brans JWM, Lindeboom R, Snoek JW, et al. Botulinum toxin versus trihexyphenidyl in cervical dystonia: a prospective, randomized, double-blind controlled trial. Neurology 1996;46:1066–1072.

45. Lew MF, Adornato BT, Duane DD, et al. Botulinum toxin type B: A double-blind, placebo-controlled, safety and efficacy study in cervical dystonia. Neurology 1997;49:701–707.

46. Poewe W, Deuschl G, Nebe A, et al. What is the optimal dose of botulinum toxin A in the treatment of cervical dystonia? Results of a double blind, placebo controlled, dose ranging study using Dysport. J Neurol Neurosurg Psychiatry 1998;64:13–17.

47. Chen R, Karp BI, Hallett M. Botulinum toxin type F for treatment of dystonia: long-term experience. Neurology 1998;51:1494–1496.

48. Greene PE, Fahn S. Response to botulinum toxin F in seronegative botulinum toxin A-resistant patients. Mov Disord 1996;11:181–184.

49. Garner CG, Straube A, Witt TN, et al. Time course effects of local injections of botulinum toxin. Mov Disord 1993;8:33–37.

50. Sampio C, Castro-Caldas A, Sales-Luis ML, et al. Brachial plexopathy after botulinum toxin administration for cervical dystonia. J Neurol Neurosurg Psychiatry 1993;56:220–221.

51. Vieregge P, Kompf D. Brachial plexopathy after botulinum toxin administration for cervical dystonia. J Neurol Neurosurg Psychiatry 1993;56:1338–1339.

52. Borodic GE, Joseph M, Fay L, et al. Botulinum A toxin for the treatment of spasmodic torticollis: dysphagia and regional toxin spread. Head Neck 1990;12:392–399.

53. Comella CL, Tanner CM, DeFoor-Hill L, et al. Dysphagia after botulinum toxin injections for spasmodic torticollis: clinical and radiologic findings. Neurology 1992;42:1307–1310.

54. Buchman AS, Comella CL, Stebbins GT, et al. Determining a dose-effect curve for botulinum toxin in the sternocleidomastoid muscle in cervical dystonia. Clin Neuropharmacol 1994;17:188–195.

55. Jankovic J. Botulinum toxin: Clinical implications of antigenicity and immunoresistance. In: Brin MF, Hallett M, Jankovic J. Scientific and Therapeutic Aspects of Botulinum Toxin. Philadelphia: Lippincott Williams & Wilkins, 2002:409–416.

56. Jankovic J, Schwartz KS. Longitudinal experience with botulinum toxin injections for treatment of blepharospasm and cervical dystonia. Neurology 1993;43:834–836.

57. Hanna PA, Jankovic J. Mouse bioassay versus Western blot assay for botulinum toxin antibodies: correlation with clinical response. Neurology 1998;50:1624–1629.

58. Jankovic J, Vuong KD, Ahsan J. Comparison of efficacy and immunogenicity of original versus current botulinum toxin in cervical dystonia. Neurology 2003;60:1186–1188.

59. Brashear A, Bergan K, Wojcieszek J, et al. Patients' perception of stopping or continuing treatment of cervical dystonia with botulinum toxin type A. Mov Disord 2000;15:150–153.

60. Sloop RR, Cole D, Patel MC. Muscle paralysis produced by botulinum toxin type A injection in treated torticollis patients compared with toxin naive individuals. Mov Disord 2001;16:100–105.

61. Dubinsky RM, Gray CS, Vetere Overfield B, et al. Electromyographic guidance of botulinum toxin treatment in cervical dystonia. Clin Neuropharm 1991;14:262–267.

62. Gelb DJ, Yoshimura DM, Olney RK, et al. Change in pattern of muscle activity following botulinum toxin injections for torticollis. Ann Neurol 1991;29:370–376.

63. Brans JWM, Aramideh M, Koelman JHTM, et al. Electromyography in cervical dystonia. Changes after botulinum and trihexyphenidyl. Neurology 1998;51:815–819.

64. O'Brien CF. Injection techniques for botulinum toxin using electromyography and electrical stimulation. Eur J Neurol 1997;4(Suppl 2):S47-S51.

65. Comella CL, Buchman AS, Tanner CM, et al. Botulinum toxin injection for spasmodic torticollis: increased magnitude of benefit with electromyographic assistance. Neurology 1992;42:878–882.

66. Braun V, Richter HP. Selective peripheral denervation for the treatment of spasmodic torticollis. Neurosurgery 1994;35:58–62.

67. Krauss JK, Toops EG, Jankovic J, et al. Symptomatic and functional outcome of surgical treatment of cervical dystonia. J Neurol Neurosurg Psychiatry 1997;63:642–648.

68. Ford B, Louis ED, Greene P, et al. Outcome of selective ramisectomy for botulinum toxin resistant torticollis. J Neurol Neurosurg Psychiatry 1998;65:472–478.

69. Krauss JK, Grossman RG, Jankovic J. Treatment options for surgery of cervical dystonia. In: Krauss JK, Jankovic J, Grossman RG, eds. Surgery for Movement Disorders. Philadelphia: Lippincott Williams & Wilkins, 2001:323–334.

70. Sanghera M, Grossman RG, Kalhorn CG, et al. Basal ganglia neuronal discharge in primary and secondary dystonia in patients undergoing pallidotomy. Neurosurgery 2003;52:1358–1373.

71. Tronnier VM, Fogel W. Pallidal stimulation for generalized dystonia. Report of three cases. J Neurosurg 2000;92:453–456.

72. Coubes P, Roubertie A, Vayssiere N, et al. Treatment of *DYT1*-generalised dystonia by stimulation of the internal globus pallidus. Lancet 2000;355:2220–2221.

73. Krauss JK, Pohle T, Weber S, et al. Bilateral stimulation of globus pallidus internus for treatment of cervical dystonia. Lancet 1999;354: 837–838.

74. Kulisevsky J, Lleo A, Gironell A, et al. Bilateral pallidal stimulation for cervical dystonia: dissociated pain and motor improvement. Neurology 2000; 55:1754–1755.

75. Parkin S, Aziz T, Gregory R, Bain P. Bilateral internal globus pallidus stimulation for the treatment of spasmodic torticollis. Mov Disord 2001;16:489–493.

76. Münchau A, Mathen D, Cox T, et al. Unilateral lesions of the globus pallidus: report of four patients presenting with focal or segmental dystonia. J Neurol Neurosurg Psychiatry. 2000;69:494–498.

CHAPTER 14

Oromandibular Dystonia

Eng-King Tan

INTRODUCTION

Oromandibular dystonia (OMD) refers to spasms of the masticatory, facial, and lingual muscles. These spasms result in repetitive and, in some patients, sustained jaw opening (JO), jaw closure (JC), jaw deviation (JD), jaw retraction (JR), or any combination of the above.[1–3]

The sixteenth century Flemish artist Pieter Brueghel the Elder painted distorted faces simulating cranial dystonia and OMD. It is not known whether the subjects of these portraits actually had any medical or neurological problems responsible for facial distortions.[4] During 1871, Horatio C. Wood established the Department of Neurology at the University of Pennsylvania. It was the first such department in the United States and among the first to draw attention in the medical literature to blepharospasm and OMD.[2] In 1899, Gowers[5] described various conditions associated with tonic and clonic contractions of the neck and jaw. In 1910, the French neurologist Henry Meige[6] published his landmark paper on blepharospasm and OMD. Various authors have ascribed the eponyms of Meige, Wood, Brueghel, and Blake (an artist who painted dystonic postures), to describe this syndrome.[4] In 1976, Marsden suggested that blepharospasm-OMD syndrome could be a variant of adult-onset torsion dystonia.[7] Since that time, OMD is widely recognized as a form of segmental cranial dystonia.

The prevalence of OMD was estimated to be 68.9 cases per 1 million persons in an American population.[8] In a survey of two large movement disorders clinics in the United States, cranial dystonias (such as blepharospasm and OMD) were reported in approximately 25% of 8,000 patients with dystonia.[9]

CLINICAL FEATURES

OMD frequently affects women more than men. The mean age of symptom onset for OMD is between 50 and 60 years of age.[10,11] OMD manifests as JC, JO, JD, JR, or combinations of these movements, caused mostly by involvement of the muscles of mastication. JC-OMD is the most common subtype.[10,11] Other repetitive, or in some patients, sustained movements may also be present including contraction of the nasalis, facial grimacing, lip pursing, lip sucking, lip smacking, chewing, tongue protrusion or other tongue dyskinesias, retraction of the corners of the mouth, or platysma contractions. These involuntary movements may cause chewing difficulties, dysarthria, dysphagia, dysphonia, breathing difficulties, and involuntary vocalizations such as humming and grunting.[1–3,10] As with other forms of dystonias, various sensory tricks have been reported to relieve patients' symptoms. These include sleeping, relaxing, talking, singing or humming, or alcohol intake. Common exacerbating factors may be elicited from personal histories; these factors include experiencing emotional stress, looking into glaring light, watching television, driving, reading, and feeling fatigued.[12] In some patients, OMD may persist during sleep or be associated with a certain specific task, such as biting into hard food. Severe OMD, accompanied by functional disability, may lead to clinical depression.

In patients with JC-OMD, dystonic spasms of the temporalis and masseter muscles may result in clenching or trismus and grinding of the teeth or bruxism. Wooten-Watts et al.[13] studied 79 patients with cranial-cervical dystonia, most of whom had symptoms of OMD. These investigators found a substantially higher prevalence of bruxism (78.5%) in this particular patient population, compared to 100 healthy controls (21%). Approximately one-fourth of bruxism patients had associated dental problems including temporomandibular joint (TMJ) dysfunction (21%) and tooth wear (5%). OMD is frequently associated with dystonia or another movement disorder in a different body parts. In a study of 162 patients with OMD, Tan and Jankovic[10] found that 57.4% of the study population had associated cervical dys-

Eng-King Tan: Consultant Neurologist, Director, Parkinson's Disease and Movement Disorder Program, Principal Investigator, Neuroscience Laboratory, Department of Neurology, National Neuroscience Institute, Singapore General Hospital, Singapore, Republic of Singapore.

The author has no affiliation to disclose.

tonia; 50% had blepharospasm; 21% had limb dystonia; 16% had tremor; and 9.9% had spasmodic dysphonia (SD). In another study of 100 patients with cranio-cervical dystonia, blepharospasm was the most frequent presenting symptom.[12] However, most patients had both blepharospasm and OMD. Many authors have described similar findings.[1,11]

ETIOLOGY

As with most forms of dystonia, most patients with OMD belong to the idiopathic category. In the series of studies by Tan and Jankovic,[10] idiopathic OMD accounted for 63% of patients, followed by drug-induced OMD at 22.8%, peripherally induced OMD at 9.3%, postanoxia OMD at 2.5%, neurodegenerative disorder-associated OMD at 1.8%, and head injury-associated OMD at 0.8% of the patient population. Many other associated neurologic and medical disorders have been reported in patients with OMD, blepharospasm, or both. Postural tremor, phenomenologically similar to essential tremor and parkinsonism, has been reported with greater than otherwise expected frequency in patients with dystonia.[14] It is not clear, however, whether other disorders such as thyroid problems, palatal myoclonus, Tourette's syndrome, or various autoimmune or psychiatric disorders are pathophysiologically linked to dystonia.[1,11,12,15] In some patients, psychiatric symptoms may precede the onset of OMD symptoms; in others, psychiatric signs may occur after symptom onset of OMD. Therefore, these observed associations are likely to be coincidental and not related to the underlying etiology of OMD.[12]

Results from other studies concur with the findings of Tan and Jankovic[11] and also suggest that the most common secondary cause of OMD is tardive dystonia. Burke et al.[16] reported that most patients with tardive dystonia also had dystonic spasms involving the orofacial muscles. Haloperidol, metoclopramide, and thioridazine are the more common neuroleptics associated with tardive OMD.[17] In addition, anticholinergics, antihistamines, long-term amphetamine ingestion, and ecstasy have been reported to cause OMD.[1,18,19] Levodopa-induced blepharospasm and lower facial spasms may occur as a result of treatment with levodopa, particularly in patients with multiple system atrophy.[20] Orofacial spasms usually occur during the "on" periods; however, these spasms may improve in response to a reduction in the dose of levodopa. Cranial dystonia (including OMD) has been reported in patients with Parkinson's disease treated with implants of fetal substantia nigra, even in patients without levodopa treatment.[21]

Tardive OMD may have different clinical features than idiopathic OMD. In a comparative study of tardive and idiopathic OMD, a relatively higher number of patients with tardive OMD manifested stereotypical orofacial-lingual features, compared to patients with idiopathic OMD.[17] Patients with OMD who also experience akathisia, stereotypic movements in the limbs, or respiratory dyskinesias are strongly suggestive of prior neuroleptic exposure. Patients with tar-

dive OMD were more likely to have their dystonia confined to the oromandibular region as compared to patients with idiopathic OMD. Blepharospasm, cervical dystonia, and spasmodic dysphonia were more commonly associated with idiopathic OMD.[17]

Peripheral trauma has been implicated in various movement disorders.[22] Sutcher et al.[23] described four patients with JO-OMD that was presumably caused by ill-fitting dentures. Other investigators have also reported OMD after tooth extraction and oral surgery.[24] Sankhla et al.[24] described the largest series of 27 patients with peripherally induced OMD in whom the onset of symptoms was anatomically and temporally related to a prior face or mouth trauma. These patients had experienced traumatic injury, underwent oromandibular surgery, or received some form of dental procedure. Sankhla et al.[24] found that the severity of symptoms and progression of disease were more prominent in patients with peripherally induced OMD, however, these patients had less symptom spread to contiguous or noncontiguous segments compared to patients with idiopathic OMD.[24]

DIFFERENTIAL DIAGNOSIS

OMD takes many forms, such as JC, JO, JR, or JD. OMD also has varying grades of severity. Its full clinical spectrum may not be appreciated even by skilled neurologists.[25] OMD is frequently misdiagnosed as TMJ dysfunction and bruxism. Delay in appropriate treatment may lead to TMJ dislocation as well as other TMJ-related problems.[26,27] Emotional disturbance worsens OMD. In some patients, this may be a factor causing delayed diagnosis because in these patients, the symptoms may be considered as psychological in origin.

The issue of whether bruxism is a separate clinical entity from OMD is sometimes debated. One problem lies in the definition of bruxism. For example, the American Academy of Orofacial Pain defines bruxism as a diurnal or nocturnal parafunctional activity including clenching, grinding, bracing, and gnashing of the teeth.[28] This definition is too general and encompassing. Prevalence estimates regarding bruxism in adult populations vary from 5–96%.[29,30] However, while some patients with OMD clench and grind their teeth,[13] these patients appear differently from nocturnal bruxors, frequently seen in the general population.[31] Wooten-Watts et al.[13] demonstrated that the majority of OMD patients had diurnal bruxism, with symptoms disappearing during sleep. Only 13% of these patients had nocturnal bruxism. Severe diurnal bruxism is frequently associated with organic brain diseases, such as Huntington's disease and Rett syndrome.[32,33]

Temporomandibular disorder refers to a group of pain conditions in the craniofacial muscles, TMJ, and associated structures.[34] Patients with these conditions may present with masseter muscle spasms associated with clenching or grinding of teeth, and clicking and crepitus of the TMJ, which is obvious on examination. This group of conditions may also be associated with other medical conditions. For instance, most patients with fibromyalgia experience headaches, facial pain, and tired jaws; approximately 50% of these patients had difficulties chewing and opening their mouth.[35] Trauma and inflammatory disorders of the TMJ and masticatory muscles may lead to jaw clenching because of pain and muscle spasm.

Hemimasticatory spasm is characterized by involuntary paroxysmal JC secondary to unilateral spasm of the muscles of mastication.[36] It may be associated with hemifacial atrophy.[37] Hemifacial spasm (HFS) is a form of segmental myoclonus involving the facial muscles innervated by the ipsilateral facial nerve.[38,39] The muscle contractions are frequently clonic in nature, which distinguishes HFS from OMD. Magnetic resonance imaging demonstrates compression of the facial nerve at its root exit zone in most patients with HFS.[40] It may also be associated with other movement disorders such as tremor and spasmodic dysphonia.[38] Focal motor seizures involving the facial muscles are abrupt in onset and may become secondarily generalized. Tetanus may lead to trismus (jaw spasm), however, involvement of other body parts gives clues to the diagnosis. Similarly, tonic spasms of facial muscles in patients with multiple sclerosis are associated with limb dystonia and other neurological signs.[41,42]

GENETICS

A GAG deletion of the *DYT1* gene on chromosome 9q34 is responsible for most cases of early limb-onset primary torsion dystonia (PTD).[43] Valente et al.[44] studied the *DYT1* mutation in 150 patients with PTD and found 4 of 22 positive for the GAG deletion had limb-onset dystonia with spread to craniocervical muscles.[44] Waddy et al.[45] found 25% of index patients with focal dystonias, including OMD, had first-degree relatives with dystonia. In a case control study, Jankovic and Nutt[46] found that 36.5% of 238 patients with craniocervical dystonia reported at least one first- or second-degree relative affected by a movement disorder. This is in comparison to only 2% in the control group who reported relatives with a movement disorder.[46] Cranial dystonia has been reported in familial diseases such as Wilson's disease[47] and X-linked dystonia-parkinsonism syndrome.[48] Steinberger et al.[49] reported a mutation of the *GCH1* gene, the gene responsible for dopa-responsive dystonia, in a 49-year-old man with adult-onset OMD. This patient reported no family history of dystonia. This evidence supports a genetic predisposition in some patients with OMD.

TREATMENT

OMD, particularly JO dystonia, is the most challenging dystonia to treat. The integral components of management include pharmacologic therapy, including drugs and botulinum toxin as well as patient educational information and available support systems. Presently there is no specific surgery for OMD.

Supportive and Alternative Treatment

Certain sensory tricks may transiently improve the symptoms of OMD. For instance, touching the lips may relieve jaw spasm; touching the chin may aid in JC. Dental assessment may be helpful in patients who have associated TMJ dysfunction, or other dental complications such as tooth wear. Speech therapy may facilitate speech and help to relieve swallowing difficulties. Various forms of relaxation and biofeedback therapies are useful in patients whose symptoms are aggravated by stress or anxiety. Acupuncture is another alternative form of treatment; however, relief of symptoms such as pain, if any, is usually transient. Encouragement from family and relatives, as well as that received from support organizations and patient educational initiatives may also be helpful in the management of OMD.

Problems in Interpreting the Results of Therapeutic Trials

Before discussing drug treatment, it is important to highlight the various problems in interpreting results of therapeutic trials in OMD. For example:

1. There are no validated clinical ratings scales to assess disease severity and functional disability for OMD. This makes assessment of therapeutic efficacy difficult to interpret and comparison of results between different centers almost impossible.
2. There are few randomized placebo-controlled trials. Therefore, results may be subject to bias or influenced by the clinical experience of the investigators.
3. Most studies have been based on small sample sizes or single case reports. This increases the risk of type I and type II statistical errors.
4. Long-term follow-up results frequently not available.
5. Most studies do not distinguish between the various etiologic forms of OMD. These various forms may respond differently to treatment.
6. The most appropriate injection sites for treatment with botulinum toxin (BTX) has not been studied in comparative trial for the various subtypes of OMD.
7. The advantage of electromyographic (EMG) guidance and the varying techniques of BTX injection have not been evaluated in controlled trials.

Drug Treatment

The rationale for drug treatment is based on postulated biochemical changes in brains of patients with dystonia. Changes in norepinephrine, serotonin, and dopamine levels have been found in the brains of patients with childhood-onset generalized dystonia and adult-onset segmental cranial dystonia.[50,51] However, the results of drug trials in patients with OMD have been largely disappointing. Anticholinergics, benzodiazepines, and tetrabenazine, among others, generally have limited efficacy in OMD.[51–55] These drugs are frequently used as adjuncts to BTX treatment. Muscle afferent block by intramuscular injection of lidocaine and alcohol has been reported to be useful, but further experience and evaluation is needed to determine the long-term efficacy and benefit of afferent blockade.[56]

Botulinum Toxin Treatment

BTX, the most powerful biologic toxin known to man, exerts its function by preventing the docking of the acetylcholine vesicles in the presynaptic neuromuscular junction.[57] Seven antigenically distinct types (A, B, C, D, E , F, and G) have been recognized. Type A cleaves the plasma protein SNAP-25 and is the most commonly used type of BTX in OMD trials.[57] The unit of measurement for botulinum toxin type A (BTX-A; BOTOX, Allergan, Inc., Irvine, CA) is the mouse unit (MU). One MU is equivalent to the amount of toxin known to kill 50% (LD_{50}) of a group of 18–20 g female Swiss-Webster mice.

Many investigators have reported the effectiveness of BTX-A in relieving symptoms of OMD.[58–70] In 1987, Jankovic and Orman[58] conducted a double-blind, placebo-controlled trial. They found that 37.5% of a small series of OMD-cervical dystonia patients improved after BTX treatment. In an open-label design study, Blitzer et al.[59] demonstrated that BTX-A yielded a 50% improvement in 20 patients with OMD patients. Most of these patients had previously failed a variety of pharmacologic treatments. Subsequent reports of BTX-A in OMD patients involved small series of patients or single case descriptions.[62–70] However, experiences at Baylor College of Medicine and Columbia University College of Physicians and Surgeons, two major movement disorder centers in the United States, enable us to analyze the effectiveness of BTX in OMD better.[10,11] Many patients were studied at these centers. BTX has been demonstrated to improve quality of life in OMD.[71]

Selection of Muscles

The Therapeutics and Technology Assessment (TTA) Subcommittee of the American Academy of Neurology has suggested numerous training guidelines for the use of BTX for the treatment of neurologic disorders.[72] One guideline states: "Physicians administrating BTX should possess the required expertise which includes a comprehension of the diagnosis, differential diagnosis, diagnostic evaluation, and treatment options with their attendant value and risk, as well as skills in the management of complications." Clearly, detailed knowledge of the anatomy and function of the various muscles in the oromandibular region along with an awareness of the potential complications of treating OMD are vital.

Spasms of different muscles give rise to different subtypes of OMD. Therefore, the importance of understanding the function of the various muscles that move the different oromandibular parts is crucial. It is equally important to recognize which muscles are most severely affected. This may be

accomplished by clinical examination as well as with EMG guidance. The masseters, temporalis, and internal pterygoid muscles are responsible for jaw closing. The external pterygoid, digastric, genohyoid and mylohyoid muscles assist in opening the jaw. In addition, the external pterygoid deviates the jaw in the opposite direction. The genioglossus and hyoglossus muscles help the tongue protrude.

Clinical examination of different jaw movements and the muscle contractions in different positions helps to determine which muscles are involved. For JC-OMD, injections of BTX in the masseters and temporalis are carried out at two to three sites into these muscles. For JO-OMD, injections are administered to the submentalis complex, comprising the digastric, genohyoid, and mylohyoid muscles. This occurs at two to three sites in the complex, approximately 1–2 cm posterior to the tip of the mandible with the jaw opened. The lateral pterygoid muscle may also be injected with the jaw opened, and under EMG guidance. In some patients, antagonistic muscles may also be actively contracting due to compensatory spasm; therefore, injections of these muscles may also be useful. For example, injecting the submentalis complex along with the masseters and temporalis muscles may be more effective in some patients with long standing JC-OMD. The doses of BTX used depend on the clinical severity and weight of patient. In most patients, the doses may have to be titrated according to clinical response and any toxin-related complications after an initial modest dose.

THE ROLE OF ELECTROMYOGRAPHY

Most masticatory muscles may be palpated by hand, hence, some investigators argue that EMG guidance is unnecessary when treating OMD.[73] This may be particularly true with experienced injectors, when ascertainment of clinical severity of muscle spasms may be relatively easy. The digastric, genohyoid, and mylohyoid are thin-layered muscles and are closely sandwiched against each other. In jaw-opening dystonia involving these muscles, it is not easy to distinguish which muscle is the most involved, even with EMG guidance. Furthermore, there have been no controlled trials in patients with OMD that compare the relative efficacy of BTX injections using EMG guidance versus clinical palpation in OMD.

However, there is a role for EMG guidance in OMD when injecting muscles such as the pterygoids, which cannot be palpated with ease. EMG may also help to localize regions of active muscle contractions in situations where the exact location of these contractions is in doubt. This situation may arise in patients who have areas of muscle wasting after repeated injections. Lastly, the use of EMG guidance to localize specific muscles may also depend on the individual injector's preference, comfort level, and skill.

RATING SCALES

Various self-rating scales have been used to assess function and degree of improvement after treatment. The Co-

TABLE 14-1. *Columbia's Global Clinical Rating Scales*

Disability Rating Scale
0 = Normal
1 = Mild discomfort or functional impairment
2 = Mild to moderate discomfort or functional impairment
3 = Moderate discomfort or functional impairment
4 = Moderate to severe discomfort or functional
    impairment
5 = Severe discomfort or functional impairment
6 = Completely disabled or incapacitated
Percentage of Normal Function Rating Scale
0% = Fully disabled, no useful function
100% = Normal

lumbia group utilized two rating scales; the Columbia University Scale, a six-point, disability ratings scale (Table 14-1); and a Global Clinical Rating Scale, a linear, self-rating scale where patients rate their function from 0% or fully disabled and no functional activity to 100% or normal function.[11]

The Baylor group used a zero- to four-point scale in which zero represented no spasm and four denoted severe incapacitating spasm (Table 14-2).[10] This group also used a peak-effect scale, where the effect was defined as the maximal benefit obtained from the injection. It was rated on a zero to four scale, where zero represented no effects and four denoted marked improvement in severity and function (Table 14-2). The rating was determined after a careful review of the patient's daily diary (a self-assessment of dystonia severity), interview of spouses and friends, and patient's own perception of response. Patients were instructed to keep the daily diary for the duration of treatment. When their response to treatment had stabilized, patients were then instructed to keep a weekly or fortnightly dairy. In those cases where there was disagreement between the self-report scores and the patient and family members, the lower score was

TABLE 14-2. *Baylor Rating Scales*

Dystonia scale
0 = No spasm
1 = Mild, barely noticeable
2 = Mild, without functional impairment
3 = Moderate spasm, moderate functional impairment
4 = Severe incapacitating spasm
Peak effect rating scale
0 = No effect
1 = Mild improvement
2 = Moderate improvement, but no change in function
3 = Moderate improvement in severity and function
4 = Marked improvement in severity and function
Global rating scale
    Peak rating score minus one point if the injection is
    associated with mild to moderate complications, and
    minus two points if associated with severe or disabling
    complications.

taken. Patients were also instructed to note any adverse events such as dysphagia or dysarthria and the duration and severity of these adverse events.

The Baylor group also used a global rating scale, which was defined as the peak score minus one point if the injection was associated with mild or moderate complications or minus two points if the injection was associated with severe or disabling complications. Validated, quantitative scales that measure degree and force of jaw closing or opening and extent of swallowing, speech, and dental abnormalities are not available. However, the rating scales discussed above do provide an indication of patients' functional disability.

RESULTS OF CLINICAL TRIALS

BOTOX was used in the two largest studies of OMD.[10,11] The conversion ratio of BOTOX and Dysport (Ipsen, Ltd., Maidenhead, Berks, United Kingdom) is approximately 1:3–1:4.[74,75] In the Baylor prospective study, which was conducted over a 10-year period, 162 of 202 patients with satisfied the inclusion criteria for analysis.[10] The inclusion criteria were as follows:

1. Dystonia causing involuntary contractions of orolingual-masticatory muscles. These contractions interfered with swallowing, speech, or chewing;
2. History of failed pharmacological therapies; and
3. BTX injection with at least one follow-up evaluation in the Baylor Clinic.

Fifty percent of the patients that were excluded were either not treated with BTX or were awaiting follow-up. The remaining patients opted for follow-up at other centers or they defaulted.

The mean age of the 162 patients was 57.9 ± 15.3 years, with an age range of 12–86 years. Of the 162 patients, 111 or 68.5% were women. The mean duration of symptoms was 9.6 ± 9.4 years with a range of 0.5–54 years. The mean follow-up period was 4.4 ± 3.8 years with a range of 0.3–10 years. In 1,213 treatment visits, the masseter muscles were injected with BTX 935 times on the right side and 934 times on the left side. Additionally, 660 injections were administered into the submentalis complex. The mean dose of BOTOX in the masseter muscles was twice the dose administered into the submentalis complex (i.e., 54.2 ± 15.2 versus 28.6 ± 16.7 units) (Table 14-3A). In this study group, 110 patients (67.9%) had a global rating of ≥ 3 (Table 14-3B). The mean time interval between BTX treatments was 5.9 ± 5.6 months, with a range of 1.5–60 months. A relatively higher number of patients with JC dystonia reported functional improvement (global rating ≥ 3) compared to JO and mixed dystonias.

Although 51 patients (31.5%) reported adverse effects with BTX on at least one treatment visit, only 135 (11.1%) of all treatment visits were complicated by some adverse effects (Table 14-3C). The most common complications included dysarthria (44 patients/124 visits) and dysphagia (7

TABLE 14-3A. *Doses of Botulinum Toxin A (BOTOX)*

Study	Muscle	Number of patients/ injections	Mean dose (units)	Range (units)
Baylor study	Masseter	135/1869	54.2 + 15.2	25–100
	Submentalis complex (digastric, genohyoid, mylohyoid)	118/660	28.6 + 16.7	10–200
			(median)	
Columbia study	Masseter	Data not available	24.5 + 17.7	2–100
	Temporalis		18.5 + 11.9	2–75
	Medial pterygoid		16.3 + 8.1	5–40
	Lateral pterygoid		15.9 + 8.7	1.5–60
	Anterior digastric		9.8 + 4.6	3.8–30

BOTOX, Allergan, Inc., Irvine, CA.

patients/11 visits). Patients categorized as JO and mixed OMD had substantially higher complication rates. BTX response of secondary OMD, such as tardive and peripherally induced OMD, appeared to be similar to that of patients with idiopathic OMD.[16]

The Columbia group studied 96 patients.[11] Of these patients, 72.9% were women, with mean age of symptom onset of 43.9 years ± 2.0 years. Median doses of BOTOX given for the jaw muscles were: masseter, 24.5; temporalis, 18.5; medial pterygoid 16.3; lateral pterygoid 15.9; and anterior digastric 9.8 units (Table 14-3A). The percentage improvement after BTX were: JC, 45%; JO, 43.9%; and JD, 37.0% (Table 14-3B). The percentage visits with adverse effects were: JC, 4.1%; JO, 9.9%; and JD, 0% (Table 14-3C). Dysphagia was the most common complaint in 13 or 40% of patients with JO-OMD, however, in patients with JC-OMD some complaints included weakened chewing, soreness and pain at injection site, facial swelling, and headache.

The different methodology and evaluation of results in the two studies make it difficult to make a comparison. However, several conclusions may be drawn:

1. BTX is an effective treatment for patients with OMD. Functional improvement, particularly with chewing and swallowing, may be seen in most OMD patients after BTX. JC-OMD tends to respond better than the other OMD subtypes.

2. BTX is generally safe for use in OMD. Adverse effects may be seen in 7–11% of treatment visits. Patients with JO and mixed OMD tend to have a relatively higher percentage of adverse events than those with JC-OMD. Dysphagia, which was the most common complaint particularly in JO-OMD, may be expected in approximately 10% of treatment visits. However, a change of diet is required in less than 1% of the visits.

2. BTX can be an effective long-term treatment for OMD, with efficacy seen up to 30 treatment visits (or over 10 years) in some patients.

3. BTX is effective when administered at 3–4 month intervals. There is no need for booster injections within 2–4 weeks after the initial treatment.

4. JO-OMD may be effectively treated by injecting the genohyoid, digastric, and mylohyoid muscles or, in addition, by injecting the lateral pterygoid muscle.

5. JC-OMD may be effectively treated by injecting the masseters alone or in combination with the temporalis muscle.

Although the two studies were large and prospective, caution is needed in interpreting the results because of their open-label design. However, most OMD patients in the Baylor study continued to report benefit from BTX after many treatment

TABLE 14-3B. *Results of Clinical Trials*

Study	Number of patients	Gender	Treatment visits	Functional improvement after BTX	Duration of benefit
Baylor study	162	68.5% females	1213	Functional improvement seen in 67.9% of patients. Mean global rating scores: JC at 3.2; JO at 2.9; JD at 2.5; mixed OMD at 2.8	Approximately 13 weeks
Columbia study	96	72.9% females	481	Patients reported 37% to 45% functional improvement: JC at 45%; JO at 43.9%; JD at 37%	Approximately 13 weeks

BTX, botulinum toxin; JC, jaw closure; JO, jaw opening; JD, jaw deviation; OMD, oromandibular dystonia.

TABLE 14-3C. *Complications of Treatment*

Study	Type of OMD	Number	Patients with adverse effects	Visits with adverse effects	Total number of treatment visits
Combined Baylor and	JC	136	22 (16.1%)	47 (5.5%)	852
Columbia series	JO	75	21 (28.0%)	57 (13.3%)	426
Total number = 258 patients	JD	8	1 (12.5%)	3 (1.1%)	27
	Mixed	39	16 (41%)	55 (14.1%)	389

OMD, oromandibular dystonia; JC, jaw closure; JO, jaw opening; JD, jaw dystonia.

visits and over a long period. This suggests that the placebo effect may not be a major confounding factor in the assessment of this patient population. Development of a quantitative rating scale to assess OMD severity, level of patient functionality, controlled trials to address the most appropriate muscles to inject for the various OMD subtypes, and the benefit of EMG guidance will be useful. However, these may not be easily achieved because of the wide and varied clinical spectrum and etiology of the disease. Ultimately, the physician's skill and experience in administrating BTX play a vital role in the clinical outcome for individual patients. A multidisciplinary team comprising the neurologist, dental surgeon, otolaryngologist, speech therapist, and supporting family members are necessary to successfully manage OMD and its related complications. Functional neurosurgery, such as pallidotomy and pallidal stimulation, has been reported to be effective in generalized dystonia.[76,77] Future trials looking at potential surgical targets will hopefully increase the armamentarium for treating this disabling form of dystonia.

ACKNOWLEDGEMENT

The author thanks Dr. Joseph Jankovic, Director of the Parkinson's Disease and Movement Disorder Clinic, Baylor College of Medicine, Houston, Texas.

REFERENCES

1. Tolosa E, Marti MJ. Blepharospasm-oromandibular dystonia (Meige's syndrome): clinical aspects. Adv Neurol 1988;49:73–84.
2. Jankovic J. Etiology and differential diagnosis of blepharospasm and oromandibular dystonia. Adv Neurol 1988;49:103–116.
3. Cardoso F, Jankovic J. Oromandibular dystonia. In: Tsui JK, Calne DB, eds. Handbook of Dystonia. New York: Marcel Dekker, 1995:181–190.
4. Parkes D, Schachter M. Meige, Brueghel or Blake. Neurology 1981;31:498.
5. Gowers WR. Manual of Diseases of Nervous System. London: Churchill, 1899:200.
6. Meige H. Les convulsions de la face: une forme clinique de convulsions faciales, bilaterale et mediane. Rev Neurol (Paris) 1910;21:437–443.
7. Marsden CD. Blepharospasm-oromandibular dystonia syndrome (Brueghel's syndrome): a variant of adult-onset torsion dystonia? J Neurol Neurosurg Psychiatry 1976;59:1204–1209.
8. Nutt JG, Muenter MD, Aronson A, et al. Epidemiology of focal and generalized dystonia in Rochester, Minnesota. Mov Disord 1988; 3:188–194.
9. Jankovic J, Fahn S. Dystonic disorders. In: Jankovic J, Tolosa E, eds. Parkinson's Disease and Movement Disorders. 3rd ed. Baltimore: Williams and Wilkins, 1998:513–551.
10. Tan EK, Jankovic J. Botulinum toxin A in patients with oromandibular dystonia: long-term follow-up. Neurology 1999;53:2102–2108.
11. Brin MF, Blitzer A, Herman S, et al. Oromandibular dystonia: treatment of 96 patients with botulinum toxin A. In: Jankovic J, Hallett M, eds: Therapy with Botulinum Toxin. New York: Marcel Dekker, 1994:429–435.
12. Jankovic J, Ford J. Blepharospasm and orofacial-cervical dystonia: clinical and pharmacological findings in 100 patients. Ann Neurol 1983;13:402–411.
13. Wooten-Watts M, Tan EK, Jankovic J. Bruxism and cranio-cervical dystonia: is there a relationship? Cranio 1999;17:196–201.
14. Jankovic J. Essential tremor: a heterogeneous disorder. Mov Disord 2002;17:638–644.
15. Morrison PJ, Patterson VH. Cranial dystonia (Meige syndrome) in postencephalitic parkinsonism. Mov Disord 1992;7:90–91.
16. Burke RE, Fahn S, Jankovic J, et al. Tardive dystonia: late-onset and persistent dystonia caused by antipsychotic drugs. Neurology 1982; 32:1335–1346.
17. Tan EK, Jankovic J. Tardive and idiopathic oromandibular dystonia: a clinical comparison. J Neurol Neurosurg Psychiatry 2000;68:186–190.
18. Jankovic J. Drug induced and other orofacial-cervical dyskinesias. Ann Intern Med 1981;94:788–793.
19. Powers JM. Decongestant-induced blepharospasm and orofacial dystonia. JAMA 1982;247:3244–3255.
20. Weiner WJ, Nausieda P. Meige's syndrome during long-term dopaminergic therapy in Parkinson's disease. Arch Neurol 1982;39:451–452.
21. Freed CR, Greene PE, Breeze RE, et al. Transplantation of embryonic dopamine neurons for severe Parkinson's disease. N Engl J Med 2001;344:710–719.
22. Jankovic J. Can peripheral trauma induce dystonia and other movement disorders? Yes! Mov Disord 2001;16:7–12.
23. Sutcher HD, Underwood RB, Beatty RA, et al. Orofacial dyskinesia: a dental dimension. JAMA 1971;216:1459–1463.
24. Sankhla C, Lai EC, Jankovic J. Peripherally induced oromandibular dystonia. J Neurol Neurosurg Psychiatry 1998;65:722–728.
25. Defazio G, Lapore V, Abbruzzese G, et al. Reliability among neurologists in the severity assessment of blepharospasm and oromandibular dystonia: a multicenter study. Mov Disord. 1994;9:616–621.
26. Gray AR, Barker GR. Idiopathic blepharospasm-oromandibular dystonia syndrome (Meige's syndrome) presenting as chronic temporomandibular joint dysfunction. Br J Oral Maxillofac Surg 1991; 29:97–99.
27. Verma RK, Gupta BK, Kochar SK, et al. Meige's syndrome. J Assoc Physicians India 1993;41:173–174.
28. McNeil C. Temporomandibular Disorders: Guidelines for Classification, Assessment, and Management. Chicago: The American Academy of Orofacial Pain, Quintessence, 1993.
29. Tan EK, Jankovic J. Treatment of severe bruxism with botulinum toxin. Am J Dent Assoc 2000;131:211–216.
30. Thompson BA, Blount BW, Krumholz TS. Treatment approaches to bruxism. Am Fam Physician 1994;49:1617–1622.
31. Rugh JD, Harlan JA. Nocturnal bruxism and temporomandibular disorders. Adv Neurol 1988;49:329–341.
32. Tan EK, Jankovic J, Ondo W. Bruxing behavior in Huntington's disease. Mov Disord 2000;15:171–173.
33. FitzGerald PM, Jankovic J, Percy AK. Rett Syndrome and associated movement disorders. Mov Disord 1990;5:195–202.
34. Blank LW. Clinical guidelines for managing mandibular dysfunction. Gen Dent 1998;46:592–597.
35. Hedenberg-Magnusson B, Ernberg M, Kopp S. Presence of orofacial pain and temporomandibular disorder in fibromyalgia. Swed Dent J 1999;23:185–192.

36. Thompson PD, Carroll WM. Hemimasticatory spasm: a peripheral paroxysmal cranial neuropathy. J Neurol Neurosurg Psychiatry 1986; 49:651–656.
37. Kaufman MD. Masticatory spasm in facial hemiatrophy. Ann Neurol 1980;7:585–587.
38. Wang A, Jankovic J. Hemifacial spasm: clinical features and treatment. Muscle Nerve 1998;21:1740–1747.
39. Tan EK, Jankovic J. Bilateral hemifacial spasm: a report of five cases and a literature review. Mov Disord 1999;14:345–349.
40. Tan EK, Chan LL, Lim SH, et al. Role of magnetic resonance imaging and magnetic resonance angiography in patients with hemifacial spasm. Ann Acad Med Singapore 1999;28:169–173.
41. Thompson PD, Obeso JA, Delgado G, et al. Focal dystonia of the jaw and the differential diagnosis of unilateral jaw and masticatory spasm. J Neurol Neurosurg Psychiatry 1986;49:651–656.
42. Berger JR, Sheremata WA, Melamed MD. Paroxysmal dystonia as the initial manifestation of multiple sclerosis. Arch Neurol 1984;41: 747–750.
43. Ozelius L, Kramer PL, Moskowitz CB, et al. Human gene for torsion dystonia located on chromosome 9q32–34. Neuron 1989;2:1427–1434.
44. Valente EM, Warner TT, Jarman PR, et al. The role of *DYT1* in primary torsion dystonia in Europe. Brain 1998;121:2335–2339.
45. Waddy HM, Fletcher NA, Harding AE, et al. A genetic study of idiopathic focal dystonias. Ann Neurol 1991;29:320–324.
46. Jankovic J, Nutt JG. Blepharospasm and cranial-cervical dystonia (Meige's syndrome): familial occurrence. Adv Neurol 1988;49: 117–123.
47. Walshe JM, Yealland M. Wilson's disease: the problem of delayed diagnosis. J Neurol Neurosurg Psychiatry 1992;55:692.
48. Lee LV, Kupke KG, Caballar-Gonzaga F, et al. The phenotype of the X-linked dystonia-parkinsonism syndrome. An assessment of 42 cases in the Philippines. Medicine 1991;70:1791–1787.
49. Steinberger D, Topka H, Fischer D, et al. *GCH1* mutation in a patient with adult-onset oromandibular dystonia. Neurology 1999;52: 877–879.
50. Hornykiewicz O, Kish SJ, Becker LE, et al. Brain neurotransmitters in dystonia musculorum deformans. N Engl J Med 1986;315:347–353.
51. Jankovic J, Svendsen CN, Bird ED. Brain neurotransmitters in dystonia. N Engl J Med 1987;316:278–279.
52. Greene P, Shale H, Fahn S. Analysis of open-label trials in torsion dystonia using high dosages of anticholinergics and other drugs. Mov Disord 1988;33:46–60.
53. Klawans HL, Tanner CM. Cholinergic pharmacology of blepharospasm with oromandibular dystonia (Meige's syndrome). Adv Neurol 1988; 49:443–449.
54. Gimenez Roldan S, Mateo D, Orbe M, et al. Acute pharmacologic tests in cranial dystonia. Adv Neurol 1988;49:451–465.
55. Jankovic J, Orman J. Tetrabenazine therapy of dystonia, chorea, tics, and other dyskinesias. Neurology 1988;38:391–394.
56. Yoshida K, Kaji R, Kubori T, et al. Muscle afferent block for the treatment of oromandibular dystonia. Mov Disord 1998;13:699–705.
57. Jankovic J, Brin F. Therapeutic uses of botulinum toxins. N Engl J Med 1991;324:1185–1194.
58. Jankovic J, Orman J. Botulinum A toxin for cranial-cervical dystonia: a double blind, placebo-controlled study. Neurology 1987;37:616–623.
59. Blitzer A, Greene PE, Brin MF, et al. Botulinum toxin for treatment of oromandibular dystonia. Ann Otol Rhinol Laryngol 1989;98:93–97.
60. Brin MF, Fahn S, Moskowitz C, et al. Localized injections of botulinum toxin for the treatment of focal dystonia and hemifacial spasm. Mov Disord 1987;2:237–254.
61. Maurri S, Brogelli S, Alfieri G, et al. Use of botulinum toxin in Meige's disease. Riv Neurol 1988;58:245–248.
62. Jankovic J, Schwartz K, Donovan DT. Botulinum toxin treatment of cranial-cervical dystonia, spasmodic dysphonia, other focal dystonias and hemifacial spasm. J Neurol Neurosurg Psychiatry 1990;53:633–639.
63. Hermanowicz N, Truong DD. Treatment of oromandibular dystonia with botulinum toxin. Laryngoscope 1991;101:1216–1218.
64. Berardelli A, Formica A, Mercuri B, et al. Botulinum toxin treatment in patients with focal dystonia and hemifacial spasm. A multicenter study of the Italian Movement Disorder Group. Ital J Neurol Sci 1993;14:361–367.
65. Behari M, Singh KK, Seshadri S, et al. Botulinum toxin A in blepharospasm and hemifacial spasm. J Assoc Physicians India 1994; 42:205–208.
66. Van den Bergh P, Francart J, Mourin S, et al. Five-year experience in the treatment of focal movement disorders with low-dose Dysport botulinum toxin. Muscle Nerve 1995;18:720–729.
67. Poungvarin N, Devahastin V, Chaisevikul R, et al. Botulinum A toxin treatment for blepharospasm and Meige syndrome: report of 100 patients. J Med Assoc Thai 1997;80:1–8.
68. Mauriello JA Jr, Dhillon S, Leone T, et al. Treatment selections of 239 patients with blepharospasm and Meige syndrome over 11 years. Br J Ophthalmol 1996;80:1073–1076.
69. Heise GJ, Mullen MP. Oromandibular dystonia treated with botulinum toxin: report of case. J Oral Maxillofac Surg 1995;53:332–335; 335–337.
70. Charles PD, Davis TL, Shannon KM, et al. Tongue protrusion dystonia: treatment with botulinum toxin. South Med J 1997;90:522–525.
71. Bhattacharyya N, Tarsy D. Impact on quality of life of botulinum toxin treatments for spasmodic dysphonia and oromandibular dystonia. Arch Otolaryngol Head Neck Surg 2001;127:389–392.
72. Assessment: the clinical usefulness of botulinum toxin-A in treating neurologic disorders. Report of the Therapeutics and Technology assessment Subcommittee of the American Academy of Neurology. Neurology 1990;40:1332–1336.
73. Jankovic J. Needle EMG guidance is rarely required. Muscle Nerve 2001;24:1568–1570.
74. Odergren T, Hjaltason H, Kaakkola S, et al. A double blind, randomised, parallel group study to investigate the dose equivalence of Dysport and Botox in the treatment of cervical dystonia. J Neurol Neurosurg Psychiatry 1998;64:6–12.
75. Sampaio C, Ferreira JJ, Simoes F, et al. DYSBOT: a single-blind, randomized parallel study to determine whether any differences can be detected in the efficacy and tolerability of two formulations of botulinum toxin type A—Dysport and Botox—assuming a ratio of 4:1. Mov Disord 1997;12:1013–1018.
76. Ondo WG, Desaloms JM, Jankovic J, et al. Pallidotomy for generalized dystonia. Mov Disord 1998;13:693–698.
77. Tronnier VM, Fogel W. Pallidal stimulation for generalized dystonia: report of three cases. J Neurosurg 2000;92:453–456.

CHAPTER 15

Laryngeal Dystonia

Jean Verheyden and Andrew Blitzer

LARYNGEAL ANATOMY

The major structures that provide the framework for the larynx are the hyoid bone, thyroid cartilage, cricoid cartilage, and arytenoid cartilages. The hyoid bone is a crescent-shaped bone located at the anterior, superior portion of the neck. It does not articulate with other bones or cartilages, however, its muscular attachments help suspend the larynx, facilitating the production of the larynx's vertical movements. The thyroid cartilage is a shield-shaped cartilage in the anterior aspect of the larynx. It is positioned inferior to the hyoid bone and provides the main support and protection for the glottis, which lies dorsally to the thyroid cartilage. The cricoid cartilage is a signet-ring-shaped cartilage that articulates at the inferior-posterior aspect of the thyroid cartilage. The cricothyroid membrane spans the inferior border of the thyroid cartilage and the superior border of the cricoid cartilage at the anterior aspect of the larynx. This membrane is easily palpable and serves as an important landmark in accessing the internal glottic musculature. The arytenoid cartilages, which are pyramidal-shaped structures, articulate in multiple vectors with the posterior superior aspect of the cricoid cartilage. The anterior prominence is the vocal process from which the vibratory aspects of the larynx are attached. The posterior prominence is the muscular process to which the majority of the muscles that move the vocal folds are attached.

The paired thyroarytenoid muscles lie between the vocal process of the arytenoid to the thyroid cartilage. The vocalis muscle is the deep portion of the thyroarytenoid muscle. These muscles adduct as well as shorten and tense the vocal folds. Adduction of these muscles changes the mass of the vocal cords, which are then able to alter the vibratory characteristics of the overlying mucosa. The paired lateral cricoarytenoid muscles lie posterior, lateral, and inferior to the thyroarytenoid muscles by inserting to the muscular process of the arytenoid cartilage and attaching to the cricoid cartilage. These muscles are also adductors, however, they are able to increase the length of the vocal folds.

Each posterior cricoarytenoid muscle inserts on the muscular process of the arytenoid cartilage and arises from the posterior surface of the cricoid cartilage. This muscle is innervated by the recurrent laryngeal nerve and is considered an intrinsic laryngeal muscle.

LARYNGEAL DYSTONIA

Spasmodic dysphonia (SD), a focal laryngeal dystonia, is a chronic neurologic disorder of central motor processing. SD is characterized by action-induced spasms of the vocal folds. The vocal folds are typically normal-appearing at rest, however, with an action-induced, task-specific movement, the muscles contract inappropriately, causing abnormal movements and muscle spasms. This typically leads to dysphonia during speaking.[1–4]

Historically, SD was considered a disorder of uncertain origin that was thought to be psychogenic in origin. This perception was fueled by the finding that patients often use sensory tricks, such as yawning or laughing when beginning to speak, to ameliorate the abnormal movements. Patients also reported that they were worse under emotional stress and often better on awakening in the morning or after having an alcoholic beverage. Many patients may laugh and sing in a normal manner. Patients are generally worse when speaking on the telephone.[2,5]

In 1871, Traube[6] coined the term "spastic dysphonia" when describing a patient with nervous hoarseness. The condition has been described as though the patient were "trying to talk whilst being choked"[7] or "stuttering with the vocal cords."[8]

Jean Verheyden: New York Center for Voice and Swallowing Disorders, St. Luke's-Roosevelt Hospital Center, New York, New York.

Andrew Blitzer: New York Center for Voice and Swallowing Disorders, St. Luke's-Roosevelt Hospital Center, New York, New York.

Disclosure Statements :

Dr. Jean Verheyden has nothing to disclose.

Dr. Andrew Blitzer receives research funding from Allergan and Elan, and is a consultant to Allergan.

Aronson et al.[9,10] documented that the Minnesota Multiphasic Personality Index (MMPI) and psychiatric interviews did not discriminate between patients with SD and those in the normal population, however, many patients were still referred to psychiatrists for treatment as the correct diagnosis was not made when the patient initially presented for treatment.

Several lines of evidence have supported the notion that SD is a form of dystonia. Fraenkel[11,12] and Gowers[13] compared the involuntary movements in SD to those of other dystonias. However, in the earlier works, a psychogenic etiology was proposed.[14] Nevertheless, SD has been compared to other dystonias, such as occupational writer's cramp[11,12] and oromandibular dystonia.[15] Jacome and Yanez[16] associated SD with Meige's disease, or segmental-cranial dystonia; other authors subsequently concurred.[1,17,18] In 1982, Marsden and Sheehy[17] stated that the body of evidence points to the conclusion that blepharospasm and oromandibular dystonia as seen in Meige's disease is another manifestation of adult-onset torsion dystonia. They further stated that dysphonia may occur in the same syndrome and dysphonia itself may be the only manifestation of dystonia. Investigators also noted that many of the phenomenological, clinical, and laboratory features of patients with focal SD were similar to the dysphonia found in many patients with focal, segmental, and more generalized disease.[1] Clinical examination and electromyographic (EMG)[19] characteristics led investigators to the conclusion that most patients with dysphonia that had been clinically diagnosed as SD actually had focal forms of cranial dystonia. Investigators recommended the term spasmodic dysphonia or focal laryngeal dystonia rather than spastic dysphonia, particularly in view of the absence of classic spastic or corticospinal signs in patients affected with the disorder.

Laryngeal dystonia presents in several forms, classified as:

- Adductor SD;
- Abductor SD;
- Adductor breathing laryngeal dystonia, and
- A combination of these forms.

Other laryngeal movement disorders that affect speech and swallowing are also discussed.

In a review of the authors' patients with dystonia (*n* = 1,448),[5] 901 patients (62%) had vocal involvement. Of these 901 patients, 744 (82.5%) had primary dystonia and 157 (17.5%) had secondary dystonia. Four hundred seventy-one patients (63%) in the primary group were women. This is similar to the female percentage (63.5%) seen in the group of all dystonias. The representation of patients with Jewish ancestry was also similar, with 20.4% in primary laryngeal dystonia and 27.8% in primary all dystonias. A positive family history was found in 12% of the patients with laryngeal dystonia.

In the group of 901 patients with laryngeal dystonia, there were 747 patients (82%) with adductor-type dysphonia and 154 (17%) patients with abductor-type dystonia. Twelve patients (1%) had adductor-breathing dystonia. The overall average age at symptom onset was 39 years.

The authors have previously reported on two other variations of presentation, including compensatory abductor dysphonia, which is found in the group of adductors that produce a breathy voice. Whispering or not contracting the vocal folds prevents spasms and broken speech patterns, thereby producing a breathy voice. The other variation is compensatory adductor dysphonia, which is a rarer entity. In this form of presentation, patients with abductor dysphonia attempt to prevent breathiness by beginning to speak with their vocal folds tightly contracted.[1–3] Cannito and Johnson[20] proposed that both adductor and abductor abnormalities exist in all patients and the symptoms depend on whether there is a preponderance of adductor or abductor activity.

Many patients also present with associated tremor. The tremor activity found in patients with SD had been described by Aronson et al.[9,10] These investigators found that the tremor was similar to that found in patients with essential tremor. They also reported that several patients had synchronous pharyngeal, lingual, velar, mandibular, facial, thoracic, and diaphragmatic tremor. Ludlow et al.[21] also observed a vocal tremor that affected amplitude; they published a paper regarding a possible link between tremor and SD. Other authors have also documented the phonatory tremor characteristics of SD.[1,22,23]

Many patients with SD present with a tremulous voice; therefore, the differential diagnosis between spasmodic vocal breaks caused by essential tremor and those caused by a dystonic tremor may be challenging. In general, dystonic tremors are irregular and have a directional preponderance; symptoms are increased when the patient postures the affected body part in a position opposed to the primary dystonic contractions. For instance, patients with torticollis often have a head tremor that may be damped by placing the head into the "preferred posture." Many patients with SD have an irregular vocal tremor that may be recorded acoustically, electromyographically,[19] and with accelerometry. Acoustic evaluation and tremor physiology evaluation may be useful in making the proper diagnosis. The clinical distinction between primary dystonia causing the tremor, and the condition of essential tremor, may be difficult in many patients, particularly when patients present with symptoms of essential tremor in other body parts.[24,25] Discriminating between tremulousness caused by essential tremor or dystonia is particularly difficult when studying voice. For example, the laryngeal muscles of phonation, as a whole, are never available for study at complete rest; one or more muscle is contracting at a given moment due to respiratory actions, and in the presence of dystonia, laryngeal muscles cannot twist or turn; the glottic muscles can only adduct or abduct in some inappropriate fashion, including the speed and rhythmicity of tremor, or myoclonus.

Patients with vocal essential tremor may have breaks and hesitations in their speech pattern. This finding is most likely the result of either hyperadduction or hyperabduction of the vocal folds that occurs during contextual speech or phonatory tasks. Lingual tremor may also contribute to a choppy speech pattern; the tongue base beats up against the posterior pharyngeal wall and interrupts the flow of air. The authors found that asking patients to speak or perform tasks in a whisper is often useful because there is less muscle activation. A subtle tremor may then become discernable.

It is arguable that if tremor, which is characteristic of essential tremor, was present in other body parts, then the laryngeal movement disorder should be classified as essential tremor and not SD caused by dystonia. This is not always the case, as in limb tremor. It is not uncommon to find limb tremor, which has the clinical characteristics of essential tremor, in patients with dystonia.[24,25] Some patients with isolated phonatory tremor with strain-strangle speech may initially be misdiagnosed and sometimes later correctly characterized.[26] A greater understanding of the pathophysiology of tremor, coupled with genetic studies may be required to make an absolute distinction.

All patients who present with dysphonia who are thought to possibly have a dystonia should have a detailed neurologic examination. This comprehensive neurologic examination should include examining patients while they perform postures and tasks to elicit the signs of dystonia. To confirm the diagnosis of the laryngeal movement disorder, patients should undergo detailed otolaryngologic and speech-language assessments. Video and voice recordings are often obtained before treatment. Fiber optic laryngoscopy is performed on every patient to evaluate for the presence of anatomic abnormalities and record abnormal vocal cord motion during connected speech and other gestures. Phonatory characteristics are documented using the Unified Spasmodic Dysphonia Rating Scale.[27]

Flexible laryngeal endoscopy is used to document and characterize laryngeal hyperfunction. Under endoscopic visualization, patients are instructed to say /i/ and perform specific vocal tasks. Spasms, hyperadduction, and disruptions may be seen during connected speech segments. Hyperadduction may be further classified into four types.[5] This classification range includes:

- Type I or forceful overcontraction of the vocal folds, with compression of the vocal process and arytenoids (Fig. 15-1);
- Type II or closure of the true and false vocal folds (Fig. 15-2);
- Type III or anterior pull of the arytenoids and aryepiglottic folds to the petiole of the epiglottis (Fig. 15-3); and
- Type IV or sphincteric closure of the glottis and supraglottis with the arytenoids tightly closed against the epiglottis (Fig. 15-4).

In the past, computed tomography (CT) and magnetic resonance imaging (MRI) examinations had been requested for many patients. After 1990, most patients have not undergone neuroimaging unless the physical or diagnostic examination suggests a symptomatic etiology or there are extenuating circumstances. For most patients, routine blood studies are performed, including chemistries, blood count, ceruloplasmin, antinuclear antibodies, thyroid function, and erythrocyte sedimentation rate.[28,29]

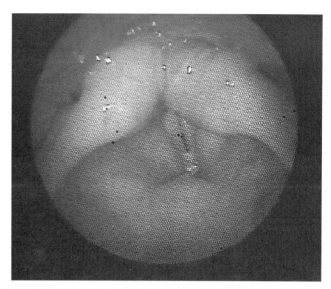
FIG. 15-1. Type 1 hyperadduction.

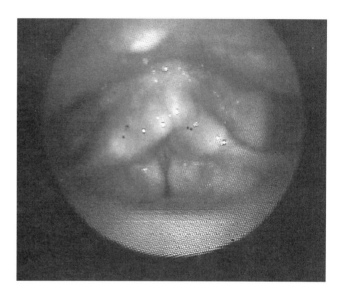
FIG. 15-2. Type 2 hyperadduction.

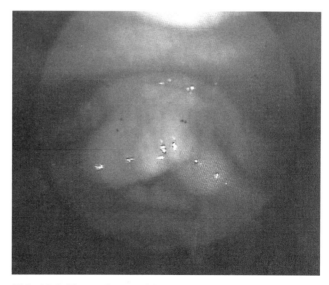
FIG. 15-3. Type 3 hyperadduction.

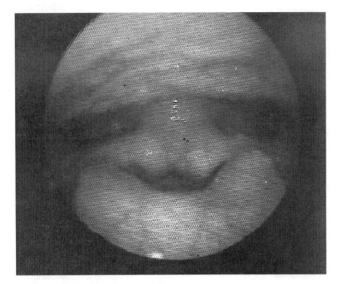

FIG. 15-4. Type 4 hyperadduction.

Most patients with the diagnosis of dystonia are classified according to primary or secondary diagnosis. The primary diagnosis represents the most likely etiologic diagnosis. For a patient to have primary dystonia, there should not be any evidence by history, examination, or laboratory studies of any cause for the dystonia symptoms (except for precipitating peripheral trauma).[30] Therefore, there must be a normal perinatal and early developmental history, no prior history of neurologic illness, or exposure to drugs that are known to cause acquired dystonia (e.g., phenothiazines). There must also be normal intellectual, pyramidal, cerebellar, and sensory examinations as well as normal diagnostic studies.[31,32] Patients who have abnormalities noted above are classified as having symptomatic or secondary dystonia. Patients of known genetic etiology, which are considered primary dystonias, present with the fundamental clinical features of dystonia. These dystonias are discussed elsewhere in this monograph (see Chapter 1).

The authors report an accepted peripheral traumatic contribution if there is:

- An anatomic relationship between the site of trauma and site of dystonia onset;
- The interval between the injury and onset or aggravation of dystonia is within 12 months, and
- Typically, if there is an interval of pain.

The patient often experiences pain at the site of the injury. As the pain resolves, dystonic symptoms become increasingly apparent, as if the resolution of pain transitions into dystonic signs. In the larynx, the most common type of injury is a symptomatic viral sore throat. This finding must be differentiated from the hoarseness that is often experienced at the onset of SD symptoms. However, the authors observed that patients develop SD after intubation, and after direct physical trauma to the larynx or neck.[29]

Patients often report the onset of SD symptoms after an emotionally traumatic or stressful event. Although stress may aggravate dystonic symptoms, no data are available to support the notion that stress can trigger dystonia. The report of a prior stressful event may represent recall bias. Nevertheless, some case histories are striking. Stress may alter the immune system[33–36] and potentially modify susceptibility to infection.[37] A viral sore throat seems the most common peripheral injury precipitating laryngeal dystonia.

Symptoms of dystonia usually begin as a focal dystonia involving a single region of the body; spread to other regions of the body is commonly seen in patients with childhood-onset dystonia. The disorder tends to remain focal in patients with adult-onset dystonia. In the authors' series, 16% of patients who had primary laryngeal involvement experienced spread to another body part. These data suggest that patients should be advised of possible spread to another body part. In addition, patients should be followed and reexamined on a regular basis for signs of other dystonic involvement.[2] Family history is also important; in the authors' series, there were 12.1% of patients with primary laryngeal dystonia who had a family history of dystonia.[2,3,5] During the 1990s, substantial advances were made in the understanding of the genetics of dystonia. These findings may prove to be a link to a possible cure or better treatment (reviewed elsewhere in this volume).

Adductor Spasmodic Dysphonia

In adductor SD, the vocal folds are normal at rest and inappropriately adduct when an action-induced, task-specific movement such as vocalization occurs. This abnormality results in dysphonia that is typically characterized by a strained, strangled voice during connected speech. In addition, patients with this form of dysphonia experience abrupt initiations and terminations of voicing, resulting in short breaks in phonation. Adductor SD is seen in approximately 90% of focal laryngeal dystonia patients in a referral practice. The median age of symptom onset is 39 years, with a slight female predominance.[5] Patients with adductor SD have a strained, strangle-choked vocal quality, with harshness, abrupt initiations and terminations in phonation.[38] Speech is produced with great effort. Vocal breaks, vocal fry, pitch variations, and disturbances in the rhythm of speech are characteristic of this disorder. Patients' speech intelligibility is often worse when speaking on the telephone or under stress. Patients report that speech is better in the morning, before their compensatory muscle action fatigues. Speaking is often better after drinking alcohol; this may be because of the effect of alcohol on brain stem motor control. In some patients, sensory tricks such as yawning, laughing, or touching the neck have been noted to improve phonation.[39] Select patients also report that laughing, yelling, and even singing may be normal.[5,40]

Approaches to treatment for SD have varied over the past few decades. In some patients, physical methods and speech therapy temporize symptoms, however, few are substantially helped with these approaches. In the authors' program, systemic pharmacotherapy provided minimal symptomatic relief. Dedo[41] described the dramatic symptomatic relief provided by sectioning the recurrent laryngeal nerve. The initial favorable reports were temporized by Aronson and DeSanto's[42] review of 33 patients who were surgically treated. At 3 years postsurgery, only 36% of patients had some persistent improvement and only 1 in 33 achieved a persistent normal voice. Adverse effects included breathiness, hoarseness, diplophonia, and falsetto. Sixty-four percent reported failed voices at 3 years; of these patients, 48% were worse than before the surgery. Failures were more common among women (77%) than men. Select patients may benefit from oral therapy as with other forms of dystonia. Speech therapy has been used to augment these pharmacologic treatments, however, as a primary modality, it does not typically adequately eradicate the symptoms.

The authors first established the treatment approach for SD with local injections of botulinum toxin type A (BTX-A) in 1984.[43,44] This treatment has emerged as the most effective treatment of the symptoms of patients with SD. In the authors' series, the average initial doses were 1 unit per 0.1 mL of BOTOX (Allergan, Inc., Irvine, CA) per vocal fold; doses ranged from 0.005 up to 10 units. Patients noted substantial improvement of speech, with an average of 90% return to normal function. Most side effects are well tolerated. Utilizing a conservative dosing regimen helps to resolve posttreatment breathiness and slight aspiration of liquids promptly. Patients with adductor SD who develop marked aspiration of liquids need further evaluation including revisiting the injected dose, technical aspects of the treatment program, or alternative treatment options. Patients with previous laryngeal nerve sections may need botulinum toxin injections into only the ipsilateral vocal cord where there is electromyographic evidence of tonic activity or contralateral muscle groups. However, in some patients, bilateral therapy results in a better voice quality.[5,29]

To effect a unilateral paralysis[45,46] or weakness in patients with adductor SD, investigators at Baylor School of Medicine and the National Institutes of Health (NIH) centers have injected higher doses of BTX-A (i.e., 15–30 units) into one vocalis complex. Investigators at both centers agreed that regardless of injection technique, there was dramatic improvement in symptoms[3,46–49] in nonsurgical patients. During therapy, patients experienced an 80–100% improvement in speech function. Adverse experiences at both centers included transient, breathy hypophonia or hoarseness (in up to 50% of patients) as well as clinically insignificant aspiration of fluids (in up to 25% of patients). Less common complications included: hyperventilation while speaking (in less than 2% of patients); brief coughing of slightly blood-tinged sputum; sore throat; pruritis without rash; and diplophonia. In more than 1,000 patients with SD who were treated in the United States there have been no reported cases of documented pneumonia; however, rare cases of bronchitis occurred.[5,29]

In most patients, multiple laryngeal muscles are affected by dystonic spasms. The lateral cricoarytenoid muscle is the strongest adductor and clinically treating the thyroarytenoid muscles improves patient's voicing. In addition, some toxin probably migrates to the lateral cricoarytenoid muscle. The improvement seen after therapy may be partially the result of a proprioceptive feedback change.

The injection technique utilized at both centers is described as follows:

- The patient is placed in a reclining position, with a pillow under the neck and shoulders to extend the head and cervical spine. This position places the larynx in an anterior position.
- A ground lead and reference lead are placed on the face and connected to an EMG machine. Most laryngeal injections are performed under EMG guidance with a 27-gauge polytetrafluoroethylene-coated (Teflon), hollow-bore EMG needle on a tuberculin syringe.
- The amount of botulinum toxin used is patient- and site-dependent.

In patients with a strong gag response, local anesthesia, which is typically administered as 0.4 mL of 2% lidocaine, is transcutaneously injected into the trachea. Because use of this anesthetic agent may attenuate recording potentials, lidocaine is used sparingly and only in hyperresponsive or coughing patients. The injection procedure is as follows:

- The monopolar EMG needle is passed through the midline of the cricothyroid membrane.
- Then needle is advanced superiorly by approximately 30° and laterally by approximately 30°. This is done until sharp potentials are visualized on the EMG tracing or heard on the EMG loudspeaker; these findings correspond to an electrically active area of the muscle. This motor activity will increase with phonation (i.e., when the patient says /i/).
- BTX-A is then injected into the thyroarytenoid muscle (Fig. 15-5).
- For adductor SD, the average starting dose of botulinum

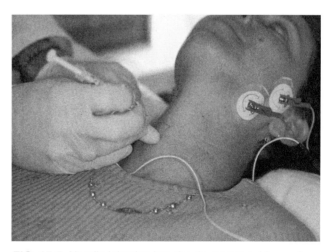

FIG. 15-5. Needle injection into the thyroarytenoid muscle.

toxin type A (BOTOX) is 1.0 unit per 0.1 mL per thyroarytenoid muscle. The volume injected into each thyroarytenoid muscle is between 0.1 and 0.15 mL. If more volume is used bilaterally, a greater risk of stridor is noted.

• The needle is withdrawn and the contralateral thyroarytenoid muscle is injected in a similar method, if needed.

• There may be bursts of motor unit potentials with needle insertion; therefore, confirmation of placement of the needle in the thyroarytenoid should be performed. The needle may be displaced from the thyroarytenoid muscle when the patient coughs or swallows.

For patients who are exquisitely sensitive to BTX-A, the authors have derived other patterns of injection. These include the administration of: relatively small doses on a more frequent basis (e.g., 0.1 unit per 0.1 mL bilaterally every 6–8 weeks); relatively small, unilateral dose (e.g., 0.25–1.0 units); or staggered doses, given 3–4 weeks apart, thus allowing partial recovery before the contralateral cord is treated.

Other authors have suggested alternative approaches to toxin delivery. Ford et al.[50] reported an indirect laryngoscopic technique for injecting the vocal folds. These investigators reported that the technique has the advantage of being "familiar to the otolaryngologist and requires no special (electromyographic) equipment or training." The onset of the response to toxin appears delayed (i.e., 9.1 days); however, the degree of benefit and the duration of efficacy appear comparable to the EMG-guided technique. Another technique was described by Rhew et al.[51] whereby the toxin injection was administered through a needle placed via an operative channel of a flexible fiber optic laryngoscope. The authors reported satisfactory results.

Regardless of technique, BTX-A injections have several advantages over surgical therapy in the management of intractable SD. For example, the patient is awake and there are no risks associated with general anesthesia. Graded degrees of weakening may be achieved with variation of the injected dose. Most adverse effects are transient and result from an extension of the toxin's pharmacology. If the patient has a strong response to the therapy and too much weakness occurs, strength gradually returns. Furthermore, the authors anticipate that increasing knowledge of molecular pathophysiology of SD will permit the development of new treatment strategies that focus on the etiology of SD and not the symptoms associated with SD. It would be unfortunate if surgery prevented the application of more efficacious therapy in the future.

Patients with adductor SD who have already undergone recurrent laryngeal nerve section and have an immobile cord may still have marked improvement with BTX-A injection therapy, however, the degree of benefit is somewhat less than in the nonsurgical patient.[52,53] When performing the EMG, either a chronic denervation pattern or a moderate-to-marked interference pattern may be found on the surgical side. The hypothesis is that there is a reinnervation from ansa

cervicalis fibers. In some patients with tonic reinnervation, BTX injections of that vocal cord may improve vocal quality. The authors experience shows that most patients obtain a better voice when the fully functional cord is treated. During an early series, mean postinjection function was 81% compared to 59% when injecting the paralyzed cord.[53,54] Similar to nonsurgical patients, treatment is individualized; occasional patients require bilateral injections.

The authors also treated three patients who had failed anterior commissure release procedures, which were not performed in the authors' institution.[5,29] These patients had intense adductor spasms, with a postoperative foreshortened appearance of the glottis. All three patients were initially treated with 2.5 units per 0.1 mL into each vocal cord. All patients experienced benefit, however, because of the laxity of the vocal cord from the release, most experienced a narrowed pitch range. These patients also experienced an extended period of breathy hypophonia after injection. Problems with restricted pitch range have persisted; breathy hypophonia has responded to treatment individualization.

In the authors' overall series of patients with SD treated with BTX-A,[5,29] the average onset of effect for botulinum toxin injection was 24–72 hours. The peak effect was at 9 days. The duration of benefit is typically 15–18 weeks. Patients frequently reported a sensation of muscle tightening within the larynx; this occurred before actual speech difficulties. On the average, patients rated their pretreatment speech intelligibility as 50% of normal function, however, after their injection, patients rated their speech intelligibility to be more than 90% of normal function. During the initial stage of toxin effect, patients may have experienced a breathy voice or a decrease in speech volume. Transient, mild aspiration on ingestion of large volumes of liquids was also reported, however, with modification of the technical aspects (e.g., dosing, injection technique, etc.) and patient education, this situation may be mitigated.

The authors recommend that most patients receiving BTX-A therapy continue with speech therapy. This may assist patients to relearn breathing strategies and the most effective use of their vocal muscles after BTX therapy. Murry and Woodson[55] demonstrated a prolonged duration of benefit when speech therapy was added to the BTX-A treatment program.

Abductor Spasmodic Dysphonia

A second less frequent form of laryngeal dystonia is primary abductor SD, which affects speech with different acoustical characteristics than adductor SD. In this form of SD, the vocal folds are typically normal at rest, however, on speaking, the vocal cords abduct in an abnormal manner. In most patients, involuntary movements and spasms cause hypophonia and breathy breaks with connected speech. This pattern is triggered by consonants, especially when they are present in the initial syllable. Similar to adductor SD, sensory tricks may ameliorate the condition and speech may worsen while patients are on the telephone or under stress.

Flexible endoscopy reveals a synchronous and untimely abduction of the true vocal folds, producing an open glottis during phonation. This abnormal movement may be easier to delineate during phrases such as "Harry's hat" and "taxi." Patients need a thorough evaluation by a neurologist as well as a complete analysis by a speech-language pathologist. Laryngeal EMG may not have a definitive pattern. Although the Unified Spasmodic Dysphonia Rating Scale was developed for adductor SD, it may be used to evaluate patients with abductor SD. The most noteworthy findings identified in abductor SD are overall severity, breathy voice quality, aphonia, and tremor. For many of these patients, botulinum toxin type A injections have also been found to be the best treatment.[56] (See also Blitzer and Brin.[57])

As with patient with adductor SD, patients with abductor dystonia require an individualized, tailored dose of BTX-A. Speech is noted to be easier and greatly improved. Approximately one-third of our patients need concomitant, low-dose systemic agents, such as Klonopin (Hoffman-LaRoche, Nutley, NJ), baclofen, and Ativan (Wyeth Pharmaceuticals, Madison, NJ).[5,29]

Since 1989, the authors have treated 154 patients with abductor SD. The average age at symptom onset was 39 years.[35] After evaluation, the patients were started with 3.75 units of BTX-A injected into the most active posterior cricoarytenoid muscle (PCA). Of the 154 patients, 31 patients (20%) developed good voices, without breathy breaks. The balance of these patients required additional toxin, which was injected into the contralateral PCA; the doses ranged from 0.625–2.5 units. Patients were injected in the contralateral cord no sooner than approximately 6 weeks after their initial treatment. The muscles were titrated based on symptom, fiber optic evaluation of motion and the airway, and the patient's development of noisy breathing or stridor. These muscles are the only abductors; substantial bilateral weakness may produce noteworthy stridor. Profound weakness of these muscles may cause the patient to require the establishment of an artificial airway (i.e., intubation or tracheotomy). This potentially fatal outcome requires that the patient's airway be evaluated before injection. In the authors' experience, at each visit, patients only receive unilateral injection of their posterior cricoarytenoid muscle. A nasal endoscopy is performed, confirming by a sniff test precisely which posterior cricoarytenoid (PCA) muscle is more active. In addition, hyperabduction is visualized on connected speech.

The injection procedure follows.

- The larynx is rotated away from the more active side, lifting the posterior edge of the thyroid lamina with the operator's thumb.
- The monopolar EMG needle is inserted along the lower half of the thyroid cartilage, traversing the inferior constrictor muscle until the cricoid cartilage is encountered.
- The needle is then withdrawn slightly. The patient is asked to sniff while the injector observes EMG-identified bursts of potentials. Muscle activity should be silent during phonation or swallowing.
- When the needle is located in an optimum position, botulinum toxin type A is injected into the PCA muscle.
- Initial starting dose of BOTOX is 3.75 units per 0.15 mL for one PCA muscle.[5]

In younger patients whose cricoid cartilage has not ossified, an alternative method may be used as follows:

- The needle is inserted into the midline of the cricothyroid membrane and traverses the airway.
- The needle is angled to the more involved side, and then passes through the cricoid cartilage into the PCA muscle, as documented by EMG.
- The needle placement is confirmed by having the patient sniff.
- Of importance to note is that some cartilage may lodge in the needle and resistance may be encountered upon injection. If this occurs, the cartilage may be extruded with increased pressure on the syringe or another needle may have to be used.
- BTX-A is injected into the active PCA muscle.[5]

The average onset of effect was 4.1 days, with the peak effect at 10.0 days. The duration of benefit was 10.5 weeks. Patients initially rated themselves at 54.8% of normal function and improved to an average 66.7% of normal function.

In addition to the PCA injections, nine patients had the cricothyroid muscles injected with 2.5 units in each muscle. These patients, despite substantial limitation of abduction, still had breathy breaks or tremor. This technique was based on the work of Ludlow et al.[58,59] who found (with EMG) that there was substantial abnormal activity in the cricothyroid muscle. In the Ludlow series of nine patients, five experienced benefit, with louder voice with fewer breaks. One patient's symptoms worsened with the injection. The authors postulated that the cricothyroid was actually involved in a compensatory strategy and the muscle was weakened; the abductor spasms were less well controlled.

In addition, 10 patients had a unilateral type I thyroplasty. During this procedure, the amount of abduction of one vocal fold was mechanically limited. The combination of BTX-A and thyroplasty raised the best average percentage of function to 82% of normal.[5,56]

When the authors' group of patients with abductor SD was analyzed, tremor was present in 30% of patients; abductor SD, in addition to segmental cranial or axial dystonia, was present in 46% of patients. Some patients experienced involvement of the respiratory muscle. With BTX-A treatment, the highest percentage improvement was reported in the group of patients with focal laryngeal involvement without tremor. These patients had an average of 43% improvement of normal function, with an average best function of 80% of normal. The worst response, which was a reported 30% improvement, was in the group with combined dystonic abnormalities.

In a series of prospectively studied abductor patients, the authors examined preinjection factors that might correlate with result. Then they devised a staging system for abductor SD patients as follows.[56]

- Stage I patients have focal symptoms.
- Stage II patients have segmental cranial or axial dystonia.
- Stage III patients have a tremor with their dysphonia and dystonia.
- Stage IV patients have a tremor with segmental axial/cranial, respiratory dyssynchrony, or both.

The authors' experience is that patients who have focal abductor SD respond better to BTX-A therapy than those with more widespread disease or vocal tremor.

When careful assessment of the airway was conducted, few adverse effects were noted, including exertional wheezing or stridor and dysphagia for solids (a possible diffusion of the botulinum toxin to the inferior constrictor muscles). In some pretreatment patients with subtle dystonic tremor, weakening the PCA muscle may permit the vocal cord to move at higher amplitude and aggravates the tremor. An underlying, unvoiced tremor becomes apparent when there is increased phonation and improved adduction.

Adductor Laryngeal Respiratory Dystonia

Adductor laryngeal respiratory dystonia is a rare disorder.[2,60,61] Patients are noted to have inspiratory stridor, which may be moderate to severe, with normal voice and cough. The stridor disappears during sleep and resumes after awakening. Exertion exacerbates the stridor. Patients may also have dysphagia secondary to difficulty breathing while eating. Most patients have no noteworthy oxygen desaturations even though they may have substantial stridor. In addition, patients may have other focal dystonias. On flexible laryngoscopy, the vocal folds have paradoxical movement during respiration. On inspiration, these abnormal movements result in a narrow glottic chink. These patients may also have primary respiratory dysrhythmia with dyssynergistic, fragmented diaphragmatic contractions, and respiratory pauses.[61] Speech therapy, biofeedback, and oral medications have provided minimal long-term benefit. BTX-A injection into bilateral thyroarytenoid muscles provides short-term relief of symptoms.

The benefit observed in the adductor SD group who were injected with BTX-A prompted the authors to attempt to reduce symptomatic adductor breathing spasms with similar doses. Patients received between 0.625 and 3.75 units BOTOX in each thyroarytenoid muscle. The dose varied and was based on the severity of the spasms. Patients used a rating scale on percent of normal function relating to the severity of their breathing. The average preinjection function was 27%; in 20 of 24 patients, pulmonary function tests showed abnormal flow volume loops with intermittent interruptions of airflow during inspiration or expiration. Most patients also had diaphragmatic dysfunction on testing. The average best post-injection function was 82% of normal, making the average percentage improvement 55% of normal function ($P = .0001$). The mean duration of relief from the stridor was 14 weeks (6–26 weeks). A breathy voice lasting 1–2 weeks occurred in 50% of the patients. Mild choking on fluids also occurred in 5 of 12 patients; this lasted for 1 week.[5,29,60,61]

CONCLUSION

Laryngeal dystonia may affect the speech and swallowing mechanisms. Several different types of laryngeal dystonia have been identified and are thought to be neurologic, motor-control disorders. Improvement of symptoms has been noted using BTX-A. The laryngeal area has complex anatomy and function. The adverse effects of BTX-A administered to the laryngeal structures warrant careful evaluation, especially in airway impairment. The use of BTX-A in the larynx is directed toward hyperfunctional muscles producing focal speech and swallowing disabilities.

REFERENCES

1. Blitzer A, Brin MF, Fahn S, et al. Clinical and laboratory characteristics of focal laryngeal dystonia: study of 110 cases. Laryngoscope 1988;98:636–640.
2. Brin MF, Fahn S, Blitzer A, et al. Movement disorders of the larynx. In: Blitzer A, Brin MF, Sasaki CT, Fahn S, Harris KS, eds. Neurological Disorders of the Larynx. New York: Thieme, 1992:248–278.
3. Blitzer A, Brin MF. Laryngeal dystonia: A series with botulinum toxin therapy. Ann Otol Rhinol Laryngol 1991;100:85–90.
4. Gibbs SR, Blitzer A. Botulinum toxin for the treatment of spasmodic dysphonia. Otolaryngol Clin North Am 2000;33:879–894.
5. Blitzer A, Brin MF, Stewart CF. Botulinum toxin management of spasmodic dysphonia (laryngeal dystonia): A 12-year experience in more than 900 patients. Laryngoscope 1998;108:1435–1441.
6. Traube L. Gesammelte Beitrage zur Pathologie und Physiologie. 2nd ed. Berlin: Verlag von August Hirschwald, 1871.
7. Critchley M. Spastic dysphonia ("inspiratory speech"). Brain 1939; 62:96–103.
8. Bellussi G. Le disfonie impercinetiche. Atti Labor Fonet Univ Padova 1952;3:1.
9. Aronson AE, Brown JR, Litin EM, et al. Spastic dysphonia. I. Voice, neurologic, and psychiatric aspects. J Speech Hear Disord 1968;33:203–218.
10. Aronson AE, Brown JR, Litin EM, Pearson JS. Spastic dysphonia. II. Comparison with essential (voice) tremor and other neurologic and psychogenic dysphonias. J Speech Hear Disord 1968;33:219–231.
11. Fraenkel B. Ueber beschaeftigungsneurosen der stimme. Leipzig: G Thieme, 1887.
12. Fraenkel B. Ueber die beschaeftigungsschwaeche der stimme: mogiphonie. Dtsch Med Wochenschr 1887;13:121–123.
13. Gowers WR. Manual of Diseases of the Nervous System. 3rd ed. London: Churchill, 1899.
14. Bloch P, Rio J. Neuro-psychiatric aspects of spastic dysphonia. Folia Phoniatr (Basel) 1965;17:301–364.
15. Gerhardt P. Bewegunggsstoerungen der stimmbaender. Nothnagels spezielle pathologie und therapie. 1896.
16. Jacome DE, Yanez GF. Spastic dysphonia and Meigs disease [Letter]. Neurology 1980;30:349.
17. Marsden CD, Sheehy MP. Spastic dysphonia, Meige disease, and torsion dystonia [Letter]. Neurology 1982;32:1202–1203.
18. Golper LAC, Nutt JG, Rau MT, et al. Focal cranial dystonia. J Speech Hear Disord 1983;48:128–134.
19. Blitzer A, Lovelace RE, Brin MF, et al. Electromyographic findings in focal laryngeal dystonia (spastic dysphonia). Ann Otol Rhinol Laryngol 1985;94:591–594.
20. Cannito MP, Johnson JP. Spastic dysphonia: a continuum disorder. J Commun Disord 1981;14:215–233.

21. Ludlow CL, Naunton RF, Bassich CJ. Procedures for the selection of spastic dysphonia patients for recurrent laryngeal nerve section. Otolaryngol Head Neck Surg 1984;92:24–31.

22. Rosenfield DB, Donovan DT, Sulek M, et al. Neurologic aspects of spasmodic dysphonia [see comments]. J Otolaryngol 1990;19:231–236.

23. Pool KD, Freeman FJ, Finitzo T, et al. Heterogeneity in spasmodic dysphonia. Neurologic and voice findings. Arch Neurol 1991;48:305–309.

24. Lou JS, Jankovic J. Essential tremor: clinical correlates in 350 patients. Neurology 1991;41:234–238.

25. Lang A, Quinn N, Marsden CD, et al. Essential tremor [Letter; comment]. Neurology 1992;42:1432–1434.

26. Aronson AE, Hartman DE. Adductor spastic dysphonia as a sign of essential (voice) tremor. J Speech Hear Disord 1981;46:52–58.

27. Briellmann-Bucher R, Bassetti C, Donati F, et al. Schlafstorungen im Kindesalter [Sleep disorders in childhood] Schweiz Med Wochenschr 1995;125:597–604.

28. Brin MF. Dystonia: Genetics and treatment with botulinum toxin. In: Smith B, Adelman G, eds. Neuroscience Year (Encyclopedia of Neuroscience). Amsterdam: Elsevier, 1997:56–58.

29. Brin MF, Blitzer A, Stewart C. Laryngeal dystonia (spasmodic dysphonia): observations of 901 patients and treatment with botulinum toxin [In Process Citation]. Adv Neurol 1998;78:237–252.

30. Jankovic J. Post-traumatic movement disorders: Central and peripheral mechanisms. Neurology 1994;44:2006–2014.

31. Marsden CD, Harrison MJG. Idiopathic torsion dystonia (dystonia musculorum deformans). A review of forty-two patients. Brain 1974;97:793–810.

32. Burke RE, Brin MF, Fahn S, et al. Analysis of the clinical course of non-Jewish, autosomal dominant torsion dystonia. Mov Disord 1986;1:163–178.

33. Bonneau RH, Sheridan JF, Feng N, et al. Stress-induced modulation of the primary cellular immune response to herpes simplex virus infection is mediated by both adrenal-dependent and independent mechanisms. J Neuroimmunol 1993;42:167–176.

34. Sternberg EM. Hypoimmune fatigue syndromes: diseases of the stress response? [Editorial; corrected] [Published erratum appears in J Rheumatol 1993;20:925] [comment]. J Rheumatol 1993;20:418–421.

35. Hermann G, Tovar CA, Beck FM, et al. Restraint stress differentially affects the pathogenesis of an experimental influenza viral infection in three inbred strains of mice. J Neuroimmunol 1993;47:83–93.

36. Dobbs CM, Vasquez M, Glaser R, et al. Mechanisms of stress-induced modulation of viral pathogenesis and immunity. J Neuroimmunol 1993;48:151–160.

37. Lee DJ, Meehan RT, Robinson C, et al. Immune responsiveness and risk of illness in U.S. Air Force Academy cadets during basic cadet training. Aviat Space Environ Med 1992;63:517–523.

38. Brin MF, Stewart C, Blitzer A, et al. Laryngeal botulinum toxin injections for disabling stuttering in adults. Neurology 1994;44:2262–2266.

39. Langeveld TP, Drost HA, Frijns JH, et al. Perceptual characteristics of adductor spasmodic dysphonia. Ann Otol Rhinol Laryngol 2000;109(8 Pt 1):741–748.

40. Almasy L, Bressman SB, Raymond D, et al. Idiopathic torsion dystonia linked to chromosome 8 in two Mennonite families. Ann Neurol 1997;42:670–673.

41. Dedo HH. Recurrent laryngeal nerve section for spastic dysphonia. Ann Otol Rhinol Laryngol 1976;85:451–459.

42. Aronson AE, DeSanto LW. Adductor spastic dysphonia: 1 1/2 years after recurrent laryngeal nerve resection. Ann Otol Rhinol Laryngol 1981;90:2–6.

43. Blitzer A, Brin MF, Fahn S, et al. Botulinum toxin (BOTOX) for the treatment of "spastic dysphonia" as part of a trial of toxin injections for the treatment of other cranial dystonias [Letter]. Laryngoscope 1986;96:1300–1301.

44. Brin MF, Fahn S, Moskowitz CB, et al. Injections of botulinum toxin for the treatment of focal dystonia [Abstract]. Neurology 1986;36(Suppl 1):120.

45. Miller RH, Woodson GE, Jankovic J. Botulinum toxin injection of the vocal fold for spasmodic dysphonia. A preliminary report. Arch Otolaryngol Head Neck Surg 1987;113:603–605.

46. Ludlow CL, Naunton RF, Sedory SE, et al. Effects of botulinum toxin injections on speech in adductor spasmodic dysphonia. Neurology 1988;38:1220–1225.

47. Jankovic J, Schwartz K, Donovan DT. Botulinum toxin treatment of cranial-cervical dystonia, spasmodic dysphonia, other focal dystonias and hemifacial spasm. J Neurol Neurosurg Psychiatry 1990;53:633–639.

48. Gacek RR. Botulinum toxin for relief of spasmodic dysphonia. Arch Otolaryngol Head Neck Surg 1987;113:1240.

49. Brin MF, Blitzer A, Fahn S, et al. Adductor laryngeal dystonia (spastic dysphonia): treatment with local injections of botulinum toxin (Botox). Mov Disord 1989;4:287–296.

50. Ford CN, Bless DM, Lowery JD. Indirect laryngoscopic approach for injection of botulinum toxin in spasmodic dysphonia. Otolaryngol Head Neck Surg 1990;103:752–758.

51. Rhew K, Fiedler DA, Ludlow CL. Technique for injection of botulinum toxin through the flexible nasolaryngoscope. Otolaryngol Head Neck Surg 1994;111:787–794.

52. Ludlow CL, Naunton RF, Fujita M, et al. Spasmodic dysphonia: botulinum toxin injection after recurrent nerve surgery. Otolaryngol Head Neck Surg 1990;102:122–131.

53. Blitzer A, Brin MF, Fahn S. Botulinum toxin therapy for recurrent laryngeal nerve section failure for adductor laryngeal dystonia. Ann Otol Rhin Laryngol 1989;98(Suppl).

54. Sulica L, Blitzer A, Brin MF, et al. Botulinum toxin management of adductor spasmodic dysphonia after failed recurrent laryngeal nerve section. Ann Otol Rhinol Laryngol 2003;112:499–505.

55. Murry T, Woodson GE. Combined-modality treatment of adductor spasmodic dysphonia with botulinum toxin and voice therapy. J Voice 1995;9:460–465.

56. Blitzer A, Brin MF, Stewart C, et al. Abductor laryngeal dystonia: a series treated with botulinum toxin. Laryngoscope 1992;102:163–167.

57. Blitzer A, Brin MF. The evaluation and management of abductor laryngeal dysphonia. In Jankovic J, Hallett M, eds. Therapy with Botulinum Toxin. New York: Marcel Dekker, 1994:451–459.

58. Ludlow CL, Naunton RF, Terada S, et al. Successful treatment of selected cases of abductor spasmodic dysphonia using botulinum toxin injection. Otolaryngol Head Neck Surg 1991;104:849–855.

59. Ludlow CL. Treating the spasmodic dysphonias with botulinum toxin: a comparison with adductor and abductor spasmodic dysphonia and vocal tremor. In: Tsui KC, Calne DB, eds. Handbook of Dystonia. New York: Marcel Dekker, 1995:431–446.

60. Grillone GA, Blitzer A, Brin MF, et al. Treatment of adductor laryngeal breathing dystonia with botulinum toxin type A. Laryngoscope 1994;104:30–32.

61. Braun N, Abd A, Baer J, et al. Dyspnea in dystonia. A functional evaluation. Chest 1995;107:1309–1316.

CHAPTER 16

Limb Dystonia

Barbara Illowsky Karp

INTRODUCTION

Limb dystonia is a movement disorder characterized by excessive and overflow muscle contraction leading to abnormal limb posture and impaired movement. Limb dystonia may be focal (i.e., limited to a single body area), segmental (i.e., affecting at least two adjacent muscle groups), or a component of generalized dystonia. As with other forms of dystonia, limb dystonia may be primary or secondary to another disorder.

Normal hand functions and gait rely on complex patterns of movement that are easily disrupted by the unwanted contractions and impaired coordination associated with dystonia. Therefore, limb dystonia may be particularly disabling. Even a minor degree of task-specific dystonia may be career ending for certain individuals such as professional musicians or others whose livelihoods depend on precise motor control.

FOCAL HAND DYSTONIA

History

Focal hand dystonia is often named by the specific function that is impaired. Thus, among other terms, this form of dystonia has been termed writer's cramp, occupational cramp, or musician's cramp. Descriptions of writer's cramp (scrivener's palsy or graphospasm), the most common focal hand dystonia, and occupational hand dystonia date at least back to 1713 when Ramazzini (1633–1714) published *De Morbis Artificum (Diseases of Workers)*.[1] In Ramazzini's section on "Disease of Scribes and Notaries," he wrote: "Furthermore, incessant driving of the pen over paper causes intense fatigue of the hand and the whole arm because of the continuous and almost tonic strain on the muscles and tendons, which in course of time results in failure of power in the right hand."

Barbara Illowsky Karp: Office of the Clinical Director, National Institute of Neurological Disorders and Stroke, National Institutes of Health, Bethesda, Maryland.

The author has no financial relationships to disclose.

In an 1864 edition of *The Lancet,* Solly provided a more complete description.[2]

> [The disease] shows itself outwardly in a palsy of the writing powers. The muscles cease to obey the mandate of the will. It comes on very insidiously, the first indication often being only a painful feeling in the thumb or forefinger of the writing hand, accompanied by some stiffness; these unnatural sensations subside during the hours of rest and sleep, to return with the writer's work on the next day.
>
> The loss of power is not sudden, as in a paralytic stroke; nor is it a complete paralysis of any group of muscles. The paralysed scrivener, though he cannot write, can amuse himself in his garden, can shoot, and cut his meat like a Christian at the dinner-table; indeed he can do almost anything he likes, except earn his daily bread as a scribbler.

W.C. Gowers' *A Manual of Diseases of the Nervous System,* which was published in 1890, also includes a section on "occupational neuroses." Gowers observed:

> After writing for some time the patient finds something unusual about his writing; the pen does not move quite as he intended it to do; a stroke now and again is irregular, extends too high or too low; a slight involuntary movement causes an unintended mark. He finds that he is grasping the pen too tightly, and cannot help doing so; that the fingers do not keep in their accustomed place; and the first finger has a tendency to slip off the pen, so that this gets between the first and second finger. He endeavors to mend matters by taking a firmer hold, but this seems to increase the difficulty, and he finds that he writes slowly, as if a weight were attached to the hand. The hand feels strangely tired and an aching pain in the finger or thumb or first metacarpal bone, or in the wrist or forearm, makes it still more difficult for him to go on writing. These symptoms may continue, with only slight impairment of the power of writing for weeks or months, but they occur after writing for a shorter time; they increase in degree, and now and then there is distinct spasm, which cannot be controlled.

Gower further notes other key features, including: typical age of onset between 20 and 50 years; the possibility of limb injury that may precipitate the onset of symptoms; and a tendency of nondominant hand involvement in individuals who switch hands for writing.

185

Although most common in scribes, similar symptoms were recorded in others whose work entailed prolonged and repetitive hand use such as seamstresses, cobblers, musicians, composers, and milkers.[2]

Epidemiology and Etiology

Focal hand dystonia usually begins during middle age. The Epidemiological Study of Dystonia in Europe Collaborative Group reported an incidence of writer's cramp of 14 in 1,000,000 population in eight countries in Europe,[3] while Nutt et al.[4] found an incidence of 2.7 in 1,000,000 population and a prevalence of 69 in 1,000,000 in Rochester, Minnesota.[4] In contrast to cervical dystonia, blepharospasm, and other focal dystonias that are more frequent in women, hand dystonia affects men and women in approximately equal numbers; however, men may have an earlier age of onset.[5]

The main factor contributing to the development of focal hand dystonia appears to be prolonged, repetitive use of the hand. Many patients report the onset of symptoms during a period of particularly intense hand use. The relationship between overt hand trauma and hand dystonia, however, is uncertain. Dystonia in the damaged limb may follow relatively minor trauma, often after recovery of full strength and sensation.[6,7] Jankovic et al.[8] noted that compared to patients with idiopathic dystonia, patients with dystonia after trauma often had local pain at the onset of the disorder and dystonia evident during periods of rest.

Despite evidence of a relationship between focal injury and limb dystonia, such traumas are common and few injured patients go on to develop dystonia. Therefore, it was proposed that the development of dystonia might require that the trauma occur in an individual with a specific predisposition.[8] This possibility was supported by a study by Schicatano et al.[9] This study showed that facial palsy could produce blepharospasm if superimposed on a mild dopamine deficiency. This deficiency was induced by the injection of 6-OH-dopamine into the basal ganglia. These study findings suggest that dystonia may follow peripheral trauma, assuming there is an underlying dopaminergic imbalance in the basal ganglia or another predisposing factor.

Although writer's cramp and occupational dystonias are largely idiopathic, the arms and hands are involved in most secondary dystonias. Focal hand dystonia may also arise with peripheral nerve damage or spinal lesions.

Genetics of Arm Dystonia

Five percent to 20% of patients with writer's cramp have a family history of dystonia,[10,11] however, the genetic underpinnings of isolated focal hand dystonia have not yet been identified. The *DYT1* mutation is an infrequent cause of idiopathic hand dystonia or musician's cramp,[12,13] although arm dystonia is frequently the presenting symptom of early onset, *DYT1*-positive dystonia. Isolated hand dystonia may also occasionally occur in family members of those with id-

iopathic generalized torsion dystonia or dopa-responsive dystonia.

Physiology

Physiologic studies of dystonia can take advantage of the task-specificity of focal hand dystonia, comparing movements that activate the dystonia with those that do not. The often unilateral nature of the dystonia also enables comparison of the dystonic hand with the nondystonic hand.

Electromyography (EMG) during writing with the dystonic hand reveals cocontraction of agonist and antagonist pairs with loss of normal alternation; prolonged muscle bursts with superimposed shorter repeated bursts; lack of muscle selectivity; overflow of contraction to muscles that are not ordinarily activated by the task being performed; tremor; and failure of some voluntary actions.[14–16] Abnormalities in long-latency reflexes,[21,22] loss of reciprocal inhibition,[23,24] cortical hyperexcitability, and defects in intracortical inhibition[14,25–31] may all contribute to the symptoms of overactivation of muscles, excessive muscle tightness, impaired movement speed and fluency, and loss of motor control. In addition to dysfunction of motor pathways, there is increasing evidence that sensory abnormalities underlie or contribute to the pathophysiology of limb dystonia. Cortical sensory mapping shows distorted finger and hand representations.[17–23] Abnormal sensory discrimination, impaired sensorimotor integration, and deficient somatosensory inhibition have all been demonstrated.[24–27] In many studies, bilateral cerebral abnormalities are found, despite unilateral symptomatology.

Signs and Symptoms

The onset of hand dystonia is insidious, with progression of symptoms over several months. After that time, the symptoms often stabilize; spontaneous remissions are rare. When hand dystonia does spread, it involves proximal muscles in the same arm or the opposite limb. Generalization in early-onset dystonia spans the course of years.[39]

The initial symptoms of hand dystonia are often vague feelings of discomfort, fatigue, or tension in the hand or forearm. These feelings become more noticeable with continued writing or limb use. As the disease progresses, there is increasing difficulty with motor control. This difficulty results in the loss of speed, motor fluency, and accuracy. Many patients develop an involuntarily tight grip on the pen, along with abnormal hand or arm posture. Symptoms generally improve with rest, however, symptoms return when the activity resumes.

In many cases, the dystonia is only present during the performance of a single activity, such as writing. In these task-specific simple cramps, the dystonia is not present with other actions, even those activities that use the same muscles. Over time, simple cramp may evolve into dystonic cramp, and the dystonia is apparent during other activities. In more severe cases, the dystonia is obvious at rest. Although both arm compartments may be affected, flexor muscles are more frequently involved than are the extensor muscles. In some patients, use of the nondominant hand elicits dystonic posturing of the dominant hand. Dystonic hand muscles become hypertrophic from excessive contraction.

Muscle strength, reflexes, and primary sensory modalities, such as light touch, pain, and vibratory sense are normal in patients with focal hand cramp. Tremor is found in up to 46% of patients with hand dystonia.[10,40] Myoclonic jerks, decreased arm swing, or a slight increase in tone in the affected arm may also be present.[10]

Differential Diagnosis

EMG demonstration of impaired reciprocal inhibition or other abnormalities characteristic of dystonia may be helpful in the diagnosis of this condition, however, the diagnosis of focal hand dystonia remains clinical. Therefore, the examination of these patients focuses on eliminating other causes of similar hand complaints and determining the nature and extent of dystonic involvement.

Repetitive stress injury (RSI) or overuse syndrome is an increasingly recognized cause of hand pain and disability.[41,42] The hallmark of RSI is pain in the affected hand and arm. Initially present only during limb use, the pain may become continuous and persists despite rest. Similar to dystonia, RSI is precipitated by repetitive use. Other identified risk factors for RSI include the use of high force, awkward joint posture, direct pressure, vibration, and prolonged, constrained postures.[43] Unlike dystonia, function is preserved with RSI unless hand and arm use is impeded by pain.

RSI is most often caused by tenosynovitis resulting from cumulative microtrauma. There may also be direct muscle damage and bone injuries such as stress fractures. Approximately 2% of patients with RSI have nerve impairment, such as pressure palsy.[41]

The therapy for RSI is aimed at decreasing pain and inflammation and preventing further damage. Rest, splinting, bracing, ice, elevation, nonsteroidal anti-inflammatory medications, and local steroid injections are all used. A change in limb posture, technique, and improved ergonomic design of work tools may also help alleviate or prevent RSI.

Nerve entrapment needs to be specifically considered in the evaluation of patients with focal hand dystonia. The initial forearm and hand discomfort of hand dystonia may easily be mistaken for carpal tunnel syndrome, however, weakness, sensory loss, Tinel's sign, and Phalen's sign should be absent. Although focal hand dystonia may sometimes precipitate a carpal tunnel syndrome,[44] carpal tunnel syndrome is an unusual cause of hand dystonia.[45] Treatment for carpal tunnel syndrome includes surgery, which offers no benefit for patients with hand dystonia.

The relationship between ulnar neuropathy and focal hand dystonia is less clear. Patients with ulnar neuropathy may develop symptoms and neurophysiologic abnormalities similar to writer's cramp.[46] The pattern of dystonic flexion of the fourth and fifth fingers is especially common in association with ulnar neuropathy. Charness et al.[46] found ulnar neuropathy in 40% of 72 musicians with occupational cramp. Surface EMG detected the ulnar nerve abnormality in only one-third of cases. Near-nerve recording was more sensitive. In some patients with dystonia and ulnar neuropathy, improvement in the dystonia paralleled that of the ulnar nerve symptoms. Ross et al.[47] found defective agonist/antagonist activation and prolonged muscle bursts on EMG in patients with ulnar neuropathy. Activation and bursts were similar to those in individuals with writer's cramp. These abnormalities were present even in muscles not innervated by the ulnar nerve, suggesting that the ulnar neuropathy altered central motor processing. Thus, even though ulnar neuropathy is not present in most patients with writer's cramp, it should be carefully excluded by physical examination. EMG with near-nerve recordings may be necessary in some patients.

The limbs are commonly involved in secondary dystonias, such as those caused by Parkinson's disease, corticobasal ganglionic degeneration or after stroke. Similar to other dystonias, when arm dystonia occurs in the presence of a central lesion, the most common location is the contralateral basal ganglia. In addition, arm dystonia has been reported with spinal cord, nerve root, and brachial plexus lesions as well.[48,49]

Reflex sympathetic dystrophy (RSD) is associated with dystonia that may precede other symptoms.[50] Dystonia is especially likely in those with severe or long-standing RSD. Early on, the dystonic symptoms may respond to sympathectomy or other RSD treatments.

Psychogenic hand dystonia is a diagnosis of exclusion, however, it may be considered when there is abrupt onset, rapid progression to fixed posture, prominent pain, other psychogenic neurologic signs, and multiple somatizations.[51]

SEGMENTAL DYSTONIA

When dystonia involves not only the limb but also the contiguous proximal limb girdle muscles, it is called segmental dystonia. Similar to hemidystonia, segmental dystonia is frequently symptomatic of an underlying basal ganglia, nerve, root, or spinal cord lesion.[52–54] The most common pattern of upper extremity segmental dystonia is shoulder elevation with adduction and internal rotation of the arm. Cervical dystonia may also be present.

LEG DYSTONIA

The most common pattern of leg dystonia is internal rotation of the lower leg and foot with extension of the great toe. Isolated, idiopathic leg dystonia is uncommon.[55,56] In rare cases, symptomatic leg dystonia is seen with spinal or radicular lesions[57,58] or after trauma.[6] However, leg dystonia is often a presenting sign of an early-onset dystonia such as idiopathic torsion dystonia and dopa-responsive dystonia. In idiopathic torsion dystonia, involvement of the trunk and arms follows within months to years. Leg dystonia in patients with dopa-responsive dystonia (DRD) improves with rest and responds to low doses of levodopa. When spasticity and hyperreflexia accompany leg dystonia, DRD may be mistaken for cerebral palsy.

In older patients, leg dystonia may be an initial sign of Parkinson's disease, occurring before the onset of bradykinesia, tremor, or rigidity. The dystonia of Parkinson's disease may respond to dopaminergic treatment. However, it is important to note that limb dystonia may also arise as a complication of levodopa therapy.

EVALUATION OF LIMB DYSTONIA

The first step in evaluating limb dystonia is to perform a complete neurologic examination. Signs of radiculopathy, peripheral neuropathy, parkinsonism, and other disorders that might require specific treatments should be sought. The examination then focuses on the dystonia itself.

To determine the full extent of dystonic involvement, patients should be examined at rest; during a sustained posture; during activities that provoke the dystonia; and while performing other activities. While most limb dystonia patients have normal resting posture, the dystonia is obvious at rest in the most severely affected patients.

Patients with writer's cramp should be examined during writing. Patients should use the task-specific grip they have developed to cope with the dystonia and while holding the pen with their premorbid grip. Musicians need to be examined while playing their instruments, both with and without any adaptations that they may have made.

In preparation for botulinum toxin injection, the first-line treatment for focal hand dystonia, it is important to delineate the specific muscles involved in the dystonia. The determination of affected muscles may not be straightforward. The performance of actions that elicit the dystonia is often complicated by the presence of compensatory movements that may not be entirely voluntary. Patients should be asked not to compensate for the dystonia; then they should be asked to perform other actions, without compensatory movements, that might evoke the dystonia. For example, in some patients, mirror dystonic posturing is present in the dominant hand when the patient writes with the nondominant hand.[59] The dystonia may sometimes be seen when patients with writer's cramp tap on a table with each finger sequentially or draw a spiral with outstretched fingers rather than while gripping the pen. Wire EMG during dystonic activation may also be used to determine the affected muscles.

Imaging and ancillary studies are only occasionally needed in patients with limb dystonia. In those with segmental dystonia, atypical features, or signs other than dystonia on examination, brain or spine imaging is indicated. Patients with sensory signs or symptoms should have an EMG or nerve conduction studies to evaluate peripheral nerve function. As previously noted, near-nerve recording may be required to detect occult neuropathies.

Treatment

The goals of treatment for patients with limb dystonia may include functional improvement, correction of abnormal posture, or relief of discomfort. Before seeking medical attention, most patients have tried nonpharmacologic measures. For example, individuals with writer's cramp try thicker pens, change their handgrip, or write with their nondominant hand. Unfortunately, up to 25% of patients who switch hands will eventually develop dystonia in the nondominant hand. Musicians often try to adapt their technique by refingering music, altering hand and wrist positions, or modifying their instruments when possible. Some patients pursue massage therapy, psychotherapy, relaxation therapy, splinting, biofeedback,[60,61] chiropractic, hypnosis, transcutaneous nerve stimulation, or acupuncture. However, these approaches rarely produce sustained relief. Herbal and alternative therapies, such as geranium oil, almond oil, and amylase enzyme treatment, are of no proven benefit.

Physical and occupational therapy, including the use of splints or other devices, is beneficial to some patients. Their use is supported by recent reports of improvement in hand dystonia with sensory retraining[62-64] or constraint-induced movement therapy.[65,66]

Peripheral nerve surgery may relieve nerve compression symptoms if present, but does not reverse the dystonia, except in some patients with ulnar nerve palsy and dystonia. In leg dystonia, tenotomy or tendon transfer may improve posture or gait. Limb amputation has been performed in severe circumstances.[67]

Stereotactic brain surgery such as pallidotomy, thalamotomy, and deep brain stimulation are being investigated as treatments for dystonia. The current experience with these procedures for focal limb dystonia is limited but promising. Iacono et al.[68] reported improvement of leg dystonia in patients with atypical parkinsonism who underwent unilateral pallidotomy.[68] Improvement in arm dystonia in a patient with writer's cramp and tremor from ventroposterior Vim nucleus thalamotomy has been documented. Goto et al.[69] reported remarkable improvement in hand function in a single patient with dystonic hand cramp from Vo-complex thalamotomy.

In limb dystonia, oral medications are largely reserved for those with severe dystonia or widespread involvement. They are seldom more than minimally helpful for focal hand dystonia and drug toxicity often outweighs the benefit. The notable exception is levodopa, which is used to treat limb symptoms in both patients with DRD and Parkinson's disease. The medications that may be tried include anticholinergics, dopamine agonists and antagonists, baclofen, clonazepam or other benzodiazepines, and muscle relaxants. Intrathecal baclofen may be especially helpful in relieving limb dystonia in patients with reflex sympathetic dystrophy.[70]

The treatment of choice for focal limb dystonias is botulinum toxin injection. There is now more than 12 years of experience using botulinum toxin for limb dystonia. It is known to be safe and effective and avoids the systemic effects of oral medications. Botulinum toxin injections may also be safely combined with oral medications and nonpharmacologic therapies.

When used for limb dystonia, the proper selection of muscles for injection is crucial. Muscles are chosen based on clinical examination, patient's report of tightness, and, if needed, EMG evidence of excessive muscle activation. When using botulinum toxin for hand dystonia, it is not always necessary to inject every dystonic muscle. Some patients respond well to injection of the main involved muscles.

There is no objective way to assess benefit in limb dystonia patients. A visual analogue scale allows patients to assess their own responses. A rating scale from zero (no improvement) to four (complete relief of the dystonia) is also commonly used.

For writer's cramp, forearm muscles and hand intrinsics are injected. Additional proximal muscles may require injection. The use of electromyographic guidance may enhance the accuracy of injections.[71] Focal hand dystonia requires a relatively low dose of toxin, such as 25–30 units of BOTOX (Allergan, Inc., Irvine, CA). This dose is divided among several muscles. High doses are rarely needed. More than 80% of patients treated for focal hand dystonia have greater than minimal improvement lasting approximately 3 months.

After the effects of botulinum toxin injection wear off, patients need to return for reinjection. After three to four injection sessions, most patients have a stable response to treatment. Other than atrophy in the injected or adjacent muscles, there have been no reports of long-term, adverse effects with repeated botulinum toxin injections. In the absence of antibody development, most patients retain their responsivity.

Although botulinum toxin helps with excessive cramping and tightness, it is less effective in improving fine motor control. Hence, musicians may not be able to continue professional performance, even if the dystonia is greatly improved.

Segmental dystonia usually takes the form of internal rotation and adduction of the arm with shoulder elevation. The muscles most frequently injected are teres major, latissimus dorsi, trapezius, and pectoralis major. A large body area is involved, so high doses, up to 500 units of BOTOX, divided among the various muscles may be required. When injecting chest and back muscles, particular care must be taken not to enter the pleural cavity.

The botulinum toxin treatment of hand and arm dystonia is usually accompanied by muscle weakness. If this weakness is excessive, it may be as disabling as the dystonia itself. Unfortunately, there is no way to predict how much weakness will be present in an individual. In addition, there is no correlation between the degree of weakness and magnitude of the benefit produced. The balance between benefit and weakness in a given individual is unpredictable. Some patients have almost complete relief of symptoms with little weakness; others have pronounced weakness with only minimal improvement in their dystonia. Therefore, the acceptability of botulinum toxin treatment lies with the patient, who needs to decide if the benefit achieved is worth tolerating the transient weakness.

Patients with symptomatic secondary dystonia, such as corticobasal ganglionic degeneration or poststroke dystonia, may develop tightly clenched fists. Even though hand function cannot be restored, botulinum toxin injection may allow the hand to be opened. Opening of the hands may provide a degree of patient comfort and improved palmar hygiene. Higher doses of toxins may be required in patients with symptomatic secondary dystonia than in patients with idiopathic hand dystonia.

For leg dystonia, the most commonly injected muscles are tibialis posterior and extensor hallucis longus. These large muscles require high doses of botulinum toxin—up to 500 units of BOTOX into the tibialis posterior alone. Despite the use of such high doses, weakness is rarely seen. Unfortunately, the results of leg injection are not as good for as for upper extremity dystonia. Only 60% of patients have more than minimal benefit. Patients with from Parkinson's disease and leg dystonia may respond less well to botulinum toxin than those with idiopathic dystonia.

SUMMARY

Limb dystonia may present as an isolated focal symptom or as part of generalized dystonia. In addition, limb dystonia may be particularly disabling. It may be idiopathic, or secondary to another process, especially in conditions that affect the contralateral basal ganglia. Writer's cramp and occupational cramp need to be distinguished from repetitive stress injury and peripheral nerve palsies, which require different therapies. Widespread or severe limb dystonia is most often treated with oral medications. Stereotactic neurosurgery may also be considered. Idiopathic limb dystonia or focal limb symptoms respond well to botulinum toxin injection.

REFERENCES

1. Ramazzini B. Diseases of Scribes and Notaries. Diseases of Workers. New York: Hafner Publishing Company, 1713:421–425.
2. Solly S. Scrivener's palsy, or the paralysis of writers. Lancet 1864;2:709–711.
3. Epidemiological Study of Dystonia in Europe (ESDE) Collaborative Group. A prevalence study of primary dystonia in eight European countries. J Neurol 2000;247:787–792.
4. Nutt JG, Muenter MD, Aronson A, et al. Epidemiology of focal and generalized dystonia in Rochester, Minn. Mov Disord 1988;3:188–194.
5. Epidemiological Study of Dystonia in Europe (ESDE) Collaborative Group. Sex-related influences on the frequency and age of onset of primary dystonia. Neurology 1999;53:1871–1873.
6. Schott GD. The relationship of peripheral trauma and pain to dystonia. J Neurol Neurosurg Psychiatry 1985;48:698–701.
7. Frucht S, Fahn S, Ford B. Focal task-specific dystonia induced by peripheral trauma. Mov Disord 2000;15:348–349.

8. Jankovic J, Van Der Linden C. Dystonia and tremor induced by peripheral trauma: predisposing factors. J Neurol Neurosurg Psychiatry 1988;51:1512–1519.

9. Schicatano EJ, Basso MA, Evinger C. Animal model explains the origins of cranial dystonia benign essential blepharospasm. J Neurophysiol 1997;77:2842–2846.

10. Sheehy MP, Marsden CD. Writer's cramp: a focal dystonia. Brain 1982;105:461–480.

11. Waddy HM, Fletcher NA, Harding AE, et al. A genetic study of idiopathic focal dystonias. Ann Neurol 1991;29:320–324.

12. Kamm C, Naumann M, Mueller J, et al. The DYT1 GAG deletion is infrequent in sporadic and familial writer's cramp. Mov Disord 2000;15:1238–1241.

13. Friedman JR, Klein C, Leung J, et al. The GAG deletion of the DYT1 gene is infrequent in musicians with focal dystonia. Neurology 2000;55:1417–1418.

14. Berardelli A, Rothwell JC, Hallett M, et al. The pathophysiology of primary dystonia. Brain 1998;121:1195–1212.

15. Cohen LG, Hallett M. Hand cramps: clinical features and electromyographic patterns in a focal dystonia. Neurology 1988;38:1005–1012.

16. Farmer SF, Sheehan GL, Mayston MJ, et al. Abnormal motor unit synchronization of antagonist muscles underlies pathological co-contraction in upper limb dystonia. Brain 1998;121:801–814.

17. Bara-Jimenez W, Catalan MJ, Hallett M, et al. Abnormal somatosensory homunculus in dystonia of the hand. Neurology 1998;44:828–831.

18. Bara-Jimenez W, Shelton P, Sanger TD, et al. Sensory discrimination capabilities in patients with focal hand dystonia. Ann Neurol 2000;47:377–380.

19. Elbert T, Candia V, Altenmuller E, et al. Alteration of digital representations in somatosensory cortex in focal hand dystonia. Neuroreport 1998;9:3571–3575.

20. Byl NN, McKenzie A, Nagarajan SS. Differences in somatosensory hand organization in a healthy flutist and a flutist with focal hand dystonia: a case report. J Hand Ther 2000;13:302–309.

21. Tamburin S, Manganotti P, Marzi CA, et al. Abnormal somatotopic arrangement of sensorimotor interactions in dystonic patients. Brain 2002;125(Pt 12):2719–2730.

22. Blake DT, Byl NN, Cheung S, et al. Sensory representation abnormalities that parallel focal hand dystonia in a primate model. Somatosens Mot Res 2002;19:347–357.

23. Pujol J, Roset-Llobet J, Rosines-Cubells D, et al. Brain cortical activation during guitar-induced hand dystonia studied by functional MRI. Neuroimage 2000;12:257–267.

24. Yoneda Y, Rome S, Sagar HJ, et al. Abnormal perception of the tonic vibration reflex in idiopathic focal dystonia. Eur J Neurol 2000;7:529–533.

25. Tinazzi M, Frasson E, Bertolasi L, et al. Temporal discrimination of somesthetic stimuli is impaired in dystonic patients. Neuroreport 1999;10:1547–1550.

26. Serrien DJ, Burgunder JM, Wiesendanger M. Disturbed sensorimotor processing during control of precision grip in patients with writer's cramp. Mov Disord 2000;15:965–972.

27. Frasson E, Priori A, Bertolasi L, et al. Somatosensory disinhibition in dystonia. Mov Disord 2001;16:674–682.

28. Panizza M, Lelli S, Nilsson J, et al. H-reflex recovery curve and reciprocal inhibition of H-reflex in different kinds of dystonia. Neurology 1990;40:824–828.

29. Naumann M, Reiners K. Long-latency reflexes of hand muscles in idiopathic focal dystonia and their modification by botulinum toxin. Brain 1997;120:409–416.

30. Panizza M, Hallett M, Nilsson J. Reciprocal inhibition in patients with hand cramps. Neurology 1989;39:85–89.

31. Chen RS, Tsai CH, Lu CS. Reciprocal inhibition in writer's cramp. Mov Disord 1995;10:556–561.

32. Chen R, Wassermann EM, Canos M, et al. Impaired inhibition in writer's cramp during voluntary muscle activation. Neurology 1997;49:1054–1059.

33. Currà A, Berardelli A, Rona S, et al. Excitability of the motor cortex in patients with dystonia. In: Fahn S, Marsden CD, DeLong M, eds. Dystonia 3: Advances in Neurology. Philadelphia: Lippincott-Raven, 1998:33–40.

34. Ikoma K, Samii A, Mercuri B, et al. Abnormal cortical motor excitability in dystonia. Neurology 1996;46:1371–1376.

35. Ibanez V, Sadato N, Karp B, et al. Deficient activation of the premotor cortical network in patients with writer's cramp. Neurology 1999;53:96–105.

36. Playford ED, Passingham RE, Marsden CD, et al. Increased activation of frontal areas during arm movement in idiopathic torsion dystonia. Mov Disord 1998;13:309–318.

37. Ridding MC, Sheean G, Rothwell JC, et al. Changes in the balance between motor cortical excitation and inhibition in focal, task specific dystonia. J Neurol Neurosurg Psychiatry 1995;59:493–498.

38. Siebner HR, Auer C, Conrad B. Abnormal increase in the corticomotor output to the affected hand during repetitive transcranial magnetic stimulation of the primary motor cortex in patients with writer's cramp. Neurosci Lett 1999;262:133–136.

39. Greene P, Kang UJ, Fahn S. Spread of symptoms in idiopathic torsion dystonia. Mov Disord 1995;10:143–152.

40. Jedynak CP, Bonnet AM, Agid Y. Tremor and idiopathic dystonia. Mov Disord 1991;6:230–236.

41. Ranney D. Work-related chronic injuries of the forearm and hand: their specific diagnosis and management. Ergonomics 1993;36:871–880.

42. Pitner MA. Pathophysiology of overuse injuries in the hand and wrist. Hand Clin 1990;6:355–364.

43. Verdon ME. Overuse syndromes of the hand and wrist. Prim Care 1996;23:305–319.

44. Drory VE, Neufeld MY, Korczyn AD. Carpal tunnel syndrome: a complication of idiopathic torsion dystonia. Mov Disord 1991;6:82–84.

45. Scherokman B, Husain F, Cuetter A, et al. Peripheral dystonia. Arch Neurol 1986;43:830–832.

46. Charness ME, Ross MH, Shefner JM. Ulnar neuropathy and dystonic flexion of the fourth and fifth digits: clinical correlation in musicians. Muscle Nerve 1996;19:431–437.

47. Ross MH, Charness ME, Lee D, et al. Does ulnar neuropathy predispose to focal dystonia? Muscle Nerve 1995;18:606–611.

48. Uncini A, Di Muzio A, Thomas A, et al. Hand dystonia secondary to cervical demyelinating lesion. Acta Neurol Scand 1994;90:51–55.

49. Choi YC, Lee MS, Choi IS. Delayed-onset focal dystonia after stroke. Yonsei Med J 1993;34:391–396.

50. Schwartzman R, Kerrigan J. The movement disorder of reflex sympathetic dystrophy. Neurology 1990;40:57–61.

51. Lang AE. Psychogenic dystonia: a review of 18 cases. Can J Neurol Sci 1995;22:136–143.

52. Munchau A, Mathen D, Cox T, et al. Unilateral lesions of the globus pallidus: report of four patients presenting with focal or segmental dystonia. J Neurol Neurosurg Psychiatry 2000;69:494–498.

53. Bhatia KP, Marsden CD. The behavioural and motor consequences of focal lesions of the basal ganglia in man. Brain 1994;117:859–876.

54. Pettigrew LC, Jankovic J. Hemidystonia: a report of 22 patients and a review of the literature. J Neurol Neurosurg Psychiatry 1985;48:650–657.

55. Marsden CD. The focal dystonias. Clin Neuropharmacol 1986;9:S49-S60.

56. Koller WC. Adult-onset foot dystonia. Neurology 1984;34:703.

57. Berardelli A, Thompson PD, Day B, et al. Dystonia of the legs induced by walking or passive movement of the big toe in a patient with cerebellar ectopia and syringomyelia. Neurology 1986;36:40–44.

58. Blunt SB, Richards PG, Khalil N. Foot dystonia and lumbar canal stenosis. Mov Disord 1996;11:723–725.

59. Jedynak PC, Tranchant C, de Beyl DZ. Prospective clinical study of writer's cramp. Mov Disord 2001;16:494–499.

60. O'Neill MA, Gwinn KA, Adler CH. Biofeedback for writer's cramp. Am J Occup Ther 1997;51:605–607.

61. Deepak KK, Behari M. Specific muscle EMG biofeedback for hand dystonia. Appl Psychophysiol Biofeedback 1999;24:267–280.

62. Byl NN, McKenzie A. Treatment effectiveness for patients with a history of repetitive hand use and focal hand dystonia: a planned, prospective follow-up study. J Hand Ther 2000;13:289–301.

63. Candia V, Schafer T, Taub E, et al. Sensory motor retuning: a behavioral treatment for focal hand dystonia of pianists and guitarists. Arch Phys Med Rehabil 2002;83:1342–1348.

64. Zeuner KE, Bara-Jimenez W, Noguchi PS, et al. Sensory training for patients with focal hand dystonia. Ann Neurol 2002;51:593–598.

65. Candia V, Elbert T, Altenmuller E, et al. Constraint-induced movement therapy for focal hand dystonia in musicians [Letter]. Lancet 1999;353:42.

66. Priori A, Pesenti A, Cappellari A, et al. Limb immobilization for the treatment of focal occupational dystonia. Neurology 2001;57: 405–409.
67. Moberg-Wolff EA. An aggressive approach to limb dystonia: a case report. Arch Phys Med Rehabil 1998;79:589–590.
68. Iacono RP, Kuniyoshi SM, Schoonenberg T. Experience with stereotactics for dystonia: case examples. Adv Neurol 1998;78:221–226.
69. Goto S, Tsuiki H, Soyama N, et al. Stereotactic selective Vo-complex thalamotomy in a patient with dystonic writer's cramp. Neurology 1997;49:1173–1174.
70. van Hilten BJ, van de Beek WJ, Hoff JI, et al. Intrathecal baclofen for the treatment of dystonia in patients with reflex sympathetic dystrophy. N Engl J Med 2000;343:625–630.
71. Molloy FM, Shill HA, Kaelin-Lang A, et al. Accuracy of muscle localization without EMG: implications for treatment of limb dystonia. Neurology 2002;58:805–807.

PART IV

Therapeutic Considerations for Related and Other Conditions

CHAPTER 17

Spastic Dystonia

Jean-Michel Gracies and David M. Simpson

INTRODUCTION

Patients affected by motor paralysis resulting from damage to the central nervous system (CNS) commonly present with abnormal postures. Such postures, which affect the upper or lower limbs, may result in prominent deformities.[1] These deformities commonly adopt classic patterns that cause socially embarrassing disfigurement. Patients are clinically recognizable at a distance (e.g., upper limb flexed and pronated, lower limb straight with ankle in equinus).[2] In addition, clinicians often note increased tone in these patients (i.e., increased resistance to passive movement), which is often assessed regardless of the movement velocity.[3] These deformities and hypertonia may result from numerous mechanisms.

Spastic dystonia is the phenomenon of stretch-sensitive tonic muscle contraction, present without volitional command, including command to neighboring or distant muscles, and without phasic stretch of the affected muscle. In other words, it is the relative inability to rest muscles, responsive to the degree and duration of the tonic stretch imposed on the muscle. In most patients, tonic stretch maintained for at least several seconds inhibits spastic dystonia and improves the ability to rest muscle (Fig. 17-1).

Pollock and Davis,[4] working in decerebrate animals, observed the presence of permanent tonic muscle contractions that persisted after limb deafferentation. This observation was made before Denny-Brown[1] confirmed these findings in monkeys with various types of brain damage. Denny-Brown[1] justified the term spastic dystonia in monkeys with specific cortical lesions by the superimposition of dystonic and spastic features in the same muscle groups. This caused abnormal muscle contractions sensitive to the degree of stretch imposed on these muscles.[1] Similar observations were made in patients with spasticity caused by cerebral or spinal lesions. The notion

Jean-Michel Gracies: Assistant Professor of Neurology, The Mount Sinai Medical Center, New York, New York.

David M. Simpson: Professor of Neurology, Director of Clinical Neurophysiology Laboratories, The Mount Sinai Medical Center, New York, New York.

Jean-Michel Gracies and David Simpson have received grant support from Allergan and Elan, and speakers honorarium from Allergan.

of spastic dystonia has then been used by other authors.[5–9] Thus, spastic dystonia is a stretch-sensitive form of muscle overactivity; it is a feature virtually constant in patients affected by paralysis resulting from damage to the CNS. Spastic dystonia is highly responsive to the degree and duration of tonic stretch imposed on the dystonic muscle, such as that applied by the load of the forearm on the elbow flexors in seated or standing patients.[1] It is an important factor of deformity and increased resistance to passive movement (hypertonia). However, deformities and hypertonia may also result from the changes in passive muscle properties caused by prolonged immobilization and overactivity.[10–14] These eventually result in decreased passive extensibility of muscle.[10]

For treatment purposes, the symptom of spastic dystonia does not occur in isolation and is commonly associated with motor weakness and muscle shortening as well as with other types of stretch-sensitive forms of muscle overactivity (e.g., spasticity, spastic cocontraction).[2] This chapter reviews the pathophysiology, classic clinical presentations, evaluation, and treatment of spastic dystonia.

PATHOPHYSIOLOGY: MECHANISMS OF FUNCTIONAL IMPAIRMENT IN PATIENTS WITH CENTRAL NERVOUS SYSTEM MOTOR DAMAGE

Spastic dystonia must be considered within the context of the complex cascade of events that occurs after CNS motor damage. The authors review here the natural history of the mechanisms of functional impairment in affected patients, which has been discussed in more detail elsewhere.[2] Severe damage to central motor pathways provokes two series of events in the neural-muscular-skeletal chain contributing to movement.

Acute Events: Paralysis, Flaccidity, and Muscle Shortening

These events occur immediately after or within hours of injury and while the patient is still at the site of the accident, in the emergency department, or in the acute care unit. If the injury to motor centers involves the corticospinal pathway

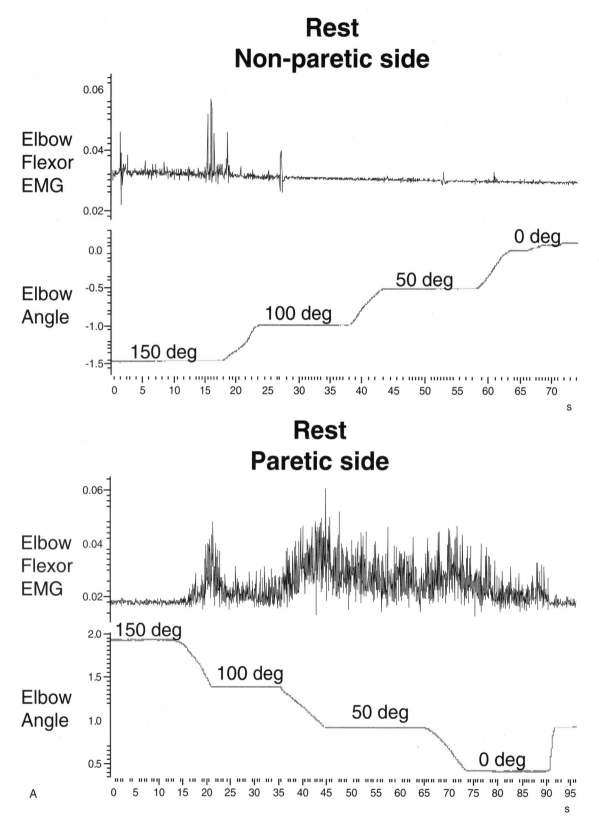

FIG. 17-1. Spastic dystonia, i.e. difficulty to rest muscle ameliorated by tonic stretch. Demonstration by a paradigm of staged stretch. The subject sits at a table with elbow and forearm supported by a rotating horizontal plate, connected to a potentiometer. The elbow is initially flexed at 150 degrees. A pair of AgCl surface electrodes 2 cm apart records elbow flexor activity. The subject is instructed to try and maintain the upper limb at absolute rest at all times, while the elbow is passively extended at slow velocity (10 deg/sec) by 50 degrees every 15-20 seconds. All analog data (elbow displacement recorded from potentiometer, sampling frequency 50Hz; surface EMG, sampling frequency 2500 Hz) are filtered (30-3KHz), converted using CED 1401 (Cambridge, UK) and recorded using Spike II software (Cambridge, UK). *Figure 1A* exemplifies a case in which the elbow flexors are at rest in the short position (muscle slack), before the initial stretch.

Rest
Non-paretic side

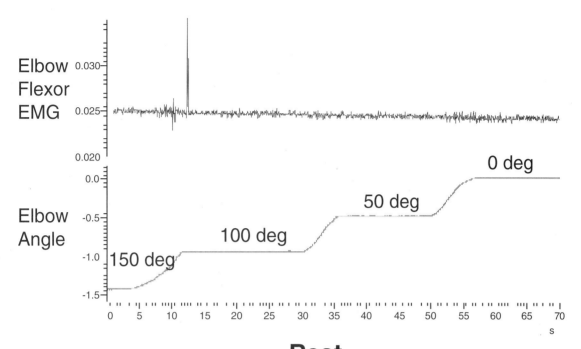

Rest
Paretic side

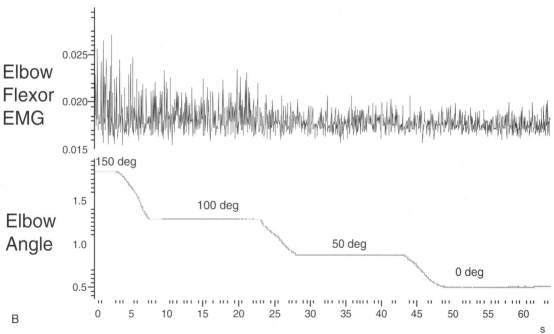

B

FIG. 17-1. *(Continued)* Despite the negative impact of each *phasic* stretch on the ability to maintain rest (due to the response to phasic stretch, or spasticity), each stage of tonic stretch is associated with gradual reduction of activity. In addition, the last potentiometer deflection at the extreme right of the figure corresponds to the elbow left free and returning to its new spontaneous resting position: this final position compatible with rest is 50 deg of flexion, a position which was associated with tonic involuntary activity prior to the stage of 0 degree stretch (full elbow extension).

Figure 1B exemplifies a case in which the elbow flexors are involuntarily active before the first stretch, and directly shows the improvement of the ability to maintain rest by *tonic* stretch (although there remains some involuntary activity after 60 seconds of staged stretch).

involved with the execution of voluntary command, the resulting paralysis immediately leaves muscles immobilized. In the acute care setting, patients are typically placed supine in stretchers, usually with the paralyzed lower limbs in full extension and the paralyzed upper limbs positioned in shoulder internal rotation, elbow flexion and pronation, and often wrist and finger flexion. Thus, among the paralyzed muscles, some are commonly immobilized in short position, and these often include extensors in the lower limbs and internal rotators, pronators, and flexors in the upper limbs. This immobilization in short position is the initial mechanism for muscle contracture, which includes loss of sarcomeres (shortening), loss of protein mass, and accumulation of connective tissue.[10,14] Most injuries to higher motor centers also disrupt other pathways that contribute to the descending flow that normally influences spinal cord reflex circuitry. This commonly results in the immediate extinction of spinal reflex responses, including stretch reflexes, with its clinical translation of flaccidity.

Subacute Events: Muscle Overactivity, Changes in Passive and Active Muscle Properties, Aggravation of Muscle, and Joint Retractions

This second set of events unfolds in the several weeks after injury. Both the CNS injury and paralysis-related disuse cause plastic neural rearrangements. As interrupted descending fibers degenerate, extensive sprouting occurs at segmental spinal levels whereby interneuronal endings branch out onto other interneurons or somatic motoneuronal membranes to occupy the spaces left empty by the missing descending fibers.[15] This causes abnormal reflex responses to peripheral inputs, such as to cutaneous stimuli[16] or to muscle stretch.[17] All contribute to global muscle overactivity,[18] including increased involuntary temporal motor unit recruitment (which thus coexists with paresis or insufficient maximal voluntary spatial motor unit recruitment). In addition to these plastic rearrangements at the spinal level, higher centers also develop replacement strategies to elicit movement, involving the remaining intact descending pathways (e.g., reticulospinal, rubrospinal, vestibulospinal), the remaining intact corticospinal fibers that may branch and sprout abnormally at the motor neurons level,[19,20] or ipsilateral motor cortex activation.[21] These cerebral mechanisms are a source of abnormal patterns of supraspinal descending drive, which also contribute to muscle overactivity.

Various Types of Muscle Overactivity

It is useful to group muscle overactivity into two categories, depending on whether or not it involves stretch sensitivity (i.e., whether the excessive involuntary motor unit recruitment is affected by the recruitment of stretch receptors in the overactive muscle).[2,22] The first category comprises the stretch-sensitive forms of muscle overactivity, which include spasticity, spastic dystonia, and spastic co-

contraction. These are distinguished by their primary triggering factor: phasic muscle stretch in spasticity; tonic muscle stretch in spastic dystonia; and volitional command in spastic concentration.[2]

- Spasticity is a velocity-dependent increase in stretch reflex (i.e., excessive muscle contraction in response to phasic stretch without volitional motor command).[23] Spasticity is thus measured at rest.
- Spastic dystonia has been defined above as involuntary tonic muscle contraction without phasic stretch or volitional command.
- Spastic cocontraction is the inappropriate recruitment of an antagonist triggered by volitional command on the agonist. This pathologic segmental cocontraction occurs in the absence of phasic stretch but is sensitive to the degree of tonic stretch of the cocontracting antagonist.[24]

Thus, spastic dystonia and spastic cocontraction are both primarily caused by an abnormal pattern of supraspinal descending drive, but can be aggravated by abnormal peripheral reflex reactions, in particular to the degree of tonic stretch imposed on the overactive muscle.

The second category of muscle overactivity comprises forms that are not prominently stretch sensitive.[2] They include pathologic extrasegmental cocontraction (i.e., features such as synkinesis, overflow, chorea, athetosis), excessive cutaneous or nociceptive responses, and inappropriate muscle recruitment during autonomic or reflex activities such as breathing, coughing, and yawning.[2] These forms of overactivity are likely to also involve some stretch-sensitivity, however, this has not been established as a major feature.

Changes in Passive and Active Muscle Properties

Increased resistance to stretch may result from changes in passive muscle properties that are caused by prolonged immobilization and overactivity.[10–14] In patients with spasticity, resting muscle passively opposes its stretch with an abnormally increased torque for the same lengthening as compared with normal muscle.[10] There are also immobilization- or overactivity-related changes in active muscle properties, which notably involve increased torque development per motor unit recruited.[25–28]

In conclusion, patients with spastic dystonia are impaired by numerous other mechanisms including muscle weakness, soft tissue contracture, and other types of muscle overactivity.

PATHOPHYSIOLOGY OF SPASTIC DYSTONIA

The pathophysiology of spastic dystonia is not completely understood.[1,4,9] The authors review here different hypotheses and the evidence supporting them. These hypotheses involve direct changes in the baseline excitability of motor neurons (MN), although these have not been directly demonstrated in humans, and changes in the excitability of spinal interneuronal pathways.

α-Motor Neuron Excitability

It was Romberg's[29] speculation that in patients with CNS damage there was an enhanced baseline activity of "α-spinal nerve cells." With the persistence of tonic permanent contractions after limb deafferentation in decerebrate animals,[1,4] Pollock and Davis, and later Denny-Brown, demonstrated that these contractions exist without stretch reflex. This reinforced Romberg's historic intuition. The hypothesis of primary α-hyperexcitability thus remained tenable because it would explain the widespread increase in motor reflex activities observed in patients with CNS lesions, whether from tendon, cutaneous, vegetative or propriospinal origin.[18] Indeed, increased α-MN excitability could be secondary to a change in membrane potential by removal of segmental inhibitory input, which is discussed below. Alternatively, this excitability could be primary, a phenomenon that has been called denervation supersensitivity. This phenomenon might be caused by spinal rearrangements that could take several forms, such as collateral sprouting of excitatory afferents or hyperexcitable areas of deafferented dendrites. Such alterations may be accompanied by anatomically demonstrable changes in numbers and kinds of synaptic endings on MNs. In animal studies, such alterations have been reported.[15]

Studies in humans have so far been unable to directly demonstrate α-hyperexcitability. The well accepted classic findings of increased Hmax/Mmax ratios,[30] increased F-wave amplitudes,[31] alterations in firing patterns,[32,33] desynchronization of motor units,[34] and increased responses to transcranial magnetic stimulation[35,36] constitute no direct evidence for α-hyperexcitability. Indeed, the preceding findings may be the result of changes in peripheral afferents, in Renshaw interneuron excitability, or in descending command, and thus are inadequate to really provide information on the excitability state of the α-MN. However, animal studies of the behavior of MN pools as well as individual MNs achieved important advances.

Motor Neuron Pools: Changes in Recruitment Gain

At any given time, the ability of a MN to generate an action potential depends on its intrinsic excitability and on the net sum of its synaptic inputs. Kernell and Hultborn[37] studied the influence of a change in synaptic input on the way the pool is recruited by a new stimulus. They introduced the term "recruitment gain" to indicate the relation between the input to a MN pool and the output (number of activated cells) from that pool.[37] If a new input situation has, for example, a different distribution to low- and high-threshold motor units (MUs), then the recruitment gain is changed. For instance, Blaschak et al.[38] and Powers and Rymer[39] have reported a compression of the recruitment order of the MUs in acute hemispinal cats. Spinal lesions acted to shift and compress the range of recruitment forces and minimum firing rates. After the lesion, all MNs tended to exhibit discharge behavior that was typical of that seen only in the lowest threshold MNs before

the lesion. In other words, there was an increase in the number of firing MNs for a low descending input after the lesion.[38,39] This is precisely in keeping with the relative inability to rest muscles characteristic of spastic dystonia.

In humans, the possibility of changes in recruitment gain has been demonstrated by Nielsen and Kagamihara,[40] in MN pools submitted to a new peripheral stimulation. However, there is as yet no evidence suggesting the contribution of increased recruitment gain to spastic dystonia in upper MN syndrome.

Individual Motor Neurons: Plateau Potentials

The studies by Hultborn and colleagues regarding modifications of discharge properties of individual MNs in chronic spinal cats (with long-term spinal cord injury), provide compelling clues for the presence and mechanism of α-hyperexcitability in spastic dystonia.[41–43] Several types of CNS neurons may generate prolonged depolarized states called plateau potentials, as first shown by Schwindt and Crill[44,45] using patch-clamp studies in spinal cats. Plateau potentials might provide a mechanism for maintaining continuous motor output despite weak tonic afferent input, for example, during the tonically maintained postures characteristic of spastic dystonia.[41,42] Using intracellular recording from MNs, Hounsgaard et al.[41] showed that a short train of excitatory synaptic potentials provoked a sustained increase in α-MN activity as a result of an all-or-none plateau depolarization. They further demonstrated that the tonic motor responses to brief stretch observed in the decerebrate cat are dependent on plateau potentials in the activated MNs.[43]

Presynaptic Inhibition on Ia Afferents and Homosynaptic Depression

Decreased presynaptic inhibition on Ia afferents and decreased homosynaptic depression at rest have been shown in patients with upper MN syndrome.[46–49] Decreased presynaptic inhibition of Ia afferents may enhance the facilitatory input from stretch receptors to MNs and thus contribute to tonic contractions for minimal tonic stretch (e.g., the stretch imposed on the elbow flexors by the load of the forearm). Decreased homosynaptic depression at rest may also contribute to enhancing contraction caused by tonic stretch, as it leads to a relative increase in the probability of transmitter release after repetitive synaptic activation.[50]

γ-Motor Neuron Excitability

The question whether enhanced fusimotor activity has a role in spastic dystonia is not resolved. Enhanced fusimotor activity, particularly of the static γ-MNs, might contribute to excessive motor responses to static stretch imposed by limb weight. From studies in the ordinary decerebrate cat, authors had claimed that γ-hyperactivity exists and contributes to maintenance of hypertonia.[51–53] However, all arguments advanced in favor of the γ-participation in human spasticity, in particular the impact of procainization[54,55] and the comparison between T and H responses,[54,56–59] were refuted or inconclusive.[60,61]

Findings based on thixotropy in human spastic muscles have shown that fusimotor drive is preserved in hemiplegia,[61] however, the most direct method to evaluate the existence of γ-hyperactivity as a factor contributing to spastic dystonia has been to directly record Ia afferents in microneurography.[62,63] Few microneurograhic studies have compared the discharge characteristics of primary spindle endings in spastics directly to those in normals.[62,63] These studies were unable to demonstrate noteworthy hyperactivity of Ia fibers in patients with spastic hemiplegia compared to normals.[62,63] However, the findings of Hagbarth et al.[62] did include a trend for increased static spindle sensitivity in the hemiplegic lower limb. Further data are required to draw definitive conclusions on γ-participation in spastic dystonia.

Nonreciprocal Ib Inhibition

Golgi tendon organs are contraction-sensitive receptors, whose response to passive changes in muscle length is comparatively small.[64] Nonreciprocal Ib inhibition, formerly called autogenic Ib inhibition (because it acts as a retrocontrol on its own muscle), is transmitted from Golgi tendon organs via large diameter group I afferents and an inhibitory interneuron called Ib.[65] Any extensor muscle contraction is normally inhibited by the Ib discharge from Golgi tendon organs of the contracting muscle, but the Ib effect is facilitatory on flexor MNs, hence the concept of nonreciprocal inhibition.[66]

Ib-mediated inhibition has been found to disappear in the decerebrate cat[67] and be reversed into facilitation in human spastic soleus.[68–72] This makes the Golgi tendon organ less effective at antagonizing muscle contraction when an extensor muscle is abnormally contracting, whether by stretch reflex or by abnormal descending contraction. Thus, this pathophysiologic mechanism might certainly play a prominent role in spastic dystonia; interestingly, it is also involved in parkinsonian rigidity.[72,73]

Recurrent Renshaw Inhibition

During their discharge, α-MNs are subject to a postsynaptic inhibition exerted by an interneuron, which is activated by a collateral branch of the motor axon (recurrent inhibition). This interneuron is called the Renshaw cell. Renshaw cells are subject to supraspinal control, which may either decrease or increase recurrent inhibition.[74] In theory, the inhibition (or dysfacilitation) of Renshaw cells after a CNS lesion could be responsible for an exaggeration in the tonic component of the stretch reflex, since a given discharge of any MN pool would be less effectively opposed by recurrent inhibition.

In decerebrate and chronic spinal cats, recurrent inhibition is increased rather than decreased, thus indicating that

changes in Renshaw cell excitation are not responsible for stretch reflex exaggeration in these preparations.[75] In humans, a method for estimating recurrent inhibition elicited by an orthodromic MN discharge has been developed.[76,77] This method was used to show that recurrent inhibition is also increased at rest in several populations of spastic patients,[78–82] except for one study in progressive paraparesis.[83] Thus, while this mechanism might not play a prominent role in spastic dystonia, it might have an important role in another type of muscle overactivity, namely spastic cocontraction, because increased Renshaw inhibition leads to decreased reciprocal Ia inhibition.

Group II Effects: Response to Small Diameter Afferent Input

The spindle secondary ending responds selectively to changes in muscle length and sends impulses to group II fibers that reach α-MNs essentially via interneurons.[84] These group II pathways have both an excitatory and inhibitory effect on homonymous MNs.[85] The enhancement in synaptic transmission from some group II muscle afferents may possibly play an important role in the development of exaggerated stretch reflexes in spastic patients.[86]

In acute spinal cat preparations, the group II afferent fibers are believed to belong to the flexor reflex afferents (FRA).[87,88] The FRAs, defined by Eccles and Lundberg,[89] are group II and III muscle afferents, cutaneous afferents, and high-threshold joint afferents that produce autogenic inhibition of extensor reflexes and autogenic facilitation of flexor reflexes. Transmission in these inhibitory pathways to extensor MNs is blocked in the decerebrate state, which could contribute to spastic dystonia in the hind limb extensors.[89]

In humans, there is no simple method to selectively explore group II pathways. Burke et al.[90,91] attempted to explore group II effects on H-reflexes of leg muscles in spastic subjects by evaluating changes after selective ischemic blockade of group I fibers and after infiltration of procain hydrochloride into the muscle (which was supposed to block small nerve fibers preferentially).[90,91] Using successive steps of tonic muscle stretch, they suggested that group II afferents might produce predominantly extensor inhibition and flexor facilitation in spastic subjects,[91] and that while the dynamic sensitivity of the primary ending determined the velocity dependence of the spastic stretch reflex, the responses to tonic changes in muscle length might be predominantly determined by inputs from the secondary ending.[91] However, these studies had no control group and the question whether inhibitory group II effects toward extensor muscles were decreased and might contribute to spastic dystonia could not be answered. Studies using different methodology, focusing on high threshold and long latency of effects from peripheral afferents, support this concept.[92] In particular, these studies suggest a potent heteronymous group II excitation of quadriceps MNs, which may contribute to spastic dystonia in hemiplegic patients.[93,94]

Contractile Muscle Properties: Immobilization- and Overactivity-Related Changes

After skeletal muscle immobilization in animals and in humans, some muscles composed predominantly of type I fibers (i.e., "red," low threshold, slow twitch, fatigue-resistant, well equipped for oxidative metabolism and semi-isometric contractions, such as soleus muscle fibers) take on properties characteristic of type II muscles (i.e., "white," fast twitch, high threshold, fatigue-sensitive).[95] These changes are also partially seen after acute CNS lesion in animals.[39] However, the immobilization and CNS lesion-induced changes may vary according to the initial motor unit type.[39,96] Despite conflicting results in the literature,[39] these changes have been shown to be concomitant with an increase in the torque developed for a given motor unit recruitment,[25,97,98] potentially a high-tension development for a moderate increase in electromyographic (EMG) activity.[27] Such increased tension development might contribute to enhancing the clinical manifestations of spastic dystonia, aggravating the postures adopted by the dystonic limbs.

In summary, the mechanisms shown in humans to potentially contribute to spastic dystonia include decreased presynaptic inhibition on Ia afferents, decreased homosynaptic depression, decreased Ib inhibition, increased facilitatory group II effects, and changes in contractile muscle properties. There is as yet no direct evidence for a role of α- and γ-MN hyperactivity.

CLASSIC CLINICAL PRESENTATIONS AND EVALUATION

The most common clinical manifestations of spastic dystonia are abnormal postures, affecting primarily the limbs. Mayer and colleagues reviewed common forms of abnormal spastic posturing elsewhere.[99] Many of the muscles involved in spastic dystonia are also involved in spastic cocontraction, and recognizing and treating an abnormal posture may help improve active movements around the corresponding joints.

Upper Limb

Extended Shoulder

Patients with upper MN syndrome often present with a slightly extended shoulder, which can be seen and measured by photographing the patient from the side while standing. While the posture itself is rarely disfiguring, it usually heralds difficulties with reaching movements, as most muscles affected with spastic dystonia are often also involved in spastic cocontraction. While reaching movements represent the majority of common upper limb movements, shoulder extensor overactivity has often been overlooked in studies of upper limb spasticity treatment.

The primary muscles involved in this pathologic posture include latissimus dorsi, long head of triceps, teres major,

and posterior deltoid. However, the posterior deltoid is also a minor external rotator of the shoulder. The clinician may want to spare this muscle in treatment if the patient is also affected by excessive shoulder internal rotation (see below). Other muscles to consider in the treatment of the extended shoulder are not shoulder extensors per se but those contributing to impeding active shoulder flexion (muscles affected by spastic cocontraction). These muscles include scapular adductors (rhomboid major and minor, middle trapezius), involved as antagonists beyond 60° of shoulder flexion, and pectoralis major, involved as an antagonist beyond 90° of shoulder flexion.[100]

Adducted and Internally Rotated Shoulder

This is another common abnormal posture in patients with upper MN syndrome, particularly frequent in patients after ischemic stroke in the territory of the middle cerebral artery. This deformity modifies sitting posture and standing balance, may lead to maceration in the armpit, and impedes certain activities such as cleaning this area and dressing. The major internal rotator of the shoulder is the subscapularis, a muscle that is difficult to reach in local treatment because of the particular anatomic location of the muscle bulk between the scapula and the rib cage. Most of the other muscles involved are the extensors outlined in the preceding paragraph (i.e., latissimus dorsi, teres major, and pectoralis major). Anterior deltoid is a minor internal rotator but should often be preserved because it is the major shoulder flexor.

Externally Rotated Shoulder

This less common abnormal posture sometimes occurs after hemorrhagic strokes or traumatic brain injuries. It may be troublesome during walking, especially in a crowded area, because the forearm and hand of the patient may inadvertently bump into objects or people. The shoulder external rotators are infraspinatus and teres minor. They are relatively easy to reach in local treatment because of their superficial anatomic location, below and lateral to the scapular spine.

Flexed Elbow

Patients often complain of the disfigurement caused by this other extremely common abnormal posture in upper MN syndrome. Beyond the cosmetic issue, this deformity may impede dressing and other activities of daily living. One way to measure elbow flexor spastic dystonia may be derived from the method of measuring elbow flexor contracture developed by O'Dwyer et al.[101] The subject lies supine with the upper arm resting horizontally on a firm bed, with the shoulder in neutral position. The arm is released and maintained in extension solely by the weight of the forearm due to gravity. The position of the arm is photographed from the side after a few seconds in this posture and spastic dystonia of the elbow flexor muscles is quantified by measuring the angle of the forearm relative to the bed from the photograph (Fig. 17-2). The muscles involved are brachialis, brachioradialis, and biceps brachii. For treatment purposes, the biceps brachii must be considered with caution because it is also a powerful supinator. Patients affected by elbow flexor spastic dystonia often have associated pronator dystonia (see below).

Pronated Elbow

Commonly associated with the flexed elbow, spastic dystonia in the pronators is less of a functional problem than the spastic cocontraction that may affect these muscles (when attempting active movements requiring supination such as reaching and grasping). The muscles involved are pronator teres and pronator quadratus. Flexor carpi radialis also exerts a minor pronator torque.

Flexed Wrist and Clenched Hand

This classic deformity causes problems with skin hygiene in the palm, splinting, and comfort. When severe and untreated, flexed wrist and clenched hand may lead to maceration of the palmar skin and a fungal infection that might eventually lead to complications such as skin dehiscence and bacterial infection of the underlying tendon sheaths.[102] The primary muscles involved are flexor carpi radialis (associated pronation), flexor carpi ulnaris (associated ulnar deviation), palmaris longus (associated cupping of hand), abductor pollicis longus (associated thumb abduction), flexor digitorum superficialis (associated flexion of the proximal interphalangeal joint), flexor pollicis longus (associated flexion of the interphalangeal joints of the thumb), and flexor digitorum profundus (associated flexion of the distal interphalangeal joints).

Metacarpophalangeal Flexion

This deformity may sometimes appear after treatment of flexed wrist and clenched hand, whether the spastic dystonia in the metacarpophalangeal (MP) flexors was an underlying problem now unmasked or a new feature brought about by CNS plasticity after relaxation of the extrinsic flexors. The muscles involved are the lumbricales, dorsal interossei, and palmar interossei. Treatment of this deformity is difficult, as selective weakening of any of these muscles might lead to weakening distal finger extension.

Thumb in Palm

The muscles involved are opponens pollicis, adductor pollicis, and flexor pollicis brevis.

Lower Limb

Adducted Hip

Hip adductor spastic dystonia is a classic cause of difficulties with perineal hygiene and urinary catheterization, particularly common in patients with spinal cord injury, advanced multiple sclerosis, or chronic cerebral palsy. The muscles involved are adductor brevis, longus and magnus, as well as pectineus and gracilis.

Flexed Hip and Knee

This abnormal posture may be seen in long-term wheelchair-bound patients with spinal cord injury. It impedes comfortable wheelchair posturing. The major muscles involved are psoas major and iliacus. Minor culprits may also include rectus femoris (hip flexion associated with knee extension), sar-

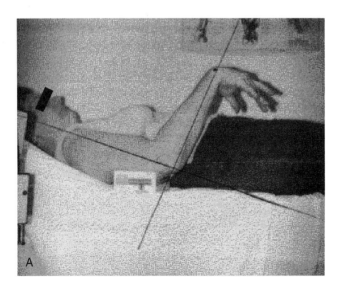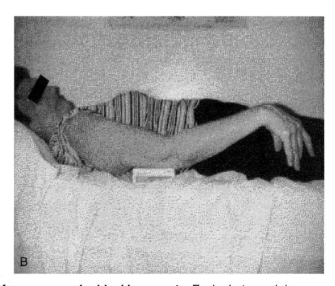

FIG. 17-2. Reduction of spastic dystonia by local injection of neuromuscular blocking agents. Each photograph is taken after a few seconds of rest in the supine position as the subject is instructed to relax completely. The subject had particularly severe elbow flexor spastic dystonia initially (photo A), probably combined with soft tissue contracture. Photo B is taken one month after injection of 160 MU of BTX-A (Botox®) into the elbow flexors.

torius (association with hip abduction and external rotation), tensor fasciae latae (association with hip abduction), and pectineus or adductor brevis, longus, and magnus (association with hip adduction). The medial hamstring group (gracilis, semitendinosus, semimembranosus) and biceps femoris may also participate in knee flexion but are also hip extensors.

Ankle Plantar Flexed (Equinus)

Equinus is the most common abnormal posture in patients with upper MN syndrome. Because the gastrocnemius muscle crosses the knee joint, flexion of the knee reduces the stretch on this muscle, thus limiting its contribution to plantar flexor torque output. Therefore, when excessive plantar flexion remains severe with knee flexed, involvement of soleus is certain. When treating this deformity, the soleus is by far the most powerful plantar flexor; even with the knee fully extended (case of maximal contribution from gastrocnemius to plantar flexion), the contribution of soleus to plantar flexor torque is close to 60% of the total plantar flexor torque and increases from there with increasing levels of knee flexion.[103] Other plantar flexors often involved in maintaining or aggravating equinus are flexor digitorum longus and flexor hallucis longus.

Inversion Associated with Plantar Flexion (Equinovarus)

Spastic dystonia in soleus alone might be indirectly responsible for an inverted posture. This is the case when compensatory dorsiflexor overactivity from tibialis anterior is diverted into inversion, as the dorsiflexor component is cancelled out by the soleus dystonia.[104] Treating tibialis anterior instead of soleus in this case might be counterproductive and simply lead to aggravate plantar flexed posture. In other patients, the main culprit is tibialis posterior. Proper treatment of a plantar flexed and inverted ankle might allow heel strike during gait and ease fitting of orthoses.

Clawed Toes

This abnormal posture may lead to pain when walking barefoot or in shoes. Muscles involved include: lumbricales, palmar, and dorsal interossei and flexor hallucis brevis (MP flexion); flexor digitorum brevis and flexor hallucis longus (proximal interphalangeal flexion); and flexor digitorum longus (distal interphalangeal flexion). Local treatment of this deformity (see below) is often rewarding.

Hitchhiking Toe

This is a relatively common deformity in patients with upper MN syndrome. Functionally, patients complain of pain at the big toe inside shoes when they initiate walking. Overactivity in extensor hallucis longus is the usual culprit. There are no systematic studies of the pathophysiology of this particular

deformity. As opposed to the deformities seen above, overactivity in extensor hallucis longus in patients with upper MN syndrome neither demonstrably nor intuitively corresponds to spastic dystonia. On the contrary, it might result from nonspastic compensatory dorsiflexor activity in patients who have severe plantar flexor spastic dystonia. Still, the problem may be extremely troublesome to patients and often requires treatment to improve footwear comfort.

EVALUATION

Two issues are intertwined in the evaluation of the patient with spastic dystonia. One issue is to measure spastic dystonia itself; such assessment may be quantitative only for limited muscle groups at the clinic. Another issue is the assessment of the functional consequences of spastic dystonia.

Measurement of Spastic Dystonia

There is no direct clinical assessment that reliably distinguishes spastic dystonia from soft tissue contracture. This measurement should always be part of the wider clinical assessment of patients with spasticity, which includes the four primary assessments of passive and active motor function: passive range of motion, spasticity, active range of motion, and rapid alternating movement (Table 17-1). The first level of assessment, passive range of motion (PROM or angle of movement arrest at slow speed), is a marker of both spastic dystonia and soft tissue contracture. Two other partial and indirect methods for evaluating spastic dystonia are available, including measurement of resting posture in the affected joints, which may be done in various body positions (e.g., standing, sitting, etc.), and the assessment of the resistance to passive movement or tone assessment as with the Ashworth Scale.[3]

Resting Posture

It is difficult to quantify resting posture for each joint and muscle group. For specific muscle groups (e.g., elbow flexors or shoulder extensors) photographs of the patient at rest, which may be repeated after treatment, may be helpful. When taking these photographs, bony landmarks may be used to place light stickers that can then be used to accurately measure joint angles on the photographs (Fig. 17-2). For most other muscle groups in routine practice, spastic dystonia should at least be assessed qualitatively, which consists of determining whether a muscle group is overactive at rest or not (i.e., whether the resting posture is abnormal or not). While the qualitative assessment of spastic dystonia may be sufficient to pose the indications for treatment, the quantitative assessment measures its effects. Outside research purposes, EMG recordings usually add little to a careful clinical examination.

However, neither resting posture nor tone assessment allows the distinction between spastic dystonia and muscle shortening or other soft tissue contracture. This distinction is a difficult task as both problems are usually intermingled.

TABLE 17-1. *Assessment of Spastic Paralysis*

Subject id: _____ Visit: _____ Date: _____

UPPER LIMB

Motion	Opposing Muscles	Passive PROM V1 Stretch	Passive Spasticity ANGLE Diff: V1-V3 (V2 or V3 Stretch)	Passive Spastic Dystonia Rest posture	Passive Ashworth	Active AROM Start	Active AROM End	Active SPASTIC cocontraction (check)	RAM
Shoulder									
Shrug	Lower trap, Rhombs								
	Scap add (>60°): Rhombs, Middle trap, LD								
Flexion	LD, TM, PD, LHT, PM>90°								
Extension	Ant Delt, Supras, CB								
Vert Abduction	Lat dorsi, Pect maj								
Hor Abduction	PD, T minor, Infras, Pmaj								
Ext rotation	SS,P maj, Lat,T maj								
Int rotation	Infraspinatus, Teres minor								
Elbow									
Extension	BB, B, BR								
Flexion	TB								
Supination	PT, PQ								
Pronation	Supinator, BB								
Wrist									
Extension	FCR, FCU, FDS, FDP								
Flexion	ECR, ECU, EDC								
Fingers									
Extension PIII/PII	FDP 2,3,4,5								
Extension PII/MC	FDS 2,3,4,5+PIO								
Extension PI/MC	PL, PIO, Lumbricals								
Thumb extension	FPL, FPB								
Thumb abduction	Thumb adductor								

PROM, passive range of motion; AROM, active range of motion; RAM, rapid alternating movement; V1, V2, V3: velocities of stretch; V1, as slow as possible; V2, velocity of the fall of the limb segment under gravity; V3: as fast as possible for the examiner; LD, latissimus dorsi; T, teres; PD, posterior deltoid; LHT, long head of triceps; PM, pectoralis major; CB, coracobrachialis; SS, supraspinatus; BB, biceps brachii; BR, brachioradialis; TB, triceps brachii; PT, pronator teres; PQ, pronator quadratus; FCR, flexor carpi radialis; FCU, flexor carpi ulnaris; FDS, flexor digitorum superficialis; FDP, flexor digitorum profundis; ECR, extensor carpi radialis; ECU, extensor carpi ulnaris; EDC, extensor digitorum communis; PIO, palmar interosseus; PL, palmaris longus; FPL, flexor pollicis longus; FPB, flexor pollicis brevis; EDC, extensor digitorum communis.

The distinction is still important because treatments specific for muscle shortening, particularly surgical treatments, are not required, and may in fact be deleterious in patients with predominant spastic dystonia. Conversely, patients with predominant muscle shortening with little or no dystonia will not be substantially improved by focal muscle weakening, a treatment specific for muscle overactivity. By definition, maximal sustained stretch at least partially releases spastic dystonia. If, despite maximal sustained stretch, the passive range of motion remains incomplete, noteworthy muscle shortening is probably associated with spastic dystonia. The ultimate test is a temporary block (local anesthetics), provided the block is complete. Otherwise, surface EMG monitoring during various resting postures may also be helpful (Fig. 17-1).

Assessment of the Functional Consequences of Spastic Dystonia

One method is to use a global subjective self-assessment of the targeted limb by the patient, such as the one shown in the Appendix 17-1, in which question 2 relates to passive functional impairment by spastic dystonia. Patients may then express their own particular problem (different from patient to patient) in this global opinion. Another option is to ask the subject to choose priority goals in a list of preselected common problems in upper limb spasticity (i.e., goal attainment scale).[105] These outcomes include the ability to put the affected arm through a sleeve (potentially impaired by spastic dystonia in elbow flexors and shoulder extensors and internal rotators), the ability to open the affected hand to clean the palm, the ability to cut the fingernails (potentially impaired by spastic dystonia in wrist and finger flexors), etc. The patient then rates the change in these priority areas after treatment.

TREATMENTS

Spastic dystonia is not evenly distributed throughout the muscles and there is always imbalance across joints between less overactive agonists and more overactive antagonists. Thus, the limb position around a joint stabilizes when the contractile forces generated by the "more spastic/dystonic" agonist are matched essentially by the soft tissue resistance from the side of the "less spastic/dystonic" antagonist. This resistance is occasionally superimposed on other forces such as the weight of the limb segment (elbow flexion/extension in a sitting or standing patient). In spastic patients, the joint stabilization at rest thus occurs at unnatural joint positions and contributes to the shortening and thus the increased spasticity (as described above) of the more overactive agonist, with the emergence of fixed deformities. The use of systemic therapies (oral or intrathecal) might improve posture and comfort in some patients but is not likely to improve active function, since these therapies tend to indiscriminately reduce motoneuronal excitability in both agonists and antagonists and may also cause additional peripheral muscle weakening.[106] Therefore, the authors recommend therapy targeting spastic dystonia in specific muscles (local treatments) as opposed to systemic approaches. The primary treatments available for spastic dystonia are chronic stretch and focal weakening. For optimal outcome, these two approaches should be used in combination.

Chronic Stretch

The effects of chronic stretch on spastic features and the various modalities available (passive range of motion exercises, dynamic splints, static splints, casting and serial casting) have been reviewed.[2] Because muscle overactivity is a factor of muscle shortening,[4,107] and because muscle shortening in turn increases spindle sensitivity,[11–13] muscle shortening

---

APPENDIX 17-1. *Patient Self-Assessment*

1. Do you have pain in your upper limb?

Worst pain imaginable ————————————————— No pain

2. Do you have any discomfort caused by the stiffness in your arm (for example when walking, getting dressed, cleaning your palm)?

Worst discomfort imaginable ————————————————— No discomfort

3. How would you rate the function of your upper limb today?

Totally useless ————————————————— Normal

and spastic dystonia are intertwined. Methods to lengthen muscles will participate in the treatment of spastic dystonia and its functional consequences. Indeed, there is a growing body of evidence for the beneficial effect of chronic stretch in spastic dystonia.

Influence of Stretch Duration

Briefly sustained stretch (i.e., a few seconds) during and immediately after contraction reduces stretch reflex responses when the muscle is tested back at its normal length (shown in animal studies).[108,109] This has been ascribed at least in part to the slack in intrafusal fibers that occurs when the muscle is returned to its normal length after being stretched; this reduces background spindle afferent discharge.[110,111] In spastic patients, as in healthy subjects, stretch reflexes are also depressed after contraction in a stretched position.[61,112] Repeated brief large amplitude joint movements also reduce spastic dystonia.[113] However, this effect disappears after only one contraction in spastic muscles, whereas it persists for at least three subsequent contractions in healthy muscles.[61] This implies that clinical use of muscle stretch to reduce spastic dystonia should be more effective if stretch is applied continuously or if a brief stretch is reapplied at frequent intervals.[61]

Maintained stretch (sessions of 30 minutes to 3 hours) was shown in open and controlled studies to reduce spastic dystonia (improvement of posture, reduction of stretch reflexes, or both) after a single session in spastic patients.[22,114–117] These effects are proportional to the degree of muscle elongation accomplished in the stretch.[116] Reduced spindle thixotropy[109] and intrinsic reduction in stretch reflex excitability at the spinal level (particularly homosynaptic depression and changes in presynaptic inhibition)[118,119] may explain these effects.

Chronic stretch (days to weeks duration) also reduces stretch reflexes.[120–126] Three controlled studies of casting or dynamic splinting show a decrease in spasticity and spastic dystonia after chronic stretch and an increase in range of motion that are greater than with traditional therapy, consisting of passive range of motion exercises.[121,123,124] Results with casting may be superior to those obtained with splinting.[124] In addition to changes in thixotropy and in stretch reflex excitability at the spinal level, the changes after chronic stretch may also be caused by true muscle lengthening, which permits decreased spindle stimulation for a given amount of stretching stimulus.

In summary, brief, sustained, and chronic stretch reduce spastic dystonia, while chronic stretch also lengthens overactive muscles or helps maintain their length.[127–129] For optimal efficacy, chronic stretch must probably be implemented as early as possible after CNS injury.[130,131] This was successful in an open study of serial leg casts implemented within 14 days of head injury for the prevention or correction of equinus.[132] In view of the extremely rapid muscle changes in patients with CNS injury, which are detectable as early as several hours after the onset of immobilization in short position (see above), quasi-immediate implementation of chronic stretch in vulnerable muscles might be beneficial after CNS injury. However, controlled evidence for the benefits of ultra-early chronic stretch in the spastic dystonia of patients with CNS injury is still lacking.

Injections of Neuromuscular-Blocking Agents

Both physiologic findings and clinical evidence indicate that spastic dystonia and muscle shortening would be best addressed simultaneously.[133,134] A physical modality primarily aimed at lengthening a muscle may have optimal results if combined with chemical or physical treatment aimed at relaxing the muscle.

Botulinum Toxin Type A

Studies of botulinum toxin type A (BTX-A) injections in spastic patients show reduction of spastic dystonia, lengthening of muscle, or both by tone reduction in the injected muscles after injection; few of these studies have directly quantified specific considerations such as resting posture.[135–157] High dilution (e.g., 20–50 U/mL of BTX-A as BOTOX [Allergan, Inc., Irvine, CA]) achieves better results, particularly in proximal muscles.[158]

Other Muscle Blocking Agents: Alcohol Compounds (Alcohol, Phenol)

Potential advantages of alcohol and phenol over BTX-A include low cost, better stability, and inability to provoke formation of antibodies. Disadvantages include tissue destruction, lack of selectivity on motor function, and adverse effects, including chronic painful dysesthesia, muscle induration and vascular reactions.[159,160] In one study, BTX-A injected intramuscularly was safer than 5% phenol injected perineurally to treat overactive calf muscles in chronic stroke patients, as complications such as common peroneal nerve palsy occurred with perineural phenol only.[161] There was no difference in effectiveness between the two techniques. However, it is possible as well as effective to restrict the alcohol administration technique to intramuscular injections, into the motor point regions (which reduces the risk of dysesthesia). There has not been a comparison of BTX-A and alcohol using a similar intramuscular technique.

Many clinicians combine local treatments, using alcohol compounds for perineural injections to block large proximal muscles, and BTX-A for smaller and more distal muscles that can be selectively targeted. However, the respective indications of neurolytic agents and BTX-A may also be based on severity and prognosis. Because of the potential for chronic adverse effects and destruction of muscle and sensory fibers, alcohol or phenol may be more appropriate than BTX-A in patients with severe symptoms in which the purpose of treatment is not recovery of active function, but rather passive function and comfort (i.e., to treat primarily spastic dystonia). Conversely, the absence of tissue destruction after repeated BTX-A injections and the specific action on efferent fibers might render this treatment preferable in situations where there is reasonable hope for functional recovery in the injected area. Pharmaco-economic considerations suggest that controlled comparative studies between neurolytic agents and BTX-A be performed in these different situations.

Treatment Strategy and Muscle Selection

In most patients, muscles presenting with spastic dystonia also cocontract inappropriately during antagonist efforts (spastic cocontraction). This common overlap between excessive contraction at rest and excessive antagonist contraction during agonist activity (spastic cocontraction), should lead clinicians to assess and treat both types of symptoms in association. The authors recommend selecting muscles according to two qualitative assessments based on inspection and palpation: one at rest and one during tests of active range of motion. The clinician may thus list the muscles presenting with spastic dystonia (overactive when examined at rest) as well as those presenting with spastic cocontraction (overactive when examined during active effort on their antagonist). Treating muscles affected with spastic dystonia primarily aims at improvement of passive function, while treating muscles affected with spastic cocontraction should improve active function.

In the case of muscles that are difficult to see and tendons difficult to palpate (e.g., shoulder extensors, obese patient), the demonstration of spastic cocontraction or spastic dystonia may be done by using a lidocaine test. Clear improvement in posture or movement after lidocaine injection in the suspected muscles demonstrates that overactivity in these muscles is functionally disabling.

Injection Technique: Stimulation Technique, Endplate Targeting

Informed consent should be obtained from all patients prior to any procedure, including injections of phenol, alcohol, lidocaine or BTX-A, and explained the potential benefits and potential risks of the procedure(s).

The authors recommend using the exploratory stimulation technique, whether targeting muscles with BTX-A or an alcohol compound. This is thought to be the most accurate technique to distinguish a muscle from its neighbors and is also the only technique that permits intramuscular localization (e.g., when injecting around motor points in an attempt to reach areas dense in endplates). In the stimulation technique, the injection needle delivers repetitive monopolar cathodal stimulation to the targeted area; the anode is a surface plate electrode, which, optimally, is taped over the opposite side of the limb to avoid confusing homonymous contractions due to anodal stimulation. When a minimal stimulation voltage elicits contraction of the target muscle (and no other neighboring muscle), as

confirmed by visual observation or tendon palpation, this indicates that the needle tip is placed inside that muscle and no other. One randomized study indicated that stimulation was superior to EMG recording in the targeting of finger flexors.[162]

It has not yet been demonstrated whether targeting motor endplates inside a muscle improves the efficacy of BTX-A injection. The authors have been conducting a controlled study to address this question in human biceps brachii, for which a cadaver study has helped define useful surface landmarks to target the endplate zone.[158] Because surface landmarks corresponding to endplate areas have not been well defined for most muscles other than biceps brachii in humans, some investigators have tried to target "motor points" in upper limb muscles,[135,136,138] which are defined physiologically by the sites of lowest percutaneous stimulation threshold which evoke muscle response, or anatomically by the sites where the motor nerve penetrates the muscle.[163] However, motor points may not always correlate with the vicinity of endplates in long muscles because axonal branching can occur up to several centimeters before motor nerve endings and neuromuscular junctions.[164]

Combination of Neuromuscular Blocking Injections with Muscle Stretch

While rigid or semi-rigid devices have been used, including rigid splints, serial casting, and dynamic splints (see above),[22,130,165] intensive home stretching programs may be the most satisfactory stretch strategy in selected subjects. Subjects instructed in a home finger flexor stretching program after long finger flexor injection with BTX-A had good results in an open study focusing on hand opening.[153] In the lower limb, the combination of selective injections of low BTX-A doses with ankle-foot taping is as effective as the injection of higher doses in reducing spastic dystonia.[166]

Combination of Neuromuscular Blocking Injections with Training of the Antagonist

Changes in training interventions in spasticity include increasing emphasis on active exercise and task-specific training, and active and passive methods of preserving muscle extensibility.[167,168] To the authors' knowledge, there is no published sham-controlled study assessing the effect of the combination of antagonist training and agonist BTX-A injection on resting posture and spastic dystonia.

Injection of Neuromuscular Blocking Agents Combined with Electrical Simulation Program

Studies by Hesse et al.[169,170] in hemiparetic patients have suggested that a program of periodic stimulation of the injected muscle and its antagonist for three 30-minute sessions per day during the 3 days after injection of BTX-A (Dysport, Ipsen Ltd., Maidenhead, Berks, United Kingdom) may improve resistance to passive movement in the injected muscles.[169,170] A lower limb study tested a program of stimulation of the injected muscle only and did not confirm these results.[171] Sham-controlled studies (e.g., with stimulation below and above sensory or motor threshold) are required to establish the advantage of combining BTX-A injections with a stimulation program, particularly on the antagonist.

Systemic Antispastic Treatments (Oral and Intrathecal)

These treatments are often effective in reducing spastic dystonia.[172] However, as the safety and efficacy of local treatments, in particular BTX-A, is becoming increasingly apparent, it is a legitimate question whether the use of systemic drugs as first-line therapy is still appropriate in patients with spasticity. The authors' review of the 29 available systemic antispasticity treatments (oral and intrathecal) yielded the following conclusions[172]:

- All systemic antispastic agents, except piracetam, have been approved by regulatory agencies or accepted by the community based only on their capacity to reduce stretch responses, much like the data generated in the first era of BTX-A studies.
- Agents that reduce response to muscle stretch are nonselective in depressing central nervous system responses. Systemic administration of these agents also causes numerous central effects on higher functions (e.g., sedation, drowsiness, hypotension, bradycardia, depression, cognitive impairment, tolerance, etc.).
- Most systemic agents that reduce response to stretch improve patient comfort, which may lead to favorable subjective patient assessments. Some have also been shown to improve passive function in controlled studies. No antispastic systemic agent has been shown to improve active function in controlled studies, except piracetam (one study); some may actually impair active function.

From these conclusions, the use of a systemic agent becomes apparent as an acceptable therapeutic option to treat spastic dystonia when passive function and comfort are prioritized. However, there is no study that has compared systemic and local treatments in these situations. When active function is prioritized, systemic treatments have the potential to be deleterious because of the lack of selectivity of their CNS action. A controlled comparative study of systemic and local BTX-A treatment, currently under development, will clarify and differentiate their respective effects.

CONCLUSION

Spastic dystonia is the inability to rest a muscle that is sensitive to stretch and that consistently improves during sustained stretch. It is a virtually constant feature in patients affected with motor paralysis resulting from CNS injury, most often associated with the other classic forms of stretch-sensitive overactivity, including spasticity and spastic cocontraction. The pathophysiology of spastic dystonia is probably multi-factorial, involving both supraspinal and spinal mechanisms. Spastic dystonia is not evenly distributed across joints and affects some muscles more than their antagonists. The main functional consequences of spastic dystonia are abnormal postures causing disfigurement, discomfort, and loss of passive function.

Controlled protocols are necessary to establish whether local treatment, combining chronic stretch and intramuscular injections of neuromuscular blocking agents (BTX-A or alcohol compounds), is a safer and more efficacious first-line therapy than systemic treatments (oral or intrathecal), in particular in those patients for whom recovery of active function is prioritized. Motor training of the antagonist and electrical stimulation in both the injected muscle and its antagonist may enhance outcomes in the treatment of spastic dystonia.

REFERENCES

1. Denny-Brown D. The Cerebral Control of Movement. Liverpool: Liverpool University Press, 1966:124–143, 171–184. Chapter IX: Spasticity resulting from cerebral lesion pp 124–143, Chapter XII: The extrapyramidal cortical system pp 171–184.
2. Gracies JM. Pathophysiology of impairment in spasticity: stretch as a treatment of spastic hypertonia. Phys Med Rehabil Clin North Am 2001;12:747–768.
3. Ashworth B. Preliminary trial of carisoprodol in multiple sclerosis. Practitioner 1964;192:540–542.
4. Pollock LJ, Davis L. Studies in decerebration. The effect of deafferentation upon decerebrate rigidity. Am J Physiol 1930;98:47–49.
5. Tardieu G. Description classique et étude critique des cinq formes d'infirmité motrice cerébrale internationalement retenues. Classifications diverses "Les Feuillets de l'Infirmité Motrice Cérébrale." Paris: Association Nationale des IMC, 1969:1–8.
6. Lance JW, McLeod JG. A Physiological Approach to Clinical Neurology. 3rd ed. London: Butterworths, 1981:145.
7. Burke D. An approach to the treatment of spasticity. Drugs 1975; 10:112–120.
8. Burke D. Spasticity as an adaptation to pyramidal tract injury. Adv Neurol 1988;47. {Functional Recovery in Neurological Disease, ed Waxman SG, Raven Press, NY, pp. 401–423 (see page 404)
9. Young RR. Spasticity: a review. Neurology 1994 Nov;44(11 Suppl 9):S12–20.
10. Tardieu C, Tardieu G, Colbeau-Justin P, et a. Trophic muscle regulation in children with congenital cerebral lesions. J Neurol Sci 1979;42:357–364.
11. Maier A, Eldred E, Edgerton VR. The effects on spindles of muscle atrophy and hypertrophy. Exp Neurol 1972;37:100–123.
12. Williams RG. Sensitivity changes shown by spindle receptors in chronically immobilized skeletal muscle. J Physiol 1980;306:26P-27P.
13. Gioux M, Petit J. Effects of immobilising the cat peroneus longus muscle on the activity of its own spindles. J Appl Physiol 1993;75: 2629–2635.
14. Tabary JC, Tabary C, Tardieu C, et al. Physiological and structural changes in cat's soleus muscle due to immobilization at different lengths by plaster casts. J Physiol 1972;224:231–244.
15. Krenz NR, Weaver LC. Sprouting of primary afferent fibers after spinal cord transection in the rat. Neuroscience 1998;85:443–458.
16. Hall M. On the Diseases and Derangements of the Nervous System. London: Baillière, 1841.
17. Little WJ. Course of lectures on the deformities of the human frame. Lecture IX. Lancet 1843;i:350–354.
18. Charcot JM. Histologie de la sclérose en plaques. Gaz Hop (Paris) 1868;41:554–555.
19. Farmer SF, Harrison LM, Ingram DA, et al. Plasticity of central motor pathways in children with hemiplegic cerebral palsy. Neurology 1991;41:1505–1510.
20. Dewald JP, Pope PS, Given JD, et al. Abnormal muscle coactivation patterns during isometric torque generation at the elbow and shoulder in hemiparetic subjects. Brain 1995;118(Pt 2):495–510.

21. Reddy H, De Stefano N, Mortilla M, et al. Functional reorganization of motor cortex increases with greater axonal injury from CADASIL. Stroke 2002;33:502–508.
22. Gracies JM, Marosszeky JE, Renton R, et al. Short-term effects of dynamic Lycra splints on upper limb in hemiplegic patients. Arch Phys Med Rehabil 2000;81:1547–1555.
23. Lance JW. Symposium synopsis. In: Feldman RG, Young RR, Koella WP, eds. Spasticity: Disordered Motor Control. Chicago: Yearbook Medical, 1980:485–494.
24. Gracies JM, Wilson L, Gandevia SC, et al. Stretched position of spastic muscles aggravates their co-contraction in hemiplegic patients. Ann Neurol 1997;42:438–439.
25. Edström L. Selective changes in the sizes of red and white muscle fibres in upper motor lesions and Parkinsonism. Neurol Sci 1970;11:537–550.
26. Williams PE, Goldspink G. Changes in sarcomere length and physiological properties in immobilised muscle. J Anat 1978;127:459–468.
27. Dietz V, Berger W. Normal and impaired regulation of muscle stiffness in gait: a new hypothesis about muscle hypertonia. Exp Neurol 1983;79:680–687.
28. Kernell D, Eerbeek O, Verhey BA, et al. Effects of physiological amounts of high- and low-rate chronic stimulation on fast-twitch muscle of the cat hindlimb. I. Speed and force related properties. J Neurophysiol 1987;58:598–613.
29. Romberg MH. Lehrbuch der Nervenkrankeiten des Menschen. Berlin: A. Dunker, 1851:542–543
30. Angel RW, Hoffman WW. The H-reflex in normal, spastic and rigid subjects. Arch Neurol 1963;8:591–596.
31. Schiller HH, Stalberg E. F responses studied with single fibre EMG in normal subjects and spastic patients. J Neurol Neurosurg Psychiatry 1978;41:45–53.
32. Dietz V, Hillesheimer W, Freund HJ. Correlation between tremor, voluntary contraction, and firing pattern of motor units in Parkinson's disease. J Neurol Neurosurg Psychiatry 1974;37:927–937.
33. Edstrom L, Grimby L, Hannerz J. Correlation between recruitment order of motor units and muscle atrophy pattern in upper motoneurone lesion: significance of spasticity. Experientia 1973;29:560–561.
34. Farmer SF, Swash M, Ingram DA, et al. Changes in motor unit synchronization following central nervous lesions in man. J Physiol 1993;463:83–105.
35. Heald A, Bates D, Cartlidge NE, et al. Longitudinal study of central motor conduction time following stroke. 1. Natural history of central motor conduction. Brain 1993;116(Pt 6):1355–1370.
36. Heald A, Bates D, Cartlidge NE, et al. Longitudinal study of central motor conduction time following stroke. 2. Central motor conduction measured within 72 h after stroke as a predictor of functional outcome at 12 months. Brain 1993;116(Pt 6):1371–1385.
37. Kernell D, Hultborn H. Synaptic effects on recruitment gain: a mechanism of importance for the input-output relations of motoneurone pools? Brain Res 1990;507:176–179.
38. Blaschak MJ, Powers RK, Rymer WZ. Disturbances of motor output in a cat hindlimb muscle after acute dorsal spinal hemisection. Exp Brain Res 1988;71:377–387.
39. Powers RK, Rymer WZ. Effects of acute dorsal spinal hemisection on motoneuron discharge in the medial gastrocnemius of the decerebrate cat. J Neurophysiol 1988;59:1540–1556.
40. Nielsen J, Kagamihara Y. Differential projection of the sural nerve to early and late recruited human tibialis anterior motor units: change of recruitment gain. Acta Physiol Scand 1993;147:385–3401.
41. Hounsgaard J, Hultborn H, Jespersen B, et al. Intrinsic membrane properties causing a bistable behaviour of alpha-motoneurones. Exp Brain Res 1984;55:391–394.
42. Conway BA, Hultborn H, Kiehn O, et al. Plateau potentials in alpha-motoneurones induced by intravenous injection of L-dopa and clonidine in the spinal cat. J Physiol 1988;405:369–384.
43. Crone C, Hultborn H, Kiehn O, et al. Maintained changes in motoneuronal excitability by short-lasting synaptic inputs in the decerebrate cat. J Physiol 1988;405:321–343.
44. Schwindt PC, Crill WE. Properties of a persistent inward current in normal and TEA-injected motoneurons. J Neurophysiol 198043:1700–1724.
45. Schwindt PC, Crill WE. Factors influencing motoneuron rhythmic firing: results from a voltage-clamp study. J Neurophysiol 1982;48:875–890.
46. Nakashima K, Rothwell JC, Day BL, et al. Reciprocal inhibition between forearm muscles in patients with writer's cramp and other occupational cramps, symptomatic hemidystonia and hemiparesis due to stroke. Brain 1989;112(Pt 3):681–697.
47. Faist M, Mazevet D, Dietz V, et al. A quantitative assessment of presynaptic inhibition of Ia afferents in spastics. Differences in hemiplegics and paraplegics. Brain 1994;117(Pt 6):1449–1455.
48. Nielsen J, Petersen N, Crone C. Changes in transmission across synapses of Ia afferents in spastic patients. Brain 1995;118(Pt 4):995–1004.
49. Aymard C, Katz R, Lafitte C, et al. Presynaptic inhibition and homosynaptic depression: a comparison between lower and upper limbs in normal human subjects and patients with hemiplegia. Brain 2000;123(Pt 8):1688–1702.
50. Lev-Tov A, Pinco M. In vitro studies of prolonged synaptic depression in the neonatal rat spinal cord. J Physiol 1992;447:149–169.
51. Granit R, Kaada B. Influence of stimulation of central nervous system structures on muscle spindles in the cat. Acta Physiol Scand 1952:27:130–160.
52. Eldred E, Granit R, Merton PA. Supraspinal control of the muscle spindles and its significance. J Physiol 1953;122:498–523.
53. Landau WM, Clare MH. Fusimotor function, part VI. H reflex, tendon jerk, and reinforcement in hemiplegia. Arch Neurol 1964;10:128–134.
54. Tardieu G, Hariga J, Tardieu C, et al. Traitemet de la spasticité par infiltration d'alcool dilué ou par injection épidurale. Rev Neurol (Paris) 1964;110:563–565.
55. Buller A, Dornhorst AC. The reinforcement of tendon reflexes. Lancet 1957;2:1260–1262.
56. Buller AJ. The ankle jerk in early hemiplegia. Lancet 1957;2:1262–1263.
57. Dietrichson P. Phasic ankle reflex in spasticity and Parkinsonian rigidity. The role of the fusimotor system. Acta Neurol Scand 1971;47:22–51.
58. Dietrichson P. The role of the fusimotor system in spasticity and Parkinsonian rigidity. In: Desmedt JE, ed. New Developments in Electromyography and Clinical Neurophysiology. Vol. 3. Karger-Basel: München, 1973:496–507.
59. Gassel MD, Diamantopoulos E. The effect of procaine nerve block on neuromuscular reflex regulation in man (an appraisal of the role of the fusimotor system). Brain 1964;87:729–742.
60. Burke D. Critical examination of the case for or against fusimotor involvement in disorders of muscle tone. In: Desmedt JE, ed. Advances in Neurology. Vol. 39. New York: Raven Press, 1983:133–150.
61. Wilson LR, Gracies JM, Burke D, et al. Evidence for fusimotor drive in stroke patients based on muscle spindle thixotropy. Neurosci Lett 1999;264:109–112.
62. Hagbarth KE, Wallin G, Löfstedt L. Muscle spindle responses to stretch in normal and spastic subjects. Scand J Rehab Med 1973;5:156–159.
63. Wilson LR, Gandevia SC, Inglis JT, et al. Muscle spindle activity in the affected upper limb after a unilateral stroke. Brain 1999;122:2079–2088.
64. Houk JC, Henneman E. Responses of Golgi tendon organs to active contractions of the soleus muscle in the cat. J Neurophysiol 1967;30:466–481.
65. Eccles JC, Eccles RM, Lundberg A. Synaptic actions on motoneurones caused by impulses in Golgi tendon organ afferents. J Physiol 1957;138:227–252.
66. Harrison PJ, Jankowska E. Sources of input to interneurones mediating group I non reciprocal inhibition of motoneurones in the cat. J Physiol 1985;361:379–401.
67. Eccles RM, Lundberg A. Supraspinal control of interneurones mediating spinal reflexes. J Physiol 1959;147:565–584.
68. Pierrot-Deseilligny E, Katz R, Morin C. Evidence for Ib inhibition in human subjects. Brain Res 1979;166:176–179.
69. Pierrot-Deseilligny E, Morin C, Bergego C, et al. Pattern of group I fibre projections from ankle flexor and extensor muscles in man. Exp Brain Res 1981;42:337–350.
70. Pierrot-Deseilligny E, Bergego C, Katz R. Reversal in cutaneous control of Ib pathways during human voluntary contraction. Brain Res 1982;233:400–403.
71. Delwaide PJ, Oliver E. Short latency autogenetic inhibition (Ib inhibition) in human spasticity. J Neurol Neurosurg Psychiatry 1988;51:1546–1550.
72. Delwaide PJ. Pathophysiological mechanisms of spasticity at the spinal cord level. In: Thilman AF, Burke D, Rymer WZ, eds. Spasticity: Mechanisms and Management. Berlin: Springer Verlag, 1993:296–308.

73. Delwaide PJ, Schoenen J, Maertens de Noordhout A. Short latency autogenetic inhibition in patients with parkinsonian rigidity. Ann Neurol 1991;30:83–89.

74. Baldissera F, Hultborn H, Illert M. Integration in spinal neuronal systems. In: Brooks VB, ed. Handbook of Physiology. Section 1. The Nervous System. Vol. II. Motor Control. Part 1. Bethesda: American Physiological Society, 1981:509–595.

75. Fedina L, Hultborn H, Illert M. Facilitation from contralateral primary afferents of interneuronal transmission in the Ia inhibitory pathway to motoneurones. Acta Physiol Scand 1975;94:198–221.

76. Pierrot-Deseilligny E, Bussel B. Evidence for recurrent inhibition by motoneurones in human subjects. Brain Res 1975;88:105–108.

77. Pierrot-Deseilligny E, Bussel B, Held JP, et al. Excitability of human motoneurones after discharge in a conditioning reflex. Electromyogr Clin Neuropysiol 1976;40:279–287.

78. Katz R, Pierrot-Deseilligny E. Recurrent inhibition of alpha-motoneurones in patients with upper motoneurone lesions. Brain 1982;105:103–124.

79. Taylor S, Ashby P, Verrier M. Neurophysiological changes following traumatic spinal cord lesions in man. J Neurol Neurosurg Psychiatry 1984;47:1102–1108.

80. Little J, Halar E. H reflex changes following spinal cord injury. Arch Phys Med Rehabil 1985;66:19–22.

81. Shefner JM, Berman SA, Sarkarati M, et al. Recurrent inhibition is increased in patients with spinal cord injury. Neurology 1992;42:2162–2168.

82. Shefner JM, Berman SA, Young RR. The effect of nicotine on recurrent inhibition in the spinal cord. Neurology 1993;43:2647–2651.

83. Mazzocchio R, Rossi A. Involvement of spinal recurrent inhibition in spasticity. Further insight into the regulation of Renshaw cell activity. Brain 1997;120(Pt 6):991–1003.

84. Matthews PB. A possible function for the secondary ending of the muscle spindle. J Physiol 1969;201):102P–103P.

85. Lundberg A, Malmgren K, Schomburg ED. Comments on reflex actions evoked by electrical stimulation of group II muscle afferents. Brain Res 1977;122:551–555.

86. Skoog B. A comparison of the effects of two antispastic drugs, tizanidine and baclofen, on synaptic transmission from muscle spindle afferents to spinal interneurones in cats. Acta Physiol Scand 1996;156:81–90.

87. Eccles RM, Lundberg A. Synaptic actions in motoneurones by afferents which may evoke the flexion reflex. Arch Ital Biol 1959;97:199–221.

88. Laporte Y, Bessou P. Modification d'excitabilité de motoneurones homonymes provoquées par l'activation physiologique de fibres afférentes d'origine musculaire du groupe II. J Physiol 1959;51:897–908.

89. Eccles RM, Lundberg A. Supraspinal control of interneurones mediating spinal reflexes. J Physiol 1959;147:565–584.

90. Burke D, Andrews CJ, Ashby P Autogenic effect of static muscle stretch in spastic man. Arch Neurol 1971;25:367–372.

91. Burke D, Lance JW. Pathophysiology of spasticity. Studies of the reflex effects of primary and secondary spindle endings in spasticity. In: Desmedt JE, ed. New Developments in Electromyography and Clinical Neurophysiology. Vol.3. Basel: Karger, 1973:475–495.

92. Cody FW, Richardson HC, MacDermott N, et al. Stretch and vibration reflexes of wrist flexor muscles in spasticity. Brain 1987;110(Pt 2):433–450.

93. Marque P, Simonetta-Moreau M, Maupas E, et al. Facilitation of transmission in heteronymous group II pathways in spastic hemiplegic patients. J Neurol Neurosurg Psychiatry 2001;70:36–42.

94. Katz R. Reevaluation of physiological mechanisms generating the stretch reflex: new hypotheses on the physiopathology of spasticity [in French]. Ann Readapt Med Phys 2001;44:268–272.

95. Booth FW. Effect of limb immobilization on skeletal muscle. J Appl Physiol 1982;52:1113–1118

96. Robinson GA, Enoka RM, Stuart DG. Immobilization-induced changes in motor unit force and fatigability in the cat. Muscle Nerve 1991;14:563–573.

97. Jakobsson F, Edstrom L, Grimby L, et al. Disuse of anterior tibial muscle during locomotion and increased proportion of type II fibres in hemiplegia. J Neurol Sci 1991;105:49–56.

98. Jakobsson F, Grimby L, Edstrom L. Motoneuron activity and muscle fibre type composition in hemiparesis. Scand J Rehabil Med 1992;24:115–119.

99. Mayer NH, Esquenazi A, Keenan MA. Patterns of upper motoneuron dysfunction in the lower limb. Adv Neurol 2001;87:311–319.

100. Hislop H, Montgomery J. Daniels and Worthingham's Muscle Testing, Techniques of Manual Examination. 6th ed. Philadelphia: WB Saunders, 1995.

101. O'Dwyer NJ, Ada L, Neilson PD. Spasticity and muscle contracture following stroke. Brain 1996;119(Pt 5):1737–1749.

102. Balakrishnan C, Bradt LM, Sylora RL, et al. Hand infection associated with clenched fist syndrome in residents of long-term care facilities. J Psychosoc Nurs Ment Health Serv 2002;40:16–19.

103. Cresswell AG, Loscher WN, Thorstensson A. Influence of gastrocnemius muscle length on triceps surae torque development and electromyographic activity in man. Exp Brain Res 1995;105:283–290.

104. Glenn MB. Nerve blocks. In: Glenn MB, White J, eds. The Practical Management of Spasticity in Children and Adults. Philadelphia: Lea & Febiger, 1990:227–258.

105. Bakheit AM, Pittock S, Moore AP, et al. A randomized, double-blind, placebo-controlled study of the efficacy and safety of botulinum toxin type A in upper limb spasticity in patients with stroke. Eur J Neurol 2001;8:559–565.

106. Nielsen JF, Sinkjaer T. Peripheral and central effect of baclofen on ankle joint stiffness in multiple sclerosis. Muscle Nerve 2000;23:98–105.

107. Ranson SW, Dixon HH. Elasticity and ductility of muscle in myostatic contracture caused by tetanus toxin. Am J Physiol 1928;86:312–319.

108. Morgan DL, Prochazka A, Proske U. The after-effects of stretch and fusimotor stimulation on the responses of primary endings of cat muscle spindles. J Physiol 1984;256:465–477.

109. Proske U, Morgan DL, Gregory E. Thixotropy in skeletal muscle and in muscle spindles: a review. Prog Neurobiol 1993;41:705–721.

110. Matthews PBC. Mammalian Muscle Receptors and their Central Actions. London: Williams & Wilkins, 1972.

111. Burke D, Gandevia SC. The muscle spindle and its fusimotor control. In: Ferrell WR, Proske U, eds. Neural Control of Movement. New York: Plenum Press, 1995:19–25.

112. Jahnke MT, Proske U, Struppler A. Measurements of muscle stiffness, the electromyogram and activity in single muscle spindles of human flexor muscles following conditioning by passive stretch or contraction. Brain Res 1989;493:103–112.

113. Schmit BD, Dewald JP, Rymer WZ. Stretch reflex adaptation in elbow flexors during repeated passive movements in unilateral brain-injured patients. Arch Phys Med Rehabil 2000;81:269–278.

114. Newman LB, Arieff AJ, Wasserman RR. Present status in the management of spasticity and spasm: preliminary report. Arch Phys Med Rehabil 1954;35:427–436.

115. Foley J. The stiffness of spastic muscle. J Neurol Neurosurg Psychiatry 1961;24:125–131.

116. Odeen I, Knutsson E. Evaluation of the effects of muscle stretch and weight load in patients with spastic paraplegia. Scand J Rehabil Med 1981;13:117–121.

117. Tremblay F, Malouin F, Richards CL, et al. Effects of prolonged muscle stretch on reflex and voluntary muscle activations in children with spastic cerebral palsy. Scand J Rehabil Med 1990;22:171–180.

118. Nielsen J, Petersen N, Ballegaard M, et al. H-reflexes are less depressed following muscle stretch in spastic spinal cord injured patients than in healthy subjects. *Exp* Brain Res 1993;97:173–176.

119. Nielsen J, Petersen N, Crone C. Changes in transmission across synapses of Ia afferents in spastic patients. Brain 1995;118(Pt 4):995–1004.

120. Kaplan N. Effect of splinting on reflex inhibition and sensorimotor stimulation treatment of spasticity. Arch Phys Med Rehabil 1962;43:565–569.

121. Otis JC, Root L, Kroll MA. Measurement of plantar flexor spasticity during treatment with tone-reducing casts. J Pediatr Orthop 1985;5:682–686.

122. McPherson JJ, Kreimeyer D, Aalderks M, et al. A comparison of dorsal and volar resting hand splints in the reduction of hypertonus. Am J Occup Ther 1982;36:664–670.

123. McPherson JJ, Becker AH, Franszczak N. Dynamic splint to reduce the passive component of hypertonicity. Arch Phys Med Rehabil 1985;66:249–252.

124. Hill J, The effects of casting on upper extremity motor disorders after brain injury. Am J Occup Ther 1994;48:219–224.

125. Lin JP, Brown JK, Walsh EG. Continuum of reflex excitability in

hemiplegia: influence of muscle length and muscular transformation after heel-cord lengthening and immobilization on the pathophysiology of spasticity and clonus. Dev Med Child Neurol 1999;41: 534–448.

126. Brouwer B, Davidson LK, Olney SJ. Serial casting in idiopathic toe-walkers and children with spastic cerebral palsy. J Pediatr Orthop 2000;20:221–225.

127. Moseley AM. The effect of casting combined with stretching on passive ankle dorsiflexion in adults with traumatic head injuries. Phys Ther 1997;77:240–247; discussion 248–259.

128. Brennan BJ. Response to stretch of hypertonic muscle groups in hemiplegia. BMJ 1959;1:1504–1507.

129. Tardieu C, Lespargot A, Tabary C, et al. For how long must the soleus muscle be stretched each day to prevent contracture? Dev Med Child Neurol 1988;30:3–10.

130. Ada L, Canning C. Anticipating and avoiding muscle shortening. In: Ada L, Canning C, eds. Key Issues in Neurological Physiotherapy. Oxford: Butterworth-Heinemann Ltd, 1990:219–236.

131. Feldman PA. Upper extremity casting and splinting. In: The Practical Management of Spasticity in Children and Adults. Glenn MB, White J, eds. Philadelphia: Lea & Febiger, 1990:149.

132. Conine TA, Sullivan T, Mackie T, et al. Effect of serial casting for the prevention of equinus in patients with acute head injury. Arch Phys Med Rehabil 1990;71:310–312.

133. McLachlan EM. Modification of the atrophic effects of tenotomy on mouse soleus muscles by various hind limb nerve lesions and different levels of voluntary motor activity. Exp Neurol 1983;81:669–682.

134. Eames NW, Baker R, Hill N, et al. The effect of botulinum toxin A on gastrocnemius length: magnitude and duration of response. Dev Med Child Neurol 1999;41:226–232.

135. Das TK, Park DM. Effect of treatment with botulinum toxin on spasticity. Postgrad Med J 1989;65:208–210.

136. Das TK, Park DM. Botulinum toxin in treating spasticity. Br J Clin Practice 1989;43:401–403.

137. Mémin B, Pollak P, Hommel M, et al. Traitement de la spasticité par la toxine botulique. Rev Neurol (Paris) 1992;148:212–214.

138. Hesse S, Friedrich H, Domasch C, et al. Botulinum toxin therapy for upper limb flexor spasticity: preliminary results. J Rehab Sci 1992; 5:98–101.

139. Konstanzer A, Ceballos-Baumann AO, et al. Lokale Injektionsbehandlung mit Botulinum-Toxin A bei schwerer Arm- und Beinspastik [Local injection treatment with botulinum toxin A in severe arm and leg spasticity]. Nervenarzt 1993;64:517–523.

140. Yablon SA, Agana BT, Ivanhoe CB, et al. Botulinum toxin in severe upper extremity spasticity among patients with traumatic brain injury: an open-labeled trial. Neurology 1996;47:939–944.

141. Simpson D, Alexander DN, O'Brien CF, et al. Botulinum toxin type A in the treatment of upper extremity spasticity: a randomized, double-blind, placebo-controlled trial. Neurology 1996;46:1306–1310.

142. Dunne JW, Heye N, Dunne S. Treatment of chronic limb spasticity with botulinum toxin A. J Neurol Neurosurg Psychiatry 1995; 58:232–235.

143. Reiter F, Danni M, Ceravolo MG, et al. Disability changes after treatment of upper limb spasticity with botulinum toxin. J Neurol Rehab 1996;10:47–52.

144. Bhakta BB, Cozens JA, Bamford JM, et al. Use of botulinum toxin in stroke patients with severe upper limb spasticity. J Neurol Neurosurg Psychiatry 1996;61:30–35.

145. Sampaio C, Ferreira JJ, Pinto AA, et al. Botulinum toxin type A for the treatment of arm and hand spasticity in stroke patients. Clin Rehabil 1997;11:3–7.

146. Corry IS, Cosgrove AP, Walsh EG, et al. Botulinum toxin A in the hemiplegic upper limb: a double-blind trial. Dev Med Child Neurol 1997;39:185–193.

147. Smith SJ, Ellis E, White S, Moore AP. A double-blind placebo-controlled study of botulinum toxin in upper limb spasticity after stroke or head injury. Clin Rehabil 2000;14:5–13.

148. Bakheit AM, Thilmann AF, Ward AB, et al. A randomized, double-blind, placebo-controlled, dose-ranging study to compare the efficacy and safety of three doses of botulinum toxin type A (Dysport) with placebo in upper limb spasticity after stroke. Stroke 2000;31: 2402–2406.

149. Richardson D, Sheean G, Werring D, et al. Evaluating the role of botulinum toxin in the management of focal hypertonia in adults. J Neurol Neurosurg Psychiatry 2000;69:499–506.

150. Bhakta BB, Cozens JA, Chamberlain MA, et al. Impact of botulinum toxin type A on disability and carer burden due to arm spasticity after stroke: a randomised double blind placebo controlled trial. J Neurol Neurosurg Psychiatry 2000;69:217–221.

151. Fehlings D, Rang M, Glazier J, et al. An evaluation of botulinum-A toxin injections to improve upper extremity function in children with hemiplegic cerebral palsy. J Pediatr 2000;137:331–337.

152. Fehlings D, Rang M, Glazier J, et al. Botulinum toxin type A injections in the spastic upper extremity of children with hemiplegia: child characteristics that predict a positive outcome. Eur J Neurol 2001; 8(Suppl 5):145–149.

153. Rodriquez AA, McGinn M, Chappell R. Botulinum toxin injection of spastic finger flexors in hemiplegic patients. Am J Phys Med Rehabil 2000;79:44–47.

154. Friedman A, Diamond M, Johnston MV, et al. Effects of botulinum toxin A on upper limb spasticity in children with cerebral palsy. Am J Phys Med Rehabil 2000;79:53–59; quiz 75–76.

155. Hurvitz EA, Conti GE, Flansburg EL, et al. Motor control testing of upper limb function after botulinum toxin injection: a case study. Arch Phys Med Rehabil 2000;81:1408–1415.

156. Panizza M, Castagna M, di Summa A, et al. Functional and clinical changes in upper limb spastic patients treated with botulinum toxin (BTX-A). Funct Neurol 2000;15:147–155.

157. Lagalla G, Danni M, Reiter F, et al. Post-stroke spasticity management with repeated botulinum toxin injections in the upper limb. Am J Phys Med Rehabil 2000;79:377–384; quiz 391–394.

158. Gracies JM, Weisz DJ, Yang BY, et al. Impact of botulinum toxin type A (BTX-A) dilution and endplate targeting technique in upper limb spasticity. Ann Neurol 2002; 52(3) Suppl 1:S87.

159. Gracies JM, Elovic E, McGuire J, Simpson D. Traditional pharmacologic treatments of spasticity—Part I. Local Treatments. Muscle Nerve 1997;20(Suppl 6):S61–S91.

160. Gracies JM, Simpson D. Neuromuscular blockers. Phys Med Rehabil Clin North Am 1999;10:357–383.

161. Kirazli Y, On AY, Kismali B, et al. Comparison of phenol block and botulinus toxin type A in the treatment of spastic foot after stroke: a randomized, double-blind trial. Am J Phys Med Rehabil 1998; 77:510–515.

162. Geenen C, Consky E, Ashby P. Localizing muscles for botulinum toxin treatment of focal hand dystonia. Can J Neurol Sci 1996;23: 194–197.

163. Del Toro DR, Park TA. Abductor hallucis false motor points: electrophysiologic mapping and cadaveric dissection. Muscle Nerve 1996; 19:1138–1143.

164. Kadrie HA, Yates SK, Milner-Brown HS, et al. Multiple point electrical stimulation of ulnar and median nerves. J Neurol Neurosurg Psychiatry 1976;39:973–985.

165. Gracies JM, Fitzpatrick R, Wilson L, et al. Lycra garments designed for patients with upper limb spasticity: mechanical effects in normal subjects. Arch Phys Med Rehab 1997;78:1066–1071.

166. Reiter F, Danni M, Lagalla G, et al. Low-dose botulinum toxin with ankle taping for the treatment of spastic equinovarus foot after stroke. Arch Phys Med Rehabil 1998;79:532–535.

167. Shepherd RB. Exercise and training to optimize functional motor performance in stroke: driving neural reorganization? Neural Plast 2001;8:121–129.

168. Dean CM, Shepherd RB. Task-related training improves performance of seated reaching tasks after stroke. A randomized controlled trial. Stroke 1997;28:722–728.

169. Hesse S, Jahnke MT, Luecke D, et al. Short-term electrical stimulation enhances the effectiveness of botulinum toxin in the treatment of lower limb spasticity in hemiparetic patients. Neurosci Lett 1995; 201:37–40.

170. Hesse S, Reiter F, Konrad M, et al. Botulinum toxin type A and short-term electrical stimulation in the treatment of upper limb flexor spasticity after stroke: a randomized, double-blind, placebo-controlled trial. Clin Rehabil 1998;12:381–388.

171. Detrembleur C, Lejeune TM, Renders A, et al. Botulinum toxin and short-term electrical stimulation in the treatment of equinus in cerebral palsy. Mov Disord 2002;17:162–169.

172. Gracies JM, Elovic E, McGuire J, et al. Traditional pharmacologic treatments of spasticity—Part II. Systemic treatments in Mayer NH, Simpson DM, eds. Spasticity: Etiology, Evaluation, Management, and the Role of Botulinum Toxin. New York: WE MOVE CME, 2002:65–93.

CHAPTER 18

Other Uses of Botulinum Toxin Type A Therapy

Mitchell F. Brin and Joseph Jankovic

INTRODUCTION

Since its introduction in the late 1970s for the treatment of strabismus and blepharospasm, botulinum toxin type A (BTX-A) has been increasingly used in the interventional treatment of numerous other disorders[1] characterized by excessive or inappropriate muscle contractions (Table 18-1).[2–6] The use of this pleuripotential agent has extended to a plethora of conditions including: focal dystonia; spasticity; inappropriate contraction in most sphincters of the body such as those associated with spasmodic dysphonia, achalasia, anal spasm, and vaginismus; eye movement disorders including nystagmus; other hyperkinetic disorders including tics and tremors; autonomic disorders such as hyperhidrosis; genitourinary disorders such as overactive and neurogenic bladder, non-bacterial prostatitis and benign prostatic hypertrophy; and aesthetically undesirable hyperfunctional facial lines (wrinkles).[7] In addition, BTX-A is being investigated for the control of pain, and for the management of tension or migraine headaches and myofascial pain syndrome.

BTX injections have several advantages over drug and surgical therapies in the management of intractable disease. Systemic pharmacologic effects are rare; permanent destruction of tissue does not occur. Graded degrees of relaxation may be achieved by varying the dose injected; most adverse effects are transient. If the patient has a strong response to therapy and too much weakness occurs, strength gradually returns. Patient acceptance is high. Although drug therapy

may be added as needed, in most patients BTX therapy is preferred to alternative pharmacotherapy.

In this chapter, the uses of BTX-A are reviewed regarding the management of dystonia-related hyperkinetic and hypokinetic disorders. In addition, its use in tardive and parkinsonism conditions, autonomic disorders (e.g., hyperhidrosis and sialorrhea), and uroanal pelvic disorders are discussed. Because there is little information on the use of botulinum toxin type B (BTX-B), this discussion is limited to the applications of BTX-A.

MOTOR DISORDERS

Tremor

Tremor refers to the periodic contraction of antagonistic muscles in either an alternating or synchronous fashion.[8] One common form of tremor is essential tremor (ET), an autosomal-dominant movement disorder that usually affects the hands, however, ET is also common in the head and neck area as well as in the larynx.[9,10] Other types of tremor include rest tremor, as observed in Parkinson's disease (PD) or other parkinsonian disorders, and cerebellar tremors. Pharmacologic remedies include β-blockers, primidone, and benzodiazepines; these often fail to provide satisfactory results, particularly for head tremor.[11] Surgery, such as thalamotomy and deep brain stimulation of the thalamus, is highly effective but carries risk of permanent neurologic deficits.[12–15]

The first pilot study of BTX-A therapy for limb tremor was motivated by the observation that BTX-A improved tremor in patients who were being treated for dystonia.[16] Of 51 patients with various forms of head or limb tremor who received BTX-A injections in cervical or forearm muscles, 35 (67%) improved. The average duration of effect was 10.5 weeks. In a follow-up, placebo-controlled study, BTX-A was injected into the forearm muscles. Reduced hand tremor amplitude was noted, however, decreased functional impairment was not reported. This finding is most likely because

Mitchell F. Brin: Senior Vice-President Development and Therapeutic Area Head, BOTOX/Neurology, Allergan, Inc., and Professor of Neurology, University of California, Irvine, Irvine, California.

Joseph Jankovic: Professor of Neurology, Director of Parkinson's Disease Center and Movement Disorders Clinic, Department of Neurology, Baylor College of Medicine, Houston, Texas.

Dr. Mitchell Brin is an employee of Allergan, Inc.

Dr. Joseph Jankovic wishes to disclose research grant funding from Allergan, Inc., Elan Biopharmaceuticals, and Ipsen Ltd.

213

TABLE 18-1. *Published and Reported Uses of Botulinum Toxin Type A*

Therapeutic	Therapeutic	Aesthetic
Skeletal Muscle: Relaxation	**Sensory: Pain**	**Skeletal Muscle: Relaxation**
Extraocular	Headache	Brow furrow
• Strabismus	• Migraine	Forehead lines
• Nystagmus	• Cluster	Crow's feet
• Oscillopsia	Back pain	Plastysma lines
Hemifacial spasm/synkinesis	Postherpetic neuralgia	
Synkinesis and myokimia (other)	Trigeminal neuralgia	
Benign eyelid fasciculation	Postsurgical spasm and pain	
Facial muscle relaxation to facilitate		
EEG recording	**Autonomic: Smooth Muscle and Gland**	
Dystonia (focal/segmental)	Esophageal-rectal	
• Blepharospasm	• Achalasia	
• Cervical	• LES spasm and synkinesis	
• Lingual	• Obesity (gastric)	
• Oromandibular	• Pylorus outlet obstruction	
• Labial	• Anal fissure/hemorrhoids (sphincters)	
• Laryngeal	• Anismus/constipation	
• Limb	Hyperhidrosis	
• Occupational cramps	• Facial (Frey's)	
• Dystonic tremor	• Axillary	
Oropharyngeal	• Palmar	
• Palatal myoclonus spasm	• Plantar	
• Cricopharyngeal spasm	• Genito-rectal-buttocks	
Stuttering	Sialorrhea	
Temporomandibular disorders	Bladder	
(spasm/deviations)	• Overactive	
Bruxism	• Neurogenic	
Headache	• Detrusor-sphincter dysinergia	
• Tension	Prostate	
Back spasm	• Prostatitis	
Spasticity (adult and pediatric)	• Benign prostatic hypertrophy	
• Poststroke		
• Traumatic brain injury		
• Spinal cord injury		
• Cerebral palsy (including club foot)		
• Multiple sclerosis		
• Multisystem atrophy		
Rectal		
• Anal fissure/hemorrhoids (external sphincter		
Pelvic floor spasm/vaginismus		
Presurgical (diagnostic/stabilization)		
Sports injuries		
Extrapyramidal rigidity		
• Parkinson's disease freezing of gait		
• Progressive supranuclear palsy		
Extrapyramidal hyperkinesias		
• Tics/Tourette's (somatic/vocal)		
• Tardive dyskinesia/dystonia		
• Drug-induced dyskinesias		
• Myoclonus		
• Tremor (essential, hereditary chin, Parkinson's,		
cerebellar, rubral symptomatic, etc.)		
Dermal wound healing		

EEG, electroencephalography; LES, lower esophageal sphincter.
  Modified from Brin MF. Treatment of dystonia. In: Jankovic J, Tolosa F, eds. Parkinson's Disease and Movement Disorders. New York: Marcel Dekker, 1998:553–578.

the rating scales could not distinguish between functional impairment caused by tremor and impairment caused by treatment-induced muscle weakness.[17] In a multicenter, double-blind study of the effect of BTX-A on ET of the hand,[18] 133 patients with ET were randomly assigned to low-dose (50 units) or high-dose (100 units) of BTX-A (BOTOX, Allergan, Inc., Irvine, CA) or to a vehicle placebo treatment. Injections were made into the wrist flexors and extensors and patients were followed for 16 weeks. After 4–16 weeks, both doses significantly reduced postural tremor on the clinical rating scales, however, kinetic tremor was significantly reduced only at the 6-week examination. Several functional measures, such as drawing a spiral or a straight line or pouring water, improved at key time points during the study. Adverse reactions consisted mainly of dose-dependent transient hand weakness.

Another early study of BTX-A for PD and essential hand tremors found little correlation between clinical and functional improvement and observed a moderate effect overall.[19] It has been observed that BTX-A improves postural but not necessarily kinetic tremor. It is kinetic tremor that is typically responsible for the disability experienced by patients with ET.[18,20] However, when proximal muscles, which are involved in the kinetic component of the tremor, are injected along with distal muscles (forearm flexor), most patients with ET experience at least some benefit.

Additional studies of the treatment of limb tremor confirmed the limiting effects of local muscle weakness on BTX-A efficacy.[20,21] These limiting effects made double-blind studies difficult. A report on a large case series estimated BTX-A efficacy to be 40%, with relatively better results for upper limbs compared to lower limbs.[21] In the same series, the level of disability was most improved for cerebellar tremor; the change in amplitude was greatest for ET. BTX-A appears to improve tremor amplitude but not frequency.[20] This is an expected effect given that amplitude is thought to be peripherally controlled while frequency is centrally controlled.

For voice tremor, there is some evidence that unilateral injections to the laryngeal muscles may improve both tremor amplitude and frequency; these benefits have a relatively short duration of less than 6 weeks.[22] One study found a greater effect of BTX-A on voice tremor with a higher dose.[23] Duration of effect has been relatively short but has been reported to be as long as 9 months for hand tremor.[24] In summary, patients with predominantly postural, dystonic, task-specific tremor (e.g., primary writing tremor) or head tremor appear to be the best candidates for BTX-A injections. Other more obscure types of tremor for which BTX-A has successfully been used include palatal tremor,[25] which causes annoying ear clicks and hereditary trembling chin.[26,27]

In addition to muscle weakness, other adverse events reported from both controlled and open trials were mild and transient and included injection pain, stiffness, cramping, hematoma, dysphagia, breathiness, coughing/choking, dry skin, and dizziness. These types of side effects may make BTX treatment for tremor less effective in the elderly, which is the population most likely to be affected by tremor.[22]

Tremor is a movement disorder that involves several different muscles in the same patient and diverse muscles across different patients. Therefore, individualized injection regimens are more critical in tremor than in BTX therapy for patients with dystonia. When BTX-A treatment was compared in nondystonic tremor and tremulous cervical dystonia, there were no differences in either efficacy or adverse events.[11] On the other hand, Pacchetti et al.[28] showed that functional improvement could be achieved by injecting only those muscles responsible for tremor disability during specific functions. These investigators observed significant functional improvement that lasted up to 3 months; finger weakness was the only adverse event.

Tardive Dyskinesia and Tardive Dystonia

Tardive dyskinesia (TD), which can be a devastating side effect of some antipsychotic medications, consists of involuntary, repetitive movements typically involving the orofacial muscles, and in some patients, the extremities and trunk. This condition occurs in approximately 30% of patients receiving dopamine-blocking agents.[29] TD may appear as early as 1–6 months after antipsychotic treatment initiation and typically follows a reduction in dose (including discontinuation) or a switch to a less potent antipsychotic or an atypical neuroleptic.[30] In younger patients in whom TD is identified early, remission rates are 50–90%.[30] There is no established treatment for TD. Systemic medications, such as benzodiazepines, neuroleptics, dopamine-depleting drugs, muscle relaxants, and anticholinergics, have been used, however, the effects of these medications are generally not sustained and carry additional mental or systemic side effects.[31–34]

BTX injections for TD may be complex because of the numerous muscle groups involved that are contracting randomly.[35] To date, data from controlled trials do not exist. However, several case reports suggest that BTX-A may be a useful treatment approach, with durations of effect from 2–6 months.[35–39] In one case series involving 12 patients, movements that responded best to BTX-A injections were grimacing, dysarthric speech, and involuntary movements of the tongue.[40] Reported adverse events were mild and transient and most commonly included neck weakness, ptosis, dysphagia, and aspiration.

An interesting phenomenon that has been reported in patients with TD who were injected with BTX-A is improvement in distant, noninjected muscle groups.[38–40] This effect may be the result of suppression of proprioceptive input from muscle spindles through Ia afferents, thus inducing a decrease in activity of nontreated muscles. This has been previously postulated as the mechanism for suppression of postural tremors in an entire limb after lidocaine injection into a single muscle;[41] this is discussed elsewhere in this chapter.

Tardive dystonia is a class of TD in which dystonic manifestations predominate[30–33,42–44] and is also reported to be as responsive to BTX-A injections.[45–49] This is an especially important observation because compared to TD, remissions of tardive dystonia are relatively rare and systemic medications are less effective.[43,50] The effect of BTX-A on tardive dystonia appears to be similar to its effect on idiopathic dystonia.[37,47,48,51,52]

Palatal and Other Types of Myoclonus

Palatal myoclonus (PM) is a rare disorder characterized by involuntary, rhythmic movements of the soft palate that result in clicking tinnitus. The clicking noise, which is often audible to the examiner, has been hypothesized to be caused by the snapping shut of the eustachian tube after being opened by the palatine muscles[53] or from the breakdown of fluid surface tension when the eustachian tube is opened by the peritubal muscles.[54] Muscular involvement may include the tensor and levator veli palatini, tensor tympani, salpingopharyngeal, or superior pharyngeal constrictor muscles.[55] The muscles of the face, pharynx, larynx, diaphragm, and arms may also be involved (called segmental cranial myoclonus). Two types of PM have been proposed: symptomatic PM, which results from a brain stem or cerebellar lesion, and essential PM, which is more common and, as the name implies, has no obvious etiology. The most widely cited theory of pathophysiology is hypertrophic degeneration of the inferior olivary nucleus,[56] although acceptance of this model is not universal.[57,58]

Spontaneous remission of PM may occur; however, this finding is rare.[59] Therefore, effective treatment is required because PM symptoms may be debilitating. Typical treatment has consisted of systemic medication to alter neurotransmitter systems in central nervous system pathways. These medications include anticholinergics, antidepressants, benzodiazepines, anticonvulsants, and neurotransmitter precursors. In addition, surgery to modify the palatal and eustachian tube function has been used to treat some patients with PM. White-noise masking appears to be more effective than medication or surgery.[54] Therefore, current treatment options offer less than satisfactory efficacy.

Results from small case reports of BTX-A injections to paralyze the levator and tensor veli palatini muscles as a treatment for PM have been described.[55,60–64] The most significant side effects appear to be paresis-induced eustachian tube obstruction and velopharyngeal insufficiency.[63] Distinguishing PM from middle ear myoclonus is important when deciding treatment. Middle ear myoclonus may be successfully treated with surgery or a stapedial and tensor tympani tendon section.[64] Interestingly, there is one case report of improvement in middle ear myoclonus after BTX-A injections for blepharospasm.[65]

Other forms of myoclonus for which successful treatment with BTX-A has been reported include painful myoclonus of the limb;[66] stimulus-sensitive spinal segmental myoclonus;[67] and segmental, generalized, and focal myoclonus in children.[68]

Dystonia of Parkinsonism

In patients with PD, dystonia is one of the most disabling symptoms of long-term levodopa therapy.[69] This form of dystonia occurs in approximately one-third of patients who are treated for longer than 3 years[70–73] and it may occur during both "peak" and "off" periods. It is hypothesized that peak dystonias are the result of overstimulation of hypersensitive, postsynaptic, dopaminergic receptors in the striatum.[74] The off dystonias result from striatal cholinergic hyperfunction and a functional dopaminergic defect.[75] Symptomatic relief

may be achieved with anticholinergics,[74] lithium carbonate,[76] baclofen,[77] or long-acting dopaminergic agonists.[78,79] Some parkinsonian conditions are characterized by prominent dystonic postures, such as nuchal posturing and foot dystonia in progressive supranuclear palsy and flexion dystonia in multisystem atrophy. Successful treatment of focal dystonias with BTX-A injections[80] led to the BTX-A treatment approach for parkinsonian dystonias.

The most common parkinsonian dystonia involves the foot and is usually correlated with the timing of levodopa intake. The symptoms typically occur during off periods, when levodopa levels are at their lowest. The authors first treated a dystonic striatal toe in 1984;[81] the patient was a man with parkinsonism. The extensor hallucis longus muscle was injected and beneficial results were obtained. Prior to treatment, this patient had developed a painful ulceration on the upper toe surface caused by chronic irritation against the inside of his shoe. After treatment, his symptoms entirely resolved. Results from case reports of treatment with BTX-A injections have been generally good with minimal side effects.[73,82]

Freezing of gait is another relatively common parkinsonian dystonia for which BTX-A treatment has been utilized.[83,84] It has been theorized that the BTX-A effect of relaxing the calf muscles interferes with the normal synchronization of leg muscle activation; this forces the brain to switch from an automatic gait mode to a different one, thus mimicking the use of sensory tricks to treat dystonias.[84] Another hypothesis is that BTX-A relaxes the toe flexors that are involved during freezing, analogous to the grasp phenomenon in the hand.

One study that treated various forms of parkinsonian dystonia reported that lower limbs responded most favorably, followed by blepharospasm, cervical dystonia, and oromandibular dystonia.[85] No functional benefit was observed for upper limb dystonia. In this study, apraxia of eyelid opening was non-responsive, whereas, in an earlier case report, this condition had responded favorably to BTX-A injection.[86] Clenched fist is a rare, late complication of PD[69,72,79,87–90] that has shown mixed levels of response to BTX-A treatment.[91]

ACQUIRED NYSTAGMUS

Therapeutic use of botulinum toxin began in ophthalmology and was designed for use in pediatric strabismus.[92] BTX has been tested as a treatment for acquired nystagmus (AN). Oscillopsia, the illusion of movement, is a debilitating manifestation of AN and is caused by excessive drift of images of stationary objects on the retina.[93] Treatments for AN have included optical devices (e.g., prisms) and medication; neither approach has been shown to be particularly effective. Surgery to shift the null point and reduce anomalous head posture may be beneficial in congenital but not acquired nystagmus.[93] The most common underlying cause of AN is multiple sclerosis.[94,95]

Two different injection sites have been used in the treatment of AN with BTX-A: the rectus muscles[93,96] and the retrobulbar space.[94,95,97,98] It has been argued that despite the risk of retrobulbar hemorrhage, the retrobulbar space is the preferable injection site. This site requires a single injection, special equipment is not needed, and ophthalmologists are familiar with this treatment.[98] On the other hand, injection into the retrobulbar space depends on diffusion of toxin into all extraocular muscles, a process that is less controlled than injection of individual muscles.[93] Injections to the superior rectus or oblique muscles increase risk of diffusion to non-injected muscles, which may result in ptosis or unwanted eye deviations.[99] Dosages used for AN treatment have been based on those used for strabismus and blepharospasm.

The few case reports on the use of BTX-A for AN suggest that while treatment may be effective[93–95,97,98] it is generally too short-lived to be satisfactory for patients.[97,98] Most patients required reinjection within 3–4 months. Considering the risk of not only retrobulbar hemorrhage but also ocular perforation and trauma to the optic nerve and other orbital structures with each injection,[98] the decision to treat or reinject must be carefully evaluated against the therapeutic effects of BTX-A.[97] As noted by Lennerstrand et al.,[99] the greatest beneficial effects have been reported in relatively immobile patients (e.g., those who are wheelchair-bound). In mobile patients, the relative ophthalmoplegia induced by the injection creates substantial problems resulting from impaired compensation for head movements. The most commonly reported adverse event has been ptosis, particularly after injections to the retrobulbar space.[94,95] Injecting with the head in an upright position, so that toxin is deposited in the lower portion of the orbit, may lessen this effect.[98] Other side effects have included diplopia and worsened movement in the nontreated eye, which may be avoided if the better eye rather than the worse one is treated.[98]

PREOPERATIVE USES

The ability of BTX-A to paralyze muscle temporarily has been a useful preoperative technique for various conditions. Usually the benefit is to eliminate involuntary spasm that could hinder healing, such as in PD[100] or cervical dystonia patients.[101] In cases of sphincter insufficiency of the larynx, laryngectomy is the most effective treatment but results in permanent voice loss. For this reason, surgical closure of the larynx is preferable, however, this closure is complicated by strong voluntary swallowing movements that interfere with the sutures.[102–104] Preoperative BTX-A injections into the posterior cricoarytenoid, aryepiglottic, medial thyroarytenoid, and lateral thyroarytenoid muscles has been shown to facilitate wound healing in these surgical patients.[105]

Cervical spondylosis with subsequent development of myelopathy is a complication of idiopathic and cerebral palsy-related cervical dystonia. In these patients, prolonged postoperative stabilization is crucial to augment fusion. It has been demonstrated that appropriate stabilization may be achieved with high-dose (500–700 units of BOTOX) BTX-A injections.[106,107] Side effects included vocal cord paraly-sis and epiglottic edema. These effects were associated with the high doses required.[106] In children with cerebral palsy, hand function may be improved through a surgical technique that lengthens the spastic muscle and tendons. However, results are highly variable and difficult to predict.[108] BTX-A may be used to simulate the effect of surgical muscle/tendon lengthening by reducing spasticity in the target muscle; thus, a preoperative evaluation and surgical outcome may be assessed.[108] In those cases in which BTX-A fails to achieve the targeted results, surgery may be eliminated as a potential remedy. BTX-A may also be used as a temporary treatment in young patients with cerebral palsy.[108]

Another reported preoperative use of BTX-A in children with cerebral palsy is to relieve postoperative pain after hip adductor-release surgery. In a double-blind, placebo-controlled study, surgical patients who were given BTX-A had substantially reduced pain scores, analgesic requirements, and hospital stays compared to patients receiving placebo.[109]

SENSORY CONDITIONS: CHRONIC MUSCULAR PAIN, MIGRAINE, AND TENSION HEADACHE

Afferent Effect with Botulinum Toxin Type A

Relevant to many movement disorders with a sensory component, BTX-A may also modify the sensory feedback loop to the central nervous system. Ludlow et al.[110] and Zwirner et al.[111] proposed that reduced muscle activity and therefore feedback to laryngeal motoneuron pools may be a primary mechanism of action of BTX-A. Brin et al.[112] offered the possibility that BTX might have a direct effect on sensory afferents by blocking intrafusal fibers, thus resulting in decreased activation of muscle spindles. This would effectively change the sensory afferent system by reducing the Ia traffic. Filippi et al.[113] supported this hypothesis by establishing that local injections of BTX-A directly reduced afferent Ia fiber traffic and thereby exerted a modulatory effect on sensory feedback. This may also account for the clinical observation that injections of BTX-A have an effect on regional noninjected muscles, most strikingly in spastic limbs.[114]

Support for this afferent mechanism derives from the cumulative work of Kaji and colleagues.[115-120] They showed that the increase in severity of dystonic writer's cramp, associated with enhancement of Ia muscle spindle activity via the tonic vibration maneuver, may be decreased by intramuscular injections of dilute lidocaine. These intramuscular injections preferentially affect the afferent innervation of the muscle spindle. Both ethanol and lidocaine block sodium channels, however, ethanol blocks the channels for a longer duration than the anesthetic lidocaine. Kaji coined the term "muscle afferent block" for this treatment of lidocaine plus ethanol. This treatment has shown effects in neck, jaw,[119] and limb dystonia,[115,116] as well as in spasticity.[118,120] The benefit for each treatment only lasts a few weeks, and therefore is of limited use in most dystonic and spastic situations.

However, this model of blocking Ia afferents supports the proposed mechanism of afferent action with BTX-A in conditions associated with excessive muscle contraction.

Analgesic Effects of Botulinum Toxin Type A

Early reports of therapeutic uses of BTX-A focused primarily on relief of muscle spasm and secondarily on pain relief. In 1985, the analgesic effects of BTX-A were first reported in a pilot study of treatment for cervical dystonia. This form of dystonia is characterized by abnormal, involuntary neck and shoulder muscle contractions and often resulting in significant, disabling musculoskeletal pain. Tsui et al.[121] described that the most marked benefit of BTX-A injections was pain relief in all six patients who reported severe neck pain caused by muscle spasm. In a small, double-blind, placebo-controlled extension of this pilot study, sixteen patients treated with BTX-A experienced substantially reduced pain compared to placebo.[122] In initial open-label, prospective studies involving larger numbers of patients, Brin et al.[81] reported pain relief in 74–84% of patients with cervical dystonia who had received BTX-A injections. Additional open-label and double-blind, placebo-controlled studies confirmed the observed effects of BTX-A on pain in patients with cervical dystonia.[123–129]

In 1992, Memin et al.[130] reported results from a pilot study for the use of BTX-A as treatment for spasticity after upper motor neuron lesion; 5 of 6 patients who had pain experienced significant pain relief. Also in 1992, Dengler et al.[131] reported analgesic effects of BTX-A among 10 patients treated for spastic drop foot. Researchers who conducted a larger prospective study of patients with chronic limb spasticity (resulting from various causes), observed that 90% of 31 patients with painful flexor spasm or passive stretching experienced at least moderate pain relief; 26% experienced complete pain resolution after BTX-A injections.[132] Investigators in Thailand conducted a prospective study and observed joint pain relief in 22 poststroke patients with spasticity.[133] Double-blind, placebo-controlled studies provided further support for the effect of BTX-A on pain relief in patients with spasticity.[134,135]

Early in its use as a therapeutic agent, BTX-A was observed to provide pain relief in disorders other than dystonia and spasticity. Published case reports detail analgesic effects of BTX-A injections for stiff-person syndrome[136] and muscle hypertrophy associated with complex repetitive discharges.[137] In a prospective study of 60 patients with achalasia, BTX-A improved chest pain associated with this disease of the esophagus.[138] Dysphagia is often accompanied by pain caused by cricopharyngeal dysfunction (i.e., hyperactivity of the upper esophageal sphincter) that is associated with prior surgical procedures or other neurologic disorders[139] including PD.[140] This dysphagia has been treated successfully with BTX-A. Among 100 patients treated for anal fissure, 78% reported pain resolution within 3 days after initial injection.[141] Painful vaginismus has also been treated with BTX-A.[142]

Brin et al.[143] have reviewed the published reports of BTX-A for the relief of pain disorders. These disorder include pain associated with myofascial pain syndrome;[144–149] blepharospasm;[150] temporomandibular disorder and bruxism;[151–157] back pain;[158] painful myoclonus;[66] prostatic pain/sterile prostatitis;[159] cervicogenic headaches;[160] cluster headaches;[161–163] tension type headaches;[163–169] and migraine headache.[163,170–174] As noted above, in a double-blind, placebo-controlled study, patients with cerebral palsy were given BTX-A for postoperative pain after adductor-release surgery. These patients had substantially reduced pain scores, analgesic requirements, and hospital stays compared to patients receiving placebo.[109] The use of BTX-A for treating various forms of headache has also been explored. Results are mixed for the most common type of headache, tension headache.[163–169,179–181] Case reports on BTX-A treatment for cluster headache have yielded inconsistent findings.[161–163] Formal studies have not been possible because of the rarity of the condition. Clinical results for the use of BTX-A for migraine headache support the use of this agent as a prophylaxis for patients with chronic symptoms.[172–174,182–185]

The association between BTX-A and pain relief was originally thought to relate only to its effect on muscle contraction; however, several studies suggest that muscle relaxation effects may not directly coincide with pain relief. This suggests alternative mechanisms for the analgesic effects of BTX-A. As noted in this chapter, there is experimental evidence that BTX-A affects afferent transmission,[113,175] which may be a factor in pain relief. There is also evidence that BTX-A inhibits the release of substance P and potentially other neuromodulators.[176] Substance P is a neuropeptide that plays a role in pain perception, vasodilation, and neurogenic inflammation. Cui and Aoki[177] have experimentally demonstrated that BTX-A relieves formalin-induced pain in laboratory animals. This is an important observation in understanding the action of BTX-A on pain because formalin does not cause pain through muscle tension. First, it stimulates nociceptors directly and then stimulates them through inflammation. It seems likely that the analgesic effects of BTX-A relate not only to its well-established effect at the neuromuscular junction but also an effect on the nociceptor system.[178]

The postulated mechanism of benefit in prophylaxis for migraine and relief of other painful conditions is not obvious. One possibility is that BTX-A interferes with any muscular trigger that could incite a migraine attack. Alternatively, there may be an indirect reduction of peripheral pain through reduced muscle contractions, mechanoreceptor stimulation, or afferent signals, which could then reduce stimulation of brain stem nociceptors. Furthermore, there are several lines of evidence that BTX-A may decrease the release of neurally active substances that mediate pain and have an effect on brain modulation of pain perception. Suzuki et al.[186] showed that acetylcholine, vasoactive intestinal polypeptide (VIP), and neuropeptide Y colocalize in parasympathetic nerves originating in the sphenopalatine, otic, and internal carotid ganglia, all of which innervate cerebral arteries. Sala et al.[187] demonstrated that BTX-A inhibits release of calcitonin gene-related peptide (CGRP) from motor nerves in rats; CGRP is thought to be important in mediating cranial headache. As noted above, Ishikawa et al.[176] showed that substance P and acetylcholine release may be blocked in the trigeminal nerve terminals in the rabbit iris dilator muscle. In an embryonic rat dorsal root ganglion model, Welch et al.[188] showed that BTX-A–cleaved SNAP-25 results in inhibition of substance P release with high sensitivity compared to other serotypes. These data suggest that BTX-A may relieve headache-associated pain through noncholinergic mechanisms.

MOTOR AND SENSORY DISORDERS: TICS AND TOURETTE'S SYNDROME

BTX-A has been tested as a therapeutic approach for chronic motor and phonic tics associated with Tourette's syndrome (TS). The etiology of TS is unknown, however, genetically determined dysfunction of the basal ganglia and limbic structures has been suggested.[189,190] Many patients experience premonitory sensations, a generalized urge or localized feeling of discomfort, that precede the tic.[191–195] This suggests that the tic itself is a voluntary (or "unvoluntary") motor response to an involuntary inner sensation. TS symptoms are often treated with antidopaminergic drugs, serotonin reuptake inhibitors, and other medications, however, these drugs are not effective in all patients[196–198] and are particularly ineffective for phonic tics.[199] BTX-A may be beneficial in disrupting the voluntary component of this sensory feedback mechanism or having a direct pharmacologic effect on the sensory component.

One socially debilitating TS-related tic is coprolalia or the shouting of profanities. This occurs in 8–50% of patients with TS at some time during their lives.[198,200] In the first case report of the use of BTX-A injection to the vocal cord to treat coprolalia, treatment improved not only the tic itself but the premonitory urges as well.[201] Other case reports found similar improvement after BTX-A treatment, with only mild adverse events (breathiness and dysphagia) and duration of effect of 9–12 weeks.[199,202]

In a longitudinal study motivated by a successful pilot study of BTX-A for dystonic tics in patients with TS,[203] 29 of 35 patients treated with BTX-A demonstrated some improvement in their tics; 23 of these showed marked improvement and 5 resolved altogether.[204,205] Tics decreased in frequency, duration, and intensity. Of 25 patients who described premonitory sensations, 21 experienced marked relief; 3 of these patients experienced complete resolution. Excluding patients with complete resolution of their tics, duration of benefit averaged approximately 14 weeks. Eyelid tics seemed to be the most responsive to treatment; cervical tics were the least responsive. The most common adverse event was neck weakness; all events were mild and

transient. While these results are encouraging, it must be noted that reduction in tic frequency and severity is well recognized as a natural course of TS; in fact, spontaneous remission occurs in 7–19% of all patients.[206]

In the first placebo-controlled study of BTX-A for TS,[207] 18 patients were randomly assigned to receive BTX-A or placebo in a double-blind, crossover design. There was significantly better response during the drug phase, however, this was not reflected in indices of overall patient well-being. The authors thought that this may have been the result of the side effects of BTX-A; the relative mildness of tics in their subjects; difficulty in measuring outcome, or; potential for unblinding because of BTX-A associated muscle weakness.

These investigators cautioned that statistically significant improvement in studies of BTX-A treatment for tics may not translate to clinically significant improvement and that BTX-A might best be reserved for patients with the most severe tics. There was no pattern to suggest that certain types of tics responded more favorably to treatment than other tics. This preliminary study lacked the power to show significant differences in several measured variables including severity score, tic suppression, pain, and patient global impression. Furthermore, the full effect of BTX may not have been appreciated at 2 weeks, a single treatment protocol does not reflect the clinical practice of evaluating patients after several adjustments in doses and sites of injections, and the patients were relatively mild because they "did not rate themselves as significantly compromised by their treated tics" at baseline.[208] A larger sample and longer follow-up are needed to evaluate the efficacy of BTX further in the treatment of tics and to demonstrate that this treatment offers clinically meaningful benefit.

AUTONOMIC GLANDULAR DISORDERS: HYPERHIDROSIS AND SIALORRHEA

Primary Focal Hyperhidrosis

Primary focal hyperhidrosis, a condition of localized excessive sweating of unknown etiology, may result in reduced health-related quality of life and occupational, physical, psychological, and social limitations for the patient.[209–212] Patients sweat 12–30 times more profusely than the healthy population.[213] Prevalence has been estimated at 0.1–1%.[214,215] Primary focal hyperhidrosis is typically symmetrical, and may affect one or more focal locations including the axillae, palms, soles of the feet, or face.[216] The exact pathogenesis of primary focal hyperhidrosis is unknown but is probably related to a dysfunctional central sympathetic nervous system, and the sweat glands of hyperhidrosis patients do not show any morphologic abnormalities.[217,218] Family pedigree research suggest evidence of genetic transmission.[219]

Diagnosis may be based on patient history and exclusion of secondary causes. Clinical tests include various staining methods (e.g., Minor's iodine-starch test) and gravimetric quantification of sweat production (milligram per minute).[213,220] Whereas Minor's iodine-starch test may be used in the clinical practice setting to define the hyperhidrotic area for treatment, gravimetric measurement is not routinely nor practically performed in clinical practice, but is often used for clinical research. Patient report via medical history or questionnaire about the effect of hyperhidrosis on quality of life or daily activities also provides valuable information in determining disease severity and management.[210] Treatments for the disorder have ranged from topical applications of antiperspirants to drastic surgical techniques. For many patients, these approaches have been unsatisfactory because of unacceptable side effects and poor results.[221]

The eccrine or sweat glands are innervated by ipsilateral postganglionic sympathetic fibers with acetylcholine as the most effective transmitter. The symptomology of botulism, which includes anhidrosis, provides evidence that BTX-A affects not only the neuromuscular junctions but also autonomic cholinergic innervated structures. Early observations of decreased sweating in response to BTX-A injections were made among patients who were treated for hemifacial spasm.[222] This finding led to a series of case reports and clinical studies that provided evidence that BTX-A is a fast-acting, extremely effective treatment for various forms of hyperhidrosis. Treatment with BTX-A not only eliminates or reduces the symptom of excessive sweating, but also markedly improves the diminished quality of life for patients.[209–212] BTX-A seems to have a longer duration of effect for hyperhidrosis than it does for neuromuscular disorders. The reasons for this clinically apparent extended duration are unclear.

Axillary Hyperhidrosis

Several clinical studies of BTX-A treatment for axillary hyperhidrosis have demonstrated BTX-A efficacy.[215,216,223–235] A BOTOX dose of 50 units appears sufficient to reduce sweating by 70–80%.[227] This dose seems to be an acceptable starting dose for most patients.[228] In a pivotal controlled clinical trial with this dose, the response rate reached 96% after the initial treatment. The mean duration between BTX-A treatments was 7 months. Twenty-eight percent of patients continued to the end of the study period (i.e., 16 months) with only one BTX-A treatment.[223] Reported adverse events have been mild and transitory for most patients, and have not generally included concomitant muscle weakness.

Palmar Hyperhidrosis

Clinical studies and reports on BTX-A treatment for palmar hyperhidrosis have demonstrated BTX-A efficacy at BOTOX dose ranges of 120–220 units, with a duration of effect between 4 and 6 months.[210,215,225,226,230,233,235–243] The doses used for palmar hyperhidrosis are generally higher than those used for axillary hyperhidrosis. Speculative explanations for the shorter duration of BTX-A effect compared to axillary treatment include problems with backflow, smaller diffusion distance in the thicker skin of the palms, a greater abundance of cholinergic nerve endings in the skin of the palms, and a quicker recovery rate in palm nerves.[213] Similar to axillary hyperhidrosis, there appear to be no differences in BTX-A efficacy for repeat treatments for palmar hyperhidrosis.[235]

The palms are the most problematic site for BTX treatment because of painful injections and the potential for inducing concomitant muscle weakness. There is a lack of consensus on how best to administer the toxin. Free nerve endings that are responsible for pain sensation reside in the papillary dermis and epidermis; sweat glands are deeply imbedded in the dermis and upper layer of subcutaneous tissue. Therefore, subcutaneous injections tend to be less painful and may deliver the toxin closer to the target organ, however, these injections carry the increased risk of inducing muscle weakness.[225,226,236–238,244] Muscle weakness may be overcome by more frequent treatments with smaller doses, however, because of the potential for antibody development, treatments administered more frequently than every 2 months are not recommended. Nerve block may be effective in reducing pain associated with treatment. Nerve block must be performed by a physician who is skilled in this procedure, thus lowering the risk of neural damage.[245] Intravenous regional anesthesia (Bier's block) has also been reported to be effective in reducing pain associated with treatment and may be an alternative to the traditional nerve block.[246]

Frey's Syndrome

Frey's syndrome is a sequela of traumatic lesions of the auriculotemporal nerve that appears to result from aberrant regrowth of postganglionic parasympathetic secretomotor fibers from the otic ganglion that normally innervate the parotid, but after transsection, regenerate and find the cholinergic receptors of the skin, innervating the sweat glands of the face upon salivary stimulation.[247] Many parotid gland surgery patients develop the syndrome,[248] and 15% of these patients consider their condition "severe."[249] Surgical techniques have been developed to treat Frey's syndrome, however these techniques often do not have acceptable risks or outcome. Thus, until recently, the recommended treatment for Frey's syndrome is simply explanation and reassurance.

Clinical reports and studies have provided conclusive evidence that BTX-A is an efficacious, well-tolerated, and long-lasting treatment for Frey's syndrome.[244,248,250–257] Reported BOTOX doses have ranged from 2.5–88.0 units. In most patients, duration of effect outlasted the observation period, some as long as 24 months.[255] The relationship between surface area of sweating and duration of effect is unclear.[248,258] Reported adverse events were mild and transitory.

Sialorrhea

There are two reported forms of sialorrhea:

1. Relative sialorrhea, which results from an impairment of the oral phase of swallowing and is a common sequela of neurologic disease and particularly associated with movement disorders, and
2. Absolute sialorrhea, which results from neurogenic abnormalities in salivary gland innervation.[259]

Sialorrhea occurs in approximately 50% of patients with amyotrophic lateral sclerosis,[260] 70–78% of patients with PD,[261] and 10–38% of patients with cerebral palsy.[262,263] Until recently, treatment options were limited to anticholinergic drugs, radiation, and surgical denervation of salivary glands, none of which are associated with acceptable risk or efficacy for most patients.

Salivary glands are controlled by the autonomic nervous system. While the function of saliva composition is under sympathetic neural control, saliva secretion is controlled by parasympathetic fibers, relying on acetylcholine to stimulate the salivary glands. It follows that saliva secretion could be susceptible to BTX inhibition. This is evidenced by dry mouth as a symptom of botulism. Also, it has been demonstrated that BTX is capable of inhibiting saliva secretion in animals.[264–267]

In 1997, Bushara[268] proposed the injection of BTX-A into the parotid glands as a treatment for ALS-associated sialorrhea. Since then, several small case reports and studies have demonstrated BTX-A efficacy not only for sialorrhea in ALS,[269] but also in PD,[270] cerebral palsy,[271,272] and various other disorders.[259,273–276]

Results reported in the literature have been generally good but somewhat variable, possibly because of differences in injection technique, specific glands injected, the precision of method used to measure outcome, and the reproducibility of study conditions from patient to patient.[270] Duration of effect ranged from 2 weeks to 6 months. While some investigators injected only the parotid or only the submandibular glands, Suskind and Tilton[272] noted better response when both sets of glands were injected. Variations in dose may have contributed to differences in results across studies, but in studies that used different dose levels, correlation between dose and response was not apparent.[270,275] Authors have recommended 20 units of BOTOX per parotid and 10 units per submandibular gland.[275] A longer duration of effect might be achieved with higher doses but may also induce reactive hypersalivation in other, noninjected salivary glands.[276,277] There were no major side effects associated with the BTX-A injections at conservative doses. Higher doses can be associated with dry mouth and secondary dysphagia. Because BTX-B (MYOBLOC, Elan Biopharmaceuticals, Dublin, Ireland) has been associated with higher frequency of dry mouth as an adverse effect of BTX-B injection in the treatment of cervical dystonia,[278,279] this type of BTX may be particularly suited for the treatment of sialorrhea. However, the overall adverse effect profile of BTX-B may limit treatment application.

TREATMENT OF SPHINCTERS OF THE LOWER GASTROINTESTINAL TRACT

BTX-A injections may treat failure of functional relaxation of many muscles involved in swallowing, peristalsis, and defecation. BTX-A has been used in both open and double-blind studies for the treatment of rectal spasms resulting in chronic constipation and anal fissures.[141,280–294] Investigators have proposed that hemorrhoids and fissures do not heal in the setting of increased rectal tone, which secondarily results in inadequate drainage of the rectal circulation. As a result, the vessels become boggy and engorged. BTX-A is proposed to weaken the rectal sphincter, which then permits an increase in venous return, thus improving circulation and promoting healing. Injections of BTX-A in both the internal (smooth muscle) and external (skeletal muscle) anal sphincters under ultrasound guidance have been used to treat anal fissures. Doses of up to 80 units of BOTOX injected either anteriorly or posteriorly to the internal anal sphincter have been reported to be safe and efficacious for the treatment of anal fissures. There have been no reports of any serious adverse event following treatment. The most common adverse event reported was flatus incontinence, which was transient in nature and in most cases resolved within 1 week. Recent reviews suggest that treating the internal sphincter is preferred with a better adverse event profile.

BLADDER DISORDERS

Experience in the use of BTX-A to treat a variety of disorders causing lower urinary tract symptoms (LUTS) is increasing. Many disorders of the genitourinary tract are related to smooth muscle dysfunction including inadequate muscle relaxation, disordered smooth muscle motility, or contraction occurring during storage. When the pathology of the underlying neurologic disorder is known it is diagnosed as detrusor-sphincter dyssynergia (DSD) or detrusor hyperreflexia (DH). If the pathology is unknown, it is referred to as detrusor instability or overactive bladder.[295]

DSD is characterized by inappropriate contractions of the sphincter during detrusor contractions, therefore causing difficulty voiding. Transperineal and transurethral injections of BTX-A into the external urethral sphincter of doses up to and including 250 units in 108 patients have been reported in the literature.[296–303] Prior to treatment, most patients were on indwelling or intermittent catheterization and experiencing various voiding dysfunctions, including incontinence. After treatment, decreases in postvoid residual volumes, mean maximal detrusor pressure, and functional detrusor capacity were accompanied by a low incidence of reported adverse events.

The successful treatment of DH with BTX-A was first reported by Schurch and colleagues.[304] Twenty-one patients with spinal cord injuries, severe detrusor hyperreflexia and incontinence were injected cystoscopically with 200–300 units of BOTOX at 20–30 sites in the detrusor. At 6-weeks postinjection, 19 of the original 21 patients returned for follow-up. Eighty-nine percent (17/19) of these patients were completely continent and anticholinergic medication need was either markedly decreased or completely abolished. Significant changes in urodynamic parameters were noted at both 6 and 36 weeks postinjection. A low incidence of adverse events was reported in these patients. Four patients had minor episodes of incontinence that were associated with a concurrent bladder infection. No other adverse events were reported. However, three patients with autonomic dysreflexia associated with DH prior to treatment had a resolution of their symptoms.

Subsequent to Schurch and colleagues, additional studies have reported treatment in both patients with and without neurologic conditions. An additional 177 patients diagnosed with DH were treated with up to 400 units injected at 20 sites across the detrusor. Significant improvements in bladder capacity and decreases in detrusor pressure were reported. Fourteen patients with urgency-frequency or urge-incontinence symptoms who were refractory to anticholinergic treatments were treated with up to 300 units of BTX-A injected at 5–15 sites across the detrusor.[305,306] Improvements in frequency, bladder capacity, first desire to void, and detrusor pressure were noted up to 20 weeks after treatment. Similar to the data from patients with DSD, a low incidence of adverse events has been reported for patients with DH and nonneurogenic voiding dysfunction injected with BTX-A in the detrusor to treat voiding dysfunction.

PROSTATITIS AND BENIGN PROSTATIC HYPERTROPHY

Patients with chronic prostatitis have been treated with BTX-A injections. Chronic nonbacterial prostatitis may be associated with pain and motor dysregulation of the pelvic floor. BTX-A may have a beneficial effect on the symptoms of chronic prostatitis-associated pain by reducing hypertonic and/or hyperreflexic sphincter activities or a direct effect on pain reflexes (see above). BTX-A injections have been administered either transurethrally or transperineally to treat chronic prostatitis in 22 patients.[159,307,308] Doses of up to 200 units were distributed in 3–4 injection sites around the external urethral sphincter. One patient reported an adverse event of mild stress incontinence that resolved within a few weeks. Significant improvements in urodynamic measures were noted after treatment. Improvements in flow rate and void volume and decreased incidences of incontinence led to satisfactory therapy in 9 of 22 patients. Pain and discomfort in the pelvic region were assessed in 11 patients.[159] Nine of these 11 (81%) patients reported an improvement in their pain levels after the injections.

Promising results of intralobar injections of BTX-A in treating patients with symptoms of benign prostatic hypertrophy (BPH) were recently reported.[309] In a double-blind study, patients received either saline or 100 units of BTX-A as BOTOX into each lobe of the prostate. One-month results of the BTX-A group showed a reduction in the American Urologic Association symptom score by 54%, serum prostate-specific–antigen by 51%, prostate volume by 54%, and postvoid residual urine volume by 60% in addition to nearly doubling the peak urinary flow rate. Further improvement was seen at 2 months.

ENHANCEMENT OF FACIAL AESTHETICS

In 1990, Carruthers and Carruthers[310] reported diminished glabellar frown lines after BTX-A injection for blepharospasm. In 1993, Blitzer et al.[311] further reported diminished forehead lines and lateral orbital lines (crow's feet) after BTX-A injection for the management of Meige's syndrome and hemifacial spasm. Subsequent to these early observations, the use of BTX-A for cosmetic enhancement has been intensely studied in the upper and lower face in reducing hyperfunctional glabellar, forehead and crow's lines, inducing brow lift, and also reducing platysmal bands and perioral lines.[312–317] BTX-A has recently been reported useful as an adjunct to other facial rejuvenation procedures.[318–320] BTX-A injections into the muscles causing facial lines to form can improve facial appearance both during muscle contraction and while at rest. Patients as well as physicians note a high degree of satisfaction with BTX-A treatment,[321,322] leading to regulatory approval in many countries.

ACKNOWLEDGMENT

This work was supported in part by the Bachmann-Strauss Dystonia and Parkinson's Disease Foundation.

REFERENCES

1. Brin MF. Interventional neurology: treatment of neurological conditions with local injection of botulinum toxin. Arch Neurobiol (Madr) 1991;54:173–189.
2. Brin MF. Botulinum toxin: new and expanded indications. Eur J Neurol 1997;4:59–66.
3. Brin MF. Treatment of dystonia. In: Jankovic J, Tolosa E, eds. Parkinson's Disease and Movement Disorders. New York: Williams & Wilkins, 1998:553–578.
4. Jankovic J, Hallett M. Therapy with Botulinum Toxin. New York: Marcel Dekker, 1994.
5. Jankovic J, Brin MF. Botulinum toxin: historical perspective and potential new indications. Muscle Nerve 1997;20:S129–S145
6. Gibbs SR, Blitzer A. Botulinum toxin for the treatment of spasmodic dysphonia. Otolaryngol Clin North Am 2000;33:879–894.
7. Blitzer A, Binder WJ, Boyd JB. Management of Facial Lines and Wrinkles. Philadelphia: Lippincott Williams & Wilkins, 1999.
8. Deuschl G, Bain P, Brin M. Consensus statement of the Movement Disorder Society on Tremor. Ad Hoc Scientific Committee. Mov Disord 1998;13(Suppl 3):2–23.
9. Lou JS, Jankovic J. Essential tremor: clinical correlates in 350 patients. Neurology 1991;41:234–238.
10. Bain PG, Findley LJ, Thompson PD, et al. A study of hereditary essential tremor. Brain 1994;117:805–824.
11. Wissel J, Masuhr F, Schelosky L, et al. Quantitative assessment of botulinum toxin treatment in 43 patients with head tremor. Mov Disord 1997;12:722–726.
12. The Deep-Brain Stimulation for Parkinson's Disease Study Group.

Deep-brain stimulation of the subthalamic nucleus or the pars interna of the globus pallidus in Parkinson's disease. N Engl J Med 2001;345:956–963.

13. Hariz MI. Complications of deep brain stimulation surgery. Mov Disord 2002;17(Suppl 3):S162–S166

14. Koller WC, Lyons KE, Wilkinson SB, et al. Long-term safety and efficacy of unilateral deep brain stimulation of the thalamus in essential tremor. Mov Disord 2001;16:464–468.

15. Pahwa R, Lyons KE, Wilkinson SB, et al. Comparison of thalamotomy to deep brain stimulation of the thalamus in essential tremor. Mov Disord 2001;16:140–143.

16. Jankovic J, Schwartz K. Botulinum toxin treatment of tremors. Neurology 1991;41:1185–1188.

17. Jankovic J, Schwartz K, Clemence W, et al. A randomized, double-blind, placebo-controlled study to evaluate botulinum toxin type A in essential hand tremor. Mov Disord 1996;11:250–256.

18. Brin MF, Lyons KE, Doucette J, et al. A randomized, double masked, controlled trial of botulinum toxin type A in essential hand tremor. Neurology 2001;56:1523–1528.

19. Trosch RM, Pullman SL. Botulinum toxin A injections for the treatment of hand tremors. Mov Disord 1994;9:601–609.

20. Henderson JM, Ghika JA, Van Melle G, et al. Botulinum toxin a in non-dystonic tremors. Eur Neurol 1996;36:29–35.

21. Pullman SL, Greene P, Fahn S, et al. Approach to the treatment of limb disorders with botulinum toxin A. Experience with 187 patients. Arch Neurol 1996;53:617–624.

22. Warrick P, Dromey C, Irish J, et al. The treatment of essential voice tremor with botulinum toxin A: a longitudinal case report. J Voice 2000;14:410–421.

23. Hertegard S, Granqvist S, Lindestad PA. Botulinum toxin injections for essential voice tremor. Ann Otol Rhinol Laryngol 2000;109:204–209.

24. Modugno N, Priori A, Berardelli A, et al. Botulinum toxin restores presynaptic inhibition of group Ia afferents in patients with essential tremor. Muscle Nerve 1998;21:1701–1705.

25. Deuschl G, Lohle E, Heinen F, et al. Ear click in palatal tremor: its origin and treatment with botulinum toxin. Neurology 1991;41:1677–1679.

26. Gordon K, Cadera W, Hinton G. Successful treatment of hereditary trembling chin with botulinum toxin. J Child Neurol 1993;8:154–156.

27. Bakar M, Zarifoglu M, Bora I, et al. Treatment of hereditary trembling chin with botulinum toxin. Mov Disord 1998;13:845–846.

28. Pacchetti C, Mancini F, Bulgheroni M, et al. Botulinum toxin treatment for functional disability induced by essential tremor. Neurol Sci 2000;21:349–353.

29. Jankovic J. Tardive syndromes and other drug-induced movement disorders. Clin Neuropharm 1995;18:197–214.

30. Tarsy D. Tardive dyskinesia. Curr Treat Options Neurol 2000; 2:205–214.

31. Burke RE, Fahn S, Jankovic J, et al. Tardive dystonia: late onset and persistent dystonia caused by antipsychotic drugs. Neurology 1982;32:1335–1346.

32. Kang UJ, Burke RE, Fahn S. Natural history and treatment of tardive dystonia. Mov Disord 1986;1:193-208.

33. Burke RE, Kang UJ. Tardive dystonia: clinical aspects and treatment. Adv Neurol 1988;49:199–210.

34. Kang UJ, Fahn S. Management of tardive dyskinesia. Ration Drug Ther 1988;22:1–7.

35. Truong DD, Hermanowicz N, Rontal M. Botulinum toxin in treatment of tardive dyskinetic syndrome. J Clin Psychopharmacol 1990;10:438–439.

36. Stip E, Faughnan M, Desjardin I, et al. Botulinum toxin in a case of severe tardive dyskinesia mixed with dystonia. Br J Psychiatry 1992; 161:867–868.

37. Kaufman DM. Use of botulinum toxin injections for spasmodic torticollis of tardive dystonia. J Neuropsychiatry Clin Neurosci 1994;6:50–53.

38. Yasufuku-Takano J, Sakurai M, Kanazawa I, et al. Successful treatment of intractable tardive dyskinesia with botulinum toxin. J Neurol Neurosurg Psychiatry 1995;58:511–512.

39. Kanovsky P, Streitova H, Bares M, et al. Treatment of facial and orolinguomandibular tardive dystonia by botulinum toxin A: evidence of a long-lasting effect. Mov Disord 1999;14:886–888.

40. Rapaport A, Sadeh M, Stein D, et al. Botulinum toxin for the treatment of oro-facial-lingual-masticatory tardive dyskinesia. Mov Disord 2000;15:352–355.

41. Rondot P, Korn H, Scherrer J. Suppression of an entire limb tremor by anesthetizing a selective muscular group. Arch Neurol 1968;19:421–429.

42. Burke RE, Fahn S, Jankovic J, et al. Tardive dystonia and inappropriate use of neuroleptic drugs. Lancet 1982;1:1299.

43. Kang UJ, Burke RE, Fahn S. Tardive dystonia. Adv Neurol 1988; 50:415–429.

44. Burke RE, Kang UJ, Jankovic J, et al. Tardive akathisia: an analysis of clinical features and response to open therapeutic trials. Mov Disord 1989;4:157–175.

45. Shulman LM, Singer C, Weiner WJ. Improvement of both tardive dystonia and akathisia after botulinum toxin injection. Neurology 1996;46:844–845.

46. Chatterjee A, Forrest GM, Giladi N, et al. Botulinum toxin in the treatment of tardive dystonia. J Clin Psychopharmacol 1997;17:497–498.

47. Tarsy D, Kaufman D, Sethi KD, et al. An open-label study of botulinum toxin A for treatment of tardive dystonia. Clin Neuropharm 1997;20:90–93.

48. Brashear A, Ambrosius WT, Eckert GJ, et al. Comparison of treatment of tardive dystonia and idiopathic cervical dystonia with botulinum toxin type A. Mov Disord 1998;13:158–161.

49. Comella CL, Shannon KM, Jaglin J. Extensor truncal dystonia: successful treatment with botulinum toxin injections. Mov Disord 1998;13:552–555.

50. Fahn S, Mayeux R. Unilateral Parkinson's disease and contralateral tardive dyskinesia: a unique case with successful therapy that may explain the pathophysiology of these two disorders. J Neural Transm Suppl 1980;179–185.

51. Molho ES, Feustel PJ, Factor SA. Clinical comparison of tardive and idiopathic cervical dystonia. Mov Disord 1998;13:486–489.

52. Tan EK, Jankovic J. Tardive and idiopathic oromandibular dystonia: a clinical comparison. J Neurol Neurosurg Psychiatry 2000;68:186–190.

53. Samant HC, Gupta SK, Gupta OP. Palatal myoclonus. Ann Otol Rhinol Laryngol 1970;79:858–861.

54. East CA, Hazell JW. The suppression of palatal (or intra-tympanic) myoclonus by tinnitus masking devices. A preliminary report. J Laryngol Otol 1987;101:1230–1234.

55. Varney SM, Demetroulakos JL, Fletcher MH, et al. Palatal myoclonus: treatment with Clostridium botulinum toxin injection. Otolaryngol Head Neck Surg 1996;114:317–320.

56. Obeso JA, Artieda J, Marsden CD. Differential clinical presentations of myoclonus. In: Jankovic J, Tolosa E, eds. Parkinson's Disease and Movement Disorders. Baltimore: Urban & Schwarzenberg, 1988: 263–274.

57. Kane SA, Thach WT. Palatal myoclonus and function of the inferior olive: are they related? In: Strata P, ed. Experimental Brain Research Series 17: The Olivocerebellar System in Motor Control. Berlin/Heidelberg: Springer, 1989:427–460.

58. Dietrichs E, Heier MS, Faye-Lund H, et al. Bulbar myoclonus without palatal myoclonus. A hypothesis on pathophysiology. Eur J Neurol 1999;6:367–370.

59. Litman RS, Hausman SA. Bilateral palatal myoclonus. Laryngoscope 1982;92:1187–1189.

60. Le Pajolec C, Marion MH, Bobin S. Objective tinnitus and palatal myoclonus. A new therapeutic approach [In French]. Ann Otolaryngol Chir Cervicofac 1990;107:363–365.

61. Saeed SR, Brookes GB. The use of clostridium botulinum toxin in palatal myoclonus. A preliminary report. J Laryngol Otol 1993; 107:208–210.

62. Giladi N, Meer J, Kidan C, et al. Interventional neurology: botulinum toxin as a potent symptomatic treatment in neurology. Isr J Med Sci 1994;30:816–819.

63. Bryce GE, Morrison MD. Botulinum toxin treatment of essential palatal myoclonus tinnitus. J Otolaryngol 1998;27:213–216.

64. Jero J, Salmi T. Palatal myoclonus and clicking tinnitus in a 12-year-old girl: case report. Acta Otolaryngol Suppl 2000;543:61–62.

65. Badia L, Parikh A, Brookes GB. Management of middle ear myoclonus. J Laryngol Otol 1994;108:380–382.

66. Polo KB, Jabbari B. Effectiveness of botulinum toxin type A against painful limb myoclonus of spinal cord origin. Mov Disord 1994;9:233–235.

67. Lagueny A, Tison F, Burbaud P, et al. Stimulus-sensitive spinal segmental myoclonus improved with injections of botulinum toxin type A. Mov Disord 1999;14:182–185.

68. Awaad Y, Tayem H, Elgamal A, et al. Treatment of childhood myoclonus with botulinum toxin type A. J Child Neurol. 1999;14: 781–786.

69. Jankovic J, Tintner R. Dystonia and parkinsonism. Parkinsonism Related Disord 2001;8:109–121.

70. Nausieda PA, Weiner WJ, Klawans HL. Dystonic foot response of Parkinsonism. Arch Neurol 1980;37:132–136.

71. Curtis L, Lees AJ, Stern GM, et al. Effect of L-dopa on course of Parkinson's disease. Lancet 1984;2:211–212.

72. Kidron D, Melamed E. Forms of dystonia in patients with Parkinson's disease. Neurology 1987;37:1009–1011.

73. Pacchetti C, Albani G, Martignoni E, et al. "Off" painful dystonia in Parkinson's disease treated with botulinum toxin. Mov Disord 1995;10:333–336.

74. Luquin MR, Scipioni O, Vaamonde J, et al. Levodopa-induced dyskinesias in Parkinson's disease: clinical and pharmacological classification. Mov Disord 1992;7:117–124.

75. Poewe WH, Lees AJ, Stern GM. Dystonia in Parkinson's disease: clinical and pharmacological features. Ann Neurol 1988;23:73–78.

76. Quinn N, Marsden CD. Lithium for painful dystonia in Parkinson's disease [Letter]. Lancet 1986;1:1377.

77. Lees AJ, Shaw KM, Stern GM. Baclofen in Parkinson's disease. J Neurol Neurosurg Psychiatry 1978;41:707–708.

78. Lees AJ, Stern GM. Bromocriptine in treatment of levodopa-induced end-of-dose dystonia. Lancet 1980;2:215–216.

79. Ilson J, Fahn S, Cote L. Painful dystonic spasms in Parkinson's disease. Adv Neurol 1984;40:395–398.

80. Jankovic J, Brin M. Therapeutic uses of botulinum toxin. N Engl J Med 1991;324:1186–1194.

81. Brin MF, Fahn S, Moskowitz C, et al. Localized injections of botulinum toxin for the treatment of focal dystonia and hemifacial spasm. Mov Disord 1987;2:237–254.

82. Yoshimura DM, Aminoff MJ, Olney RK. Botulinum toxin therapy for limb dystonias. Neurology 1992;42:627–630.

83. Giladi N, Honigman S. Botulinum toxin injections to one leg alleviate freezing of gait in a patient with Parkinson's disease. Mov Disord 1997;12:1085–1086.

84. Giladi N, Gurevich T, Shabtai H, et al. The effect of botulinum toxin injections to the calf muscles on freezing of gait in parkinsonism: a pilot study. J Neurol 2001;248:572–576.

85. Limousin P, Memin B, Pollak P. Treatment of dystonia occurring in parkinsonian syndromes by botulinum toxin. Eur Neurol 1997;37:66–67.

86. Defazio G, Lepore V, Lamberti P, et al. Botulinum A toxin treatment for eyelid spasm, spasmodic torticollis and apraxia of eyelid opening. Ital J Neurol Sci 1990;11:275–280.

87. Reynolds F, Petropoulous G. Hand deformities in parkinsonism. J Chronic Dis 1965;18:593–595.

88. LeWitt PA, Burns RS, Newman RP. Dystonia in untreated parkinsonism. Clin Neuropharm 1986;9:293–297.

89. Kyriakides T, Hewer RL. Hand contractures in Parkinson's disease. J Neurol Neurosurg Psychiatry 1988;51:1221–1223.

90. Hu MT, Bland J, Clough C, et al. Limb contractures in levodopa-responsive parkinsonism: a clinical and investigational study of seven new cases. J Neurol 1999;246:671–676.

91. Cordivari C, Misra VP, Catania S, et al. Treatment of dystonic clenched fist with botulinum toxin. Mov Disord 2001;16:907–913.

92. Scott AB. Botulinum toxin injection into extraocular muscles as an alternative to strabismus surgery. Ophthalmology. 1980;87:1044–1049.

93. Leigh RJ, Tomsak RL, Grant MP, et al. Effectiveness of botulinum toxin administered to abolish acquired nystagmus. Ann Neurol 1992;32:633–642.

94. Ruben S, Dunlop IS, Elston J. Retrobulbar botulinum toxin for treatment of oscillopsia. Aust NZ J Ophthalmol 1994;22:65–67.

95. Ruben ST, Lee JP, O'Neil D, et al. The use of botulinum toxin for treatment of acquired nystagmus and oscillopsia. Ophthalmology 1994;101:783–787.

96. Crone RA, de Jong PT, Notermans G. Treatment of nystagmus using injections of botulinum toxins into the eye muscles [in German]. Klin Monatsbl Augenheilkd 1984;184:216–217.

97. Helveston EM, Pogrebniak AE. Treatment of acquired nystagmus with botulinum A toxin. Am J Ophthalmol 1988;106:584–586.

98. Repka MX, Savino PJ, Reinecke RD. Treatment of acquired nystagmus with botulinum neurotoxin A. Arch Ophthalmol 1994;112:1320–1324.

99. Lennerstrand G, Nordbo OA, Tian S, et al. Treatment of strabismus and nystagmus with botulinum toxin type A. An evaluation of effects and complications. Acta Ophthalmol Scand 1998;76:27.

100. Gasser T, Fritsch K, Arnold G, et al. Botulinum toxin A in orthopaedic surgery. Lancet 1991;338:761.

101. Adler CH, Zimmerman RS, Lyons MK, et al. Perioperative use of botulinum toxin for movement disorder-induced cervical spine disease. Mov Disord 1996;11:79–81.

102. Montgomery WW. Surgical laryngeal closure to elminiate chronic aspiration. N Engl J Med 1975;292:1390–1391.

103. Levine HL, Wood BG, Batza E, et al. Recurrent layngeal nerve section for spasmodic dysphonia. Ann Otol Rhinol Laryngol 1979;88:527–530.

104. Habal MB, Murray JE. Surgical treatment of life-endangering chronic aspiration pneumonia. Use of an epiglottic flap to the arytenoids. Plast Reconstr Surg 1972;49:305–311.

105. Pototschnig CA, Schneider I, Eckel HE, et al. Repeatedly successful closure of the larynx for the treatment of chronic aspiration with the use of botulinum toxin A. Ann Otol Rhinol Laryngol 1996;105:521–524.

106. Racette BA, Lauryssen C, Perlmutter JS. Preoperative treatment with botulinum toxin to facilitate cervical fusion in dystonic cerebral palsy. Report of two cases. J Neurosurg 1998;88:328–330.

107. Basciani M, Intiso D, Cioffi RP, et al. Preoperative treatment with botulinum A toxin in patients with cervical disk herniation secondary to dystonic cerebral palsy. Neurol Sci 2000;21:63.

108. Autti-Ramo I, Larsen A, Peltonen J, et al. Botulinum toxin injection as an adjunct when planning hand surgery in children with spastic hemiplegia. Neuropediatrics 2000;31:4–8.

109. Barwood S, Baillieu C, Boyd R, et al. Analgesic effects of botulinum toxin A: a randomized, placebo- controlled clinical trial. Dev Med Child Neurol 2000;42:116–121.

110. Ludlow CL, Hallett M, Sedory SE, et al. The pathophysiology of spasmodic dysphonia and its modification by botulinum toxin. In: Berardelli A, Benecke R, Manfredi M, et al., eds. Motor Disturbances II. New York: Academic Press, 1990:273–288.

111. Zwirner P, Murry T, Swenson M, et al. Effects of botulinum toxin therapy in patients with adductor spasmodic dysphonia: acoustic, aerodynamic, and videoendoscopic findings. Laryngoscope 1992;102:400–406.

112. Brin MF, Blitzer A, Stewart C, et al. Treatment of spasmodic dysphonia (laryngeal dystonia) with local injections of botulinum toxin: review and technical aspects. In: Blitzer A, Brin MF, Sasaki CT, et al., eds. Neurological Disorders of the Larynx. New York: Thieme, 1992:214–228.

113. Filippi GM, Errico P, Santarelli R, et al. Botulinum A toxin effects on rat jaw muscle spindles. Acta Otolaryngol (Stockh) 1993;113:400–404.

114. Borg-Stein J, Pine ZM, Miller JR, et al. Botulinum toxin for the treatment of spasticity in multiple sclerosis. New observations. Am J Phys Med Rehabil 1993;72:364–368.

115. Kaji R, Rothwell JC, Katayama M, et al. Tonic vibration reflex and muscle afferent block in writer's cramp. Ann Neurol 1995;38:155–162.

116. Kaji R, Kohara N, Katayama M, et al. Muscle afferent block by intramuscular injection of lidocaine for the treatment of writer's cramp. Muscle Nerve 1995;18:234–235.

117. Kaji R, Shibasaki H, Kimura J. Writer's cramp: a disorder of motor subroutine? [Editorial; comment]. Ann Neurol 1995;38:837–838.

118. Kaji R, Mezaki T, Kubori T, et al. Treatment of spasticity with botulinum toxin and muscle afferent block [in Japanese]. Rinsho Shinkeigaku 1996;36:1334–1335.

119. Yoshida K, Kaji R, Kubori T, et al. Muscle afferent block for the treatment of oromandibular dystonia. Mov Disord 1998;13:699–705.

120. Mezaki T, Kaji R, Hirota N, et al. Treatment of spasticity with muscle afferent block. Neurology 1999;53:1156–1157.

121. Tsui JK, Eisen A, Mak E, et al. A pilot study on the use of botulinum toxin in spasmodic torticollis. Can J Neurol Sci 1985;12:314–316.

122. Tsui JKC, Eisen A, Stoessl AJ, et al. Double-blind study of botulinum toxin in spasmodic torticollis. Lancet 1986;2:245–247.

123. Greene P, Kang U, Fahn S, et al. Double-blind, placebo-controlled trial of botulinum toxin injections for the treatment of spasmodic torticollis. Neurology 1990;40:1213–1218.

124. Blackie JD, Lees AJ. Botulinum toxin treatment in spasmodic torticollis. J Neurol Neurosurg Psychiatry 1990;53:640–643.

125. Lorentz IT, Subramaniam SS, Yiannikas C. Treatment of idiopathic

spasmodic torticollis with botulinum toxin A: a double-blind study on twenty-three patients. Mov Disord 1991;6:145–150.

126. Lu CS, Chen RS, Tsai CH. Double-blind, placebo-controlled study of botulinum toxin injections in the treatment of cervical dystonia. J Formos Med Assoc 1995;94:189–192.

127. Tsui JKC, Fross RD, Calne S, et al. Local treatment of spasmodic torticollis with botulinum toxin. Can J Neurol Sci 1987;14:533–535.

128. Jankovic J, Schwartz K. Botulinum toxin injections for cervical dystonia. Neurology 1990;40:277–280.

129. Poewe W, Schelosky L, Kleedorfer B, et al. Treatment of spasmodic torticollis with local injections of botulinum toxin. One-year follow-up in 37 patients. J Neurol 1992;239:21–25.

130. Memin B, Pollack P, Hommel M, et al. Effects of botulinum toxin on spasticity. Rev Neurol (Paris) 1992;148:212–214.

131. Dengler R, Neyer U, Wohlfarth K, et al. Local botulinum toxin in the treatment of spastic foot drop. J Neurol 1992;239:375–378.

132. Dunne JW, Heye N, Dunne SL. Treatment of chronic limb spasticity with botulinum toxin A. J Neurol Neurosurg Psychiatry 1995;58:232–235.

133. Viriyavejakul A, Vachalathiti R, Poungvarin N. Botulinum treatment for post-stroke spasticity: low dose regime. J Med Assoc Thai 1998;81:413–422.

134. Grazko MA, Polo KB, Jabbari B. Botulinum toxin A for spasticity, muscle spasms, and rigidity. Neurology 1995;45:712–717.

135. Hyman N, Barnes M, Bhakta B, et al. Botulinum toxin (Dysport) treatment of hip adductor spasticity in multiple sclerosis: a prospective, randomised, double blind, placebo controlled, dose ranging study. J Neurol Neurosurg Psychiatry 2000;68:707–712.

136. Davis D, Jabbari B. Significant improvement of stiff-person syndrome after paraspinal injection of botulinum toxin-A. Mov Disord 1993;8:371–373.

137. Nix WA, Butler IJ, Roontga S, et al. Persistent unilateral tibialis anterior muscle hypertrophy with complex repetitive discharges and myalgia: report of two unique cases and response to botulinum toxin. Neurology 1992;42:602–606.

138. Fishman VM, Parkman HP, Schiano TD, et al. Symptomatic improvement in achalasia after botulinum toxin injection of the lower esophageal sphincter. Am J Gastroenterol 1996;91:1724–1730.

139. Schneider I, Thumfart WF, Pototschnig C, et al. Treatment of dysfunction of the cricopharyngeal muscle with botulinum A toxin: introduction of a new, noninvasive method. Ann Otol Rhinol Laryngol 1994;103:31–35.

140. Restivo DA, Palmeri A, Marchese-Ragona R. Botulinum toxin for cricopharyngeal dysfunction in Parkinson's disease. N Engl J Med 2002;346:1174–1175.

141. Jost WH. One hundred cases of anal fissure treated with botulin toxin: early and long-term results. Dis Colon Rectum 1997;40:1029–1032.

142. Brin MF, Vapnek JM. Treatment of vaginismus with botulinum toxin injections. Lancet 1997;349:252–253.

143. Brin MF, Binder WJ, Blitzer A, et al. Botulinum toxin type A for pain and headache. In: Brin MF, Hallett M, Jankovic J, eds. Scientific and Therapeutic Aspects of Botulinum Toxin. New York: Lippincott Williams & Wilkins, 2002:233–250

144. Acquadro MA, Borodic GE. Treatment of myofascial pain with botulinum A toxin [Letter]. Anesthesiology 1994;80:705–706.

145. Diaz JH, Gould HJ. Management of post-thoracotomy pseudoangina and myofascial pain with botulinum toxin. Anesthesiology 1999;91:877–879.

146. Cheshire WP, Abashian SW, Mann JD. Botulinum toxin in the treatment of myofascial pain syndrome. Pain 1994;59:65–69.

147. Porta M. A comparative trial of botulinum toxin type A and methylprednisolone for the treatment of myofascial pain syndrome and pain from chronic muscle spasm. Pain 2000;85:101–105.

148. Wheeler AH. Botulinum toxin A, adjunctive therapy for refractory headaches associated with pericranial muscle tension. Headache 1998;38:468–471.

149. Monsivais JJ, Monsivais DB. Botulinum toxin in painful syndromes. Hand Clin 1996;12:787–789.

150. Johnstone SJ, Adler CH. Headache and facial pain responsive to botulinum toxin: an unusual presentation of blepharospasm. Headache 1998;38:366–368.

151. Girdler NM. Use of botulinum toxin to alleviate facial pain. Br J Hosp Med 1994;52:363.

152. von Lindern JJ, Niederhagen B, Berge S, et al. Type A botulinum toxin in the treatment of chronic facial pain associated with masticatory hyperactivity. J Oral Maxillofac Surg 2003;61:774–778.

153. Van Zandijcke M, Marchau MM. Treatment of bruxism with botulinum toxin injections [Letter]. J Neurol Neurosurg Psychiatry 1990;53:530.

154. Ivanhoe CB, Lai JM, Francisco GE. Bruxism after brain injury: successful treatment with botulinum toxin-A. Arch Phys Med Rehabil 1997;78:1272–1273.

155. Rijsdijk BA, van ES RJ, Zonneveld FW, et al. De toepassing van botuline A toxine bij cosmetisch storende M.- masseterhypertrofie [Botulinum toxin type A treatment of cosmetically disturbing masseteric hypertrophy]. Ned Tijdschr Geneeskd 1998;142:529–532.

156. Tan EK, Jankovic J. Treating severe bruxism with botulinum toxin. J Am Dent Assoc 2000;131:211–216.

157. Freund B, Schwartz M, Symington JM. Botulinum toxin: new treatment for temporomandibular disorders. Br J Oral Maxillofac Surg 2000;38:466–471.

158. Foster L, Clapp L, Erickson M, et al. Botulinum toxin A and chronic low back pain: a randomized, double-blind study. Neurology 2001;56:1290–1293.

159. Zermann D, Ishigooka M, Schubert J, et al. Perisphincteric injection of botulinum toxin type A. a treatment option for patients with chronic prostatic pain? Eur Urol 2000;38:393–399.

160. Freund BJ, Schwartz M. Treatment of chronic cervical-associated headache with botulinum toxin A: a pilot study. Headache 2000;40:231–236.

161. Ginies PR, Fraimount JL, Siou DK, et al. Treatment of cluster headache by subcutaneous injection of botulinum toxin [Abstract]. In: Jensen TS, ed. Progress in Pain Research and Management. 8th. ed. Seattle: IASP Press, 1996:501.

162. Freund BJ, Schwartz M. The use of botulinum toxin A in the treatment of refractory cluster headache: case reports. Cephalalgia 2000;20:329–330.

163. Smuts JA, Barnard PWA. Botulinum toxin type A in the treatment of headache syndromes: a clinical report of 79 patients. Cephalalgia 2000;20:332.

164. Zwart JA, Bovim G, Sand T, et al. Tension headache: botulinum toxin paralysis of temporal muscles. Headache 1994;34:458–462.

165. Relja M. Treatment of tension-type headache by local injection of botulinum toxin. Eur J Neurol 1997;4(Suppl 2):S71–S74.

166. Relja MA. Treatment of tension-type headache by local injection of botulinum toxin: 1-year followup. Cephalalgia 2000;20:336.

167. Schulte-Mattler WJ, Wieser T, Zierz S. Treatment of tension-type headache with botulinum toxin: a pilot study. Eur J Med Res 1999;4:183–186.

168. Porta M. A comparative trial of botulinum toxin type A and methylprednisolone for the treatment of tension-type headache. Curr Rev Pain 2000;4:31–35.

169. Carruthers A, Langtry JA, Carruthers J, et al. Improvement of tension-type headache when treating wrinkles with botulinum toxin A injections. Headache 1999;39:662–665.

170. Binder W, Brin MF, Blitzer A, et al. Botulinum toxin type A (BTX-A) for migraine: an open label assessment [Abstract]. Mov Disord 1998;13:241.

171. Mauskop A, Basedo R. Botulinum toxin A is an effect prophylactic therapy of migraines. Cephalalgia 2000;20:422.

172. Binder WJ, Brin MF, Blitzer A, et al. Botulinum toxin type A (BOTOX) for treatment of migraine headaches: an open-label study. Otolaryngol Head Neck Surg 2000;123:669–676.

173. Silberstein S, Mathew N, Saper J, et al. Botulinum toxin type A as a migraine preventive treatment. For the BOTOX Migraine Clinical Research Group. Headache 2000;40:445–450.

174. Brin MF, Swope DM, Abassi S, et al. BOTOX for migraine: double-blind, placebo-controlled, region-specific evaluation [Abstract]. Cephalalgia 2000;20:421–422.

175. Rosales RL, Arimura K, Takenaga S, et al. Extrafusal and intrafusal muscle effects in experimental botulinum toxin-a injection. Muscle Nerve 1996;19:488–496.

176. Ishikawa H, Mitsui Y, Yoshitomi T, et al. Presynaptic effects of botulinum toxin type A on the neuronally evoked response of albino and pigmented rabbit iris sphincter and dilator muscles. Jpn J Ophthalmol 2000;44:106–109.

177. Cui M, Aoki KR. Botulinum toxin type A (BTX-A) reduces inflam-

matory pain in the rat formalin model [Abstract]. Cephalalgia 2000;
20:414.

178. Aoki KR. Pharmacology and immunology of botulinum toxin serotypes. J Neurol 2001;248(Suppl 1):3–10.

179. Gobel H, Lindner V, Krack P, et al. Treatment of chronic tension-type
headache with botulinum toxin. Cephalalgia 1999;19:455.

180. Rollnik JD, Tanneberger O, Schubert M, et al. Treatment of tension-
type headache with botulinum toxin type A: a double-blind, placebo-
controlled study. Headache 2000;40:300–305.

181. Schmitt WJ, Slowey E, Fravi N, et al. Effect of botulinum toxin a injections in the treatment of chronic tension-type headache: a double-
blind, placebo-controlled trial. Headache 2001;41:658–664.

182. Blumenfeld A. Botulinum toxin type a as an effective prophylactic
treatment in primary headache disorders. Headache 2003;43:853–860.

183. Evans RW, Blumenfeld A. Botulinum toxin injections for headache.
Headache 2003;43:682–685.

184. Blumenfeld AM, Binder W, Silberstein SD, et al. Procedures for administering botulinum toxin type A for migraine and tension-type
headache. Headache 2003;43:884–891.

185. Ashkenazi A, Silberstein SD. The evolving management of migraine.
Curr Opin Neurol 2003;16:341–345.

186. Suzuki N, Hardebo JE, Kahrstrom J, et al. Neuropeptide Y co-exists
with vasoactive intestinal polypeptide and acetylcholine in parasympathetic cerebrovascular nerves originating in the sphenopalatine,
otic, and internal carotid ganglia of the rat. Neuroscience 1990;36:
507–519.

187. Sala C, Andreose JS, Fumagalli G, et al. Calcitonin gene-related peptide: possible role in formation and maintenance of neuromuscular
junctions. J Neurosci 1995;15:520–528.

188. Welch MJ, Purkiss JR, Foster KA. Sensitivity of embryonic rat dorsal
root ganglia neurons to Clostridium botulinum neurotoxins. Toxicon
2000;38:245–258.

189. Peterson B, Riddle MA, Cohen DJ, et al. Reduced basal ganglia volumes in Tourette's syndrome using 3-dimensional reconstruction techniques from magnetic resonance images. Neurology 1993;43:941–949.

190. Jankovic J. Tourette's syndrome. N Engl J Med 2001;345:1184–1192.

191. Kurlan R. Tourette's syndrome: current concepts. Neurology 1989;
39:1625–1630.

192. Cohen AJ, Leckman JF. Sensory phenomena associated with Gilles de
la Tourette's syndrome. J Clin Psychiatry 1992;53:319–323.

193. Leckman JF, Grice DE, Boardman J, et al. Symptoms of obsessive-
compulsive disorder. Am J Psychiatry 1997;154:911–917. .

194. Scahill LD, Leckman JF, Marek KL. Sensory phenomena in
Tourette's syndrome. Adv Neurol 1995;65:273–280.

195. Chee KY, Sachdev P. A controlled study of sensory tics in Gilles de la
Tourette syndrome and obsessive-compulsive disorder using a structured interview. J Neurol Neurosurg Psychiatry 1997;62:188–192.

196. Singer HS, Walkup JT. Tourette syndrome and other tic disorders. Diagnosis, pathophysiology, and treatment. Medicine 1991;70:15–31.

197. Lees AJ, Abbott R, Banerji N, et al. Comparisons of therapeutic effects of levodopa, levodopa and selegiline, and bromocriptine in patients with early, mild Parkinson's disease: three-year interim report.
BMJ 1993;307:469–472.

198. Goldenberg JN, Brown SB, Weiner WJ. Coprolalia in younger patients with Gilles de la Tourette syndrome. Mov Disord 1994;
9:622–625.

199. Trimble MR, Whurr R, Brookes G, et al. Vocal tics in Gilles de la
Tourette syndrome treated with botulinum toxin injections. Mov Disord 1998;13:617–619.

200. Lees AJ, Robertson M, Trimble MR, et al. A clinical study of Gilles
de la Tourette syndrome in the United Kingdom. J Neurol Neurosurg
Psychiatry 1984;47:1–8.

201. Scott BL, Jankovic J, Donovan DT. Botulinum toxin injection into vocal cord in the treatment of malignant coprolalia associated with
Tourette's syndrome. Mov Disord 1996;11:431–433.

202. Salloway S, Stewart CF, Israeli L, et al. Botulinum toxin for refractory vocal tics. Mov Disord 1996;11:746–748.

203. Jankovic J. Botulinum toxin in the treatment of tics. In: Jankovic J,
Hallett M, eds. Therapy with Botulinum Toxin. New York: Marcel
Dekker, 1994:503–509.

204. Kwak C, Jankovic J. Tics in Tourette syndrome and botulinum toxin.
J Child Neurol 2000;15:631–634.

205. Kwak CH, Hanna PA, Jankovic J. Botulinum toxin in the treatment of
tics. Arch.Neurol 2000;57:1190–1193.

206. Shapiro AK, Shapiro ES, Brovn RD, et al., eds. Gilles de la Tourette
syndrome. New York: Raven Press, 1978.

207. Marras C, Andrews D, Sime E, et al. Botulinum toxin for simple motor tics: a randomized, double-blind, controlled clinical trial. Neurology 2001;56:605–610.

208. Kurlan R. New treatments for tics? Neurology 2001;56:580–581.

209. Naumann MK, Lowe NJ. Effect of botulinum toxin type A on quality
of life measures in patients with excessive axillary sweating: a randomized controlled trial. Br J Dermatol 2002;147:1218–1226.

210. Swartling C, Naver H, Lindberg M. Botulinum A toxin improves life
quality in severe primary focal hyperhidrosis. Eur J Neurol
2001;8:247–252.

211. Tan SR, Solish N. Long-term efficacy and quality of life in the treatment of focal hyperhidrosis with botulinum toxin A. Dermatol Surg
2002;28:495–499.

212. Campanati A, Penna L, Guzzo T, et al. Quality-of-life assessment in
patients with hyperhidrosis before and after treatment with botulinum
toxin: results of an open-label study. Clin Ther 2003;25:298–308.

213. Glogau RG. Treatment of palmar hyperhidrosis with botulinum toxin.
Semin Cutan Med Surg 2001;20:101–108.

214. Adar R, Kurchin A, Zweig A, et al. Palmar hyperhidrosis and its surgical treatment: a report of 100 cases. Ann Surg 1977;186:34–41.

215. Goldman A. Treatment of axillary and palmar hyperhidrosis with botulinum toxin. Aesthetic Plast Surg 2000;24:280–282.

216. Naver H, Aquilonius SM. The treatment of focal hyperhidrosis with
botulinum toxin. Eur J Neurol 1997;4(Suppl 2):S75–S80.

217. Sato K, Kang WH, Saga K, et al. Biology of sweat glands and their
disorders. II. Disorders of sweat gland function. J Am Acad Dermatol
1989;20:713–726.

218. Sato K, Kang WH, Saga K, et al. Biology of sweat glands and their
disorders. I. Normal sweat gland function. J Am Acad Dermatol
1989;20:537–563.

219. Ro KM, Cantor RM, Lange KL, et al. Palmar hyperhidrosis: evidence
of genetic transmission. J Vasc Surg 2002;35:382–386.

220. Leung AK, Chan PY, Choi MC. Hyperhidrosis. Int J Dermatol
1999;38:561–567.

221. Naumann M, Hamm H. Treatment of axillary hyperhidrosis. Br J Surg
2002;89:259–261.

222. Bushara KO, Park DM. Botulinum toxin and sweating. Neurol Neurosurg Psychiatry 1994;57:1437–1438.

223. Naumann M, Lowe NJ, Kumar CR, et al. Botulinum toxin type a is a
safe and effective treatment for axillary hyperhidrosis over 16 months:
a prospective study. Arch Dermatol 2003;139:731–736.

224. Glogau RG. Botulinum A neurotoxin for axillary hyperhidrosis. No
sweat Botox. Dermatol Surg 1998;24:817–819.

225. Naumann M, Hofmann U, Bergmann I, et al. Focal hyperhidrosis: effective treatment with intracutaneous botulinum toxin. Arch Dermatol 1998;134:301–304.

226. Naumann M, Bergmann I, Hofmann U, et al. Botulinum toxin for focal hyperhidrosis: technical considerations and improvements in application. Br J Dermatol 1998;139:1123–1124.

227. Odderson IR. Axillary hyperhidrosis: treatment with botulinum toxin
A. Arch Phys Med Rehabil 1998;79:350–352.

228. Odderson IR. Hyperhidrosis treated by botulinum A exotoxin. Dermatol Surg 1998;24:1237–1241.

229. Schnider P, Binder M, Kittler H, et al. A randomized, double-blind,
placebo-controlled trial of botulinum A toxin for severe axillary hyperhidrosis. Br J Dermatol 1999;140:677–680.

230. Naver H, Swartling C, Aquilonius SM. Palmar and axillary hyperhidrosis treated with botulinum toxin: one-year clinical follow-up. Eur
J Neurol 2000;7:55–62.

231. Heckmann M, Schaller M, Breit S, et al. Evaluation of therapeutic success of hyperhidrosis therapy. Arch Dermatol 2001;137:94.

232. Heckmann M, Ceballos-Baumann AO, Plewig G. Botulinum toxin A
for axillary hyperhidrosis (excessive sweating). N Engl J Med
2001;344:488–493.

233. Naumann M. Evidence-based medicine: botulinum toxin in focal hyperhidrosis. J Neurol 2001;248(Suppl 1):31–33.

234. Naumann M, Lowe NJ. Botulinum toxin type A in treatment of bilateral primary axillary hyperhidrosis: randomised, parallel group, double blind, placebo controlled trial. BMJ 2001;323:596–599.

235. Schnider P, Moraru E, Kittler H, et al. Treatment of focal hyperhidrosis with botulinum toxin type A: long-term follow-up in 61 patients.
Br J Dermatol 2001;145:289–293.

236. Schnider P, Binder M, Auff E, et al. Double-blind trial of botulinum A toxin for the treatment of focal hyperhidrosis of the palms. Br J Dermatol 1997;136:548–552.

237. Schnider P, Binder M, Kittler H, et al. Uses of botulinum toxin. Lancet 1997;349:953.

238. Shelley WB, Talanin NY, Shelley ED. Botulinum toxin therapy for palmar hyperhidrosis. J Am Acad Dermatol 1998;38:227–229.

239. Solomon BA, Hayman R. Botulinum toxin type A therapy for palmar and digital hyperhidrosis. J Am Acad Dermatol 2000;42:1026–1029.

240. Saadia D, Voustianiouk A, Wang AK, et al. Botulinum toxin type A in primary palmar hyperhidrosis: randomized, single-blind, two-dose study. Neurology 2001;57:2095–2099.

241. Swartling C, Farnstrand C, Abt G, et al. Side-effects of intradermal injections of botulinum A toxin in the treatment of palmar hyperhidrosis: a neurophysiological study. Eur J Neurol 2001;8:451–456.

242. Vadoud-Seyedi J, Heenen M, Simonart T. Treatment of Idiopathic palmar hyperhidrosis with botulinum toxin. Report of 23 cases and review of the literature. Dermatology 2001;203:318–321.

243. Wollina U, Karamfilov T. Botulinum toxin A for palmar hyperhidrosis. J Eur Acad Dermatol Venereol 2001;15:555–558.

244. Naumann M, Flachenecker P, Brocker EB, et al. Botulinum toxin for palmar hyperhidrosis. Lancet 1997;349:252.

245. Hernot S, Samii K. Different types of nerve injuries in locoregional anesthesia [in French]. Ann Fr Anesth Reanim 1997;16:274–281.

246. Blaheta HJ, Vollert B, Zuder D, et al. Intravenous regional anesthesia (Bier's block) for botulinum toxin therapy of palmar hyperhidrosis is safe and eEffective. Dermatol Surg 2002;28:666–672.

247. Ford FR, Woodhall B. Phenomena due to misdirection of regenerating fibers of cranial, spinal and automatic nerves. Clinical observations. Acta Otolaryngol 1958;49:132–143.

248. Beerens AJ, Snow GB. Botulinum toxin A in the treatment of patients with Frey syndrome. Br J Surg 2002;89:116–119.

249. May JS, McGuirt WF. Frey's syndrome: treatment with topical glycopyrrolate. Head Neck 1989;11:85–89.

250. Drobik C, Laskawi R. Frey's syndrome: treatment with botulinum toxin. Acta Otolaryngol 1995;115:459–461.

251. Schulze-Bonhage A, Schroder M, Ferbert A. Botulinum toxin in the therapy of gustatory sweating. J Neurol 1996;243:143–146.

252. Bjerkhoel A, Trobbe O. Frey's syndrome: treatment with botulinum toxin. J Laryngol Otol 1997;111:839–844.

253. Laskawi R, Drobik C, Schonebeck C. Up-to-date report of botulinum toxin type A treatment in patients with gustatory sweating (Frey's syndrome). Laryngoscope 1998;108:381–384.

254. Laccourreye O, Muscatelo L, Naude C, et al. Botulinum toxin type A for Frey's syndrome: a preliminary prospective study. Ann Otol Rhinol Laryngol 1998;107:52–55.

255. Arad-Cohen A, Blitzer A. Botulinum toxin treatment for symptomatic Frey's syndrome. Otolaryngol Head Neck Surg 2000;122:237–240.

256. Dulguerov P, Quinodoz D, Cosendai G, et al. Frey syndrome treatment with botulinum toxin. Otolaryngol Head Neck Surg 2000;122:821–827.

257. von Lindern JJ, Niederhagen B, Berge S, et al. Frey syndrome: treatment with type A botulinum toxin. Cancer 2000;89:1659–1663.

258. Laccourreye O, Akl E, Gutierrez-Fonseca R, et al. Recurrent gustatory sweating (Frey syndrome) after intracutaneous injection of botulinum toxin type A: incidence, management, and outcome. Arch Otolaryngol Head Neck Surg 1999;125:283–286.

259. Ellies M, Laskawi R, Rohrbach-Volland S, et al. Botulinum toxin to reduce saliva flow: selected indications for ultrasound-guided toxin application into salivary glands. Laryngoscope 2002;112:82–86.

260. Rose FC. The management of motor neurone disease. Adv Exp Med Biol 1987;209:167–174.

261. Eadie MJ, Tyrer JH. Alimentary disorder in parkinsonism. Aust Ann Med 1965;14:13–22.

262. Ekedahl C, Mansson I, Sandberg N. Swallowing dysfunction in the brain-damaged with drooling. Acta Otolaryngol 1974;78:141–149.

263. Van de Heyning PH, Marquet JF, Creten WL. Drooling in children with cerebral palsy. Acta Otorhinolaryngol Belg 1980;34:691–705.

264. Dickson EC, Shevky R. Studies upon the manner in which the toxin of clostridium botulinum acts upon the body. I. The effect upon the autonomic nervous system. J Exp Med 1923;37:711–731.

265. Ekstrom J, Kemplay SK, Garrett JR, et al. Effect of botulinum toxin on the choline acetyltransferase activity in salivary glands of cats. Experientia 1977;33:1458–1460.

266. Shaari CM, Wu BL, Biller HF, et al. Botulinum toxin decreases salivation from canine submandibular glands. Otolaryngol Head Neck Surg 1998;118:452–457.

267. Ellies M, Laskawi R, Gotz W, et al. Immunohistochemical and morphometric investigations of the influence of botulinum toxin on the submandibular gland of the rat. Eur Arch Otorhinolaryngol 1999;256:148–152.

268. Bushara KO. Sialorrhea in amyotrophic lateral sclerosis: a hypothesis of a new treatment—botulinum toxin A injections of the parotid glands. Med Hypotheses 1997;48:337–339.

269. Giess R, Naumann M, Werner E, et al. Injections of botulinum toxin A into the salivary glands improve sialorrhoea in amyotrophic lateral sclerosis. J Neurol Neurosurg Psychiatry 2000;69:121–123.

270. Pal PK, Calne DB, Calne S, et al. Botulinum toxin A as treatment for drooling saliva in PD. Neurology 2000;54:244–247.

271. Jongerius PH, Rotteveel JJ, van den HF, et al. Botulinum toxin A: a new option for treatment of drooling in children with cerebral palsy. Presentation of a case series. Eur J Pediatr 2001;160:509–512.

272. Suskind DL, Tilton A. Clinical study of botulinum-A toxin in the treatment of sialorrhea in children with cerebral palsy. Laryngoscope 2002;112:73–81.

273. Glickman S, Deaney CN. Treatment of relative sialorrhoea with botulinum toxin type A: description and rationale for an injection procedure with case report. Eur J Neurol 2001;8:567–571.

274. Friedman A, Potulska A. Quantitative assessment of parkinsonian sialorrhea and results of treatment with botulinum toxin. Parkinsonism Related Disord 2001;7:43–46.

275. Porta M, Gamba M, Bertacchi G, et al. Treatment of sialorrhoea with ultrasound guided botulinum toxin type A injection in patients with neurological disorders. J Neurol Neurosurg Psychiatry 2001;70:538–540.

276. Guntinas-Lichius O, Eckel HE. Temporary reduction of salivation in laryngectomy patients with pharyngocutaneous fistulas by botulinum toxin A injection. Laryngoscope 2002;112:187–189.

277. Reichel G. Botulinum toxin A therapie bei sialorrho. Aktuelle Neurol 1999;26:325–326.

278. Brashear A, Lew MF, Dykstra DD, et al. Safety and efficacy of NeuroBloc (botulinum toxin type B) in type A- responsive cervical dystonia. Neurology 1999;53:1439–1446.

279. Brin MF, Lew MF, Adler CH, et al. Safety and efficacy of NeuroBloc (botulinum toxin type B) in type A-resistant cervical dystonia. Neurology 1999;53:1431–1438.

280. Joo JS, Agachan F, Wolff B, et al. Initial north american experience with botulinum toxin type a for treatment of anismus. Dis Colon Rectum 1996;39:1107–1111.

281. Hallan RI, Williams NS, Melling J, et al. Treatment of anismus in intractable constipation with botulinum A toxin. Lancet 1988;2:714–717.

282. Albanese A, Maria G, Bentivoglio AR, et al. Severe constipation in Parkinson's disease relieved by botulinum toxin. Mov Disord 1997;12:764–766.

283. Langer JC, Birnbaum E. Preliminary experience with intrasphincteric botulinum toxin for persistent constipation after pull-through for Hirschsprung's disease. J Pediatr Surg 1997;32:1059–1061.

284. Langer JC, Birnbaum EE, Schmidt RE. Histology and function of the internal anal sphincter after injection of botulinum toxin. J Surg Res 1997;73:113–116.

285. Maria G, Brisinda G, Bentivoglio AR, et al. Influence of botulinum toxin site of injections on healing rate in patients with chronic anal fissure. Am J Surg 2000;179:46–50.

286. Mason PF, Watkins MJ, Hall HS, et al. The management of chronic fissure in-ano with botulinum toxin. J R Coll Surg Edinb 1996;41:235–238.

287. Jost WH, Schimrigk K. Botulinum toxin in therapy of anal fissure [Letter; comment]. Lancet 1995;345:188–189.

288. Albanese A, Bentivoglio AR, Cassetta E, et al. Review article: the use of botulinum toxin in the alimentary tract. Aliment Pharmacol Ther 1995;9:599–604.

289. Gui D, Cassetta E, Anastasio G, et al. Botulinum toxin for chronic anal fissure. Lancet 1994;344:1127–1128.

290. Maria G, Brisinda G, Bentivoglio AR, et al. Botulinum toxin injections in the internal anal sphincter for the treatment of chronic anal fissure: long-term results after two different dosage regimens. Ann Surg 1998;228:664–669.

291. Maria G, Cassetta E, Gui D, et al. A comparison of botulinum toxin and saline for the treatment of chronic anal fissure. N Engl J Med 1998;338:217–220.

292. Brisinda G, Maria G, Bentivoglio AR, et al. A comparison of injections of botulinum toxin and topical nitroglycerin ointment for the treatment of chronic anal fissure. N Engl J Med 1999;341:65–69.

293. Fernandez-Lopez F, Conde FR, Rios RA, et al. Botulinum toxin for the treatment of anal fissure. Dig Surg 1999;16:515–518.

294. Minguez M, Melo F, Espi A, et al. Therapeutic effects of different doses of botulinum toxin in chronic anal fissure. Dis Colon Rectum 1999;42:1016–1021.

295. DeLancey JO, Fowler CJ, Keane D, et al. Pathophysiology. In: Abrams P, Khoury S, Wein A, eds. Incontinence. United Kingdom: Health Publication Ltd., 1999:227–294.

296. Schwartz J, Defabiani N, Castanier M, et al. Efficiency of intrasphincteric botulinum toxin injections for detrusor-sphincter-dyssynergia [Abstract]. Eur Urol 2001;39(Suppl 5):128.

297. Petit H, Wiart L, Gaujard E, et al. Botulinum A toxin treatment for detrusor-sphincter dyssynergia in spinal cord disease. Spinal Cord. 1998;36:91–94.

298. Phelan MW, Franks M, Somogyi GT, et al. Botulinum toxin urethral sphincter injection to restore bladder emptying in men and women with voiding dysfunction. J Urol 2001;165:1107–1110.

299. Wheeler JSJ, Walter JS, Chintam RS, et al. Botulinum toxin injections for voiding dysfunction following SCI. J Spinal Cord Med 1998; 21:227–229.

300. Gallien P, Robineau S, Verin M, et al. Treatment of detrusor sphincter dyssynergia by transperineal injection of botulinum toxin. Arch Phys Med Rehabil 1998;79:715–717.

301. Dykstra DD, Sidi AA. Treatment of detrusor-sphincter dyssynergia with botulinum A toxin: a double-blind study. Arch Phys Med Rehabil 1990;71:24–26.

302. Schurch B, Hauri D, Rodic B, et al. Botulinum-A toxin as a treatment of detrusor-sphincter dyssynergia: a prospective study in 24 spinal cord injury patients. J Urol 1996;155:1023–1029.

303. Strasser G, Schima W, Schober E, et al. Cervical osteophytes impinging on the pharynx: importance of size and concurrent disorders for development of aspiration. AJR Am J Roentgenol 2000;174:449–453.

304. Schurch B, Stohrer M, Kramer G, et al. Botulinum-A toxin for treating detrusor hyperreflexia in spinal cord injured patients: a new alternative to anticholinergic drugs? Preliminary results. J Urol 2000;164:692–697.

305. Radziszewski P, Dobronski P, Borkowski A. Treatment of the non-neurogenic storage and voiding disorders with the chemical denervation caused by botulinum toxin type A: a pilot study. Neurourol Urodyn 2001;20:410–412.

306. Zermann DH, Ishigooka M, Schubert J, et al. Trigonum and bladder base injection of botulinum toxin A (BTX) in patients with severe urgency-frequency-syndrome refractory to conservative medical treatment and electrical stimulation. Neurourol Urodyn 2001;20:412–413.

307. Maria G, Destito A, Lacquaniti S, et al. Relief by botulinum toxin of voiding dysfunction due to prostatitis [Letter]. Lancet 1998;352:625.

308. Bentivoglio A, Maria G, Destito A, et al. Type A botulinum toxin in the striated urethral sphincter for the treatment of voiding dysfunction due to chronic nonbacterial prostatits [Abstract]. Mov Disord 2000;15(Suppl 5):42–43.

309. Maria G, Brisinda G, Civello IM, et al. Relief by botulinum toxin of voiding dysfunction due to benign prostatic hyperplasia: results of a randomized, placebo-controlled study. Urology 2003;62:259–264.

310. Carruthers A, Carruthers J. The treatment of glabellar furrows with botulinum A exotoxin [Abstract]. J Dermatol Surg Oncol 1990;16:63.

311. Blitzer A, Brin MF, Keen MS, et al. Botulinum toxin for the treatment of hyperfunctional lines of the face. Arch Otolaryngol Head Neck Surg 1993;119:1018–1022.

312. Carruthers JA, Lowe NJ, Menter MA, et al. A multicenter, double-blind, randomized, placebo-controlled study of the efficacy and safety of botulinum toxin type A in the treatment of glabellar lines. J Am Acad Dermatol 2002;46:840–849.

315. Niamtu J III. Botulinum toxin A: a review of 1,085 oral and maxillofacial patient treatments. J Oral Maxillofac Surg 2003;61:317–324.

316. Flynn TC, Carruthers JA, Carruthers JA, et al. Botulinum A toxin (BOTOX) in the lower eyelid: dose-finding study. Dermatol Surg 2003;29:943–950.

317. Carruthers JD, Lowe NJ, Menter MA, et al. Double-blind, placebo-controlled study of the safety and efficacy of botulinum toxin type a for patients with glabellar lines. Plast Reconstr Surg 2003;112:21S–30S.

318. Fagien S. Botox for the treatment of dynamic and hyperkinetic facial lines and furrows: adjunctive use in facial aesthetic surgery. Plast Reconstr Surg 1999;103:701–713.

319. Fagien S, Brandt FS. Primary and adjunctive use of botulinum toxin type A (Botox) in facial aesthetic surgery: beyond the glabella. Clin Plast Surg 2001;28:127–148.

320. West TB, Alster TS. Effect of botulinum toxin type A on movement-associated rhytides Following CO2 laser resurfacing. Dermatol Surg 1999;25:259–261.

321. Sommer B, Zschocke I, Bergfeld D, et al. Satisfation of patients after treatment with botulinum toxin for dynamic facial lines. Dermatol Surg 2003;29:456–460.

322. Cox SE, Finn JC, Stetler L, et al. Development of the facial lines treatment satisfaction questionnaire and initial results for botulinum toxin type A-treated patients. Dermatol Surg 2003;29:444–449.

CHAPTER 19

Smooth Muscle Spasms and Sphincters

Giuseppe Brisinda, Giorgio Maria, Anna Rita Bentivoglio, and Alberto Albanese

INTRODUCTION

More than 50 years after the discovery that botulinum neurotoxins (BoNT) inhibit neuromuscular transmission,[1] these powerful poisons have become drugs with multiple indications. Scott[2] first used botulinum neurotoxin type A (BoNT/A) to treat strabismus, but local injections of BoNT/A are now considered a safe and efficacious treatment for many neurologic and nonneurologic conditions. One achievement in the field is the observation that BoNT/A is also a treatment for diseases of the gastrointestinal tract. BoNT/A is potent in blocking skeletal neuromuscular transmission; in addition, it is also effective in blocking cholinergic nerve endings in the autonomic nervous system.[3,4] Its capability to inhibit contractions of gastrointestinal tract smooth muscles was first suggested based on in vitro observations; the same capability was later demonstrated in vivo.[5]

It has also been shown that BoNT/A does not block nonadrenergic, noncholinergic responses that are mediated by nitric oxide (NO). This finding promoted interest in the use of BoNT/A as a treatment for overactive smooth muscles and sphincters, including the lower esophageal sphincter (LES) in achalasia and the internal anal sphincter (IAS) in anal fissure.

Familiarity with the anatomic and functional organization of gastrointestinal tract innervation is a prerequisite to understanding the many features of BoNT/A action on the gastrointestinal tract and the effects of injections placed into specific sphincters (Table 19-1). This review presents current data on the use of BoNT/A to treat diseases of the gastrointestinal tract and summarizes knowledge on the pathogenesis of gastrointestinal tract disorders that occur because of dysfunction of the enteric nervous system (ENS).

NEUROMYOGENIC PROPERTIES OF THE GASTROINTESTINAL TRACT SMOOTH MUSCLES

Motility of a gut segment depends on its extrinsic and intrinsic innervation. Preganglionic parasympathetic nerves and postganglionic sympathetic nerves, which constitute the autonomic nervous system, provide extrinsic innervation.[6,7] The enteric nervous system provides the intrinsic innervation. It is a highly complex system, responsible for the coordination of motility, secretion, and microcirculation in the gastrointestinal tract. This system is also responsible for the regulation of the local response to immune inflammatory processes. The ENS can function independently of the central nervous system (CNS), which maintains a coordinating role for the diverse functions of gastrointestinal tract neurons. The CNS coordinates via sympathetic and parasympathetic motor and sensory pathways (Fig. 19-1).[6] A deficiency

Giuseppe Brisinda: Istituto di Clinica Chirurgica, Università Cattolica del Sacro Cuore, Rome, Italy.

Giorgio Maria: Istituto di Clinica Chirurgica, Università Cattolica del Sacro Cuore, Rome, Italy.

Anna Rita Bentivoglio: Istituto di Neurologia, Università Cattolica del Sacro Cuore, Rome, Italy.

Alberto Albanese: Istituto di Neurologia, Università Cattolica del Sacro Cuore, Rome, Italy, and Istituto Nazionale Neurologico Carlo Besta, Milano, Italy.

The authors have nothing to disclose.

TABLE 19-1. *Target Site for the Injection of Botulinum Neurotoxins in Different Conditions*

Condition	Muscle
Achalasia	LES
Cricopharyngeal dysphagia	Cricopharyngeal muscle
Diffuse esophageal spasm	LES
Isolated hypertensive LES	LES
Obesity	Gastric antrum
Delayed gastric emptying	Pylorus
Infantile hypertrophic pyloric stenosis	Pylorus
Sphincter of Oddi dysfunction	Sphincter of Oddi
Chronic anal fissure	IAS
Outlet-type constipation	Puborectalis muscle or EAS
Anterior rectocele	Puborectalis muscle and EAS

LES, lower esophageal sphincter; IAS, internal anal sphincter; EAS, external anal sphincter.

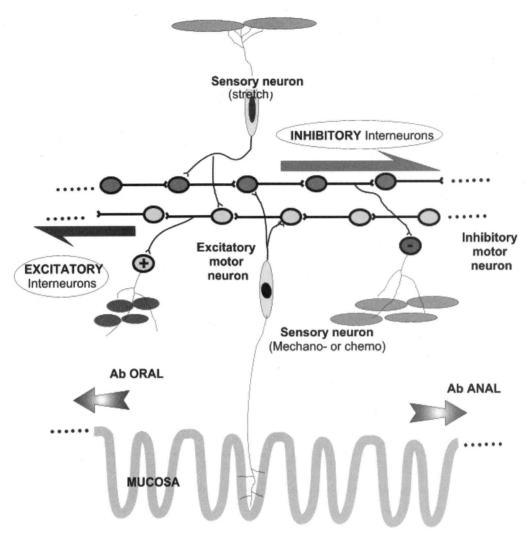

FIG. 19-1. Organization of neurons located in the enteric nervous system.

of enteric neurons causes obstruction and lack of intestinal propulsion.

Functional Organization of the Enteric Nervous System

The ENS is composed of nerve cell bodies and their processes, which are embedded in the gut wall. These form two main ganglionated plexuses: Auerbach's myenteric plexus and Meissner's submucous plexus. Other nonganglionated plexuses supply the gastrointestinal tract layers (Fig. 19-2). These include:

- The longitudinal muscle plexus;
- The circular muscle plexus;
- The plexus of the muscularis mucosae; and
- The mucosal plexus.

In addition, perivascular plexuses are found around arteries and arterioles in the gut wall.[6-8]

In the ENS, intraparietal neurons (which are located within the gastrointestinal wall) encompass excitatory and inhibitory motor neurons, interneurons, and intrinsic sensory

neurons. Sympathetic and parasympathetic neurons also innervate the gastrointestinal tract. Excitatory motor neurons innervate longitudinal muscles, circular muscles, and the muscularis mucosae. Their primary transmitter is acetylcholine (ACh); however, they also release tachykinins, substance P, neurokinin A, and neuropeptides K and Y.[6-9] Inhibitory motor neurons relax smooth muscles and are involved in reflexes that facilitate the passage of food along the gastrointestinal tract. Inhibitory neurons release a combination of at least three transmitters: NO, adenosine triphosphate (ATP), and vasoactive intestinal polypeptide (VIP).[6-9] In most neurons, NO is the primary transmitter; the roles of ATP and VIP may vary. A neuronal NO synthase is expressed in ENS neurons where it is typically colocalized with VIP. During nerve stimulation, NO regulates the release of VIP and diffuses to muscle cells to participate in relaxation. In turn, VIP acts on smooth muscle cells to regenerate NO, which constitutes the predominant component, or up to 60%, of NO produced during nerve stimulation.[6]

Sympathetic pathways to the gastrointestinal tract are noradrenergic. These pathways inhibit motility, constrict the

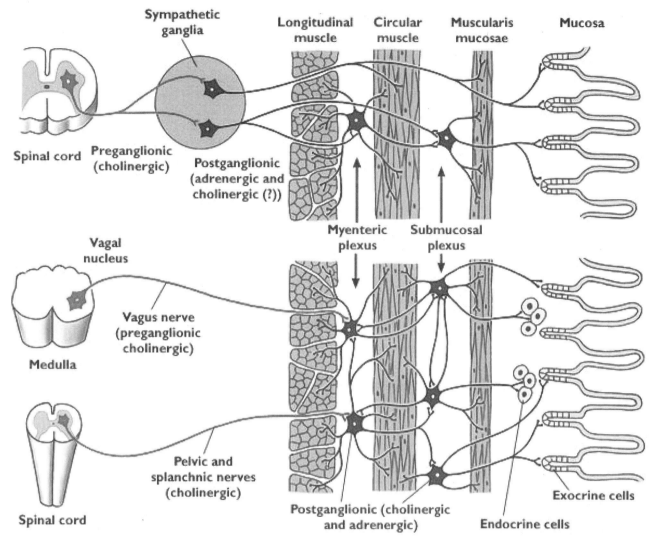

FIG. 19-2. Sympathetic and parasympathetic control of smooth muscles in the gastrointestinal tract.

sphincters, and generally inhibit contractile activity. This is accomplished by a presynaptic action on the myenteric plexus. The vagus nerve includes the axons of neurons located in the brain stem. A variety of central effects are mediated by the vagus nerve. These include: relaxation of the proximal stomach, enhancement of gastric peristalsis, secretion of acid, and promotion of gastrin secretion. Vagal neurons form synaptic connections with neurons whose cell bodies are in the intrinsic ganglia of the gastrointestinal tract. They are involved in complex circuits integrating various enteric reflexes with signals that derive from the CNS and from other gastrointestinal tract regions. For the most part, ACh mediates this transmission.[6]

Smooth Muscle Contraction

Smooth muscle contraction is regulated by changes in cytosol calcium levels. Calcium regulation is affected by a variety of regulatory proteins, including myosin light chains, calmodulin, and calponin.[10–12] Contraction is de-

pendent on an increase in cellular calcium. The activation of myosin may induce relaxation or allow cross bridges to enter a state of prolonged contraction, the so-called latch state. The precise mechanisms responsible for the maintenance of smooth muscle tone are still not entirely known. Relaxation of smooth muscles occurs when there is a resulting decrease in cytosolic calcium. These functions depend on the intrinsic electrical and mechanical properties of gastrointestinal tract smooth muscles. In addition, these functions are regulated by the ENS as well as sympathetic and parasympathetic influences.[7] An increase in cellular calcium may be produced by an influx of calcium through membrane channels or by stimulation of a_1-adrenoceptors. This influx results in the release of calcium from the sarcoplasmic reticulum, which is mediated by inositol triphosphate. Stimulation of a_2-adrenoceptors brings about cyclic adenosine monophosphate (cAMP)-mediated return of calcium to the sarcoplasmic reticulum. Stimulation of NO induces a cyclic guanine monophosphate (cGMP)-mediated decrease in cellular calcium.

Hormones and autacoids also regulate muscle activity and influence gastrointestinal tract motility.[6–8] The interstitial cells of Cajal act as local pacemakers to generate the rhythmic activity of the gastrointestinal tract's circular muscle layer. Motor neurons control the musculature in an indirect manner. This control is accomplished through the neurons action on Cajal's cells, which are innervated by the myenteric plexus in the stomach and small intestine and by the submuscular plexus in the colon.[13] Cajal's cells are lost in patients with Hirschsprung's disease and in infantile pyloric stenosis[14,15]; their deficiency contributes to the motor abnormalities associated with such diseases.

For the most part, hormonal influences on smooth muscle activity occur during meals and between meals. Chemical substances such as histamine, serotonin, adenosine, and eicosanoids, which are produced by nonneural cells in the muscle layers, may influence smooth muscle activity. Receptors for these agents have been identified on gastrointestinal tract smooth muscle cells. These receptors may act directly and indirectly on muscle cells by stimulating or inhibiting the release of neurotransmitters.[8]

Muscle tone of the LES results from the interaction of neurogenic and myogenic conditions.[16] In humans, neurogenic tone is caused in part by cholinergic innervation. Various other excitatory and inhibitory neurotransmitters are present in the sphincter, however, their physiologic importance is unclear. Myogenic tone is mediated by shifts of intracellular stores of calcium in the sphincter muscle. The modulation of LES tone, which occurs with activity of migrating motor complex (MMC), is largely mediated through the vagus nerve. Relaxation of the sphincter induced by swallowing is mediated through the dorsal nucleus of the vagus. Efferent stimuli travel to the sphincter via the vagus nerve and myenteric plexus. ACh is the presynaptic neurotransmitter. Postsynaptic transmission is mediated by NO; however, VIP is also thought to contribute.[6]

At the anal level, the sphincter complex consists of two overlapping sphincters.[10,17] The external anal sphincter (EAS), which forms the outer layer of the complex, is composed of a voluntary, striated skeletal muscle. The IAS is an inner, involuntary, smooth muscle component of the anal sphincter complex. The IAS is in a state of continuous maximal contraction and functions as a natural barrier to the involuntary loss of stool and gas. This state of contraction is caused by a combination of intrinsic myogenic and extrinsic autonomic, neurogenic properties.[6,11,18] The IAS is responsible for 50–85% of resting anal tone. The IAS is of visceral origin and is supplied by both sympathetic and parasympathetic nerves; in addition, the ENS modulates its tonic activity. Noradrenergic sympathetic nerves are considered excitatory; parasympathetic nerves are considered inhibitory to the IAS. Sympathetic neurons that supply the IAS are noradrenergic. Vagal neurons do not act directly but rather form synaptic connections with neurons whose cell bodies are in the intrinsic gastrointestinal tract ganglia. This transmission is mediated principally by ACh, which acts on nicotinic receptors.[6]

It has been demonstrated that the longitudinal and circular smooth muscle layers of the human rectum receive intrinsic NO-mediated inhibitory innervation.[19,20] The exact site of involvement remains to be determined; however, data suggest that carbon monoxide and heme oxygenase pathways may have a role in the neurally mediated relaxation of the IAS.[21]

In vitro studies on strips of human IAS have revealed excitatory α-adrenergic receptors; inhibitory α-adrenergic receptors; excitatory or biphasic cholinergic receptors; and inhibitory nonadrenergic noncholinergic receptors. Experimental evidence suggests that norepinephrine induces contraction of isolated IAS strips. Adrenaline has a variable response and isoprenaline induces relaxation.[12] Furthermore, in patients with anal fissure or in healthy subjects, blockade of a_1-adrenoceptor causes a lasting reduction in resting pressure along the length of the anal canal.[22] This blockade is accomplished with a single dose of indoramin.

ACHALASIA

Achalasia is a failure of the LES to relax, causing it to remain tonically contracted. This results in a functional obstruction of the esophagus. The lower two-thirds of the esophagus, which contains smooth musculature (Fig. 19-3), is affected and peristaltic contractions are absent.

The cause of achalasia may be a generalized loss of enteric neurons. The cause may also be a selective loss or dysfunction of the inhibitory VIP- and NO-containing neurons, which are located in esophageal myenteric plexus.[23,24] NO synthase is not detectable in the myenteric plexus or the nerve fibers reaching the esophagus, the cardias, and the gastric fundus.[25] Esophageal ganglion cells and neurons of the vagus's dorsal motor nucleus are decreased in number. In addition, the vagus nerves degenerate.[7] The etiology is not known. NO-containing neurons are primarily involved, however, cholinergic neurons may be spared. The preserved cholinergic innervation to LES induces increased sphincter pressure, which is a characteristic feature of this disorder. A postulated autoimmune reaction may cause achalasia; two-thirds of patients have autoantibodies against DARPP-32, a dopamine carrier protein located on the cell surface in the myenteric plexus.[26] The degenerative neural lesions of achalasia cannot be corrected; therefore, treatment is symptomatic. Peristalsis rarely recovers and treatment is aimed at reducing LES pressure with drug therapy or by forceful dilatation or surgical myotomy.

Some diseases may cause ENS dysfunction, resulting in secondary achalasia. These diseases include: paraneoplastic syndromes, Chagas' disease, and Parkinson's disease. Herpes infections have been reported with increased frequency in the myenteric plexus of patients with achalasia[6,7]; this virus has a preferred tropism for the squamous epithelium that lines the esophagus.

Familial achalasia occurs in some genetic disorders; clinical severity may vary among family members. A positive

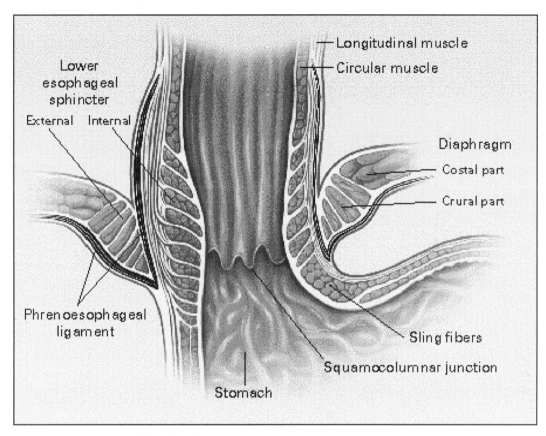

FIG. 19-3. Drawing of the lower esophageal sphincter.

association with the HLA allele DQw1 has been reported in several populations; the allele DRw53 is also reduced among Caucasians.[27,28]

Treatment

Classic therapies for achalasia are aimed at mechanically reducing LES tone by pneumatic dilation or surgical myotomy.[29-45] These procedures are efficacious in most patients (65–90%), however, these procedures carry a substantial risk of complications. Perforation occurs in 2–5% of patients and gastroesophageal reflux is reported in 10–50% of patients after myotomy (Table 19-2). In addition, repeated procedures are sometimes required after dilation. In addition, the therapeutic benefit declines after 10–20 years after surgery. The limitations of classic surgical procedures prompted the use of injections of BoNT/A into the LES.[46] The use of BoNT/A was based on the rationale that BoNT/A injections would inhibit an unbalanced cholinergic influence on the sphincter and improve esophageal emptying.

Results of Botulinum Neurotoxin Type A Treatment

During an upper endoscopy, the LES of patients with achalasia is easily injected using a 5-mm sclerotherapy needle. Endoscopic ultrasonography has been used to guide injections to maximize the amount of BoNT/A delivered to LES.[4]

During the injection, the infiltration appears as an enlarging anechoic zone around the needle.

Short-term symptomatic relief occurs in 70–100% of patients (Table 19-3).[46–62] The occurrence of vigorous achalasia has been described as the principal determinant of the response to BoNT/A.[60] LES pressure decreases and esophageal emptying improves in parallel to symptomatic relief but to a lesser degree than after dilation. Other drawbacks of the treatment with BoNT/A have been observed. Classic surgical procedures and BoNT/A treatment have equal success rates; however, the long-term efficacy of BoNT/A is substantially shorter than the duration of benefit from balloon dilation.[55] BoNT/A may be more expensive than pneumatic dilation, particularly because of the need for repeated treatments.[56] Another limitation of BoNT/A treatment is the lack of an initial symptomatic response and a high residual LES pressure (≥18 mm Hg).

On the other hand, there are obvious advantages of BoNT/A treatment. For example, the procedure is endoscopic and there is reasonable long-term efficacy. BoNT/A therapy is safe in older patients who may have tortuous megaesophagus or epiphrenic diverticulum or in whom pneumatic dilation is extremely risky.[58] BoNT/A is also noted as efficacious on pediatric patients with achalasia. In 43% of patients in this population, the response is sustained beyond 6 months.[59] However, in one-half of these young patients, an additional injection is required approximately 7

TABLE 19-2. *Review of Experience Using Surgical Myotomy for the Treatment of Achalasia*

Procedure	Patients	Improved %	Dysphagia %	GE reflux %	Mortality %	Morbidity %	Esophageal perforation %	Follow-up (months)	Citation
Laparotomy									
M + Toupet	722	95	NR	NR	0	NR	NR	6-180	Ref. 29
M + Dor	206	94	4	9	0	2	0	64	Ref. 30
M + Dor	72	87	13	10	NR	NR	NR	87	Ref. 31
M	83	48	7	23	NR	NR	NR	193	Ref. 31
M + Nissen	36	47	53	20	NR	NR	NR	72	Ref. 32
Thoracotomy									
M	468	85	3	3	1	NR	1	77	Ref. 33
M	103	91	5	4	0	10	0	81	Ref. 34
M	60	90	17	21	0	5	NR	57	Ref. 35
M	30	54	20	23	NR	NR	NR	137	Ref. 31
Laparoscopy									
M + Dor	43	88	7	2	0	0	NR	12	Ref. 36
M + Toupet	20	90	15	10	0	10	25	12	Ref. 37
M + Toupet	40	88	12	5	0	7	0	12	Ref. 38
M + Dor	61	98	12	NR	0	3	11	21	Ref. 39
M	30	89	11	14	0	4	0	18	Ref. 40
M + Dor	133	93	NR	17	NR	NR	NR	NR	Ref. 41
M + Dor	24	88	NR	NR	NR	NR	NR	16.5	Ref. 42
M	78	91	18	NR	0	7.7	7	NR	Ref. 43
Thoracoscopy									
M	22	88	12	NR	0	18	0	24	Ref. 44
M	21	80	10	30	0	0	5	22	Ref. 45
M	35	85	NR	60	NR	NR	NR	NR	Ref. 41

GE, gastroesophageal; NR, not reported; M, myotomy; Dor, anterior fundoplication; Toupet, partial fundoplication; Nissen, complete fundoplication.

months after the first treatment. For this reason, BoNT/A is recommended for use only in those children with achalasia who are poor candidates for pneumatic dilation or surgical myotomy.[59]

The effect of BoNT/A inevitably wanes over time, usually some months after treatment (Fig. 19-4A and 19-4B). Only three studies report on a follow-up longer than 1 year. A decline in beneficial effects from 65–30% has been observed. This decline occurred despite repeat injections in 31 patients followed for 2.4 years.[49] One year after treatment, 36% of 33 patients had a good to excellent response after a single injection; 39% of patients required subsequent treatment.[50] Another study, with an observational period of 18 months, reported that 72% of 57 patients had a good to excellent response, provided that therapy was repeated upon symptom relapse.[47] Both commercial preparations of BoNT/A (BOTOX, Allergan, Inc., Irvine, CA and Dysport, Ipsen, Ltd., Maidenhead, Berks, United Kingdom) have been used and results were comparable.[54]

The injection of BoNT/A in achalasia is remarkably safe and well tolerated. Mild chest pain, which has been observed in some patients (<10%) shortly after the injection, does not require a specific treatment. A single case of esophageal ulceration and hematemesis has been observed 2 weeks after the injection. Moreover, a failure of BoNT/A treatment does not influence the efficacy of subsequent surgical myotomy or dilation. BoNT/A diffuses from the injection site into the surrounding tissues; the effects diminish as the distance from

injection site increases. Spread to nearby muscles is possible, particularly when high volumes are injected; however, weakness of distant muscles or generalized weakness is very rare. Diffusion of BoNT/A was postulated to be responsible for the detection of abnormalities of cardiovascular reflexes and occurrence of a heart block after a single patient's treatment for achalasia. Conversely, this 91-year-old patient had a preexisting history of first-degree atrioventricular block, right bundle branch block, and incomplete left bundle branch block; the patient was also taking digoxin.[63]

The available data on the endoscopic injection of BoNT/A into the LES are promising but many issues are raised that remain to be addressed. These issues include: identification of predictors of outcome; definition of the optimal dosage; identification of treatment schedule; methods to prolong BoNT/A efficacy; long-term evaluation of cost effectiveness and quality of life; and a more thorough explanation of the action of BoNT/A on smooth muscles.

CRICOPHARYNGEAL DYSPHAGIA

The cricopharyngeal muscle, or upper esophageal sphincter (UES), constitutes a sphincter separating the hypopharynx from the esophagus.[6] It is activated during swallowing to prevent the inlet of air into the esophagus and to prohibit esophageal reflux to the pharynx during inspiration. Cricopharyngeal dysphagia derives from a dysfunction of the cricopharyngeal muscle, which may be primary or sec-

TABLE 19-3. *Review of Experience Using Botulinum Toxin for the Treatment of Achalasia*

Description	Patients	Results/conclusions	Citation
BoNT vs. placebo	21	67% were improved at 6 weeks.	Ref. 46
BoNT vs. placebo vs. dilation	16	100% were improved at 1 month; 88% required repeated injections; BoNT is as effective as pneumatic dilation.	Ref. 47
BoNT vs. placebo	13	72% were improved at 3 months.	Ref. 48
BoNT	31	60% (82% of those aged >50) were improved at 3 months.	Ref. 49
BoNT	65	60 idiopathic cases: BoNT treatment improved symptoms of dysphagia, chest pain and regurgitation in the majority of patients. Five secondary cases: there was no response to BoNT in 4 patients. Patients who respond to a first BoNT injection but relapse may respond to a second treatment.	Ref. 50
BoNT	55	60% were improved at 6 months.	Ref. 51
BoNT in Chagas' disease	3	Clinical improvement occurred in all patients. Mean LES pressure dropped by 29%.	Ref. 52
BoNT	30	Symptomatic improvement for >3 months was seen in 77% of patients. Seven patients had a sustained response after a single injection; 16 relapsed and required re-treatment.	Ref. 53
BOTOX vs. Dysport	78	Type A BoNT has comparable efficacy in esophageal achalasia after up to 6 months after treatment.	Ref. 54
BoNT vs. balloon dilation	24	The two treatments had equal initial success rate (dilation 83%, BoNT 75%). In the long term the efficacy of BoNT injection was statistically significantly and shorter than that of balloon dilation.	Ref. 55
BoNT vs. balloon dilation	NR	Intrasphincteric BoNT injection was more costly than pneumatic dilation (USD $5,033 compared to USD $3,608). BoNT treatment may be less costly if life expectancy is less than 2 years.	Ref. 56
BoNT	11	The relapse rate was 73% within 2 years from treatment. There was a beneficial effect on dysphagia, no improvement in chest pain or regurgitation scores, and no reduction of mean LES pressure.	Ref. 57
BoNT in high risk patients	20	80% were improved at 6 weeks. Mean cardia diameter was increased from 2.1 mm to 3.2 mm. The patients who initially had a symptomatic relapse after an average of 5 months. BoNT re-injections were efficacious.	Ref. 58
BoNT in children	23	The mean duration of effect in 19 responders was 4.2 months. Fifty percent of the patients required an additional procedure (pneumatic dilation, surgery) on average 7 months after the first treatment.	Ref. 59
BoNT dose-raging study	118	82% were responders at 1 month. No dose-related effect was observed. Vigorous achalasia was the main determinant of the response to BoNT.	Ref. 60
BoNT in children	7	100% were improved at 4 months. Sustained response beyond 6 months occurred in 43% of patients.	Ref. 61
BoNT plus pneumatic dilation	3	Propulsive peristalsis of the esophagus was restored in all patients.	Ref. 62

BoNT, botulinum toxin; LES, lower esophageal sphincter.
BOTOX, Allergan, Inc., Irvine, CA.

ondary to several conditions. These conditions include cerebrovascular accidents, amyotrophic lateral sclerosis (ALS), oculopharyngeal muscular dystrophy, and lesions of the skull base. Proximal dysphagia is the typical clinical presentation; pharyngeal or Zenker's diverticula are possible aftermaths.

Increased function of the cricopharyngeal muscle has traditionally been treated with myotomy, mechanical dilatation, or neurectomy of the oropharyngeal plexus.[64] Localized BoNT/A injections have also been used successfully.[65] The outcomes of swallowing disorders caused by UES spasticity, hypertonus, or delayed relaxation have been documented with cinematic radiograms and manometry in seven patients.[65] The dose range, which was decided based on symptom severity, was between 80 and 120 units

of BOTOX per patient. After identification of the UES by direct esophagoscopy and under electromyographic (EMG) guidance, the injections were performed into the dorsomedial part of the UES and on either side of the UES, into the ventrolateral portion of the muscle. The procedure required general anesthesia and admittance to hospital for an average of 2 days. Except for two patients, all patients experienced a marked improvement or complete relief of symptoms. This benefit lasted up to 5 months. BoNT injection (16 units of BOTOX) provided marked functional recovery in an 86-year-old man with multifocal dystonia and severe dysphagia. This patient had persistent tonic UES activity.[66]

In addition, BoNT/A injections were used to reduce pharyngoesophageal spasms in five postlaryngectomy patients.[67] The injection site was identified using EMG under

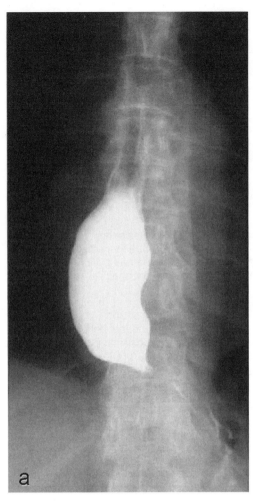
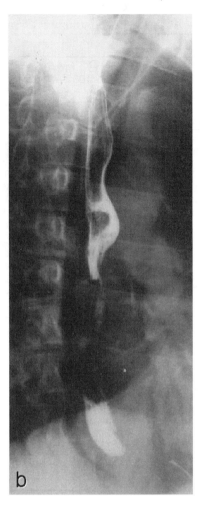

FIG. 19-4. A: Esophagogram of a patient with achalasia before treatment. **B**: Twelve weeks after treatment with botulinum toxin type A.

fluoroscopic control. With one exception, swallowing or voice function improved in all patients.

The treatment of cricopharyngeal dysphagia has been performed in nonanesthetized outpatients using computed tomography (CT)-guided injections.[68] In one patient, appropriate intramuscular placement could not be achieved; however, in the remaining patients, the dose of BoNT/A was progressively increased until good symptom control occurred. A dose as low as 5 units of BOTOX produced onset of benefit after approximately 10 days. The benefit lasted for approximately 2 weeks; it was proposed to identify patients who can benefit from BoNT/A treatment by starting with a lower test dose. Higher doses resulted in improvement for up to 3 months.

A simplified percutaneous technique with EMG guidance has also been developed to inject the UES.[69] The muscle is reached after manual rotation of the larynx. This is accomplished by inserting an EMG recording needle through the skin and advancing it behind the thyroid lamina. This is done until muscle motor unit potentials are recorded. In six patients, two injections of 2.5 units of BOTOX were administered on each side; in one patient with unsatisfactory re-

sponse, endoscopic injection under general anesthesia had to be performed. The best results were obtained in the patients with pure cricopharyngeal spasm and Zenker's diverticula.[70]

Local injections of BoNT/A into the UES are a relatively simple, safe, and effective means of improving dysphagia. Injections may be used during diagnostic evaluation to ascertain the role played by cricopharyngeal spasm in determining the patient's clinical picture. In addition, this approach assists in selecting those patients who are more likely to benefit from myotomy. If BoNT/A fails to improve the symptoms, despite evidence of cricopharyngeal muscle weakening, myotomy will be unlikely to provide benefit. If BoNT/A improves symptoms, the patient could be treated with repeated injections or undergo myotomy.

Secondary oropharyngeal dysphagia may occur in 14–50% of patients who receive BoNT/A injections for cervical or oromandibular dystonia.[71] Female patients who have a thin neck or patients who have received large doses into the sternocleidomastoid (SCM) muscles are thought to be more likely to experience dysphagia. The symptoms are transient, however, in some patients, the symptoms are severe enough to require a liquid diet. Whether BoNT/A injections into the cricopharyngeal muscle can accelerate recovery in such cases has not been tested.

OTHER INDICATIONS FOR THE USE OF BOTULINUM NEUROTOXINS IN THE UPPER GASTROINTESTINAL TRACT

Interest is being focused on the use of BoNT to treat esophageal motility disorders other than achalasia or cricopharyngeal dysphagia (Fig. 19-5A and 19-5B). BoNT may have a potential for treating these motility disorders. These conditions are not as debilitating as achalasia, and in such patients, surgery may be judged too invasive and pneumatic dilation too risky.

Diffuse Esophageal Spasm

Diffuse esophageal spasm, a poorly understood hypermotility disorder, is characterized by chest pain or dysphagia because of repetitive, simultaneous, high-amplitude esophageal contractions. The etiology is unknown. A history of some other functional gastrointestinal tract complaints is common, suggesting an involvement of the ENS. Antispasmodic drugs such as anticholinergics or benzodiazepines are occasionally

helpful. The response to sublingual nitroglycerin is variable, and in some patients, dramatic. Calcium channel blockers may also be of benefit. Dilation may relieve dysphagia and chest pain for several weeks to several months; if required, dilation may need to be repeated. In patients with unresponsive spasm, thoracic esophagomyotomy has been performed, however, the results are less reliable and favorable than in patients with achalasia.[6] A small series of patients with manometrically proven, diffuse esophageal spasm has been treated with BoNT/A injections into the LES.[72] Two months after treatment, 80% of patients had scored a 50% or greater decrease in a scale for dysphagia, chest pain, and regurgitation.

Isolated Hypertensive Lower Esophageal Sphincter

Isolated hypertensive LES is a rare esophageal motor disorder characterized by high LES pressure, LES relaxation, and normal esophageal peristalsis. In these patients, the mechanism of dysphagia remains unclear, however, in some patients, incomplete LES relaxation may play a role. Pneumatic dilation has been utilized with good results in those patients with noteworthy dysphagia who failed conservative therapy. Most patients with dysphagia caused by hyperten-

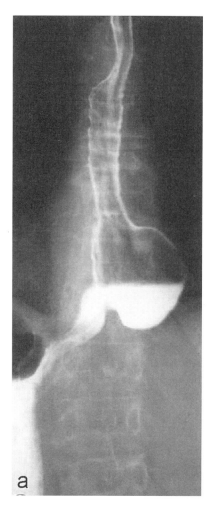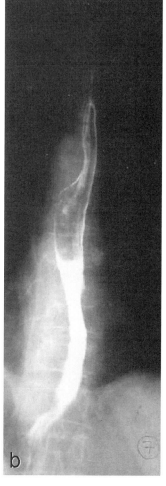

FIG. 19-5. A: Esophagogram of a patient with dysphagia, showing an epiphrenic esophageal diverticulum. **B**: Twelve weeks after treatment with botulinum toxin in the internal esophageal sphincter. A reduction of the diverticulum is observed.

sive LES do not experience progressive symptoms or weight loss, and dilation carries an appreciable risk for esophageal perforation. Therefore, dilation is indicated only in the most extreme cases. Attention has focused on endoscopic injection of BoNT/A directly into the LES as a means of reducing LES pressure and improving dysphagia.[73] A 45-year-old woman with a 3-year history of intermittent solid food dysphagia was treated with 80 units of BOTOX into the LES. The patient had a 75% subjective improvement in dysphagia for 8 months.[73] Short-term responses have been favorable and without any noteworthy complication. Long-term studies are needed to fully evaluate the efficacy of this treatment for patients with isolated hypertensive LES.

Obesity

BoNT/A injection into the gastric antrum may be used to decrease gastric emptying transiently as a treatment for obesity. Preliminary data in rats have shown a substantial loss of body weight associated with a reduction of dietary intake in the BoNT/A-treated group.[74] Experiments in humans are under consideration.

Delayed Gastric Emptying

BoNT/A has been used to facilitate gastric emptying in patients who underwent pylorus-preserving duodenopancreatectomy.[75] Six patients were treated with 80 units of BOTOX. At the end of these patients' surgeries, they received injections into the pylorus. During the postoperative period, only one patient reported symptoms related to delayed gastric emptying.

Infantile Hypertrophic Pyloric Stenosis

Infantile hypertrophic pyloric stenosis is a congenital hereditary disorder characterized by a functional gastric outlet obstruction. This disorder occurs in 1 in 750 births. Pyloric obstruction is the result of a gradual hypertrophy of the circular smooth muscle of the pylorus. Myenteric neurons have a normal appearance; neurons that innervate the circular muscle layer of the pyloric sphincter lack NO synthase. In two patients with pyloric stenosis, there was an observed lack of response to BoNT/A injection.[76]

Sphincter of Oddi Dysfunction

Recurrent upper abdominal pain is a common clinical problem affecting 10% or more of patients undergoing cholecystectomy. Sphincter of Oddi dysfunction has been implicated in the etiology of 10–20% of these patients. Unfortunately, it is difficult to diagnose this dysfunction without performing a manometry of the sphincter; this procedure carries the potential risk of pancreatitis. Sphincterotomy is considered the most effective treatment because response to medical therapy is poor,[77] however, it is not easy to establish a direct

relationship between Oddi dysfunction and pain before sphincterotomy.

Experimental studies have demonstrated that local injections of BoNT/A substantially reduce wave amplitude and phasic contractile activities in the sphincter of Oddi. This reduction is achieved by a selective inhibition of cholinergic influences. At least two potential uses of BoNT/A may be hypothesized:

1. An intrasphincteric injection may serve as a test to select patients whose pain is related directly to Oddi dysfunction.[78]
2. Repeated BoNT treatments may provide a treatment modality alternative to sphincterotomy.[79,80]

Further prospective studies are needed to investigate the potential use of BoNT/A in these patients.

Fifteen consecutive patients who experienced 6 months of frequent attacks of acute pancreatitis as well as manometrically proven pancreatic sphincter of Oddi dysfunction were treated by endoscopy with 100 units of BOTOX into the major papilla.[81] No side effects occurred. Twelve patients (80%) remained asymptomatic for 3 months after BoNT/A treatment. One of the 3 patients (who had no symptomatic benefit) experienced continued, elevated, pancreatic sphincter pressure; eventually, this patient did benefit from pancreatic sphincterotomy. Eleven of the 12 patients (who initially responded to BoNT/A) had a symptomatic relapse that occurred an average of 6 months after BoNT/A treatment. These patients then achieved long-term, clinical remission when treated with pancreatic or combined sphincterotomy.

Chronic Anal Fissure

A chronic anal fissure is a cut or crack in the anal canal or anal verge that may extend from the mucocutaneous junction to the dentate line (Fig. 19-6).[10,18,82] This common complaint in young adults, which has a roughly equal incidence in both sexes, shows a great reluctance to heal without appropriate intervention. Classic symptoms of chronic anal fissure include pain on or after defecation; the pain is often severe and may last from a few minutes to several hours. Often there is bright blood on the toilet paper. The patient may report constipation as the antecedent event, however, once pain develops, the fear of the act of defecation and refusal of the call to stool may exacerbate this problem.[10]

The majority of fissures occur in the posterior midline of the anal canal; fissures are located in the anterior midline in 10% of women and 1% of men. Multiple fissures or fissures occurring in the lateral position raise suspicion of other diseases including Crohn's disease, ulcerative colitis, tuberculosis, human immunodeficiency virus, or syphilis.[10,82]

The fissure may be seen as the buttocks are parted. Chronic anal fissure is often suspected because there is marked spasm of the anus, thus making examination difficult. Digital or proctoscopic examination is often impossible because of pain experienced by the patient. Under general anesthesia, the fissure is seen as a linear or pear-shaped

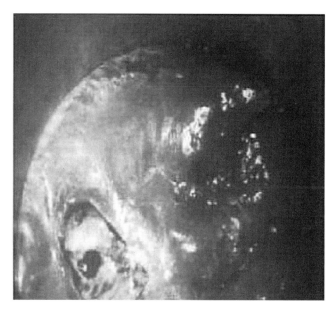

FIG. 19-6. Direct observation of a chronic anal fissure with sharp borders and exposure of fibers of the internal anal sphincter.

breach in the lining of the anal canal, below the dentate line. Spasm of the IAS has been noted in association with chronic fissure and, for many years, treatment has focused on alleviating IAS hypertonia.

Pathophysiology of Chronic Fissure

The cause of chronic fissure and reasons for their failure to heal remains unclear. Also unexplained are the main characteristics of this painful condition, including the predilection for posterior midline and lack of granulation tissue at the fissure site. Several theories have been advanced to unravel the underlying cause of anal fissure. Most of these theories are conflicting and none gives a satisfactory explanation for the characteristic features of chronic fissure.

The passage of a hard stool bolus has traditionally been thought to cause anal fissure. Fibers of the superficial EAS decussate to form a Y-shape posteriorly; the overlying skin has been said to be poorly supported and prone to tearing on passage of a large stool. However, a history of constipation preceding the onset of anal fissure is obtained only in 1 of 4 patients; diarrhea is seen to be a predisposing factor in approximately 6% of patients.[82]

In 3–10% of patients, fissures that commonly occur in the anterior midline are associated with childbirth.[10,82] Shearing forces on the anal mucosa from the fetal head or mucosal tethering after childbirth may render the anterior midline more susceptible to trauma; both of these shearing forces have been incriminated; in addition, postpartum anal fissure is associated with reduced anal canal pressures.[83]

IAS spasm has been noted for many years in association with anal fissure; thus, surgical treatment has been generally aimed at overcoming the spasm. The IAS of patients with

anal fissure is fibrotic, as compared with the nonfibrotic IAS of controls.[84] A postulated myositis might occur early in the course of a fissure and that myositis is the underlying cause of both spasm and fibrosis. Although the cause of the spasm remains obscure, resting anal pressure is consistently higher in the patients with anal fissure than in normal controls. This finding suggests that the high resting pressure is related to IAS hypertonicity. Interestingly, the resting pressure of patients healed by conservative treatment tends to increase to pretreatment level while patients remain symptom free. This probably means that sphincter hypertonus does not directly cause pain.

It has been postulated that the increased incidence of fissure in the anterior and posterior midline positions is related to the distribution of vessels supplying blood to the anal canal. Relief of symptoms and healing induced by treatment could be attributed to a decrease in anal pressure. This decrease in pressure would increase the mucosal blood flow and relieve ischemia. The inferior rectal arteries, which branch from the internal pudendal artery, provide blood supply to the distal anal canal. These vessels cross the ischiorectal fossa; their divisions pass through the anal sphincters to reach the mucosa. Post-mortem angiography of the inferior rectal artery has revealed a paucity of inferior rectal artery branches at the posterior commissure in 85% of 41 subjects.[85] A morphologic study of the capillaries revealed that in most subjects, there was reduced density in the sub-anodermal space as well as within IAS in the posterior midline. The predilection of anal fissures for the posterior midline and the lack of granulation tissue seen in the base of a chronic fissure may be explained by ischemia.[85,86]

Decreased anodermal blood flow may be promoted by endothelial cell dysfunction associated with reduced NO synthesis. This dysfunction is known to be involved in the regulation of local blood flow. Interruption of the endothelial continuity removes the anticoagulant and vasodilator functions of the endothelium; it also exposes the subendothelium, which has several procoagulant functions. In addition, even without detectable microscopic changes, endothelial function may change from vasodilator to vasoconstrictor and from anticoagulant to procoagulant. These changes may be induced by inflammatory or immune cytokines. Activation of the endothelium may express antigens and these endothelial cells may act as antigen-presenting cells. Antiendothelial cell antibodies have been found in many patients with anal fissure, but not in healthy controls.[87] In antibody-positive patients, higher resting anal tone, with no change of maximum voluntary contraction, has been observed.[87] This supports a role of the endothelium in the pathogenesis of anal ischemia. Circulating antibodies may activate the endothelium to produce vasoactive autacoids; these, in turn, could contribute to the increased basal tone and aggravate the ischemia at the level of the posterior anal commissure. The observation that, in up to 60% of patients, topical application of nitroglycerin ointment may induce anal fissure healing supports a pathogenic role of endothelial NO synthesis.[88]

A primary IAS disturbance may be a contributing etiologic factor. IAS supersensitivity to α_2-agonists has been observed in the patients with chronic fissure.[89] This hypersensitivity may be induced by:

- Prolonged absence of the neurotransmitter;
- Abnormalities at the neurotransmitter level;
- Abnormalities at the metabolic level; and
- A modification of cholinergic and adrenergic receptors.

Increased IAS adrenergic or cholinergic activity is likely to occur in patients with chronic fissure. This is demonstrated by the efficacy of BoNT/A in inducing fissure healing and reduction of resting tone following injection into the IAS.[90–98]

Conservative Therapies

The passage of a hard stool is thought to contribute to the development of anal fissure. Therefore, for many years, the control of constipation has been considered the main treatment. Patients with a history suggestive of anal fissure (with recent onset) are often treated successfully with conservative measures, such as stool softeners, bulking agents, a high-fiber diet, and sitz baths.[10,82] To prevent recurrence, a patient should be encouraged to continue with the diet and the use of bulked laxative agent. If required, these measures may be continued even after symptoms have resolved.

For many years, anal dilators have been used in the treatment of anal fissure. These dilators were popular for some time; however, their use has been criticized as being merely a way of applying an anesthetic ointment. Dilators have not been helpful in treating anal fissure. Furthermore, the addition of an anal dilator was not found to be more useful than stool softeners or topical anesthesia alone. More than 50% of patients were initially cured using this technique; however, half of these patients eventually relapsed.[82]

Surgical Treatment

If symptoms fail to resolve or have been present for a long period, resolution without surgery becomes increasingly less likely. Since the 1950s, lateral internal sphincterotomy has been the most commonly used surgical treatment for chronic fissure.[99] This procedure may be performed under local or general anesthesia, through a radial or circumferential incision, or using a subcutaneous approach. Open or subcutaneous methods produce adequate and equivalent falls in anal pressure. The IAS may be divided from medial to lateral or vice versa. The results of lateral sphincterotomy have been reported from many centers. Surgery is associated with several complications, most of which may be prevented by the use of a judicious technique and, of course, by familiarity with anorectal anatomy. Although lateral internal sphincterotomy heals and relieves symptoms of chronic fissure in nearly all patients (96%),[100,101] the incidence of incontinence varies. The largest studies report impairment of continence in up to 30% of patients. Although most episodes of incon-

tinence are minor and transient, in a subset of patients, incontinence is permanent.[102]

An incision of the IAS throughout its entire length is inadvisable. However, it is uncertain how much of the sphincter should be divided. A common practice is to divide the sphincter for the length of the fissure. The length of sphincterotomy reportedly does not affect the incidence of recurrence and alterations of continence. There is, however, some disagreement on this point.[103] A prospective study with anal endosonography has revealed that more of the IAS than intended was divided by sphincterotomy, particularly in multiparous women, who were thought to have an unrecognized, obstetric-related sphincter injury.[104]

Treatment with Nitro-Derivate

NO donors may promote healing of anal fissure by increasing local blood flow in two ways: (1) they reduce intra-anal pressure or (2) they are vasodilators to the anal vessels. The indication for use of NO donors has been documented. Local application of nitro-derivates reduces anal pressures; improves anodermal blood flow; and substantially reduces pain within 5 minutes of application. These improvements were assessed during clinical trials with the use of a linear analogue pain score.[88] Many patients (from 19–44%) have experienced transient headache when using topical nitrate preparations and have reported a burning sensation in the anus.[88,105–111] The benefit of glyceryl trinitrate is not always permanent. In a review of 23 patients with chronic anal fissure, it was demonstrated that, after 3 months of successful healing with glyceryl trinitrate ointment, 8 patients (35%) experienced a recurrence, 6 patients had spontaneous healing, and 2 patients healed with a further course of treatment.[110] Treatment with topical glyceryl trinitrate ointment is reportedly less efficacious than in previous accounts.[109] This study emphasized issues related to poor patient compliance, and reported that 62% of the patients had relevant side effects that interfered with their quality of life. In addition, high doses of glyceryl trinitrate are not more efficacious in inducing healing.[111] An important issue is the development of drug tolerance, which is well documented, as when the same drugs are used to treat cardiovascular diseases. Nitrates have a short duration of action, thus, their frequent application is necessary. Side effects, such as headaches and tachyphylaxis, limit the utility of nitrates to the point that glyceryl trinitrate ointment seemingly causes headaches more often than it treats the symptoms of fissure.[111]

Botulinum Neurotoxin Type A Treatment

BoNT/A may be used to treat anal fissure, particularly when a patient is at high risk of incontinence (Table 19-4). With patients lying on their side (usually their left side, when the operator is right handed), the IAS can be easily palpated and injected. The lower, rounded edge of the IAS may be felt on physical examination, approximately 1–1.5 cm from the dentate line all around the circumference. The groove be-

TABLE 19-4. *Comparison of Published Results on the Treatment of Two Hundred Thirty-Two Patients with Anal Fissure*

Reference (chronological order)	Patients	Dose (units)	Healing rate at 6 weeks	Temporary incontinence	Recurrence	Complications
Ref. 90	10	15 units of Botox	70%	10%	20%	10%
Ref. 91	12	5 units of Dysport	83%	0%	8%	0%
Ref. 112	54	5 units of Dysport	78%	6%	6%	11%
Ref. 92	5	NR	60%	0%	0%	0%
Ref. 93	100	5 units of Dysport	82%	7%	6%	0%
Ref. 94	15	20 units of Botox	73%	0%	0%	0%
Ref. 97	69	10–21 units of Botox	48–70%	0%	37–52%	0%

NR, not reported
BOTOX, Allergan, Inc., Irvine, CA.
Dysport, Ipsen Ltd., Maidenhead, Berks, UK.

tween the internal and the external sphincters may be visualized or easily palpated.

In an open-label study,[90] the authors observed that 60% of 10 patients healed after a single infiltration of 15 units of BOTOX into the IAS. In a subsequent double-blind study, a success rate of 76% was achieved after a single treatment with 20 units.[94] A prospective comparison between two dose regimens (15 and 20 units) showed negligible side effects and no complications. Symptomatic improvement was achieved in both groups of patients, but the healing rate was higher in the group that received 20 units.[95] The authors also demonstrated that fissure healing was induced more effectively by BoNT/A treatment than by glyceryl trinitrate treatment and that IAS hypertonia was also alleviated more effectively.[96] Compared to baseline values, 1 month posttreatment resting pressure was reduced by 26.2% in BoNT/A-treated patients and 16.6% in the nitrate ointment-treated patients. Two months after treatment, resting anal pressure was reduced by 28.4% in the BoNT/A-treated group and 13.7% in the nitrate-treated group.

The therapeutic efficacy of different doses of BoNT/A has been reported in patients with chronic anal fissure.[97] The healing rates do not differ substantially when the total dose and number of injection sites are varied. The healing rate was 83% in the patients who were treated with 10 units of BOTOX; 78% in those treated with 15 units; and 90% in the group treated with 21 units of BOTOX. Between-group comparisons did not reveal significant differences. The injections were administered through the intersphincteric groove in the direction of the IAS, however, 1 month after treatment, the mean squeeze pressure was reduced more than resting pressure. This finding suggests some diffusion of the toxin to the external sphincter.[97]

Based on the theory that low anodermal perfusion at the fissure's base contributes to pathophysiology, additional infiltration of BoNT/A has been performed at this point.[97] In the authors' experience, patients with a posterior chronic fissure have better results when BoNT/A is injected anteriorly into the IAS.[96,98] These beneficial results are represented by a lowering of resting anal tone as well as early development of a healing scar. Anterior placement of the injections induces a relatively greater decrease in resting pressure and

improves the clinical outcome. Fibrosis of the IAS, which is more prominent at the fissure's site than elsewhere in the smooth muscle, may reduce IAS compliance and limit BoNT/A intramuscular diffusion. The myenteric plexus with myenteric ganglia is located between the circular and longitudinal smooth muscle layers along the entire extent of the IAS. A chronic reduction of perfusion in the anus's posterior part may affect the myenteric nervous fibers at this location, making them less sensitive to the action of BoNT/A.

It was observed that BoNT/A injections into the striated EAS are also effective for treating fissure.[93,112] The mechanism is probably mediated by diffusion to the IAS; this is demonstrated by the observation that maximum squeeze pressure and resting pressure are both reduced with this procedure. Because the fundamental pathogenic event in chronic fissure is IAS spasm, injection into the EAS is not the first choice for treatment. In addition, the IAS is readily visible and easier to inject than the EAS.

In conclusion, BoNT/A seems to be a safe treatment for patients with chronic anal fissure. It is less expensive and easier to perform than surgical treatment and does not require anesthesia. It is also more efficacious than nitrate therapy. In patients with a posterior chronic fissure, results are more beneficial when BoNT/A is injected anteriorly into the IAS (Table 19-5). No adverse effects or permanent IAS damage have resulted from BoNT injection.

OTHER APPLICATIONS IN THE LOWER GATROINTESTINAL TRACT

Chronic Constipation Caused by Pelvic Floor Dysfunction

Constipation is a common primary presenting symptom of pelvic floor dysfunction and one of the most common chronic complaints. A diagnosis of constipation includes fewer than three bowel movements per week and at least one of the following occurring on a minimum of 25% of occasions:

- Hard bowel movements,
- Difficulty passing the bowel movement, and
- Sense of inadequate defecation.[14]

TABLE 19-5. *Variables Affecting the Outcome of Treatment with Botulinum Toxin for Anal Fissure*

Item	Influence of dose regimens[95]		Influence of site of injections[98]	
	15 units	20 units	Posterior injections	Anterior injections
Number of patients	23	34	25	24
Baseline characteristics				
Age (yr)	45 ± 17	41 ± 13	40 ± 13	46 ± 15
M/F ratio	10/13	18/16	14/11	11/14
Duration of symptoms (months)	11 ± 8	13 ± 12	17 ± 16	16 ± 15
Baseline anal pressures				
Resting tone (mm Hg)	94 ± 35	111 ± 30	109 ± 30	101 ± 27
Voluntary contraction (mm Hg)	66 ± 34	84 ± 40	83 ± 38	84 ± 31
One month evaluation				
Fissure healing	5	17	12	22
Symptomatic improvement	12	24	—	—
Resting tone (mm Hg)	68 ± 26	80 ± 23	84 ± 24	69 ± 18
Voluntary contraction (mm Hg)	54 ± 28	72 ± 36	79 ± 43	83 ± 40
Two month evaluation				
Fissure healing	10	23	15	22
Symptomatic improvement	13	24	—	—
Resting tone (mm Hg)	80 ± 34	79 ± 28	84 ± 29	69 ± 14
Voluntary contraction (mm Hg)	58 ± 0	74 ± 35	79 ± 37	83 ± 39
Rescue treatment	5 (20 units)	7 (25 units)	6 (posterior injections)	3 (anterior injections)
Healing	13	30	20	25

Patients with chronic idiopathic constipation can be classified in two pathophysiologic groups: slow transit constipation and pelvic floor dysfunction.

Pelvic floor dysfunction is characterized by a failure of the puborectalis muscle to relax during efforts to defecate or its paradoxical contraction. With an effort to evacuate the rectum, the puborectalis and the EAS normally relax to straighten the anorectal angle and open the anal canal. The diagnosis of pelvic floor dysfunction is suggested by demonstration of a persistent impression of the puborectalis on the anal canal's posterior surface during attempted evacuation of barium paste (Figs. 19-7 and 19-8). This may be demonstrated with greater reliability by EMG evidence of increased electrical activity in the puborectalis muscle during straining.

The etiology of pelvic floor dysfunction is unclear. As in other forms of constipation, the patients are commonly women, who developed constipation as adolescents or young adults. Prolonged efforts to empty the rectum may aggravate the condition. Paradoxical puborectalis contraction during straining reportedly represents a focal dystonia that is characterized by excessive recruitment of synergistic and antagonistic muscle groups during voluntary activity along with lack of reciprocal inhibition.[113] Signs of anismus have been noted in normal subjects,[114] in patients with anorectal pain,[115] and even in patients with fecal incontinence.[114,116]

In patients who are constipated, BoNT/A has been used to selectively weaken the EAS and puborectalis muscle. BoNT/A relaxes the puborectalis muscle;[117] consequently, the anorectal angle increases during straining and evacuation becomes possible. However, despite good results, the effect of BoNT/A injections is short term. From 6–15 units of BOTOX were injected under EMG guidance into the EAS or the puborectalis muscle.[118] This injection brought about short-term improvement in all four patients. These patients had failed to respond to conventional biofeedback treatment; however, in the long-term, only half of the patients experienced sustained benefit.

In a 1998 study, a symptomatic improvement was noted in 13 of 15 patients after injections of 25 units of BOTOX into the EAS.[119] Improvement was maintained for a mean duration of 5 months, and reinjection was necessary. In a group of 50 patients with chronic outlet obstruction constipation, 4 patients with a puborectalis syndrome were studied using anorectal manometry, defecography, and EMG. These patients were treated with 30 units of BOTOX, which was injected into two sites on either side of the puborectalis muscle (under ultrasonographic guidance).[120] One patient was lost to follow-up; in the remaining 3 patients, the frequency of natural bowel movements increased from 0–6 per week; only 1 patient required laxatives. Anorectal manometry demonstrated decreased tone during straining: at 4 weeks with a decrease from 96 ± 12 mm Hg to 42 ± 13 mm Hg ($P = .003$) and at 8 weeks with a decrease to 63 ± 22 mm Hg ($P = .009$).

Defecography performed 8 weeks after treatment showed improvement in evacuation of barium paste and an increase in the anorectal angle (from $94° \pm 11°$ to $114° \pm 13°$ [$P = .01$]). EMG demonstrated that the puborectalis muscle was still capable of producing a mild paradoxical contraction. Still, at 16 weeks posttreatment, one patient experienced a symptomatic recurrence. The patient was re-treated with 50 units of BOTOX and 8 months later received 60 units of BOTOX. Seven months after the last injection, the patient had normal daily bowel movements, without the use of laxatives.

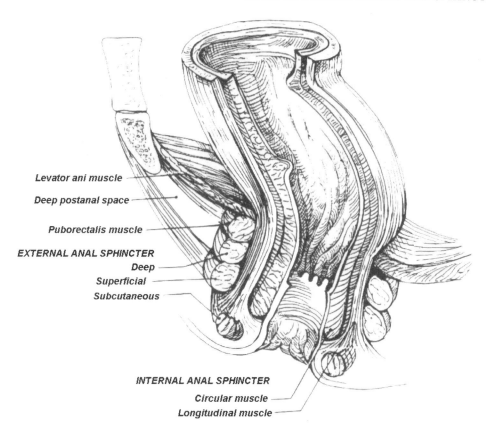

FIG. 19-7. View of the external and the internal anal sphincters, pelvic floor, and anal canal.

Outlet-type constipation may also occur in Parkinson's disease (PD). The authors observed dramatic improvement in a patient with PD with outlet-type constipation who was treated with BoNT/A injections into the puborectalis muscle.[121] The authors performed a prospective study to identify the prevalence of this condition among outpatients with PD. Patients with a diagnosis of PD completed an inventory-type questionnaire regarding their gastrointestinal function. The questionnaire evaluated the number of bowel movements and defecatory function. These patients also received a proctological evaluation. Of the 138 patients who met the inclusion criteria for chronic constipation, 18 (13%) had isolated or combined outlet-type constipation. Ten of these patients (1 woman and 9 men) were enrolled in the prospective study. They were evaluated by manometry, defecography, and EMG. In addition, these patients received BoNT/A injections into the puborectalis. The total dose per session was 100 units of BOTOX in 10 patients. The results indicate a reduction in tone during straining and an improvement of the anorectal angle (Fig. 19-9A–19-9C).

Anterior Rectocele

Rectocele is a hernia of the anterior rectal wall into the lumen of the vagina (Fig. 19-10). It is a frequent finding in women and its clinical relevance is questionable. From 20–81% of nonsymptomatic women and constipated individuals may present with a rectocele.[122,123] If a rectocele is less than 2 cm in diameter, it is considered a normal finding in constipated or healthy subjects. When the diameter is greater than 2 cm, the rectocele may cause outlet obstruction and rectal emptying difficulties.[122–124]

It has been suggested that in some instances, a rectocele is caused by failure of relaxation or a dystonic-like, paradoxi-

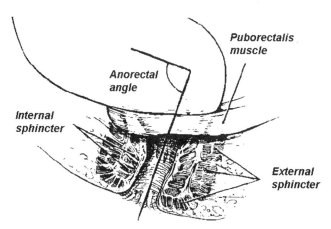

FIG. 19-8. Schematic drawing of the muscles of the anal canal, including the puborectalis and surrounding structures. The anorectal angle is also shown. The anterior-bound pull of the puborectalis contributes to the reduction of the anorectal angle (i.e., between the rectum and the anal canal).

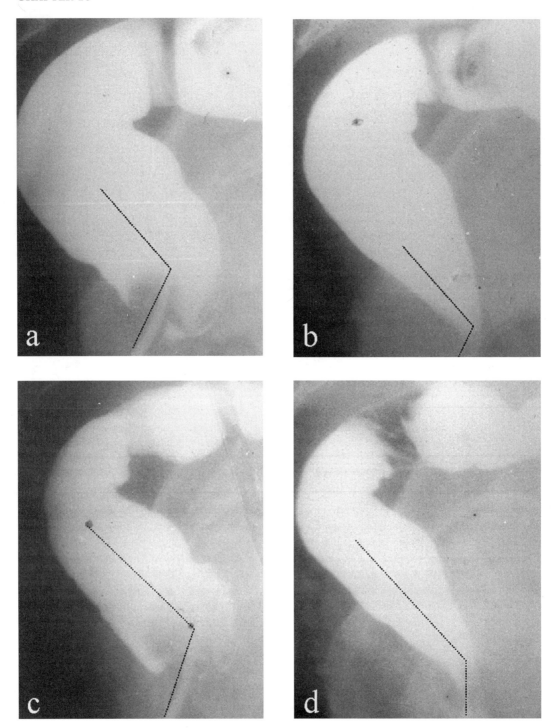

FIG. 19-9. A and **B**: Pretreatment of outlet-type constipation in Parkinson's disease (PD) with injection of botulinum toxin in the puborectalis muscle. **C** and **D**: Posttreatment with botulinum toxin. Note: Defecographies (A) and (C) represent the resting condition; defecographies (B) and (D) were taken during straining. After treatment, during straining, the pelvic floor descends approximately 3 cm and the anorectal angle becomes obtuse (compare B and D).

cal contraction of the puborectalis muscle occurring during attempted evacuation, however, the exact reason for its establishment is not clear. It is important to identify a rectocele when it is the primary cause of intractable obstructed evacuation. A rectocele may cause mild to severe anorectal symptoms, which are usually associated with chronic constipa-tion. Straining possibly aggravates the rectocele, enlarges it, and makes evacuation more difficult. When there is a recto-cele or a paradoxical sphincter reaction, defecation has to oc-cur through the nonrelaxed pelvic floor.[122–124]

Although simple to diagnose, the rectocele has proven dif-ficult to treat. The initial phase of management usually in-

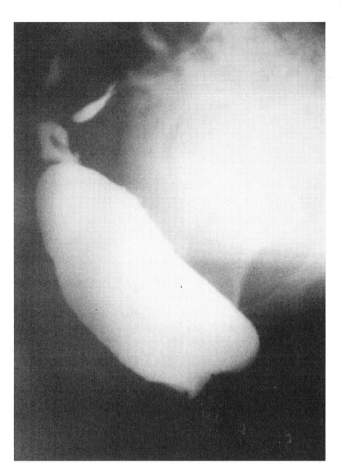

FIG. 19-10. Defecography during straining, showing an anterior rectocele and lack of relaxation of the puborectalis muscle and the pelvic floor.

volves a high-fiber diet, in an attempt to elicit rectal voiding. The next step is to use increasing doses of laxatives as well as enemas. Neither procedure is effective in resolving the problem. Wide varieties of surgical approaches have been proposed to ensure rectal emptying by reducing the dimension of the rectocele. However, the results of these surgical approaches are often disappointing with regard to emptying difficulties. Vaginal, transperineal, or transanal surgical repair does not always alleviate symptoms; in some patients, surgery may cause impaired fecal continence. Furthermore, transanal repair may compromise anal sphincter pressures. When the anal sphincter is lax, an alternative approach should be considered. From 30–72% of patients continued to experience difficulties with evacuation during the postoperative period. After the surgical procedure, 54% of patients complained of constipation, which was often severe. Seventeen percent of patients noted persistent anorectal pain and 34% had impaired fecal continence. Six months after successful transanal repair, noteworthy impairment in resting and squeezing anal pressures were noted.[125] These findings probably correlated with the stretch of the anal sphincters. When the transvaginal approach was used, reports included the occurrence of increased incidence of rectovaginal fistulas, vaginal narrowing, and substantial postoperative pain.

Recently, 14 women, with a mean age of 55 ±11 years, were treated with a total of 30 units of BOTOX. These injections were evenly divided into three sites: two on either side of the puborectalis muscle and the third anteriorly in the EAS.[126] At 1 month, examination revealed a symptomatic improvement in 7 patients. Incomplete evacuation was resolved in 7 patients and reduced in 2 patients. In 7 patients who previously reported blood or mucus discharge, this finding was no longer present. The pressure during straining was reduced by 41% (compared to baseline value), and pressure was substantially lower than the previously recorded resting pressure. At the 2-month evaluation, a symptomatic improvement was found in 9 patients. Defecographic results revealed that the depth of the rectocele was reduced from 4.3 ± 0.6 cm to 1.8 ± 90.5 cm ($P < .001$) and that the rectocele area was reduced from 9.2 ± 1.3 cm^2 to 2.8 ± 1.6 cm^2 ($P < .001$). The anorectal angle measured during straining increased from a mean of 98° ± 15° before treatment to a mean of 121° ± 19° ($P = .001$). At the 1-year evaluation, there were no reports of digitally assisted rectal voiding and rectocele were not found on physical examination.

CONCLUSION

The demonstration that smooth muscles are responsive to BoNT has opened an entirely new field of indications related to diseases of the gastrointestinal tract. The complex functional anatomy of gastrointestinal tract motor control allows for multiple interactions after BoNT injections that have not been fully explored. New treatments and new indications are expected in this vast field of clinical practice. The few striated muscles that affect gastrointestinal tract motility and function are located in the pelvic floor. At this level BoNT may relieve focal dystonia or paradoxical muscle activity.

REFERENCES

1. Burgen ASV, Dickens F, Zatman LJ. The action of botulinum toxin on the neuromuscular junction. J Physiol Lond 1949;109:10–24.
2. Scott AB. Botulinum toxin injection into extraocular muscles as an alternative to strabismus surgery. Ophthalmology 1980;87:1044–1049.
3. Simpson LL. The origin, structure, and pharmacological activity of botulinum toxin. Pharmacol Rev 1981;33:155–188.
4. Bhutani MS. Gastrointestinal uses of botulinum toxin. Am J Gastroenterol 1997;92:929–933.
5. MacKenzie I, Burnstock G, Dolly JO. The effects of purified botulinum neurotoxin type A on cholinergic, adrenergic and non-adrenergic, atropine-resistant autonomic neuromuscular transmission. Neuroscience 1982;7:997–1006.
6. Albanese A, Brisinda G, Mathias CJ. The autonomic nervous system and gastrointestinal disorders. In: Appenzeller O, ed. The Autonomic Nervous System. Part II. Dysfunctions. Amsterdam, The Netherlands: Elsevier, 2001:613–663.
7. Goyal RK, Hirano I. The enteric nervous system. N Engl J Med 1996;334:1106–1115.
8. Furness JB, Bornstein JC. The enteric nervous system and its extrinsic connections. In: Yamada T, ed. Textbook of Gastroenterology. Philadelphia: Lippincott, 1995:2–24.
9. Brookes SJ, Steele PA, Costa M. Identification and immunohistochemistry of cholinergic and non-cholinergic circular muscle motor neurons in the guinea-pig small intestine. Neuroscience 1991;42: 863–878.

10. Corman ML. Colon and Rectal Surgery. 4th ed. Philadelphia: Lippincott, 1998.

11. Jorge JM, Wexner SD. Anatomy and physiology of the rectum and anus. Eur J Surg 1997;163:723–731.

12. Bhardwaj R, Vaizey CJ, Boulos PB, et al. Neuromyogenic properties of the internal anal sphincter: therapeutic rationale for anal fissures. Gut 2000;46:861–868.

13. Der-Silaphet T, Malysz J, Hagel S, et al. Interstitial cells of Cajal direct normal propulsive contractile activity in the mouse small intestine. Gastroenterology 1998;114:724–736.

14. Vanderwinden JM, Rumessen JJ, Liu H, et al. Interstitial cells of Cajal in human colon and in Hirschsprung's disease. Gastroenterology 1996;111:901–910.

15. Vanderwinden JM, Liu H, De Laet MH, et al. Study of the interstitial cells of Cajal in infantile hypertrophic pyloric stenosis. Gastroenterology 1996;111:279–288.

16. Mittal RK, Balaban DH. The esophagogastric junction. N Engl J Med 1997;336:924–932.

17. Sangwan YP, Solla JA. Internal anal sphincter: advances and insights. Dis Colon Rectum 1998;41:1297–1311.

18. Beck DE, Wexner SD. Fundamentals of Anorectal Surgery. 2nd ed. London: W.B. Saunders, 1998.

19. Stebbing JF, Brading AF, Mortensen NJ. Nitrergic innervation and relaxant response of rectal circular smooth muscle. Dis Colon Rectum 1996;39:294–299.

20. Stebbing JF, Brading AF, Mortensen NJ. Role of nitric oxide in relaxation of the longitudinal layer of rectal smooth muscle. Dis Colon Rectum 1997;40:706–710.

21. Chakder S, Cao GY, Lynn RB, et al. Heme oxygenase activity in the internal anal sphincter: effects of nonadrenergic, noncholinergic nerve stimulation. Gastroenterology 2000;118:477–486.

22. Pitt J, Craggs MM, Henry MM, et al. Alpha-1 adrenoceptor blockade: potential new treatment for anal fissures. Dis Colon Rectum 2000;43:800–803.

23. Mearin F, Mourelle M, Guarner F, et al. Patients with achalasia lack nitric oxide synthase in the gastro-oesophageal junction. Eur J Clin Invest 1993;23:724–728.

24. Goldblum JR, Rice TW, Richter JE. Histopathologic features in esophagomyotomy specimens from patients with achalasia. Gastroenterology 1996;111:648–654.

25. Lui H, Vanderwinden JM, Ji P, et al. Nitric oxide synthase distribution in the enteric nervous system of children with cardiac achalasia. Chin Med J (Engl) 1997;110:358–361.

26. Singaram C, Sweet MA, Belcaster CM. A novel autoantibody exists in patients with esophageal achalasia [Abstract]. Gastroenterology 1994;106:A566.

27. Verne GN, Hahn AB, Pineau BC, et al. Association of HLA-DR and -DQ alleles with idiopathic achalasia. Gastroenterology 1999;117:26–31.

28. Wong RK, Maydonovitch CL, Metz SJ, et al. Significant DQw1 association in achalasia. Dig Dis Sci 1989;34:349–352.

29. Pinotti HW, Felix VN, Zilberstein B, et al. Surgical complications of Chagas' disease: megaesophagus, achalasia of the pylorus, and cholelithiasis. World J Surg 1991;15:198–204.

30. Bonavina L, Nosadini A, Bardini R, et al. Primary treatment of esophageal achalasia. Long-term results of myotomy and Dor fundoplication. Arch Surg 1992;127:222–226.

31. Mattioli S, Di Simone MP, Bassi F, et al. Surgery for esophageal achalasia. long-term results with three different techniques. Hepatogastroenterology 1996;43:492–500.

32. Cosentini E, Berlakovich G, Zacherl J, et al. Achalasia. Results of myotomy and antireflux operation after failed dilatations. Arch Surg 1997;132:143–147.

33. Okike N, Payne WS, Neufeld DM, et al. Esophagomyotomy versus forceful dilation for achalasia of the esophagus: results in 899 patients. Ann Thorac Surg 1979;28:119–125.

34. Ellis FH, Crozier RE, Watkins E. Operation for esophageal achalasia. Results of esophagomyotomy without an antireflux operation. J Thorac Cardiovasc Surg 1984;88:344–351.

35. Ferguson MK, Reeder LB, Olak J. Results of myotomy and partial fundoplication after pneumatic dilation for achalasia. Ann Thorac Surg 1996;62:327–330.

36. Anselmino M, Zaninotto G, Costantini M, et al. One-year follow-up after laparoscopic Heller-Dor operation for esophageal achalasia. Surg Endosc 1997;11(1):3-7.

37. Vogt D, Curet M, Pitcher D, et al. Successful treatment of esophageal achalasia with laparoscopic Heller myotomy and Toupet fundoplication. Am J Surg 1997;174:709–714.

38. Hunter JG, Trus TL, Branum GD, et al. Laparoscopic Heller myotomy and fundoplication for achalasia. Ann Surg 1997;225:655–664.

39. Rosati R, Fumagalli U, Bona S, et al. Evaluating results of laparoscopic surgery for esophageal achalasia. Surg Endosc 1998;12:270–273.

40. Wang PC, Sharp KW, Holzman MD, et al. The outcome of laparoscopic Heller myotomy without antireflux procedure in patients with achalasia. Am Surg 1998;64:515–520.

41. Patti MG, Pellegrini CA, Horgan S, et al. Minimally invasive surgery for achalasia: an 8-year experience with 168 patients. Ann Surg 1999;230:587–593.

42. Yamamura MS, Gilster JC, Myers BS, et al. Laparoscopic Heller myotomy and anterior fundoplication for achalasia results in a high degree of patient satisfaction. Arch Surg 2000;135:902–906.

43. Bloomston M, Boyce W, Mamel J, et al. Videoscopic Heller myotomy for achalasia—results beyond short-term follow-up. J Surg Res 2000;92:150–156.

44. Pellegrini CA, Leichter R, Patti M, et al. Thoracoscopic esophageal myotomy in the treatment of achalasia. Ann Thorac Surg 1993;56:680–682.

45. Maher JW. Thoracoscopic esophagomyotomy for achalasia: maximum gain, minimal pain. Surgery 1997;122:836–840.

46. Pasricha PJ, Ravich WJ, Hendrix TR, et al. Intrasphincteric botulinum toxin for the treatment of achalasia. N Engl J Med 1995;332:774-778.

47. Annese V, Basciani M, Perri F, et al. Controlled trial of botulinum toxin injection versus placebo and pneumatic dilation in achalasia. Gastroenterology 1996;111(6):1418-1424.

48. Fiorini A, Corti RE, Valero JL, et al. Botulinum toxin is effective in the short-term treatment of esophageal achalasia. Preliminary results of a randomized trial [in Spanish]. Acta Gastroenterol Latinoam 1996; 26:155–157.

49. Pasricha PJ, Rai R, Ravich WJ, et al. Botulinum toxin for achalasia: long-term outcome and predictors of response. Gastroenterology 1996;110:1410–1415.

50. Fishman VM, Parkman HP, Schiano TD, et al. Symptomatic improvement in achalasia after botulinum toxin injection of the lower esophageal sphincter. Am J Gastroenterol 1996;91:1724-1730.

51. Cuilliere C, Ducrotte P, Zerbib F, et al. Achalasia: outcome of patients treated with intrasphincteric injection of botulinum toxin. Gut 1997;41:87–92.

52. Brant CQ, Nakao F, Ardengh JC, et al. Echoendoscopic evaluation of botulinum toxin intrasphincteric injections in Chagas' disease achalasia. Dis Esophagus 1999;12:37–40.

53. Kolbasnik J, Waterfall WE, Fachnie B, et al. Long-term efficacy of Botulinum toxin in classical achalasia: a prospective study. Am J Gastroenterol 1999;94:3434–3439.

54. Annese V, Bassotti G, Coccia G, et al. Comparison of two different formulations of botulinum toxin A for the treatment of oesophageal achalasia. The Gismad Achalasia Study Group. Aliment Pharmacol Ther 1999;13:1347–1350.

55. Muehldorfer SM, Schneider TH, Hochberger J, et al. Esophageal achalasia: intrasphincteric injection of botulinum toxin A versus balloon dilation. Endoscopy 1999;31:517–521.

56. Panaccione R, Gregor JC, Reynolds RP, et al. Intrasphincteric botulinum toxin versus pneumatic dilatation for achalasia: a cost minimization analysis. Gastrointest Endosc 1999;50:492–498.

57. Greaves RR, Mulcahy HE, Patchett SE, et al. Early experience with intrasphincteric botulinum toxin in the treatment of achalasia. Aliment Pharmacol Ther 1999;13:1221–1225.

58. Wehrmann T, Kokabpick H, Jacobi V, et al. Long-term results of endoscopic injection of botulinum toxin in elderly achalasic patients with tortuous megaesophagus or epiphrenic diverticulum. Endoscopy 1999;31:352–358.

59. Hurwitz M, Bahar RJ, Ament ME, et al. Evaluation of the use of botulinum toxin in children with achalasia. J Pediatr Gastroenterol Nutr 2000;30:509–514.

60. Annese V, Bassotti G, Coccia G, et al. A multicentre randomised study of intrasphincteric botulinum toxin in patients with oesophageal achalasia. GISMAD Achalasia Study Group. Gut 2000;46:597–600.

61. Ip KS, Cameron DJ, Catto-Smith AG, et al. Botulinum toxin for achalasia in children. J Gastroenterol Hepatol 2000;15:1100–1104.

62. Hep A, Dolina J, Dite P, et al. Restoration of propulsive peristalsis of the esophagus in achalasia. Hepatogastroenterology 2000;47:1203–1204.

63. Malnick SD, Metchnik L, Somin M, et al. Fatal heart block following treatment with botulinum toxin for achalasia. Am J Gastroenterol 2000;95:3333–3334.

64. McKenna JA, Dedo HH. Cricopharyngeal myotomy: indications and technique. Ann Otol Rhinol Laryngol 1992;101:216–221.

65. Schneider I, Pototschnig C, Thumfart WF, et al. Treatment of dysfunction of the cricopharyngeal muscle with botulinum a toxin: introduction of a new, noninvasive method. Ann Otol Rhinol Laryngol 1994; 103:31–35.

66. Dunne J, Hayes M, Cameron D. Botulinum toxin A for cricopharyngeal dystonia. Lancet 1993;342:559.

67. Crary MA, Glowasky AL. Using botulinum toxin A to improve speech and swallowing function following total laryngectomy. Arch Otolaryngol Head Neck Surg 1996;122:760–763.

68. Atkinson SI, Rees J. Botulinum toxin for cricopharyngeal dysphagia: case reports of CT- guided injection. J Otolaryngol 1997;26:273–276.

69. Blitzer A, Brin MF. Use of botulinum toxin for diagnosis and management of cricopharyngeal achalasia. Otolaryngol Head Neck Surg 1997;116:328–330.

70. Ahsan SF, Meleca RJ, Dworkin JP. Botulinum toxin injection of the cricopharyngeus muscle for the treatment of dysphagia. Otolaryngol Head Neck Surg 2000;122:691–695.

71. Jankovic J, Schwartz K. Botulinum toxin injections for cervical dystonia. Neurology 1990;40:277–280.

72. Miller LS, Parkman HP, Schiano TD, et al. Treatment of symptomatic nonachalasia esophageal motor disorders with botulinum toxin injection at the lower esophageal sphincter. Dig Dis Sci 1996;41:2025–2031.

73. Jones MP. Botulinum toxin in hypertensive lower esophageal sphincter [Letter]. Am J Gastroenterol 1996;91:1283–1284.

74. Gui D, De Gaetano A, Spada PL, et al. Botulinum toxin injected in the gastric wall reduces body weight and food intake in rats. Aliment Pharmacol Ther 2000;14:829–834.

75. Wiesel PH, Bettschart V, Suter M, et al. Prevention of delayed gastric emptying after pylorus-preserving pancreatoduodenectomy with intrapyloric injection of botulinum toxin [Abstract]. Gastrointest Endosc 1997;45:44.

76. Heinen F, Mall V, Ruckauer KD, et al. Lack of response to botulinum toxin A in patients with hypertrophic pyloric stenosis. Eur J Pediatr 1999;158:436.

77. Geenen JE, Hogan WJ, Dodds WJ, et al. The efficacy of endoscopic sphincterotomy after cholecystectomy in patients with sphincter-of-Oddi dysfunction. N Engl J Med 1989;320:82–87.

78. Pasricha PJ, Miskovsky EP, Kalloo AN. Intrasphincteric injection of botulinum toxin for suspected sphincter of Oddi dysfunction. Gut 1994;35:1319–1321.

79. Sand J, Nordback I, Arvola P, et al. Effects of botulinum toxin A on the sphincter of Oddi: an in vivo and in vitro study. Gut 1998;42:507–510.

80. Muehldorfer SM, Hahn EG, Ell C. Botulinum toxin injection as a diagnostic tool for verification of sphincter of Oddi dysfunction causing recurrent pancreatitis. Endoscopy 1997;29:120–124.

81. Wehrmann T, Schmitt TH, Arndt A, et al. Endoscopic injection of botulinum toxin in patients with recurrent acute pancreatitis due to pancreatic sphincter of Oddi dysfunction. Aliment Pharmacol Ther 2000;14:1469–1477.

82. Lund JN, Scholefield JH. Aetiology and treatment of anal fissure. Br J Surg 1996;83:1335–1344.

83. Corby H, Donnelly VS, O'Herlihy C, et al. Anal canal pressures are low in women with postpartum anal fissure. Br J Surg 1997;84:86–88.

84. Brown AC, Sumfest JM, Rozwadowski JV. Histopathology of the internal anal sphincter in chronic anal fissure. Dis Colon Rectum 1989;32:680–683.

85. Klosterhalfen B, Vogel P, Rixen H, et al. Topography of the inferior rectal artery: a possible cause of chronic, primary anal fissure. Dis Colon Rectum 1989;32:43–52.

86. Schouten WR, Briel JW, Auwerda JJ, et al. Ischaemic nature of anal fissure. Br J Surg 1996;83:63–65.

87. Maria G, Brisinda D, Ruggieri MP, et al. Identification of anti-endothelial cell antibodies in patients with chronic anal fissure. Surgery 1999;126:535–540.

88. Lund JN, Scholefield JH. A randomised, prospective, double-blind, placebo-controlled trial of glyceryl trinitrate ointment in treatment of anal fissure [published erratum appears in Lancet 1997;349:656]. Lancet 1997;349:11–14.

89. Regadas FS, Batista LK, Albuquerque JL, et al. Pharmacological study of the internal and sphincter in patients with chronic anal fissure. Br J Surg 1993;80:799–801.

90. Gui D, Cassetta E, Anastasio G, et al. Botulinum toxin for chronic anal fissure. Lancet 1994;344:1127–1128.

91. Jost WH, Schimrigk K. Therapy of anal fissure using botulinum toxin. Dis Colon Rectum 1994;37:1321–1324.

92. Mason PF, Watkins MJ, Hall HS, et al. The management of chronic fissure in-ano with botulinum toxin. J R Coll Surg Edinb 1996;41:235–238.

93. Jost WH. One hundred cases of anal fissure treated with botulinum toxin: early and long-term results. Dis Colon Rectum 1997;40:1029–1032.

94. Maria G, Cassetta E, Gui D, et al. A comparison of botulinum toxin and saline for the treatment of chronic anal fissure. N Engl J Med 1998;338:217–220.

95. Maria G, Brisinda G, Bentivoglio AR, et al. Botulinum toxin injections in the internal anal sphincter for the treatment of chronic anal fissure: long-term results after two different dosage regimens. Ann Surg 1998;228:664–669.

96. Brisinda G, Maria G, Bentivoglio AR, et al. A comparison of injections of botulinum toxin and nitroglycerin ointment for the treatment of chronic anal fissure. N Engl J Med 1999;341:65–69.

97. Minguez M, Melo F, Espi A, et al. Therapeutic effects of different doses of botulinum toxin in chronic anal fissure. Dis Colon Rectum 1999;42:1016–1021.

98. Maria G, Brisinda G, Bentivoglio AR, et al. Influence of botulinum toxin site of injections on healing rate in patients with chronic anal fissure. Am J Surg 2000;179:46–50.

99. Eisenhammer S. Surgical correction of chronic internal anal sphincter contracture. S Afr Med J 1951;25:486–489.

100. Hananel N, Gordon PH. Lateral internal sphincterotomy for fissure-in-ano—revisited. Dis Colon Rectum 1997;40:597–602.

101. Argov S, Levandovsky O. Open lateral sphincterotomy is still the best treatment for chronic anal fissure. Am J Surg 2000;179:201–202.

102. Nyam DC, Pemberton JH. Long-term results of lateral internal sphincterotomy for chronic anal fissure with particular reference to incidence of fecal incontinence. Dis Colon Rectum 1999;42:1306–1310.

103. Garcia-Aguilar J, Belmonte MC, Perez JJ, et al. Incontinence after lateral internal sphincterotomy: anatomic and functional evaluation. Dis Colon Rectum 1998;41:423–427.

104. Sultan AH, Kamm MA, Nicholls RJ, et al. Prospective study of the extent of internal anal sphincter division during lateral sphincterotomy. Dis Colon Rectum 1994;37:1031–1033.

105. Watson SJ, Kamm MA, Nicholls RJ, et al. Topical glyceryl trinitrate in the treatment of chronic anal fissure. Br J Surg 1996;83:771–775.

106. Bacher H, Mischinger HJ, Werkgartner G, et al. Local nitroglycerin for treatment of anal fissures: an alternative to lateral sphincterotomy? Dis Colon Rectum 1997;40:840–845.

107. Oettle GJ. Glyceryl trinitrate vs. sphincterotomy for treatment of chronic fissure-in-ano: a randomized, controlled trial. Dis Colon Rectum 1997;40:1318–1320.

108. Kennedy ML, Sowter S, Nguyen H, et al. Glyceryl trinitrate ointment for the treatment of chronic anal fissure: results of a placebo-controlled trial and long-term follow-up. Dis Colon Rectum 1999;42:1000–1006.

109. Dorfman G, Levitt M, Platell C. Treatment of chronic anal fissure with topical glyceryl trinitrate. Dis Colon Rectum 1999;42:1007–1010.

110. Lund JN, Armitage NC, Scholefield JH. Use of glyceryl trinitrate ointment in the treatment of anal fissure. Br J Surg 1996;83:776–777.

111. Carapeti EA, Kamm MA, McDonald PJ, et al. Randomised controlled trial shows that glyceryl trinitrate heals anal fissures, higher doses are not more effective, and there is a high recurrence rate. Gut 1999;44:727–730.

112. Jost WH, Schanne S, Mlitz H, et al. Perianal thrombosis following injection therapy into the external anal sphincter using botulinum toxin. Dis Colon Rectum 1995;38:781.

113. Mathers SE, Kempster PA, Swash M, et al. Constipation and paradoxical puborectalis contraction in anismus and Parkinson's disease: a dystonic phenomenon? J Neurol Neurosurg Psychiatry 1988;51:1503–1507.

114. Voderholzer WA, Neuhaus DA, Klauser AG, et al. Paradoxical sphincter contraction is rarely indicative of anismus. Gut 1997;41:258–262.

115. Schouten WR, Briel JW, Auwerda JJ, et al. Anismus: fact or fiction? Dis Colon Rectum 1997;40:1033–1041.
116. Wexner SD, Marchetti F, Salanga VD, et al. Neurophysiologic assessment of the anal sphincter. Dis Colon Rectum 1991;34:606–612.
117. Hallan RI, Williams NS, Melling J, et al. Treatment of anismus in intractable constipation with botulinum A toxin. Lancet 1988;2:714–717.
118. Joo JS, Agachan F, Wolff B, et al. Initial North American experience with botulinum toxin type A for treatment of anismus. Dis Colon Rectum 1996;39:1107–1111.
119. Shafik A, El Sibai O. Botulin toxin in the treatment of nonrelaxing puborectalis syndrome. Dig Surg 1998;15:347–351.
120. Maria G, Brisinda G, Bentivoglio AR, et al. Botulinum toxin in the treatment of outlet obstruction constipation caused by puborectalis syndrome. Dis Colon Rectum 2000;43:376–380.
121. Albanese A, Maria G, Bentivoglio AR, et al. Severe constipation in Parkinson's disease relieved by botulinum toxin. Mov Disord 1997;12:764–766.
122. Siproudhis L, Dautreme S, Ropert A, et al. Dyschezia and rectocele—a marriage of convenience? Physiologic evaluation of the rectocele in a group of 52 women complaining of difficulty in evacuation. Dis Colon Rectum 1993;36:1030–1036.
123. Van Laarhoven CJ, Kamm MA, Bartram CI, et al. Relationship between anatomic and symptomatic long-term results after rectocele repair for impaired defecation. Dis Colon Rectum 1999;42:204–210.
124. Karlbom U, Graf W, Nilsson S, et al. Does surgical repair of a rectocele improve rectal emptying? Dis Colon Rectum 1996;39:1296–1302.
125. Ho YH, Ang M, Nyam D, et al. Transanal approach to rectocele repair may compromise anal sphincter pressures. Dis Colon Rectum 1998;41:354–358.
126. Maria G, Brisinda G, Bentivoglio AR, et al. Anterior rectocele due to obstructed defecation relieved by botulinum toxin. Surgery 2001;129:524–529.

Index